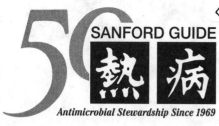

# THE SANFORD GUIDE
## To Antimicrobial Therapy
## 2019

**50 Years
1969-2019**

David N. Gilbert, M.D.
Henry F. Chambers, M.D.
George M. Eliopoulos, M.D.
Michael S. Saag, M.D.
Andrew T. Pavia, M.D.

Douglas Black, Pharm.D.
David O. Freedman, M.D.
Kami Kim, M.D.
Brian S. Schwartz, M.D.

# THE SANFORD GUIDE
## To Antimicrobial Therapy
2019

**50 Years**
**1969-2019**

## Editors

**David N. Gilbert, M.D.**
Chief of Infectious Diseases,
Providence Portland Medical Center, Oregon
Professor of Medicine,
Oregon Health Sciences University

**George M. Eliopoulos, M.D.**
Beth Israel Deaconess Hospital
Professor of Medicine,
Harvard Medical School, Boston, Massachusetts

**Henry F. Chambers, M.D.**
San Francisco General Hospital
Professor of Medicine Emeritus
University of California, San Francisco

**Michael S. Saag, M.D.**
Associate Dean for Global Medicine
Director, UAB Center for AIDS Research
Professor of Medicine and Director,
Division of Infectious Diseases,
University of Alabama, Birmingham

**Andrew T. Pavia, M.D.**
George & Esther Gross Presidential Professor
Chief, Division of Pediatric Infectious Diseases,
University of Utah, Salt Lake City

## Publisher

**Antimicrobial Therapy, Inc.**

## Contributing Editors

**Douglas Black, Pharm.D.**
Professor of Pharmacy,
University of Washington, Seattle

**Brian S. Schwartz, M.D.**
Associate Professor of Medicine,
University of California, San Francisco

**David O. Freedman, M.D.**
Emeritus Professor of Medicine,
University of Alabama, Birmingham

**Kami Kim, M.D.**
Professor of Internal Medicine,
Division of Infectious Diseases
and International Medicine,
Morsani College of Medicine,
University of South Florida, Tampa

## Managing Editor

**Jeb C. Sanford**

## Memoriam

**Jay P. Sanford, M.D.**
1928-1996
**Merle A. Sande, M.D.**
1939-2007
**Robert C. Moellering, Jr., M.D.**
1936-2014

**The GUIDE TO ANTIMICROBIAL THERAPY is published by:**

**ANTIMICROBIAL THERAPY, INC.**
11771 Lee Highway, P.O. Box 276
Sperryville, VA 22740-0276 USA
Tel 540-987-9480 Fax 540-987-9486
**Email: info@sanfordguide.com**
**www.sanfordguide.com**

**Acknowledgements**
Thanks to Silvina Trapé, Jonatan Bohman and their team for manuscript design and layout of this edition of the SANFORD GUIDE.

**Note to Readers**
Since 1969, the SANFORD GUIDE has been independently prepared and published. Decisions regarding the content of the SANFORD GUIDE are solely those of the editors and the publisher. We welcome questions, comments and feedback concerning the SANFORD GUIDE. All of your feedback is reviewed and taken into account in updating the content of the SANFORD GUIDE.

Every effort is made to ensure accuracy of the content of this guide. However, current full prescribing information available in the package insert for each drug should be consulted before prescribing any product. The editors and publisher are not responsible for errors or omissions or for any consequences from application of the information in this book and make no warranty, express or implied, with respect to the currency, accuracy, or completeness of the contents of this publication. Application of this information in a particular situation remains the professional responsibility of the practitioner.

**For the most current information, subscribe to webedition.sanfordguide.com**
**or Sanford Guide mobile device applications**

Printed in the United States of America
**ISBN 978-1-944272-09-8**
Pocket Edition (English)

—TABLE OF CONTENTS—

## ABBREVIATIONS

3TC = lamivudine
AB,% = percent absorbed
ABC = abacavir
ABCD = amphotericin B colloidal dispersion
ABLC = ampho B lipid complex
ABSSSI = acute bacterial skin & skin structure infection
AD = after dialysis
ADF = adefovir
AG = aminoglycoside
AIDS = Acquired Immune Deficiency Syndrome
AM-CL = amoxicillin-clavulanate
AM-CL-ER = amoxicillin-clavulanate extended release
AMK = amikacin
Amox = amoxicillin
AMP = ampicillin
Ampho B = amphotericin B
Ampho-SB = ampicillin-sulbactam
AP = atovaquone proguanil
APAG = antipseudomonal aminoglycoside
ARDS = acute respiratory distress syndrome
ARF = acute rheumatic fever
ASA = aspirin
ATS = American Thoracic Society
ATV = atazanavir
AUC = area under the curve
Azithro = azithromycin
bid = 2x per day
BL/BLI = beta-lactam/beta-lactamase inhibitor
BSA = body surface area
BW = body weight
C&S = culture & sensitivity
C/S = culture & sensitivity
CABP = community-acquired bacterial pneumonia
CAPD = continuous ambulatory peritoneal dialysis
CARB = carbapenems
CDC = U.S. Centers for Disease Control

Cefpodox = cefpodoxime proxetil
Ceftaz = ceftazidime
Ceph = cephalosporin
CFB = ceftobiprole
CFP = cefepime
Chloro = chloramphenicol
CIP = ciprofloxacin; CIP-ER = CIP extended release
Claritho = clarithromycin; ER = extended release
Clav = clavulanate
Clinda = clindamycin
CLO = clofazimine
Clot = clotrimazole
CMV = cytomegalovirus
Cobi = cobicistat
CQ = chloroquine phosphate
CrCl = creatinine clearance
CrCln = CrCl normalized for BSA
CRBSI = catheter-related bloodstream infection
CRRT = continuous renal replacement therapy
CSD = cat-scratch disease
CSF = cerebrospinal fluid
CXR = chest x-ray
d4T = stavudine
Dapto = daptomycin
DBPCT = double-blind placebo-controlled trial
dc = discontinue
ddC = zalcitabine
ddI = didanosine
Diclox = Dicloxacillin
div = divided
DLV = delavirdine
DORI = doripenem
DOT = directly observed therapy
Doxy = doxycycline
DR = delayed release

DRSP = drug-resistant S. pneumoniae
DBRPCT = Double blind, randomized, placebo-controlled trial
DS = double strength
EBV = Epstein-Barr virus
EES = erythromycin ethyl succinate
EFZ = efavirenz
ELV = elvitegravir
EMB = ethambutol
ENT = entecavir
ER = extended release
ERTA = ertapenem
Erythro = erythromycin
ESBLs = extended spectrum β-lactamases
ESR = erythrocyte sedimentation rate
ESRD = endstage renal disease
Flu = fluconazole
Flucyt = flucytosine
FOS-APV = fosamprenavir
FQ = fluoroquinolone
FTC = emtricitabine
G = generic
GAS = Group A Strep
Gati = gatifloxacin
GC = gonorrhea
Gemi = gemifloxacin
Gent = gentamicin
gm = gram
GNB = gram-negative bacilli
Grazo = grazoprevir
Griseo = griseofulvin
Gtts = drops
H/O = history of
HEMO = hemodialysis
HHV = human herpesvirus
HIV = human immunodeficiency virus
HLR = high-level resistance

# ABBREVIATIONS (2)

HSCT = hematopoietic stem cell transplant
HSV = herpes simplex virus
IA = injectable agent/anti-inflammatory drugs
IDV = indinavir
IFN = interferon
IM = intramuscular
IMP = imipenem-cilastatin
INH = isoniazid
Inv = investigational
IP = intraperitoneal
IT = intrathecal
Itra = itraconazole
IV = intravenous
IVDU = intravenous drug user
IVIG = intravenous immune globulin
Keto = ketoconazole
kg = kilogram
LAB = liposomal ampho B
LCM = lymphocytic choriomeningitis virus
LCR = ligase chain reaction
Levo = levofloxacin
LP/R = lopinavir/ritonavir
mcg (or µg) = microgram
MDR = multi-drug resistant
MER = meropenem
Metro = metronidazole
Mino = minocycline
mL = milliliter
Moxi = moxifloxacin
MQ = mefloquine
MSM = men who have sex with men
MSSA/MRSA = methicillin-sensitive/resistant S. aureus
MTB = Mycobacterium tuberculosis
NAF = Nafcillin
NAI = not FDA-approved (indication or dose)
NB = name brand

NF = nitrofurantoin
NFR = nelfinavir
NNRTI = non-nucleoside reverse transcriptase inhibitor
NRTI = nucleoside reverse transcriptase inhibitor
NSAIDs = non-steroidal
NUS = not available in the U.S.
NVP = nevirapine
O Ceph = oral cephalosporins
Oflox = ofloxacin
P Ceph = parenteral cephalosporins
PCR = polymerase chain reaction
PEP = post-exposure prophylaxis
PI = protease inhibitor
PIP-TZ = piperacillin-tazobactam
po = oral dosing
PQ = primaquine
PRCT = Prospective randomized controlled trials
Pts = patients
PTLD = post-transplant lymphoproliferative disease
PZA = pyrazinamide
q wk = dose weekly
q[x]h = every [x] hours, e.g., q8h = every 8 hrs
qid = 4x per day
QS = quinine sulfate
Quinu-dalfo = Q-D = quinupristin-dalfopristin
R = resistant
RDBPCT = randomized double blind placebo controlled trial
RFB = rifabutin
RFP = rifapentine
Rick = rickettsia
RIF = rifampin
RSV = respiratory syncytial virus
RTI = respiratory tract infection
RTV = ritonavir
rx = treatment

SA = Staph. aureus
sc = subcutaneous
SSPE = Subacute sclerosing panencephalitis
SD = serum drug level after single dose
Sens = sensitive (susceptible)
SM = streptomycin
Sofos = sofosbuvir
SQV = saquinavir
SS = steady state serum level
STD = sexually transmitted disease
subcut = subcutaneous
Sulb = sulbactam
Sx = symptoms
TAF = tenofovir alafenamide
Tazo = tazobactam
TBc = tuberculosis
TDF = tenofovir
TEE = transesophageal echocardiography
Teico = teicoplanin
Telithro = telithromycin
Tetra = tetracycline
tid = 3x per day
TMP-SMX = trimethoprim-sulfamethoxazole
TNF = tumor necrosis factor
Tobra = tobramycin
TPV = tipranavir
TST = tuberculin skin test
UTI = urinary tract infection
Vanco = vancomycin
Velpat = velpatasvir
VISA = vancomycin intermediately resistant S. aureus
VL = viral load
Vori = voriconazole
VZV = varicella-zoster virus
ZDV = zidovudine

## ABBREVIATIONS OF JOURNAL TITLES

**AAC:** Antimicrobial Agents & Chemotherapy
**Adv PID:** Advances in Pediatric Infectious Diseases
**AHJ:** American Heart Journal
**AIDS Res Hum Retrovir:** AIDS Research & Human Retroviruses
**AAP:** American Academy of Pediatrics
**AJG:** American Journal of Gastroenterology
**AJM:** American Journal of Medicine
**AJRCCM:** American Journal of Respiratory Critical Care Medicine
**AJTMH:** American Journal of Tropical Medicine & Hygiene
**Aliment Pharmacol Ther:** Alimentary Pharmacology & Therapeutics
**Am J Transpl:** American Journal of Transplantation
**AnEM:** Annals of Emergency Medicine
**AnIM:** Annals of Internal Medicine
**Ann Pharmacother:** Annals of Pharmacotherapy
**AnSurg:** Annals of Surgery
**Antivir Ther:** Antiviral Therapy
**ArDerm:** Archives of Dermatology
**ArIM:** Archives of Internal Medicine
**ARRD:** American Review of Respiratory Disease
**BMJ:** British Medical Journal
**BMT:** Bone Marrow Transplantation
**Brit J Derm:** British Journal of Dermatology
**Can JID:** Canadian Journal of Infectious Diseases
**Canad Med J:** Canadian Medical Journal
**CCM:** Critical Care Medicine
**CCTID:** Current Clinical Topics in Infectious Disease
**CDSR:** Cochrane Database of Systematic Reviews
**CID:** Clinical Infectious Diseases
**Clin Micro Inf:** Clinical Microbiology and Infection
**CMN:** Clinical Microbiology Newsletter
**Clin Micro Rev:** Clinical Microbiology Reviews
**CMAJ:** Canadian Medical Association Journal

**COID:** Current Opinion in Infectious Disease
**Curr Med Res Opin:** Current Medical Research and Opinion
**Derm Ther:** Dermatologic Therapy
**Dermatol Clin:** Dermatologic Clinics
**Dig Dis Sci:** Digestive Diseases and Sciences
**DMID:** Diagnostic Microbiology and Infectious Disease
**EID:** Emerging Infectious Diseases
**EJCMID:** European Journal of Clin. Micro. & Infectious Diseases
**Eur J Neurol:** European Journal of Neurology
**Exp Mol Path:** Experimental & Molecular Pathology
**Exp Rev Anti Infect Ther:** Expert Review of Anti-Infective Therapy
**Gastro:** Gastroenterology
**Hpt:** Hepatology
**ICHE:** Infection Control and Hospital Epidemiology
**IDC No. Amer:** Infectious Disease Clinics of North America
**IDCP:** Infectious Diseases in Clinical Practice
**IJAA:** International Journal of Antimicrobial Agents
**Inf Med:** Infections in Medicine
**J AIDS & HR:** Journal of AIDS and Human Retrovirology
**J All Clin Immun:** Journal of Allergy and Clinical Immunology
**J Am Ger Soc:** Journal of the American Geriatrics Society
**J Chemother:** Journal of Chemotherapy
**J Clin Micro:** Journal of Clinical Microbiology
**J Clin Virol:** Journal of Clinical Virology
**J Derm Treat:** Journal of Dermatological Treatment
**J Hpt:** Journal of Hepatology
**J Inf:** Journal of Infection
**J Med Micro:** Journal of Medical Microbiology
**J Micro Immunol Inf:** Journal of Microbiology, Immunology, & infection
**J Ped:** Journal of Pediatrics
**J Viral Hep:** Journal of Viral Hepatitis
**JAC:** Journal of Antimicrobial Chemotherapy
**JACC:** Journal of American College of Cardiology

**JAIDS:** JAIDS Journal of Acquired Immune Deficiency Syndromes
**JAMA:** Journal of the American Medical Association
**JAVMA:** Journal of the Veterinary Medicine Association
**JCI:** Journal of Clinical Investigation
**JCM:** Journal of Clinical Microbiology
**JIC:** Journal of Infection and Chemotherapy
**JID:** Journal of Infectious Diseases
**JNS:** Journal of Neurosurgery
**JPIDS:** Journal of Pediatric Infectious Diseases Society
**JTMH:** Journal of Tropical Medicine and Hygiene
**Ln:** Lancet
**LnID:** Lancet Infectious Disease
**Mayo Clin Proc:** Mayo Clinic Proceedings
**Med Lett:** Medical Letter
**Med Mycol:** Medical Mycology
**MMWR:** Morbidity & Mortality Weekly Report
**NEJM:** New England Journal of Medicine
**Neph Dial Transpl:** Nephrology Dialysis Transplantation
**OFID:** Open Forum Infectious Diseases
**Ped Ann:** Pediatric Annals
**Peds:** Pediatrics
**Pharmacother:** Pharmacotherapy
**PIDJ:** Pediatric Infectious Disease Journal
**QJM:** Quarterly Journal of Medicine
**Scand J Inf Dis:** Scandinavian Journal of Infectious Diseases
**Sem Resp Inf:** Seminars in Respiratory Infections
**SGO:** Surgery Gynecology and Obstetrics
**SMJ:** Southern Medical Journal
**Surg Neurol:** Surgical Neurology
**Transpl Inf Dis:** Transplant Infectious Diseases
**Transpl:** Transplantation
**TRSM:** Transactions of the Royal Society of Medicine

# TABLE 1 – CLINICAL APPROACH TO INITIAL CHOICE OF ANTIMICROBIAL THERAPY*

Treatment based on presumed site or type of infection. In selected instances, treatment and prophylaxis based on identification of pathogens.
Regimens should be reevaluated based on pathogen isolated, antimicrobial susceptibility determination, and individual host characteristics. *(Abbreviations on 2)*

| ANATOMIC SITE/DIAGNOSIS/ MODIFYING CIRCUMSTANCES | ETIOLOGIES (usual) | SUGGESTED REGIMENS* | | ADJUNCT DIAGNOSTIC OR THERAPEUTIC MEASURES AND COMMENTS |
|---|---|---|---|---|
| | | PRIMARY | ALTERNATIVE§ | |
| **ABDOMEN:** *See Peritoneum, page 49; Gallbladder, page 18; and Pelvic Inflammatory Disease, page 28* | | | | |
| **BONE: Osteomyelitis. Microbiologic diagnosis is essential.** If blood culture negative, need culture of bone *(Eur J Clin Microbiol Infect Dis 33:371, 2014).* Culture of sinus tract drainage not predictive of bone culture. For comprehensive review of antimicrobial penetration into bone, see *Clinical Pharmacokinetics 48:89, 2009.* | | | | |
| **Hematogenous Osteomyelitis** *(see IDSA guidelines for vertebral osteo: CID July 29, 2015)* | | | | |
| **Empiric therapy—Collect bone and blood cultures before empiric therapy** | | | | |
| Newborn (<4 mos.) | S. aureus, Gm-neg. bacilli, Group B Strep, Kingella kingae in children. | **MRSA possible: Vanco + (Ceftaz or CFP)** | **MRSA unlikely: (Nafcillin or Oxacillin) + (Ceftaz or CFP)** | Severe allergy or toxicity: **(Linezolid^NAI 10 mg/kg IV/po q8h + Aztreonam).** |
| Children (>4 mos.) – Adult: Osteo of extremity *(NEJM 370:352, 2014)* | S. aureus, Group A strep, Gm-neg. bacilli rare, Kingella kingae in children | **MRSA possible: Vanco** 40 mg/kg/day div q6h **Add Ceftaz or CFP** if Gm-neg. bacilli on Gram stain | **MRSA unlikely: (Nafcillin or Oxacillin)** 150 mg/kg/day div q6h (max 12 gm) | Severe allergy or toxicity: **Clinda** or **TMP-SMX** or **Linezolid^NAI** Adults: **Ceftaz** 2 gm IV q8h, **CFP** 2 gm IV q12h. *See Table 10B for adverse reactions to drugs.* |
| Adult (>21 yrs) Vertebral osteo ± epidural abscess *(see IDSA guidelines for vertebral osteo: CID 61:859, 2015)* **Blood & bone cultures essential.** | S. aureus most common but variety other organisms. Brucella, M. tuberculosis, Coccidioides important in regions of high endemicity for the organisms | **Adult doses below.** Vanco 15-20 mg/kg IV q 8-12h for trough of 15-20 µg/mL + **(Ceftriaxone** 2 gm q24h OR CFP 2 gm q8h OR **Levo** 750 mg q24h) | **Dapto** 8-10 mg/kg IV q24h OR Linezolid 600 mg q12h + **(Ceftriaxone** 2 gm q24h OR **Levo** 750 mg q24h) | **Ceftriaxone** should not be used if pseudomonas suspected. **Piperacillin/Tazobactam** another option for pseudomonas or other Gram-negative coverage. **Dx: MRI diagnostic test of choice, indicated to rule out epidural abscess. Risk factors for recurrence:** end-stage renal disease, MRSA infection, undrained paravertebral or psoas abscess; pathogen-specific therapy for >8 wks recommended if any of these are present *(CID 62:1262, 2016);* 6 wks of pathogen-specific therapy comparable to 12 wks for less complicated infection *(CID 62:1262, 2016 and Lancet 385:875, 2015).* Whenever possible empirical therapy should be administered after cultures are obtained. |

\* **PRIMARY REGIMENS SUGGESTED are for adults** (unless otherwise indicated) with clinically severe (often life-threatening) infections. Dosages also assume normal renal function, and not severe hepatic dysfunction.
§ **ALTERNATIVE REGIMENS INCLUDE** these considerations: allergy, pregnancy, pharmacology/pharmacokinetics, compliance, costs, local resistance profiles.

**TABLE 1 (2)**

| ANATOMIC SITE/DIAGNOSIS/ MODIFYING CIRCUMSTANCES | ETIOLOGIES (usual) | SUGGESTED REGIMENS* | | ADJUNCT DIAGNOSTIC OR THERAPEUTIC MEASURES AND COMMENTS |
|---|---|---|---|---|
| | | PRIMARY | ALTERNATIVE§ | |
| **BONE/Hematogenous Osteomyelitis** (continued) | | | | |
| **Specific therapy**—Culture and in vitro susceptibility results known. See CID Jul 29, 2015 for IDSA Guidelines | | | | |
| | MSSA | **Nafcillin** or **Oxacillin** 2 gm IV q4h or **Cefazolin** 2 gm IV q8h | **Vanco** 15-30 mg/kg IV q 8-12h for trough or 15-20 μg/mL, OR **Dapto** 8-10 mg/kg IV q24h OR **Linezolid** 600 mg IV/po q12h | **Other options if susceptible in vitro and in allergy/toxicity issues (see NEJM 382:17, 2010):** 1) **TMP-SMX** 8-10 mg/kg/d po/IV div q8h + **RIF** 300-450 mg bid; limited data, particularly for MRSA (see AAC 53:2672, 2009); 2) **Levo** 750 mg po q24h) + **RIF** 600 mg po q24h; 3) **Fusidic acid**[NUS] 500 mg IV q8h + **RIF** 300 mg po bid. (CID 42:394, 2006); 4) **Ceftriaxone** 2 gm IV q24h (CID 54-585, 2012) |
| | MRSA—See Table 6, page 90; IDSA Guidelines CID 52:e18-55, 2011; CID 52:285-92, 2011 | **Vanco** 15-20 mg/kg IV q 8-12h for trough of 15-20 μg/mL ± **RIF** 300-450 mg bid. | **Linezolid** 600 mg po/IV q12h/po ± **RIF** 300 mg po/IV bid OR **Dapto** 8-10 mg/kg q24h IV ± **RIF** 300-450 mg po/IV bid | (MSSA only): Duration of therapy: 6 weeks, provided that epidural or paravertebral abscesses can be drained; consider longer course in those with extensive infection or abscess particularly if not amenable to drainage because of increased risk of treatment failure (OFID Dec 5:1, 2014) (although data are lacking that this approach improves efficacy versus a 6 wks course) and >8 weeks in patients undergoing device implantation (CID 60:1330, 2015). |
| **Hemoglobinopathy:** Sickle cell/thalassemia | Salmonella; other Gm-neg. bacilli | **CIP** 400 mg IV q12h OR **CIP** 750 mg po bid | **Levo** 750 mg IV po q24h | Thalassemia: transfusion and iron chelation risk factors. Because of decreasing levels of susceptibility to fluoroquinolones among Salmonella sp. and growing resistance among other gram-negative bacilli, would add a second agent (e.g., third-generation cephalosporin) until susceptibility test results available. Alternative for salmonella is Ceftriaxone 2 gm IV q24h if nalidixic acid resistant which is predictive of fluoroquinolone resistance. |
| **Contiguous Osteomyelitis Without Vascular Insufficiency** | | | | |
| **Empiric therapy: Get cultures!** | | | | |
| Foot bone osteo due to nail through tennis shoe | P. aeruginosa | **CIP** 750 mg po bid or **Levo** 750 mg po q24h | **Ceftaz** 2 gm IV q8h or **CFP** 2 gm IV q8h | See Skin—Nail puncture, page 60. Need debridement to remove foreign body. |
| Long bone, post-internal fixation of fracture | S. aureus, Gm-neg. bacilli, P. aeruginosa | **Vanco** 15-20 mg/kg q8-12h IV q 8-12h for trough of 15-20 μg/mL + [**Ceftaz** or **CFP**]. See Comment | **Linezolid** 600 mg IV/po bid[NAI] + (**Ceftaz** or **CFP**). See Comment | Often necessary to remove hardware after union to achieve eradication. May need revascularization. Regimens listed are empiric. Adjust after culture data available. If susceptible Gm-neg. bacillus, **CIP** 750 mg po bid or **Levo** 750 mg po q24h. For other S. aureus options: See Hem. Osteo. Specific Therapy. |
| Osteonecrosis of the jaw | Probably rare adverse reaction to bisphosphonates | Infection may be secondary to bone necrosis and loss of overlying mucosa. Treatment: minimal surgical debridement, chlorhexidine rinses, antibiotics (e.g., PIP-TZ). Evaluate for concomitant actinomycosis, for which specific long-term antibiotic treatment would be warranted | | |
| Prosthetic joint | See prosthetic joint, page 35 | | | |
| Spinal implant infection | S. aureus, coag-neg staphylococci, gram-neg bacilli | Onset within 30 days: culture, treat for 3 mos. Onset after 30 days remove implant, culture & treat | | See CID 55:1481, 2012 |
| Sternum, post-op | S. aureus, S. epidermidis, occasionally, gram-negative bacilli | **Vanco** 15-20 mg/kg q8-12h IV for trough of 15-20 μg/mL recommended for serious infections. | **Linezolid** 600 mg po/IV[NAI] bid | Sternal debridement for cultures & removal of necrotic bone. For S. aureus options: Hem. Osteo. Specific Therapy, page 6. If setting or gram stain suggests possibility of gram-negative bacilli, add appropriate coverage based on local antimicrobial susceptibility profiles (e.g., cefepime, PIP-TZ). |

Abbreviations on page 2.    *NOTE: All dosage recommendations are for adults (unless otherwise indicated) and assume normal renal function. § Alternative dosage recommendations consider allergy, PK, compliance, local resistance, cost.

**TABLE 1 (3)**

| ANATOMIC SITE/DIAGNOSIS/ MODIFYING CIRCUMSTANCES | ETIOLOGIES (usual) | SUGGESTED REGIMENS* | | ADJUNCT DIAGNOSTIC OR THERAPEUTIC MEASURES AND COMMENTS |
|---|---|---|---|---|
| | | PRIMARY | ALTERNATIVE§ | |
| **BONE** *(continued)* | | | | |
| **Contiguous Osteomyelitis with Vascular Insufficiency.** | | | | |
| Most pts are diabetics with peripheral neuropathy & infected skin ulcers *(See Diabetic foot, page 18)* | Polymicrobic [Gm+ cocci (to include MRSA) (aerobic & anaerobic), and Gm-neg. bacilli (aerobic & anaerobic)] | Debride overlying ulcer & submit bone for histology & culture. Select antibiotic based on culture results & treat for 6 weeks. **No empiric therapy unless acutely ill.** If acutely ill, *see suggestions, Diabetic foot, page 18.* Revascularize if possible. | | **Diagnosis of osteo:** Culture bone biopsy (gold standard). Poor concordance of culture results between swab of ulcer and bone – need bone. Sampling by needle puncture inferior to biopsy *(CID 47:888, 2009).* Osteo likely if ulcer >2 cm², positive probe to bone, ESR >70 & abnormal plain x-ray *(JAMA 299:806, 2008).* **Treatment:** (1) **Revascularize if possible;** (2) Culture bone; (3) Specific antimicrobial(s). |
| **Chronic Osteomyelitis: Specific Therapy** By definition, implies presence of dead bone. **Need valid cultures** | S. aureus, Enterobacteriaceae, P. aeruginosa | Empiric rx not indicated. Base systemic rx on results of culture, sensitivity testing. If acute exacerbation of chronic osteo, rx as acute hematogenous osteo. Surgical debridement important. | | **Important adjuncts:** removal of orthopedic hardware, surgical debridement; vascularized muscle flaps, distraction osteogenesis (Ilizarov) techniques. Antibiotic-impregnated cement & hyperbaric oxygen are adjunctive. **NOTE: RIF + (Vanco or β-lactam)** effective in animal model and in a clinical trial of S. aureus chronic osteo. |
| **BREAST: Mastitis**–Obtain culture: need to know if MRSA present. *Review of breast infections: (Cochrane Review: Cochrane Database Syst Rev 2013 Feb 28;2:CD005458; see also CID 54:71, 2012)* | | | | |
| Postpartum mastitis | | | | |
| Mastitis without abscess | S. aureus; less often, S. pyogenes (Gp A or B), E. coli, bacteroides species, maybe Corynebacterium sp., & selected coagulase-neg. staphylococci (e.g., S. lugdunensis) | **NO MRSA: Outpatient:** Diclox 500 mg po qid or **Cephalexin** 500 mg po qid. **Inpatient: Nafcillin** or **Oxacillin** 2 gm IV q4-6h | **MRSA Possible: Outpatient:** TMP-SMX-DS tabs 1-2 po bid or, if susceptible, **Clinda** 300 mg po tid **Inpatient: Vanco** 1 gm IV q12h; if over 100 kg, 1.5 gm IV q12h. | If no abscess & controllable pain, ↑ freq of nursing may hasten response. |
| Mastitis with abscess | | | | For painful abscess I&D is standard; needle aspiration reported successful. Resume breast feeding from affected breast as soon as pain allows. *(Breastfeed Med 9:239, 2014)* |
| Non-puerperal mastitis with abscess | S. aureus; less often Bacteroides sp., peptostreptococcus (Peptoniphilus sp.), & selected coagulase-neg. staphylococci | See regimens for Postpartum mastitis, page 7. | | Smoking and diabetes may be risk factors *(BMJ 342:d396, 2011).* **If subareolar & odoriferous,** most likely anaerobes; need to **add Metro 500 mg** IV/po tid. If not subareolar, staph. Need pretreatment aerobic/anaerobic cultures. Surgical drainage for abscess. **I&D standard.** Corynebacterium sp. assoc. with chronic granulomatous mastitis *(JCM 53:2895, 2015).* **Consider TB IS chronic infections.** |
| Breast implant infection | Acute: S. aureus, S. pyogenes. TSS reported. Chronic: Look for rapidly growing Mycobacteria | Acute: **Vanco** 15-20 mg/kg IV q8-12h. | Chronic: Await culture results. See Table 12A for mycobacteria treatment. | Risk of complications higher with late-onset infection (>30 days post implantation). Antibiotics alone may be sufficient for minor infections; explantation often required for more serious infections. *Plast. Reconstr. Surg 139:20, 2017.* |

*Abbreviations on page 2.    *NOTE: All dosage recommendations are for adults (unless otherwise indicated) and assume normal renal function. § Alternatives consider allergy, PK, compliance, local resistance, cost.*

**TABLE 1 (4)**

| ANATOMIC SITE/DIAGNOSIS/ MODIFYING CIRCUMSTANCES | ETIOLOGIES (usual) | SUGGESTED REGIMENS* | | ADJUNCT DIAGNOSTIC OR THERAPEUTIC MEASURES AND COMMENTS |
|---|---|---|---|---|
| | | PRIMARY | ALTERNATIVE† | |
| **CENTRAL NERVOUS SYSTEM** | | | | |
| **Brain abscess** | | | | |
| Primary or contiguous source. Review: *NEJM 371:447, 2014.* | Streptococci (60–70%), bacteroides (20–40%), Enterobacteriaceae (25–33%), S. anginosus grp. Rare: Nocardia (*below*), Listeria. See *S. aureus* Comment | (**Cefotaxime** 2 gm IV q4h or **Ceftriaxone** 2 gm IV q12h) + (**Metro** 7.5 mg/kg IV q6h or 15 mg/kg IV q12h). Add **Vanco** 15-20 mg/kg IV q8-12h or **Linezolid** 600 mg IV/po q12h to the regimen if S. aureus is a possibility | **Pen G** 3-4 million units IV q4h or + **Metro** 7.5 mg/kg IV q6h or 15 mg/kg IV q12h | If CT suggests cerebritis or abscesses <2.5 cm and pt neurologically stable and conscious, start antibiotics and observe. Otherwise, surgical drainage necessary. If blood cultures or other clinical data do not yield a likely etiologic agent, aspirate even small abscesses for diagnosis if this can be done safely. S. anginosus grp. esp. prone to produce abscess. Ceph/metro does not cover listeria. |
| | | Duration of rx unclear: usually 4-6 wks or until resolution by neuro-imaging (CT/MRI) | | |
| Post-surgical, post-traumatic. Review: *NEJM 371:447, 2014.* | S. aureus, Enterobacteriaceae | For MSSA: (**Nafcillin** or **Oxacillin**) 2 gm IV q4h + (**Ceftriaxone** or **Cefotaxime**) | For MRSA: **Vanco** 15-20 mg/kg IV q8-12h for trough of 15-20 mcg/mL + (**Ceftriaxone** or **Cefotaxime**) | Empiric coverage, de-escalated based on culture results. **Aspiration of abscess usually necessary for dx & rx. If P. aeruginosa suspected, substitute (Cefepime or Ceftazidime) for (Ceftriaxone or Cefotaxime).** |
| HIV-1 infected (AIDS) | Toxoplasma gondii | See *Table 13A, page 166* | | |
| Nocardia: Haematogenous abscess | N. farcinica, N. asteroides & N. brasiliensis. See *AAC 58:795, 2014* for other species. | **TMP-SMX:** 15 mg/kg/day of TMP, 6.75 mg/kg/day of SMX, IV/po divided q6h, later switch to po therapy. Immunocompetent pts: **TMP-SMX, minocycline** or **AM-CL** x 3+ months. Immunocompromised pts: Treat with 2 drugs x 1 yr. | **Linezolid** 600 mg q12h + **meropenem** 2 gm q8h | **Linezolid** 600 mg po bid reported effective. For in vitro susceptibility testing: Wallace (+) 903-877-7690 or U.S. CDC (+) 404-639-3158. **TMP-SMX** remains a drug of choice for Nocardia infection. In vitro resistance to TMP-SMX may be increasing (*CID 51:1445, 2010*), but whether this is associated with worse outcomes is not known and a recent study casts doubt on this with only 2.5% of 552 isolates resistant; difficulties with end-point determinations might account for discrepancies in reported rates of resistance (*JCM 50:670, 2012*). **If sulfonamide resistant or sulfa-allergic, Amikacin plus one of: IMP, MER, Ceftriaxone or Cefotaxime. N. farcinica is resistant to third-generation cephalosporins, which should not be used for treatment of infection caused by this organism. If TMP-SMX resistance reported (*JCM 50:670, 2012* before stopping TMP-SMX).** |
| | | *N. farcinica:* add **Amikacin** 7.5 mg/kg q12h. After 3-6 wks of IV therapy, switch to po therapy. | | |
| **Subdural empyema:** In adult 60–90% is extension of sinusitis or otitis media. Rx same as primary brain abscess. Surgical emergency; must drain. Review in *IDID 7:62, 2007.* | | | | |
| Encephalitis/encephalopathy IDSA Guideline: *CID 47:303, 2008; Intl diagnosis consensus: CID 57:1114, 2013.* (For Herpes; see *Table 14A, page 181* and for rabies, *Table 20B, page 254*) | H. simplex (42%), VZV (15%), M. TB (15%), Listeria (10%). Other: arbovirus, West Nile, rabies, Parvo B19, Cat-scratch, Mycoplasma, EBV and others. | Start IV **Acyclovir** while awaiting results of CSF PCR for H. simplex. For dx of amebic encephalitis see *Table 13A*. Start **Doxy** 100 mg q12h if setting suggests R. rickettsii, Anaplasma, Ehrlichia or Mycoplasma. **Ceftriaxone** 2 gm IV q24h or **Doxy** 100 mg q12h x 14 days for Lyme encephalitis. | **Linezolid** 600 mg IV or po q12h + **meropenem** 2 gm q8h | Increasing recognition of autoimmune antibody-mediated encephalitis, e.g., anti-N-methyl aspartate receptors & others. Dx: CSF antibody panel. Ref: *NEJM 2018;378:840.* Review of acute viral encephalitis (*NEJM 2018;379:557*) |
| Meningitis, "Aseptic:" Pleocytosis of up to 100s of cells, CSF glucose normal, neg. culture for bacteria (See *Table 14A, page 178*) Ref: *CID 47:783, 2008* | Enteroviruses, HSV-2, LCM, HIV, VZV, other viruses, syphilis, drugs [NSAIDs, metronidazole, carbamazepine, lamotrigine TMP-SMX, IVIG, (e.g., detuximab, infliximab)], rarely leptospirosis, Lyme. | For all but leptospirosis, IV fluids and analgesics. D/C drugs that may be etiologic. For lepto: **Doxy** 100 mg IV/po q12h) or (**Pen G** 5 million units IV q6h) or **AMP** 0.5-1 gm IV q6h). Repeat LP if suspect partially-treated bacterial meningitis. **Acyclovir** 5-10 mg/kg IV q8h sometimes given for HSV-2 meningitis (**NOTE:** distinct from HSV encephalitis where early rx is mandatory). | | If available, PCR of CSF for enterovirus. VZV, HSV-2: concurrent or history of prior genital lesions often absent (*Ann J Neurovirol 19:166, 2013*). For lepto, positive epidemiologic history and concomitant hepatitis, conjunctivitis, dermatitis, nephritis. For list of implicated drugs: *Inf Med 25:331, 2008.* CNS Lyme: Varies – palsy, encephalitis, aseptic meningitis; see page 62. Etiologies: *Med 95:e2372, 2016.* |

*NOTE: All dosage recommendations are for adults (unless otherwise indicated) and assume normal renal function. § Alternatives consider allergy; PK, compliance, local resistance, cost.

Abbreviations on page 2.

**TABLE 1 (5)**

| ANATOMIC SITE/DIAGNOSIS/ MODIFYING CIRCUMSTANCES | ETIOLOGIES (usual) | SUGGESTED REGIMENS* | | ADJUNCT DIAGNOSTIC OR THERAPEUTIC MEASURES AND COMMENTS |
|---|---|---|---|---|
| | | PRIMARY | ALTERNATIVE§ | |
| **CENTRAL NERVOUS SYSTEM** (continued) | | | | |
| **Meningitis, Bacterial, Acute. Goal is empiric therapy, then CSF analysis.** If focal neurologic deficit, give empiric therapy, then head CT. If no focal deficit, empiric therapy, LP & then head CT (CID 2018;66:e32). For distribution of pathogens by age group, see NEJM 364:2016, 2011. | | | | |
| **Empiric Therapy—CSF Gram stain is negative—immunocompetent** | | | | |
| **Age: Preterm to <1 mo** LnID 10:32, 2010 | Group B strep 49%, E. coli 18%, listeria 7%, misc. Gm-neg. 10%, misc. Gm-pos. 10% | AMP 75-100 mg/kg IV q6h + Cefotaxime 75 mg/kg IV q6h + Gent 2.5 mg/kg IV q8h | AMP 75-100 mg/kg IV q6h + Cefotaxime 75 mg/kg IV q6h + Gent 2.5 mg/kg IV q8h 5-7 mg/kg IV q24h | Regimens active vs. Group B strep, most coliforms, & listeria. If premature infant with long nursery stay, S. aureus, enterococci, and resistant coliforms potentially pathogens. **If high risk of MRSA,** use vanco + cefotaxime. Alter regimen after culture/ sensitivity data available. |
| | | Intraventricular treatment not recommended. | | |
| **Age: 1 mo– 50 yrs** Recent review: Lancet Infect Dis 16:339, 2016. | S. pneumo, meningococci, H. influenzae now uncommon; **listeria unlikely if young adult & immunocompetent** (add Ampicillin if suspect listeria 2 gm IV q4h) | Adult: [(Cefotaxime 2 gm IV q4-6h OR Ceftriaxone 2 gm IV q12h)] + Dexamethasone + Vanco Dexamethasone 0.15 mg/kg IV q6h x 2-4 days. **Give with, or just before, 1st dose of antibiotic.** (see Comment, See footnote1 for Vanco Adult dosage and§ for ped. dosage | (Peds: 40 mg/kg IV q6h)] + Dexamethasone + Vanco1 | For patients with severe β-lactam allergy, see below (Empiric Therapy— positive gram stain and Specific Therapy) for alternative therapies. |
| **Age: >50 yrs or alcoholism or other debilitating assoc diseases or impaired cellular immunity** | S. pneumo, listeria, meningococci, Gm-neg. bacilli | (AMP 2 gm IV q4h) + (Ceftriaxone 2 gm IV q12h or Cefotaxime 2 gm IV q4-6h) + Vanco1 + Dexamethasone. **For Vanco dose, see footnote1. Dexamethasone** 0.15 mg/kg IV q6h x 2-4 days; 1st dose before, or concomitant with, 1st dose of antibiotic. | MER 2 gm IV q8h + Vanco + IV Dexamethasone For severe Pen allergy, see Comment. | For patients with severe β-lactam allergy, see below (Empiric Therapy— positive gram stain and Specific Therapy): alternative agents that can be substituted to cover likely pathogens. LP without CT for patients with altered level of consciousness and non-focal neurological exam associated with earlier treatment and improved outcome (CID 60:1162, 2015) |
| **Post-neurosurgery Ventriculostomy/lumbar catheter; ventriculoperitoneal (atrial) shunt or penetrating trauma w/o basilar skull fracture** Shunt-related meningitis IDSA Guidelines: CID 64:e34, 2017. | S. epidermidis, S. aureus, Cutibacterium acnes, Facultative and aerobic gram-neg bacilli, including: P. aeruginosa & A. baumannii (may be multi-drug resistant) | Vanco (to achieve trough level of 15-20 mg/kg IV q8h) + (Cefepime or Ceftaz 2 gm IV q8h) • **If severe Pen/Ceph allergy,** substitute either: Aztreonam 2 gm IV q6-8h or CIP 400 mg IV q12h. **Intraventricular antibiotic dosing** (lower dose for slit ventricles, intermediate dose for normal size ventricles, higher dose for enlarged ventricles): **Amikacin** 30 mg, **Gent** 4-8 mg in adults, 1-2 mg in infants, children, **Polymyxin E** (Colistin) 10 mg, **Tobra** 5-20 mg, **Vanco** 5-20 mg, **Dapto** 5 mg. **Frequency of administration** depends on drainage output: < 50 mL/24h: every 3rd day, 50-100 mL/24h: every second day, 100-150 mL/day: once daily, 150-200 mL/24h: increase dose of vancomycin by 5 mg, gentamicin by 1 mg, increase dose of vancomycin by 5 mg, gentamicin by 1 mg | Vanco (to achieve trough level of 15-20 mg/mL) + (MER 2 gm IV q8h) | Remove infected shunt and place external ventricular catheter for drainage or pressure control. Intraventricular therapy used if the shunt cannot be removed or cultures fail to clear with systemic therapy. **Shunt reimplantation:** If coagulase-negative staphylococci, diphtheroids, or C. acnes: next no CSF abnormalities, day 3 after external ventricular cultures are negative at 48h; if CSF abnormalities present: 7-10 days after the last positive CSF culture. If S. aureus or Gram-negative organism: 10 days after last positive CSF culture. |

1 Vanco adult dose: 15-20 mg/kg IV q8-12h to achieve trough level of 15-20 µg/mL.
2 Dosage of drugs used to treat children age ≥1 mo: **Cefotaxime** 50 mg/kg per day IV q6h; **Ceftriaxone** 50 mg/kg IV q6h to achieve trough level of 15-20 µg/mL; **Vanco** 15 mg/kg q6h to achieve trough level of 15-20 µg/mL

§ Alternatives consider allergy, PK, compliance, local resistance, cost.

Abbreviations on page 2.    * NOTE: All dosage recommendations are for adults (unless otherwise indicated) and assume normal renal function.

**TABLE 1 (6)**

| ANATOMIC SITE/DIAGNOSIS/ MODIFYING CIRCUMSTANCES | ETIOLOGIES (usual) | SUGGESTED REGIMENS* | | ADJUNCT DIAGNOSTIC OR THERAPEUTIC MEASURES AND COMMENTS |
|---|---|---|---|---|
| | | **PRIMARY** | **ALTERNATIVE§** | |
| **CENTRAL NERVOUS SYSTEM/Meningitis, Bacterial, Acute/Empiric Therapy—CSF Gram stain is negative—immunocompetent** *(continued)* | | | | |
| **Trauma with basilar skull fracture** | S. pneumoniae, H. influenzae, S. pyogenes | **Vanco** (to achieve trough level of 15-20 mg/mL) + (**Ceftriaxone** 2 gm IV q12h or **Cefotaxime** 2 gm IV q4-6h) | (**Ceftriaxone** 2 gm IV q12h or **Cefotaxime** 2 gm IV q4-6h) + **Dexamethasone** 0.15 mg/kg IV q6h x 2-4 d (1st dose w/or before 1st antibiotic dose)). See *Clin Micro Rev* 21:519, 2008. | |
| **Empiric Therapy—Positive CSF Gram stain** | | | | |
| Gram-positive diplococci | S. pneumoniae | (**Ceftriaxone** 2 gm IV q12h or **Cefotaxime** 2 gm IV q4-6h) + **Vanco** 15-20 mg/kg IV q8-12h (to achieve 15-20 µg/mL trough) + **Dexamethasone** 0.15 mg/kg IV q6h; first dose is given 15-20 minutes prior to first antibiotic dose, and then continued for 4 days for confirmed pneumococcal infection. | **Alternatives: MER** 2 gm IV q8h or **Moxi** 400 mg IV q24h. | |
| Gram-negative diplococci | N. meningitidis | (**Ceftriaxone** 2 gm IV q4-6h or **Ceftriaxone** 2 gm IV q12h) | | **Alternatives: Pen G** 4 mill units IV q4h or **AMP** 2 gm q4h or **Moxi** 400 mg IV q24h or **Chloro** 1 gm IV q6h (chloro less effective than other alternatives; see *JAC* 70:979, 2015) |
| Gram-positive bacilli or coccobacilli | Listeria monocytogenes | **AMP** 2 gm IV q4h ± **Genta** 2 mg/kg IV loading dose then 1.7 mg/kg IV q8h | | If pen allergic: use **TMP/SMX** 5 mg/kg (TMP component) q6-8h. Use of meropenem associated with increased 30-day mortality (*Clin Microbiol Infect* 22: 725, 2016). Data showing beneficial effect of gentamicin combination therapy are inconclusive. |
| Gram-negative bacilli | H. influenzae, enterics, P. aeruginosa | (**Ceftazidime** or **Cefepime** 2 gm IV q8h) + **Genta** 2 mg/kg IV 1st dose then 1.7 mg/kg IV q8h | | **Alternatives: MER** 2 gm IV infused over 4h q8h (covers ESBLs); **Aztreonam** 2 gm IV q6-8h (safe in beta-lactam allergic patient). **Dexamethasone not recommended for Gram-negatives other than suspected H. influenzae** administered as 0.15 mg/kg IV q6h; first dose is given 15-20 minutes prior to first antibiotic dose, and then continued for 4 days if H. influenza infection is confirmed. |
| **Specific Therapy—Positive culture of CSF with in vitro susceptibility results available** | | | | |
| H. influenzae | β-lactamase positive | **Ceftriaxone** 2 gm IV q12h (adult), 50 mg/kg IV q12h (peds) + **Dexamethasone** 0.15 mg/kg IV q6h; first dose is given 15-20 minutes prior to first antibiotic dose, and then continued for 4 days in microbiologically confirmed cases. | | **Pen. allergic: Chloro** 12.5 mg/kg IV q6h (max. 4 gm/day.) (Chloro less effective than other alternatives; see *JAC* 70:979, 2015). **CIP** 400 mg IV q8-12h; **Aztreonam** 2 gm q6-8h. |
| Listeria monocytogenes (*CID* 43:1233, 2006) | | **AMP** 2 gm IV q4h ± **Genta** 2 mg/kg IV loading dose, then 1.7 mg/kg IV q8h | | If pen allergic: use **TMP/SMX** 5 mg/kg (TMP component) q6-8h. Use of meropenem associated with increased 30-day mortality (*Clin Microbiol Infect* 22: 725, 2016). Data showing beneficial effect of gentamicin combination therapy are inconclusive. |
| N. meningitidis | | **Pen G** (adult dose 4 million units q4h) x 7 days or **Ceftriaxone** 2 gm IV q12h x 7 days (preferred if MIC is 0.1 to 1.0 µg/ml); if β-lactam allergic, **Chloro** 12.5 µg/kg (up to 1 gm) IV q6h (but chloro less effective than other alternatives; see *JAC* 70:979, 2015). | | Other alternatives: **MER** 2 gm IV q8h or **Moxi** 400 mg IV q24h. Rare isolates resistant to Chloro. FQ-resistant isolates encountered rarely. Increased risk of invasive meningococcal infection in recipients of eculizumab (*MMWR* 66:734, 2017). |

*MOTE: All dosage recommendations are for adults (unless otherwise indicated) and assume normal renal function. §Alternatives consider allergy, PK, compliance, local resistance, cost.

Abbreviations on page 2.

**TABLE 1 (7)**

| ANATOMIC SITE/DIAGNOSIS/ MODIFYING CIRCUMSTANCES | ETIOLOGIES (usual) | SUGGESTED REGIMENS* | | ADJUNCT DIAGNOSTIC OR THERAPEUTIC MEASURES AND COMMENTS |
|---|---|---|---|---|
| | | PRIMARY | ALTERNATIVE§ | |
| **CENTRAL NERVOUS SYSTEM/Meningitis, Bacterial, Acute/Specific Therapy—Positive culture of CSF with in vitro susceptibility results available** *(continued)* | | | | |
| **S. pneumoniae** Notes: 1. Dexamethasone 0.15 mg/kg IV q6h times 2-4 days, 15-20 minutes prior to first antibiotic dose, and then continued for 4 days. If MIC ≥1, repeat CSF exam after 24-48h. 3. Treat for 10-14 days. | Pen G MIC <0.1 mcg/mL | Pen G 4 million units IV q4h or AMP 2 gm IV q4h | Alternatives: Ceftriaxone 2 gm IV q12h, Chloro 1 gm IV q6h (Chloro less effective than other alternatives; see JAC 70:979, 2015) | |
| | 0.1–1 mcg/mL | Ceftriaxone 2 gm IV q12h or Cefotaxime 2 gm IV q4-6h | Alternatives: Cefepime 2 gm IV q8h; MER 2 gm IV q8h | |
| | ≥2 mcg/mL | Vanco 15-20 mg/kg IV q8-12h (15-20 µg/mL trough target) + (Ceftriaxone or Cefotaxime as above) | Alternatives: Moxi 400 mg IV q24h | |
| | Ceftriaxone MIC ≥1 mcg/mL | Vanco 15-20 mg/kg IV q8-12h (15-20 µg/mL trough target) + (Ceftriaxone or Cefotaxime as above) | If MIC to Ceftriaxone >2 mcg/mL, add RIF 600 mg po/IV 1x/day to Vanco + (Ceftriaxone or Cefotaxime). | |
| **E. coli, other coliforms, or P. aeruginosa** | **Consultation advised**— need susceptibility results | (Ceftazidime or Cefepime 2 gm IV q8h) + Genta 2 mg/kg IV × 1 dose, then 1.7 mg/kg IV q8h x 21 days. | Alternatives: MER 2 gm IV infused over 4h q8h; CIP 400 mg IV q8h (need to confirm susceptibility) Reculture CSF after 4-5 days of therapy. If culture is still positive, may need adjunctive intrathecal or intraventricular antibiotic therapy. | |
| **Prophylaxis for H. influenzae and N. meningitidis** | | | | |
| **Haemophilus influenzae type B** Household or close contact group defined as persons who reside with the patient or a nonresident who has spent 4 hours or more with the index patient for at least 5 of the 7 days preceding the day of hospitalization of the patient. | | **RIF** 20 mg/kg (not to exceed 600 mg) once daily × 4 days for individuals ≥1 mo; 10 mg/kg once daily × 4 days for age <1 mo. | | **Household or Close Contacts:** RIF chemoprophylaxis recommended for index patients (unless treated with Cefotaxime or Ceftriaxone) and all household contacts in households with members aged <4 years who are not fully vaccinated or members aged <18 years who are immunocompromised, regardless of their vaccination status. **Child Care Contacts:** RIF chemoprophylaxis recommended in child care settings when two or more cases of invasive Hib disease have occurred within 60 days and unimmunized or underimmunized children attend the facility, when prophylaxis is indicated, it should be prescribed and administered regardless of age or vaccine status, and for child care providers. |
| **Prophylaxis for Neisseria meningitidis exposure** (close contact) | | **RIF** 10 mg/kg (max dose 600 mg) q12h × 2 days (adult or child ≥1 mo); 5 mg/kg q12h × 2 dose child <1 mo OR **Ceftriaxone** single IM dose of 250 mg (adult) or 125 mg (child age <15 years) OR **CIP** single po 500 mg dose (age ≥18; not recommended in pregnant or lactating women, or if CIP resistant isolates circulating in the local community). | | ↑ risk if close contact for at least 4 hrs during wk before illness onset Spread by respiratory droplets, not aerosols, hence close contact req. (e.g., housemates, day care contacts, cellmates) or exposure to pt's nasopharyngeal secretions (e.g., kissing, mouth-to-mouth resuscitation, intubation, nasotracheal suctioning). |
| **Meningitis, chronic** Defined as symptoms + CSF pleocytosis for 24 wks | MTB cryptococcosis, other fungal, neoplastic, Lyme, syphilis, Whipple's disease | Treatment depends on etiology. No urgent need for empiric therapy, but when TB suspected treatment should be expeditious. | | Long list of possibilities: bacteria, parasites, fungi, viruses, neoplasms, vasculitis, and other miscellaneous etiologies—see Neurol Clin 28:1061, 2010. See NEJM 370:2408, 2014 for diagnosis of neuroleptospirosis by next generation sequencing technologies. |
| **Meningitis, eosinophilic** *Hawaii J Med Public Health, 72(6 Suppl 2):52, 2013* | Angiostrongyliasis, gnathostomiasis, baylisascaris | Corticosteroids | Anti-helminthic therapy probably not beneficial | 1/3 lack peripheral eosinophilia. Need serology to confirm diagnosis. Steroid ref: Cochrane Database Syst Rev. 2015 Feb 17;(2):CD009088 |
| **Meningitis, HIV-1 infected (AIDS)** See Table 11, SANFORD GUIDE TO HIV/AIDS THERAPY | As in adults, >50 yrs: also consider cryptococci. M. tuberculosis, syphilis, HIV aseptic meningitis, Listeria monocytogenes | If etiology not identified: treat as adult >50 yrs + obtain CSF/serum crypto-coccal antigen (see Comments) | For crypto rx, see Table 11A, page 136 | C. neoformans most common etiology in AIDS patients. H. influenzae, pneumococci, listeria, TBc, syphilis, viral, Histoplasma & coccidiodes also need to be considered. Obtain blood cultures. |

*Abbreviations on page 2.*   *NOTE: All dosage recommendations are for adults (unless otherwise indicated) and assume normal renal function. § Alternatives consider allergy, PK, compliance, local resistance, cost.*

**TABLE 1 (8)**

| ANATOMIC SITE/DIAGNOSIS/ MODIFYING CIRCUMSTANCES | ETIOLOGIES (usual) | SUGGESTED REGIMENS° PRIMARY | ALTERNATIVE§ | ADJUNCT DIAGNOSTIC OR THERAPEUTIC MEASURES AND COMMENTS |
|---|---|---|---|---|
| **EAR** | | | | |
| **External otitis** | | | | |
| Acute external otitis: "Swimmer's ear", ear buds, headsets. Ref: *JAMA 2018;320:1375* | S. aureus, P. aeruginosa | Ear drops: 1) CIP + (dexamethasone or hydrocortisone) bid x 7 days; 2) Oflox qd x 7 days; 3) CIP single dose | | In Cochrane meta-analysis, antiseptics, acidifying agents, glucocorticoids & topical antibiotics have similar outcomes (*Coch Sys Rev 2010;1:CD004740*). Topical antibiotic therapy favored with cure rates of 65-90%; all are expensive ($70-300). |
| Chronic | Usually 2° to seborrhea | Eardrops: [(Polymyxin B + Neomycin + hydrocortisone) qid) + selenium sulfide shampoo] | | Control seborrhea with dandruff shampoo containing selenium sulfide (Selsun) or [(ketoconazole shampoo) + (medium potency steroid solution, triamcinolone 0.1%)]. |
| Fungal | Candida species | Fluconazole 200 mg po x 1 dose & then 100 mg po q 3-5 days. | | |
| "Necrotizing (malignant) otitis externa" Risk groups: Diabetes mellitus, AIDS, chemotherapy. See *Am J Otolaryngol 37:425, 2016.* | Pseudomonas aeruginosa in >95% (*Otol & Neurotology 34:620, 2013*) | CIP 400 mg IV q8h; 750 mg po q8-12h only for early disease | PIP-TZ 3.375 gm q8h or extended infusion (3.375 gm over 4 hrs q8h) + Tobra | Very high ESRs are typical. Debridement usually required. R/O osteomyelitis: CT or MRI scans. If bone involved, treat for 6-8 wks. Other alternatives if P. aeruginosa is susceptible: IMP 0.5 gm q6h or MER 1 gm IV q8h or CFP 2 gm IV q12h or Ceftaz 2 gm IV q8h. |
| **Otitis media—infants, children, adults** (*Cochrane review: Cochrane Database Syst Rev. Jan 31;1:CD000219, 2013); American Academy of Pediatrics Guidelines: Pediatrics 131:e964, 2013*) | | | | |
| **Acute** Two RCTs indicate efficacy of antibiotic rx if age <36 mos & definite AOM (*NEJM 364:105, 116 & 168, 2011*) | Overall detection in middle ear fluid:<br>No pathogen 4%<br>Virus 70%<br>Bact + virus 66%<br>Bacteria 92%<br>Bacterial pathogens from middle ear: S. pneumo 49%, H. influenzae 29%, M. catarrhalis 28%. Ref: *CID 43:1417 & 1423, 2006.* Children 6 mos-3 yrs, 2 episodes AOM/yrs & 63% are virus positive (*CID 46:815 & 824, 2008*) | | | |
| **Initial empiric therapy of acute otitis media (AOM)**<br>**NOTE:** Treat children <2 yrs old. If >2 yrs old, afebrile, no ear pain, neg./questionable examination—consider analgesic treatment without antimicrobials. Favorable results in mostly afebrile pts with waiting 48hrs before deciding on antibiotic use (*JAMA 296:1235, 1290, 2006*) | | **If NO antibiotics in prior month:**<br>Amox 80-90 mg/kg/d divided q8h or q12h (**preferred regimen**) OR<br>AM-CL 90/6.4 mg/kg/d divided bid<br>Options for nonIgE PCN allergy:<br>Cefdinir 14 mg/kg/d divided q12h or once q24h<br>Cefpodoxime proxetil 10 mg/kg/d divided q12h or once q24h<br>Cefprozil 15 mg/kg/d divided q12h<br>Cefuroxime axetil 30 mg/kg/d divided q12h | **Received antibiotics in prior month:** AM-CL 90/6.4 mg/kg/d divided bid OR Ceftriaxone 50 mg/kg IV or IM once daily for 3 days<br>Other options include oral Cefdinir, Cefpodoxime proxetil, Cefprozil, or Cefuroxime axetil but these may be less effective for pen-non-susceptible S. pneumoniae. For adults also: Levo or Moxi<br><br>**All doses are pediatric**<br>**Duration of rx:** <2 yrs old x 10 days; ≥2 yrs x 5-7 days. Appropriate duration unclear 5 days may be inadequate for severe disease (*NEJM 347:1169, 2002*)<br><br>For adult doses, see **Sinusitis, page 53, and Table 10A** | β-lactam allergy: If history unclear or rash, oral ceph OK; avoid ceph if IgE-mediated allergy, e.g., anaphylaxis.<br>TMP-SMX: high failure rate if etiology is DRSP or H. influenzae<br>Macrolides: limited efficacy against S. pneumo and H. influenzae, use only if β-lactam not an option.<br>Drug-resistant S. pneumo: Risk ↑ if age <2 yrs, antibiotics last 3 mos, &/or daycare attendance. Selection of drug based on (1) effectiveness against β-lactamase producing H. influenzae & M. catarrhalis & (2) effectiveness against S. pneumo, inc. DRSP. Cefaclor, Loracarbef, & Ceftibuten less active vs. S. pneumo (Pen resistant) than other β-lactams.<br>Otitis media with effusion: no benefit of antibiotics (*Cochrane Database Syst Rev. Sep 12;9:CD009163, 2012).*<br>Persistent otorrhea with PE tubes: Hydrocortisone/Bacitracin/Colistin eardrops 5 drops IU x 7 d more effective than po AM-CL (*NEJM:370:723, 2014).*<br>Refractory or recurrent AOM, age 6 months to 5 years: Levofloxacin 20 mg/kg/d in divided doses q12h if other options have failed. Tympanostomy tubes may prevent recurrent AOM. |

°NOTE: All dosage recommendations are for adults (unless otherwise indicated) and assume normal renal function. § Alternatives consider allergy, PK, compliance, local resistance, cost.

**TABLE 1 (9)**

| ANATOMIC SITE/DIAGNOSIS/ MODIFYING CIRCUMSTANCES | ETIOLOGIES (usual) | SUGGESTED REGIMENS* PRIMARY | ALTERNATIVE§ | ADJUNCT DIAGNOSTIC OR THERAPEUTIC MEASURES AND COMMENTS |
|---|---|---|---|---|
| **EAR/Otitis media—infants, children, adults** *(continued)* | | | | |
| Treatment for clinical failure after 3 days | Drug-resistant S. pneumoniae main concern | **NO antibiotics in month prior to last 3 days:** **AM-CL HD** or **Cefinir** or **Cefpodoxime** or **Cefprozil** or **Cefuroxime Axetil** or **IM Ceftriaxone** x 3 days | **Antibiotics in month prior to last 3 days:** [(IM **Ceftriaxone**) or (**Clinda**)] and/or tympanocentesis] *See Comments* *For dosage, see footnote[3]* **All doses are pediatric** | **Clindamycin** not active vs. H. influenzae or M. catarrhalis. S. pneumo resistant to macrolides is usually also resistant to clindamycin. Definition of failure: no change in ear pain, fever, bulging TM or otorrhea after 3 days of therapy. Tympanocentesis will allow culture. **Levo** 20 mg/kg/d in divided doses q12h if other options have failed (not FDA approved). |
| After **>48 hrs** of nasotracheal intubation | Pseudomonas sp., klebsiella, enterobacter | **Ceftazidime** or **CFP** or **IMP** or **MER** or (**PIP-TZ**) or **CIP** *(For dosages, see Ext. Ear, Necrotizing (malignant) otitis externa, page 12)* | **Duration of rx as above** | With nasotracheal intubation >48 hrs, about ½ pts will have otitis media with effusion. |
| **Prophylaxis:** acute otitis media **Antimicrobial Stewardship: Use of antibiotics to prevent otitis media is a major contributor to emergence of antibiotic-resistant S. pneumo.** | | **Antimicrobial prophylaxis is not recommended.** | Pneumococcal protein conjugate vaccine decreases frequency of acute otitis media infections. Tympanostomy tube may prevent recurrent. AOM *(Otolaryn Head Neck Surg 156(4S):S88, 2017)*. Evidence supporting benefits of adenoidectomy are inconclusive *(Cochrane Database Syst Rev 2010;CD006282)*. Avoid FQ ear drops post-T-tubes; increased risk of chronic perforation *(NEJM 2017;64-1052)* | |
| **Mastoiditis:** Complication of acute or chronic otitis media. If chronic, look for cholesteatoma (Keratoma) | | | | |
| **Acute** Generally too ill for outpatient therapy. | 1st episode: S. pneumoniae H. influenzae M. catarrhalis *If secondary to chronic otitis media:* S. aureus P. aeruginosa S. pneumoniae | Obtain cultures, then empiric therapy. 1st episode: **Ceftriaxone** 2 gm IV once daily | 1st episode: **Ceftriaxone** 2 gm IV once daily OR **Levo** 750 mg | • Diagnosis: CT or MRI • Look for complication: osteomyelitis, suppurative lateral sinus thrombophlebitis, purulent meningitis, brain abscess • ENT consultation for possible mastoidectomy Acute exacerbation of chronic otitis media: Surgical debridement of auditory canal, then [**Vanco** (dose to achieve tough of 15-20 mcg/mL) + **PIP-TZ** 3.375 gm IV q6h] OR [**Vanco** (dose as above) + **CIP** 400 mg IV q8h] |
| **Chronic** Generally not ill enough for parenteral antibiotics | As per 1st episode and: S. aureus P. aeruginosa Anaerobes Fungi | Culture ear drainage. May need surgical debridement. Topical Fluoroquinolone ear drops. | Obtain cultures, then empiric therapy. ENT consult. | • Diagnosis: CT or MRI |

---

[3] **Drugs & peds dosage** (all po unless specified) for acute otitis media: **Amoxicillin UD (usual dose)** = 40 mg/kg per day div q12h or q8h. **Amoxicillin HD (high dose)** = 90 mg/kg per day div q12h or q8h. **AM-CL HD** = 90 mg/kg per day of amox component. **Extra-strength AM-CL oral suspension** (Augmentin ES-600) available with 600 mg AM & 42.9 mg CL / 5 mL—dose: 90/6.4 mg/kg per day div bid. **Cefuroxime axetil** 30 mg/kg per day div q12h. **Ceftriaxone** 50 mg/kg IM x 3 days. **Clindamycin** 20-30 mg/kg per day div q8h (may be effective vs. DRSP but no activity vs. H. influenzae). **Other drugs suitable for drug (e.g., Penicillin) - sensitive S. pneumo:** TMP-SMX 4 mg/kg of TMP q12h. **Erythro-sulfisoxazole** 50 mg/kg per day of erythro div q6-8h. **Clarithro** 15 mg/kg per day div q12h; **Cefpodoxime proxetil** 10 mg/kg per day as single dose; **Cefaclor** 40 mg/kg per day div q8h. **Cefdinir** 7 mg/kg q12h or 14 mg/kg q24h. **Azithro** 10 mg/kg per day x 1 & then 5 mg/kg per day x 4 days 2-5. Other FDA-approved regimens: 10 mg/kg q24h x 3 days & 30 mg/kg x 1. **Cefprozil** 15 mg/kg q12h;

*Abbreviations on page 2.*        *NOTE: All dosage recommendations are for adults (unless otherwise indicated) and assume normal renal function. § Alternatives consider allergy, PK, compliance, local resistance, cost.*

**TABLE 1 (10)**

| ANATOMIC SITE/DIAGNOSIS/ MODIFYING CIRCUMSTANCES | ETIOLOGIES (usual) | SUGGESTED REGIMENS* | | ADJUNCT DIAGNOSTIC OR THERAPEUTIC MEASURES AND COMMENTS |
|---|---|---|---|---|
| | | **PRIMARY** | **ALTERNATIVE§** | |
| **EYE** | | | | |
| **Eyelid:** (See Cochrane Database Syst Rev 5:CD005556, 2012) | | | | |
| **Blepharitis** | Etiol. unclear. Factors include Staph. aureus & Staph epidermidis, seborrhea, rosacea, & dry eye | Lid margin care with baby shampoo & warm compresses q24h. Artificial tears if assoc. dry eye (see Comment). | | Topical ointments of uncertain benefit (Cochrane Database Syst Rev 2017 Feb 7;2:CD011965). If associated rosacea, add doxy 100 mg po bid for 2 wks and then q24h. |
| **Hordeolum (Stye)** Cochrane review of effectiveness of non-surgical interventions found no evidence for or against non-surgical interventions for treatment of acute internal hordeola (Cochrane Database Syst Rev 2017 Jan 9;1:CD00774). | | | | |
| External (eyelash follicle) | Staph. aureus. Will drain spontaneously | Hot packs only. Will drain spontaneously | | Infection of superficial sebaceous gland. |
| Internal (Meibomian glands): Can be acute, subacute or chronic. | Staph. aureus, MSSA | Oral **Diclox** + hot packs | | Also called acute meibomianitis. Rarely drain spontaneously; may need I&D and culture. MRSA often |
| | Staph. aureus, MRSA | **TMP-SMX-DS**, tabs ii po bid | | resistant to lower conc.; may be susceptible to higher concentration of FQ |
| | Staph. aureus, MRSA (MDR) | **Linezolid** 600 mg po bid | | in ophthalmologic solutions of gati, levo or moxi. |
| **Conjunctiva:** Review: JAMA 310:1721, 2013. | | | | |
| **Conjunctivitis of the newborn (ophthalmia neonatorum):** by day of onset post-delivery—all dose pediatric | | | | |
| Onset 1st day | Chemical due to silver nitrate prophylaxis. | None | | Usual prophylaxis is erythro ointment; hence, silver nitrate irritation rare. |
| Onset 2–4 days | N. gonorrhoeae | **Ceftriaxone** 25–50 mg/kg IV x 1 dose (see Comment), not to exceed 125 mg | | Treat mother and her sexual partners. Hyperpurulent. Topical rx inadequate. **Treat neonate for concomitant Chlamydia trachomatis.** |
| Onset 3–10 days | Chlamydia trachomatis | **Erythro base or ethylsuccinate syrup** 12.5 mg/kg q6h x 14 days. No topical rx needed. | | Diagnosis by NAAT. Alternative: **Azithro suspension** 20 mg/kg po q24h x 3 days. Treat mother & sexual partner. |
| Onset 2–16 days | Herpes simplex types 1, 2 | Topical anti-viral rx under direction of ophthalmologist. | | Also give Acyclovir 60 mg/kg/day IV div 3 doses (Red Book online, accessed Jan 2017). |
| Ophthalmia neonatorum prophylaxis: **Erythro** 0.5% ointment x 1 or **Tetra** 1% ointment** x 1 application; effective vs. gonococcus but not C. trachomatis | | | | |
| **Pink eye** (viral conjunctivitis) Usually unilateral | Adenovirus (types 3 & 7 in children; 8, 11 & 19 in adults) | No treatment. If symptomatic, artificial tears may help. (some studies show 2 day reduction of symptoms with steroids; not recommended) | | Highly contagious. Onset of ocular pain and photophobia in an adult suggests associated keratitis--rare. |
| **Inclusion conjunctivitis (adult)** Usually unilateral & concomitant genital infection | Chlamydia trachomatis | **Azithro** 1 gm once | **Doxy** 100 mg po bid x 7 days | Oculogenital disease. Diagnosis NAAT. Urine NAAT for both GC & chlamydia. Treat sexual partner. May need to repeat dose of azithro. |
| **Trachoma** —a chronic bacterial keratoconjunctivitis linked to poverty | Chlamydia trachomatis | **Azithro** 20 mg/kg po single dose--78% effective in children; Adults: 1 gm po. | **Doxy** 100 mg po bid x minimum of 21 days or **Tetracycline** 250 mg po qid x 14 days. | Starts in childhood and can persist for years with subsequent damage to cornea. Topical therapy of marginal benefit. Avoid doxy/tetracycline in young children. Mass treatment works. |
| **Suppurative conjunctivitis**, bacterial: Children and Adults (Eyedrops speed resolution of symptoms: Cochrane Database Syst Rev. Sep 12;9:CD001211, 2012) | | | | |
| JAMA 310:1721, 2013 | Staph. aureus, S. pneumoniae, H. influenzae, Viridans Strep., Moraxella sp. | FQ ophthalmic solns: **CIP** (generic); others expensive (**Besi, Levo, Moxi**) All 1-2 gtts q2h while awake 1st 2 days, then q4-8h up to 7 days. | **Polymyxin B + TMP** solution 1-2 gtts q3-6h x 7-10 days. | Broad-spectrum for empiric therapy. High concentrations ↑ likelihood of activity vs. S. aureus--even MRSA. **TMP** spectrum may include MRSA. Polymyxin B spectrum only Gm-neg. bacilli but no ophthal. prep of only **TMP**. Most S. pneumo resistant to Gent & Tobra. |
| Gonococcal (peds/adults) | N. gonorrhoeae | **Ceftriaxone** 25–50 mg/kg IV/IM (not to exceed 125 mg) as one dose in children; 1 gm IM/IV as one dose in adults | | **FQs** best spectrum for empiric therapy. High concentrations ↑ likelihood |

Abbreviations on page 2.   *NOTE: All dosage recommendations are for adults (unless otherwise indicated) and assume normal renal function. § Alternatives consider allergy, PK, compliance, local resistance, cost.

**TABLE 1 (11)**

**EYE** *(continued)*

**Cornea (keratitis): Usually serious and often sight-threatening. Prompt ophthalmologic consultation essential for diagnosis, antimicrobial and adjunctive therapy! Herpes simplex most common etiology in developed countries; bacterial and fungal infections more common in underdeveloped countries.**

| ANATOMIC SITE/DIAGNOSIS/ MODIFYING CIRCUMSTANCES | ETIOLOGIES (usual) | SUGGESTED REGIMENS* | | ADJUNCT DIAGNOSTIC OR THERAPEUTIC MEASURES AND COMMENTS |
|---|---|---|---|---|
| | | PRIMARY | ALTERNATIVE§ | |
| **Viral** | | | | |
| H. simplex *(See Clin Exp Ophthalmol 44:824, 2016)* | H. simplex, types 1 & 2 | **Trifluridine** ophthalmic soln, one drop q2h up to 9 drops/day until re-epithelialized, then one drop q4h up to 5x/day, for total not to exceed 21 days. *See Comment* | **Ganciclovir** 0.15% ophthalmic gel: Indicated for acute herpetic keratitis. One drop 5 times per day while awake until corneal ulcer heals; then, one drop three times per day for 7 days. | **For severe infection or immunocompromised host**, consider adding **acyclovir** 400 mg po 5x daily or **valacyclovir** 1000 mg bid. Topical acyclovir 3% ointment 5x daily is a first-line treatment for HSV epithelial keratitis outside the United States. Approx 30% recurrence rate within one year; consider prophylaxis with acyclovir 400 mg bid for 12 months or valacyclovir 500 mg once daily to prevent recurrences. |
| Varicella-zoster ophthalmicus | Varicella-zoster virus | **Famciclovir** 500 mg po tid or **Valacyclovir** 1 gm po tid x 10 days | **Acyclovir** 800 mg po 5x/day x 10 days | Clinical diagnosis most common: dendritic figures with fluorescein staining in patient with varicella-zoster of ophthalmic branch of trigeminal nerve. |
| **Bacterial** | **All treatment listed for bacterial, fungal, protozoan is topical unless otherwise indicated** | | | |
| Acute: No comorbidity | S. aureus, S. pneumo, S. pyogenes, Haemophilus sp. | **Moxi** ophthalmic (0.5%): 1 drop q3h for the first 48h then taper according to response | **CIP** 0.3% ophthal or **Levo** 0.5% ophthal: 1-2 gtts/hr x 24-72 hrs, then taper based on clinical response. **Gati** eye drops: 1-2 gtts q2h while awake x 2 days, then q4h x 3-7 days | Regimens vary: some start rx by applying drops q5 min for 5 doses; some apply drops q15-30 min for several hours; some extend interval to q2h during waking hours. In a clinical trial drops were applied q1h for 48-72h, then q2h through day 6, then q2h during waking hours on days 7-9, then q6h until healing *(Cornea 29:751, 2010)*. **NOTE:** despite high concentrations, may fail vs. MRSA. Prior use of fluoroquinolones associated with increased MICs *(JAMA Ophthalmol. 131:310, 2013)*; high MICs associated with poorer outcome *(Clin Infect Dis 54:1381, 2012)*. |
| Contact lens users | P. aeruginosa | **CIP** 0.3% ophthalmic solution or **Levo** 0.5% ophthalmic solution 1-2 gtts hourly x24-72h, taper based on response | **Gent** or **Tobra** 0.3% ophthalmic solution 1-2 gtts hourly q24h then taper based on clinical response. | Recommend alginate swab culture and susceptibility testing; refer to ophthalmologist. **Cornea abrasions:** treated with Tobra, Gent, or CIP gtts qid for 3-5 days; referral to ophthalmologist recommended corneal infiltrate or ulcer, visual loss, lack of improvement or worsening symptoms *(Am Fam Physician, 87:114, 2013)*. |
| Dry cornea, diabetes, immunosuppression | Staph. aureus, S. epidermidis, S. pneumoniae, S. pyogenes, Enterobacteriaceae, listeria | **CIP** 0.3% ophthalmic solution 1-2 gtts hourly x24-72h, then taper based on clinical response. | **Vanco** (50 mg/mL) + **Ceftaz** ophthalmic solution 1-2 gtts hourly q24-72h, taper depending upon response. See *Comment*. | Specific therapy guided by results of alginate swab culture. |
| **Fungal** | Aspergillus, fusarium, candida and others. | **Natamycin** (5%): 1 drop q1-2h for several days; then q3-4h for several days; can reduce frequency depending upon response | **Amphotericin B** (0.15%): 1 drop q1-2h for frequency several days; can reduce frequency depending upon response. | Obtain specimens for fungal wet mount and cultures. Numerous other treatment options (**Itra** 1% topical x 6 wks, **Itra** 100 mg po bid x 3 wks, **Vori** 1% topical x 2 wks, **Miconazole** 1% topical 5x daily, **silver sulphadiazine** 0.5-1% topical 5x daily) appear to have similar efficacy *(Cochrane Syst Rev 2004:241, 2012)* |

*Abbreviations on page 2.*   *§NOTE: All dosage recommendations are for adults (unless otherwise indicated) and assume normal renal function. § Alternatives consider allergy, PK, compliance, local resistance, cost.*

**TABLE 1 (12)**

| ANATOMIC SITE/DIAGNOSIS/ MODIFYING CIRCUMSTANCES | ETIOLOGIES (usual) | SUGGESTED REGIMENS* | | ADJUNCT DIAGNOSTIC OR THERAPEUTIC MEASURES AND COMMENTS |
|---|---|---|---|---|
| | | PRIMARY | ALTERNATIVE§ | |
| **EYE/Cornea (keratitis)** (continued) | | | | |
| **Mycobacteria:** Post-refractive eye surgery | M. chelonae; M. abscessus | **Gati** or **Moxi** eye drops: 1 gtt qid in conjunction with other active antimicrobial eyedrops (**Amikacin** 50 mg/L and **Clarithro** 10 mg/L). | | **Alternative:** systemic rx: **Doxy** 100 mg po bid + **Clarithro** 500 mg po bid (*PLoS One* 10:do10236, 2015). |
| **Protozoan** — Soft contact lens users. Ref: *CID* 35:434, 2002. Uncommon. Trauma and soft contact lenses are risk factors. | Acanthamoeba, sp. | Topical 0.02%–0.2% biguanide chlorhexidine or 0.02%–0.06% Polyhexamethylene biguanide (PHMB) in combination with propamidine (0.1 %) or hexamidine (0.1 %). Start with lower dose of PHMB and titrate to clinical response. | | Initially, drops should be applied up to hourly day and night for the first 48 hours then hourly during the daytime for the first week, then with subsequent taper over 3 - 4 weeks. Debridement may also be warranted (*https://www.cdc.gov/parasites/acanthamoeba/health_professionals/acanthamoeba_keratitis_hcp.html*). |
| **Lacrimal apparatus** | | | | |
| Canaliculitis | Actinomyces Staph., Strept. Rarely, Arachnia, fusobacterium, nocardia, candida | Apply hot packs to punctal area 4x/day. Refer to ophthalmologist for removal of granules and local irrigation with an antibiotic solution. | | Digital pressure produces exudate at punctum; Gram stain confirms diagnosis. |
| Dacryocystitis (lacrimal sac) | S. pneumo, S. aureus, H. influenzae, S. pyogenes, P. aeruginosa | Often consequence of obstruction of lacrimal duct. Empiric systemic antimicrobial therapy based on Gram stain of aspirate—*see Comment.* | | Need ophthalmologic consultation. Surgery may be required. Can be acute or chronic. Culture to detect MRSA. |

**Endophthalmitis:** Endogenous (secondary to bacteremia or fungemia) and exogenous (post-injection, post-operative) types. **Ophthalmologic consult imperative.**
Bacterial: Haziness of vitreous key to diagnosis. Needle aspirate of both vitreous and aqueous humor for culture prior to therapy. Intravitreal administration of antimicrobials essential.

| ANATOMIC SITE/DIAGNOSIS/ MODIFYING CIRCUMSTANCES | ETIOLOGIES (usual) | PRIMARY | ALTERNATIVE§ | ADJUNCT DIAGNOSTIC OR THERAPEUTIC MEASURES AND COMMENTS |
|---|---|---|---|---|
| **Postocular surgery (cataracts)** | | | | |
| Early, acute onset (incidence 0.05%) | S. epidermidis 60%, Staph. aureus, streptococci, & enterococci each 5–10%, Gm-neg. bacilli 6% | **Immediate ophthal. consult.** If only light perception or worse, immediate vitrectomy + intravitreal **vanco** 1 mg & intravitreal ceftazidime 2.25 mg. | Referral to ophthalmologist for intravitreal **Vanco** 1 mg + **Ceftaz** 2.25 mg and a topical ophthalmic antimicrobial. | |
| Low grade, chronic | Cutibacterium acnes, S. epidermidis, S. aureus | Intraocular **Vanco.** Usually requires vitrectomy, lens removal. | Referral to ophthalmologist for intravitreal **Vanco** 1 mg + **CIP** 400 mg [V/po q12h]. Vitrectomy may be required. | |
| **Post filtering blebs for glaucoma** | Strep. species (viridans & others), H. influenzae | Referral to ophthalmologist for intravitreal **Vanco** 1 mg + (**Ceftaz** 1 g iv q8h or **CIP** 400 mg IV/po q12h) + systemic **Vanco** 15–20 mg/kg IV q8-12h + (**Ceftaz** 2.25 mg or **Amikacin** 0.4 mg). | | |
| Post-penetrating trauma | Bacillus sp., S. epidermidis (rare) | Referral to ophthalmologist for intravitreal **Vanco** 1 mg + (**Ceftaz** 2.25 mg or **Amikacin** 0.4 mg) + systemic **Vanco** 15–20 mg/kg IV q8-12h + **Ceftaz** 1 g iv q8h or **CIP** 400 mg IV/po q12h). | | |
| Hematogenous | S. pneumoniae, N. meningitidis, Staph. aureus, Grp B Strep, K. pneumo | Referral to ophthalmologist for intravitreal **Vanco** 1 mg + (**Cefotaxime** 2 gm IV q4h or **Ceftriaxone** 2 gm IV q24h) + **Vanco** 30-60 mg/kg/day IV in 2-3 div doses to achieve target trough serum concentration of 15-20 mcg/mL, pending cultures. Intravitreal antibiotics as with early postocular surgery. Urgent ophthalmological consultation. | | |
| IV heroin abuse | S. aureus, Bacillus cereus, Candida sp. | Empirically, as above for hematogenous with definitive therapy based on etiology and antimicrobial susceptibility. Urgent ophthalmological consultation. | | |

Abbreviations on page 2.   *NOTE: All dosage recommendations are for adults (unless otherwise indicated) and assume normal renal function. § Alternatives consider allergy, PK, compliance, local resistance, cost.

**TABLE 1 (13)**

| ANATOMIC SITE/DIAGNOSIS/ MODIFYING CIRCUMSTANCES | ETIOLOGIES (usual) | SUGGESTED REGIMENS* | | ADJUNCT DIAGNOSTIC OR THERAPEUTIC MEASURES AND COMMENTS |
|---|---|---|---|---|
| | | **PRIMARY** | **ALTERNATIVE§** | |
| **EYE/Endophthalmitis** *(continued)* | | | | |
| **Mycotic (fungal).** Broad-spectrum antibiotics, often corticosteroids, indwelling venous catheters | Candida sp., Aspergillus sp. | Intravitreal **Ampho B** 0.005–0.01 mg in 0.1 mL. *Also see Table 11A, page 135 for concomitant systemic therapy. See Comment.* | | Patients with *Candida* spp. chorioretinitis usually respond to systemically administered antifungals *(Clin Infect Dis 53:262, 2011)*. Intravitreal ampho and/or vitrectomy may be necessary for those with vitritis or endophthalmitis. *(IDSA guidelines CID 62:e09, 2016)*. |
| **Retinitis** | | | | |
| Acute retinal necrosis | Varicella zoster virus (VZV), Herpes simplex | IV **Acyclovir** 10–12 mg/kg IV q8h x 5–7 days, then **Acyclovir** 800 mg po 5 x/day OR **Valacyclovir** 1000 mg po tid OR **Famciclovir** 500 mg po tid | | Strong association of VZ virus with atypical necrotizing herpetic retinopathy. Ophthalmology consultation. |
| HIV+ (AIDS) CD4 usually <100/mm³ | Cytomegalovirus | See Table 14A, page 180 | | Occurs in 5–10% of AIDS patients |
| Progressive outer retinal necrosis | VZV, H. simplex, CMV (rare) | **Acyclovir** 10–12 mg/kg IV q8h for 1–2 weeks, then **Valacyclovir** 1000 mg po tid, or **Famciclovir** 500 mg po tid, or **Acyclovir** 800 mg po tid. Ophthalmology consultation imperative: approaches have also included intra-vitreal injection of anti-virals (foscarnet, ganciclovir implant). In rare cases due to CMV use **Ganciclovir/Valganciclovir** (see CMV retinitis, Table 14A). | | Most patients are highly immunocompromised (HIV with low CD4 or transplantation). In contrast to Acute Retinal Necrosis, lack of intraocular inflammation or arteritis. May be able to stop oral antivirals when CD4 recovers with ART *(Ocul Immunol Inflammation 15:425, 2007)*. |
| **Orbital cellulitis** *(See page 57 for erysipelas, facial)* | S. pneumoniae, H. influenzae, M. catarrhalis, S. aureus, anaerobes, group A strep, occ. Gm-neg. bacilli post-trauma | **Vanco** 15–20 mg/kg IV q8–12h (target trough serum concentrations of 15–20 µg/mL) + ([**Ceftriaxone** 2 gm IV q24h + **Metro** 1 gm IV q12h] OR **PIP-TZ** 3.375 gm IV q6h | | **If Penicillin/Ceph allergy: Vanco + Moxi** 400 mg IV q24h. Problem is frequent inability to make microbiologic diagnosis. Image orbit (CT or MRI). Risk of cavernous sinus thrombosis. If vanco intolerant, another option for S. aureus is dapto 8–10 mg/kg IV q24h. |

Abbreviations on page 2.   *NOTE: All dosage recommendations are for adults (unless otherwise indicated) and assume normal renal function. § Alternatives consider allergy, PK, compliance, local resistance, cost.

**TABLE 1 (14)**

| ANATOMIC SITE/DIAGNOSIS/ MODIFYING CIRCUMSTANCES | ETIOLOGIES (usual) | SUGGESTED REGIMENS* | | ADJUNCT DIAGNOSTIC OR THERAPEUTIC MEASURES AND COMMENTS |
|---|---|---|---|---|
| | | PRIMARY | ALTERNATIVE§ | |
| **FOOT** | | | | |
| **"Diabetic foot"**—Two thirds of patients have triad of neuropathy, deformity and pressure-induced trauma. IDSA Guidelines *CID 54:e132, 2012.* | | | | |
| Ulcer without inflammation | Colonizing skin flora | No antibacterial therapy. | | **General:** |
| Mild infection | S. aureus (assume MRSA), S. agalactiae (Gp B), S. pyogenes predominate | Oral therapy: **Diclox** or **Cephalexin** or **AM-CL** (not MRSA). **Doxy** or **TMP-SMX-DS** (MRSA). **Clinda** (covers MSSA, MRSA, strep) *Dosages in footnote[4]* | | 1. Glucose control, eliminate pressure on ulcer 2. **Assess for peripheral vascular disease** 3. Caution in use of TMP-SMX in patients with diabetes, as many have risk factors for hyperkalemia (e.g., advanced age, reduced renal function, concomitant medications) (*Arch Intern Med 170:1045, 2010*). 4. Improved outcomes in healing of diabetic foot ulcer using negative-pressure wound therapy (*See Curr Opin Infect Dis 29:145, 2016* for review). |
| Moderate infection. **Osteomyelitis** *See Comment.* | As above, plus coliforms possible | Oral: As above Parenteral therapy: [based on prevailing susceptibilities: (**AM-SB** or **PIP-TZ** or **ERTA** or other carbapenem) plus [**Vanco** (or alternative anti-MRSA drug as below)] until MRSA excluded]. *Dosages in footnotes[5,6]* | | **Principles of empiric antibacterial therapy:** 1. Obtain culture; cover for MRSA in moderate, more severe infections pending culture data, local epidemiology. 2. Severe limb and/or life-threatening infections require initial parenteral therapy with predictable activity vs. Gm-positive cocci including MRSA, coliforms & other aerobic Gm-neg. rods, & anaerobic Gm-neg. bacilli. |
| Extensive local inflammation plus systemic toxicity. | As above, plus anaerobic bacteria. Role of enterococci unclear. | Parenteral therapy: (**Vanco** plus β-lactam/β-lactamase inhibitor) or (**vanco** plus [**DORI** or **IMP** or **MER**]). Other alternatives: 1. **Dapto** or **Linezolid** for vanco 2. **CIP** or **Levo** or **Aztreonam**) plus **Metronidazole** for β-lactam/β-lactamase inhibitor **Assess for arterial insufficiency!** *Dosages in footnote[6]* | | 3. **NOTE:** The regimens listed are suggestions consistent with above principles. Other alternatives exist & may be appropriate for individual patients. 4. Risk of associated osteomyelitis is increased if ulcer area >2 cm², positive to probe to bone (*CID 2016;63:944*), ESR >70 and abnormal plain x-ray. Negative MRI reduces likelihood of osteomyelitis (*JAMA 299:806, 2008*). MRI is best imaging modality (*CID 47:519 & 528, 2008*). |
| Onychomycosis: See *Table 11, page 138,* fungal infections | | | | *Osteomyelitis; page 5.* 1–2% evolves to osteo. |
| Puncture wound: Nail/Toothpick | P. aeruginosa (Nail), S. aureus Strept (Toothpick) | Cleanse. Tetanus booster. Observe. | | |
| **GALLBLADDER** | | | | |
| **Cholecystitis, cholangitis, biliary sepsis,** or **common duct obstruc-tion** (partial: 2nd° to tumor, stones, stricture). | Enterobacteriaceae 68%, enterococci 14%, bacteroides 10%, Clostridium sp. 7%, rarely candida | (**PIP-TZ** or **AM-SB**) if life-threatening: **IMP** or **MER** or **DORI** *Dosages in footnote[6] on page 18.* | (**P Ceph 3[3]** + **Metro**) or (**Aztreonam**† + **Metro**) or (**CIP** + **Metro**) or **Moxi** * Add **Vanco** for empiric activity vs. enterococci | In severely ill pts, antibiotic therapy complements adequate biliary drainage. 15–30% pts will require decompression: surgical, percutaneous or ERCP-placed stent. Gallbladder bile is culture pos. in 40–60% (*J Infect 51:128, 2005*). No benefit to continuation of antibiotics after surgery in pts with acute calculous cholecystitis (*JAMA 3312:145, 2014*). |

[4] **TMP-SMX-DS** 1–2 tabs po bid. **Minocycline** 100 mg po bid. **Pen VK** 500 mg po qid. (O Ceph 2, 3; **Cefprozil** 500 mg po q12h, **Cefuroxime axetil** 500 mg po q12h, **Cefdinir** 300 mg po q12h or 600 mg po q24h, **Cefpodoxime** 200 mg po q12h). **CIP** 750 mg po q12h. **Levo** 750 mg po bid. **Diclox** 500 mg po qid. **Cephalexin** 500 mg po qid. **AM-CL** 875/125 bid. **Doxy** 100 mg bid (now considered safe, regardless of age, for rx ≤21 days). **Clinda** 300–450 mg t.id.

[5] **AM-CL-ER** 2000/125 po q12h. **TMP-SMX-DS** 1–2 tabs po bid. **CIP** 750 mg po bid, **Levo** 750 mg po q24h, **CIP** 400 mg IV q12h, **Moxi** 400 mg po q24h, **Linezolid** 600 mg po bid.

[6] **Vanco** 1 gm IV q12h, **(parenteral β-lactam/β-lactamase inhibitors: AM-SB** 3 gm IV q6h, **PIP-TZ** 3.375 gm IV q6h or 4.5 gm IV q8h or 4 hr infusion of 3.375 gm q8h); **carbapenems: Doripenem** 500 mg (1-hr infusion) q8h, **ERTA** 1 gm IV q24h, **IMP** 0.5 gm IV q6h, **MER** 1 gm IV q8h, **Dapto** 6 mg per kg IV q24h, **Linezolid** 600 mg IV q12h, **Aztreonam** 2 gm IV q12h, **Levo** 750 mg IV q24h, **Moxi** 400 mg IV q24h, **Metro** 1 gm IV loading dose & then 0.5 gm IV q6h or 1 gm IV q12h.

*Abbreviations on page 2.*     *\*NOTE: All dosage recommendations are for adults (unless otherwise indicated) and assume normal renal function. § Alternatives consider allergy, PK, compliance, local resistance, cost.*

**TABLE 1 (15)**

| ANATOMIC SITE/DIAGNOSIS/ MODIFYING CIRCUMSTANCES | ETIOLOGIES (usual) | SUGGESTED REGIMENS* | | ADJUNCT DIAGNOSTIC OR THERAPEUTIC MEASURES AND COMMENTS |
|---|---|---|---|---|
| | | PRIMARY | ALTERNATIVE§ | |
| **GASTROINTESTINAL** | | | | |
| **Gastroenteritis—Empiric Therapy** (laboratory studies not performed or culture, microscopy, toxin results NOT AVAILABLE) *NEJM 370:16, 2014;* IDSA Guideline (Diarrhea): *CID 2017;65:1963 & e45.* | | | | |
| **Premature infant** with necrotizing enterocolitis | Associated with intestinal flora | Treatment should cover broad range of intestinal bacteria using drugs appropriate to the age and local susceptibility patterns, rationale as in diverticulitis/peritonitis, *page 24.* | | Pneumatosis intestinalis, if present on x-ray confirms diagnosis. Bacteremia-peritonitis in 30–50%. If Staph. epidermidis isolated, add vanco (IV). For review and general management, *see NEJM 364:255, 2011.* |
| **Mild diarrhea** (≤3 unformed stools/day, minimal associated symptomatology) | Bacterial (*see Severe, below*), viral (norovirus), parasitic. Viral usually causes mild to moderate disease. | Fluids only + lactose-free diet, avoid caffeine | | **Rehydration: For po fluid replacement,** *see Cholera, page 21.* **Antimotility:** Do not use if fever, bloody stools, or suspicion of HUS); Loperamide (Imodium) 4 mg po, then 2 mg after each loose stool to max. of 16 mg per day. Bismuth subsalicylate (Pepto-Bismol) 2 tablets (262 mg) po qid. |
| **Moderate diarrhea** (≥4 unformed stools/day &/or systemic symptoms) | For traveler's diarrhea, *see page 22.* | Antimotility agents (*see Comments*) + fluids | | **Hemolytic uremic syndrome (HUS):** Risk in **children** infected with E. coli 0157:H7 is 6–10%. Early treatment with TMP-SMX or FQs ↑ risk of HUS. |
| **Severe diarrhea** (≥6 unformed stools/day, &/or temp ≥101°F, tenesmus, blood, or fecal leukocytes). **NOTE: Severe afebrile bloody diarrhea should ↑ suspicion of Shiga-toxin E. coli O157:H7 & others** (*MMWR 58 (RR-12):1, 2009*). | Shigella, salmonella, C. jejuni, Shiga toxin + E. coli, toxin-positive C. difficile, Klebsiella oxytoca, E. histolytica. | Azithro 1000 mg po x 1 dose or 500 mg po q12h x 3 days | CIP 750 mg po x 1 dose, continue for 3 days if not resolved OR 500 mg po q12 x 3 days | **Norovirus:** Etiology of over 90% of non-bacterial diarrhea (± nausea/ vomiting). Lasts 12-60 hrs. Hydrate. No effective antiviral. **Other potential etiologies (parasitic):** Cryptosporidia—no treatment in immunocompetent host. Cyclospora—usually chronic diarrhea, responds to TMP-SMX (*see Table 13A*). Klebsiella oxytoca identified as cause of antibiotic-associated hemorrhagic colitis (cytotoxin positive): *NEJM 355:2418, 2006.* |
| | If recent antibiotic therapy (C. difficile toxin colitis possible): promptly test stool for C. diff. toxin | | | |
| | For typhoid fever, *see page 65* | | | |
| **Gastroenteritis—Specific Therapy** (results of culture, microscopy, toxin assay AVAILABLE) Ref. *NEJM 370:1532, 2014;* IDSA Infectious diarrhea guideline (*CID 2017;65:1963*). | | | | |
| **If culture negative, probably Norovirus** (Norwalk) other virus (*EID 17:1381, 2011*) — see Norovirus, page 186 | | CIP 750 mg po bid x 3 days. | TMP-SMX DS tab 1 po bid x 3 days | Aeromonas ref: *Eur J Clin Microbiol 36:1393, 2017.* |
| **Aeromonas/Plesiomonas** | | | | |
| **Amebiasis (Entamoeba histolytica, Cyclospora, Cryptosporidia and Giardia),** *see Table 13A.* | | | | |
| **Campylobacter jejuni** History of fever in 53-83%. Self-limited diarrhea in normal host. | | Azithro 500 mg po q24h x 3 days OR 1000 mg po one dose | Erythro stearate 500 mg po qid x 5 days or CIP 500 mg po bid (CIP resistance increasing) (*CID 2017;65:1624*). | **Post-Campylobacter Guillain-Barré:** assoc. 15% of cases (*Ln 366:1653, 2005*). Assoc. with small bowel lymphoproliferative disease; may respond to antimicrobials (*NEJM 350:239, 2004*). **Reactive arthritis** another potential sequelae. See *Traveler's Diarrhea, page 22.* |
| **Campylobacter fetus** Diarrhea uncommon. More systemic disease in debilitated hosts | | Genta (*see Table 10D*) | AMP 100 mg/kg/day IV div q6h or IMP 500 mg IV q6h | Draw blood cultures. In bacteremic pts, FQ resistance common in C. fetus. Meropenem inhibits C. fetus at low concentrations in vitro. Clinical review: *CID 56:1579, 2014.* |

**NOTE:** WBC >15,000 suggestive of C. difficile in hospitalized patient.

**TABLE 1 (16)**

| ANATOMIC SITE/DIAGNOSIS/ MODIFYING CIRCUMSTANCES | ETIOLOGIES (usual) | SUGGESTED REGIMENS* | | ADJUNCT DIAGNOSTIC OR THERAPEUTIC MEASURES AND COMMENTS |
|---|---|---|---|---|
| | | PRIMARY | ALTERNATIVE§ | |
| **GASTROINTESTINAL/Gastroenteritis—Specific Therapy (results of culture, microscopy, toxin assay AVAILABLE)** *(continued)* | | | | |
| Differential diagnosis of toxin-producing diarrhea: <br>• C difficile <br>• Klebsiella oxytoca <br>• S. aureus <br>• Shiga toxin producing E. coli (STEC) <br>• Enterotoxigenic B. fragilis | **C. difficile toxin positive antibiotic-associated colitis.** Cochrane review found moderate quality evidence the probiotics prevents C. diff. associated diarrhea *(Cochrane Database Syst Rev. 2017 Dec 19;12:CD006095).* | | | |
| | po meds okay; WBC <15,000; no increase in serum creatinine. | Metro 500 mg po qid x 10 days | *See Comment* | **D/C antibiotic if possible: avoid antimotility agents, hydration, enteric isolation.** Recent review suggests antimotility agents can be used cautiously in certain pts who are receiving rx *(CID 48: 598, 2009)*. **Relapse in 10-20%.** Note: **Metro 500 mg tid no longer recommended as first-line therapy and should be used only if resources preclude access to Vanco or Fidaxomicin.** |
| IDSA Guidelines (C. diff): *CID 2018;66:987* | po meds okay; Sicker; WBC >15,000; ≥50% increase in baseline creatinine | Vanco 125 mg po qid x 10 days. <br>For oral rx of IV Vanco, see Table 10A, page 117. | Fidaxomicin 200 mg po bid x 10 days | **Vanco superior to metro** in sicker pts. Relapse in 10-20%. Fidaxomicin had lower rate of recurrence than Vanco for diarrhea with non-NAP1 strains *(N Engl J Med 364:422, 2011).* Bezlotoxumab 1 dose IV + standard rx reduced relapse rate 11-14% *(NEJM 2017, 376:305).* |
| | Post-treatment relapse | Vanco 125 mg po bid x 10-14 days, then immediately start taper *(See Comments)* | Fidaxomicin 200 mg po bid x 10 days | **Vanco taper** (all doses 125 mg po): week 1 - tid, week 2 - bid week 3 - q24h week 4 - q48h, week 5 - q72h. Ref: *CID 2017:65-1624.* <br>**Fecal transplant** more efficacious than Vanco (15/16 [93%]) versus 7/26 [27%]) in curing recurrent C. difficile infection *(New Engl J Med 368:407, 2013).* Pre-transplant Vanco taper increases success of fecal transplants *(CID 2017:65:721).* Bezlotoxumab anti-C. diff toxin B antibody decreases recurrence 10% but very expensive *NEJM 376-381 2017.* If Metro used for initial therapy can use standard 10-day course of Vanco. <br>For vanco instillation into bowel, add 500 mg vanco to 500 mL of saline. **NOTE: IV vanco not effective.** Indications for colectomy, see *ICHE 31:431, 2010.* |
| | **Enterohemorrhagic E. coli (EHEC):** O157:H7 & O104:H4 & others. Hemolytic uremic syndrome complicates 6-9% *(See Comment)* | Treatment: <br>1. If afebrile, bloody diarrhea: <br>   a. Hydration <br>   b. Avoid antiperistaltic drugs <br>   c. No antibiotics <br>2. If febrile, bloody diarrhea, risk of bacteremia: Azithro 500 mg IV/po once daily x 3 d | | **Risk of antibiotic therapy is HUS due to Shiga toxin production.** HUS = renal failure, hemolytic anemia, thrombocytopenia. Risk of HUS with antibiotic use for EHEC: OR 2.24 (CI 1.45-3.46). Hence, restrict antibiotics to patients with increased risk of, or documentation of, bacteremia due to EHEC. Refs: *CID 2016,62:1251 & 1259; CID 2012,55-33; Infection 1992,20:25; JID 2000,181:664.* |
| | **Klebsiella oxytoca— antibiotic-associated diarrhea** | Responds to stopping antibiotic | | Suggested that stopping NSAIDs helps. Ref: *NEJM 355:2418, 2006.* |
| | **Listeria monocytogenes** | Usually self-limited. Value of oral antibiotics (e.g., AMP or TMP-SMX) unknown, but their use might be reasonable in populations at risk for serious listeria infections. Those with bacteremia/meningitis require parenteral therapy. *see pages 10 & 65.* | | Recognized as a cause of febrile gastroenteritis. Populations at 1 risk of severe systemic disease: pregnant women, neonates, the elderly, and immunocompromised hosts *(MMWR 57:1097, 2008).* Not detected in standard stool cultures. |

(Continued on next page)

*NOTE: All dosage recommendations are for adults (unless otherwise indicated) and assume normal renal function. § Alternatives consider allergy, PK, compliance, local resistance, cost.

**TABLE 1 (17)**

| ANATOMIC SITE/DIAGNOSIS/ MODIFYING CIRCUMSTANCES | ETIOLOGIES (usual) | SUGGESTED REGIMENS* | | ADJUNCT DIAGNOSTIC OR THERAPEUTIC MEASURES AND COMMENTS |
|---|---|---|---|---|
| | | PRIMARY | ALTERNATIVE§ | |
| *(Continued from previous page)* **GASTROINTESTINAL/Gastroenteritis—Specific Therapy (results of culture, microscopy, toxin assay AVAILABLE)** *(continued)* | | | | |
| *Salmonella*, non-typhi— For typhoid fever (enteric) fever, see page 65 Fever in 71–91%, history of bloody stools in 34% | | **If asymptomatic or illness mild, antimicrobial therapy not indicated. Treat if** age <1 yr or >50 yrs, immunocompromised, vascular grafts or prosthetic joints, bacteremic, hemoglobinopathy, or hospitalized *(see typhoid fever, page 65)*. **CIP** 500 mg bid) or (**Levo** 500 mg q24h) x 7–10 days (14 days if immunocompromised). | ↑ resistance to TMP-SMX and chloro. Ceftriaxone, cefotaxime usually active if ↑ resistance required *(see footnote on page 27, for dosage)*. **Azithro** 500 mg po once daily x 7 days (14 days if immunocompromised). | Clinical labs have established new interpretive breakpoints to CIP: susceptible strains, MIC ≤0.06 μg/mL *(Clin Infect Dis 55:1107, 2012)*. **Primary treatment of enteritis is fluid and electrolyte replacement.** |
| *Shigella* Fever in 58%, history of bloody stools | | **CIP** 750 mg qd or po bid x 3 days **Pockets of resistance** *(see Comment)* **Peds doses: Azithro** 10 mg/kg/day once daily x 3 days. For severe disease, **Ceftriaxone** 50–75 mg/kg per day x 2–5 days. **CIP** suspension 10 mg/kg bid x 5 days. | **Azithro** 500 mg po once daily x 3 days | Immunocompromised children & adults: Treat for 7–10 days. Pockets of resistance: *S. flexneri* resist to CIP & Ceftriaxone *(MMWR 59:1619, 2010)*; *S. sonnei* resist to CIP in travelers *(MMWR 64:318, 2015)*; *S. sonnei* suscept to CIP but resist to azithro in MSM *(MMWR 64:597, 2015)*. CDC recommends avoiding CIP if MIC ≥0.12 μg/mL *(CDC Health Alert Network, Apr 18, 2017)*. For most healthy, treatment not necessary. May be associated with traveler's diarrhea, where one dose of treatment may be sufficient. |
| **Spirochetosis (*Brachyspira pilosicoli*)** | | Benefit of treatment unclear. Susceptible to **Metro**, **Ceftriaxone**, and **Moxi**. | | Anaerobic intestinal spirochete that colonizes colon of domestic & wild animals plus humans. Called enigmatic disease due to uncertain status *(Digest Dis & Sci 58:202, 2013)*. |
| **Vibrio cholerae** (*classic, -O1 & O39*) Treatment decreases duration of disease, volume losses, & duration of excretion | | **Primary therapy is rehydration.** Select antibiotics based on susceptibility & locally prevailing isolates. Options include: **Doxy** 300 mg po single dose, **Azithro** 1 gm po single dose, **Tetra** 500 mg po qid x 3 days. **Erythro** 500 mg po qid x 3 days. | **Pregnancy:** **Azithro** 1 gm po single dose OR **Erythro** 500 mg po qid x 3 days **Peds:** **Azithro** 20 mg/kg as single dose; for other age-specific alternatives, see CDC website http:// www.cdc.gov/haiti/cholera/ hcp_goinghot.htm | **Antimicrobial therapy shortens duration of illness, but rehydration is paramount.** When IV hydration is needed, use Ringer's lactate. Switch to po fluids. Oral Rehydration Salts (ORS) as soon as able to take oral fluids. ORS are commercially available for reconstitution in potable water. If not available, WHO suggests a substitute can be made by dissolving ½ teaspoon salt and 6 level teaspoons of sugar per liter of potable water *(http://www.who.int/cholera/technical/en/)*. CDC recommendations for other aspects of management developed for Haiti outbreak can be found at http://www.cdc.gov/haiti/cholera/ hcp_goinghot.htm |
| **Vibrio parahaemolyticus, V. mimicus, V. fluvialis** | | **Antimicrobial rx does not shorten course. Hydration.** | | Isolates from this outbreak demonstrate reduced susceptibility to ciprofloxacin and resistance to sulfisoxazole, nalidixic acid and furazolidone. Vaccine for cholera available *(Med Lett Drugs Ther. 55:113, 2013)*. |
| **Vibrio vulnificus** Usual presentation is skin lesions & bacteremia; life-threatening | | Adult: (**Doxy** or **Minocycline** 100 mg IV/po bid) + (**Ceftriaxone** (max 200 mg/day). Alternatives: **Levo** or **CIP**. Ref: *Epidemiol Infect. 142:878, 2014.* | **Ceftaz** 1 gm IV q8h). Peds: **Doxy** 4.4 mg/kg/day div bid | Shellfish exposure common. Treat severe disease: **FQ, Doxy, P Ceph 3** |
| **Yersinia enterocolitica** Fever in 68%, bloody stools in 26% | | **No treatment unless severe.** If severe, **Doxy** 100 mg IV bid + **TMP-SMX** or **FQs** are alternatives. | **Tobra** or **Gent** 5 mg/kg per day once (q24h). **TMP-SMX** | Mesenteric adenitis pain can mimic acute appendicitis. Lab diagnosis difficult: requires "cold enrichment" and/or yersinia selective agar. Desferrioxamine therapy increases severity, discontinue if on it. Iron overload states predispose to yersinia. |

*NOTE: All dosage recommendations are for adults (unless otherwise indicated) and assume normal renal function. § Alternatives consider allergy, PK, compliance, local resistance, cost.

Abbreviations on page 2.

**TABLE 1 (18)**

| ANATOMIC SITE/DIAGNOSIS/ MODIFYING CIRCUMSTANCES | ETIOLOGIES (usual) | SUGGESTED REGIMENS* | | ADJUNCT DIAGNOSTIC OR THERAPEUTIC MEASURES AND COMMENTS |
|---|---|---|---|---|
| | | PRIMARY | ALTERNATIVE§ | |
| **GASTROINTESTINAL** (continued) | | | | |
| **Gastroenteritis—Specific Risk Groups–Empiric Therapy** | | | | |
| **Anoreceptive intercourse** | | | | |
| Proctitis (distal 15 cm only) | Herpes viruses, gonococci, chlamydia, syphilis. *See Genital Tract, page 24* | | | *See specific GI pathogens, Gastroenteritis, above.* |
| Colitis | Shigella, salmonella, campylobacter, E. histolytica *(see Table 13A)* | | | |
| **HIV-1 infected (AIDS); >10 days diarrhea** | G. lamblia | | | See Table 13A |
| | Acid fast: Cryptosporidium parvum, Cyclospora cayetanensis | | | |
| | Other: Isospora belli, microsporidia (Enterocytozoon bieneusi, Septata intestinalis) | | | |
| **Neutropenic enterocolitis or "typhlitis"** *(CID 56:711, 2013) (World J Gastroenterol 23: 42, 2017).* | Mucosal invasion by **Clostridium septicum** and others. Occasionally caused by C. sordellii or P. aeruginosa | Bowel rest and **PIP-TZ** 4.5 gm IV q6h or **IMP** 500 mg IV q6h + **Metro** 500 mg IV q8h or **MER** 2 gm IV q8h | **Cefepime** 2 gm IV q8h + **Metro** 500 mg IV q8h | Tender right lower quadrant may be the clue, but may be diffuse or absent in immunocompromised. Need surgical consult. Surgical resection controversial but may be necessary. **NOTE:** Resistance of clostridia to clindamycin reported. PIP-TZ, IMP, MER, DORI should cover most pathogens. |
| **Traveler's diarrhea**, self-medication. Patient often afebrile | **Acute:** 60% due to diarrheagenic E. coli; shigella, salmonella, or campylobacter. | **Adult: Azithro** 1000 mg po once or 500 mg po q24h for 3 days in stool, **CIP** 750 mg po x 1 dose or 500 mg po x 3 days **OR** **Levo** 500 mg po q24h for 1-3 days **OR** | | **Antimotility agent:** For non-pregnant adults with no fever or blood in stool, add **loperamide** 4 mg po x 1, then 2 mg po after each loose stool to a maximum of 16 mg per day. |
| **Single dose therapy** is the recommended guideline. *(Am J Gastro 111:602, 2016; J Trav Med 24:S63, 2017; JAMA 2017;318:957)* | C. difficile, amebiasis *(see Table 13A).* **If chronic:** cyclospora, crypto-sporidia, giardia, Isospora | **Oflox** 300 mg po bid for 3 days **OR** **Rifaximin** 200 mg po tid for 3 days **OR** **Peds: Azithro** 10 mg/kg/day as a single dose for 3 days or **Ceftriaxone** 50 mg/kg/day as single dose for 3 days. Avoid FQs. | | **Comments:** Rifaximin approved only for ages 12 and older. Works only for diarrhea due to non-invasive E. coli; do not use if fever or bloody stool. **Ref:** *NEJM 361:1560, 2009; Clin Micro Inf 21:744, 2015.* **NOTE:** Self treatment with FQs associated with acquisition of resistant Gm-neg bacilli *(CID 60:837, 847, 872, 2015).* Increasing resistance of Campylobacter to FQ, particularly in Asia. Azithro now first line choice. |
| Advise patient: 1 dose usually sufficient, continue for 3d if not resolved after 1 dose | | **Pregnancy:** Use Azithro. Avoid FQs. **For loperamide,** see Comment. | | |
| **Prevention of Traveler's diarrhea** | | Not routinely indicated. Current recommendation is to take Imodium with 1st loose stool. | | |

*NOTE: All dosage recommendations are for adults (unless otherwise indicated) and assume normal renal function. § Alternatives consider allergy, PK, compliance, local resistance, cost.

TABLE 1 (19)

| ANATOMIC SITE/DIAGNOSIS/ MODIFYING CIRCUMSTANCES | ETIOLOGIES (usual) | SUGGESTED REGIMENS* PRIMARY | ALTERNATIVE§ | ADJUNCT DIAGNOSTIC OR THERAPEUTIC MEASURES AND COMMENTS |
|---|---|---|---|---|
| **GASTROINTESTINAL** *(continued)* | | | | |
| **Gastrointestinal Infections by Anatomic Site: Esophagus to Rectum** | | | | |
| Esophagitis. | Candida albicans, HSV, CMV | *See Table 11A and Table 14A.* | | |
| **Duodenal/Gastric ulcer:** gastric cancer, MALT lymphomas (not 2° NSAIDs). Comparative effectiveness & tolerance of treatment (*Amer J Gastroenterol 2017;112:212*) | **Helicobacter pylori** *See Comment.* Prevalence of pre-treatment resistance increasing, especially clarithro (*AAC 2017;61:e02530-16*). Ask about previous antibiotics and try to avoid prior antibiotic given. Consensus recs slightly different but rec all H.pylori + should be treated. Test & treat without EGD if age <45 yrs. | **Quadruple therapy:** (**Bismuth subsalicylate** 2 tabs qid + **Tetra** 500 mg qid + **Metro** 500 mg tid + **PPI**) x 14 days. For doses, see *footnote⁷ & Comments* | (**PPI + Amox** 1000 mg bid + **Metro** 500 mg bid + **Clarithro** 500 mg bid) x 14 days. | **Comments:** Any one of these **proton pump inhibitors (PPI)** may be used: omeprazole 20 mg bid, esomeprazole 20 mg bid, lansoprazole 30 mg bid, pantoprazole 40 mg bid, rabeprazole 20 mg bid. In many locations, 20% failure rates with previously recommended *triple regimens* (**PPI + Amox + Clarithro**). Exercise caution regarding potential interactions with other drugs, contraindications in pregnancy and warnings for other special populations. **Dx: Stool antigen**—Monoclonal EIA >90% sens. & 92% specific. Other tests: if endoscoped, rapid urease &/or histology &/or culture; serology less sens & spec; urea breath test, but some office-based tests underperform. Testing ref: *BMJ 344:d4, 2012.* **Test of cure:** Repeat stool antigen and/or urea breath test >8 wks post-treatment. **Treatment outcome:** Failure rate of triple therapy 20% due to clarithro resistance. |
| **Small intestine:** **Whipple's disease** (*NEJM 356:55, 2007; LnID 8:179, 2008*) Treatment: (*JAC 69:219, 2014.* See *Infective endocarditis, culture-negative, page 32.* | Tropheryma whipplei | (**Doxy** 100 mg po bid + **Hydroxychloroquine** 200 mg po tid x 1 year, then **Doxy** 100 mg po bid for life (Pelys) see *Comment* Immune reconstitution inflammatory response (IRIS) reactions occur. Thalidomide therapy may be better than steroids for IRIS reaction (*J Infect 60:79, 2010*) | **Doxy** 100 mg po bid for life see *Comment* | In vitro susceptibility testing and collected clinical experience (*JAC 69:219, 2014*). In vitro resistance to TMP-SMX plus frequent clinical failures & relapses. Frequent in vitro resistance to carbapenems. Ceftriaxone demonstrates high MICs against intracellular organisms in vitro (*AAC 48: 747, 2004*). **Doxy** considered safe regardless of age for duration of 21 days or less: 4.4 mg/kg div bid (*AAP Redbook 2018*). |

⁷ **Bismuth preparations:** (1) In U.S., **bismuth subsalicylate (Pepto-Bismol)** 262 mg tabs; adult dose for helicobacter is 2 tabs (524 mg) qid. (2) Outside U.S., **colloidal bismuth subcitrate (De-Nol)** 120 mg chewable tablets; dose is 1 tablet qid. In the U.S., bismuth subcitrate is available in combination cap only (Pylera): each cap contains bismuth subcitrate 140 mg + Metro 125 mg + Tetracycline 125 mg), given as 3 caps po 4x daily for 10 days **together with** a twice daily PPI.

*NOTE: All dosage recommendations are for adults (unless otherwise indicated) and assume normal renal function. § Alternatives consider allergy, PK, compliance, local resistance, cost.

*Abbreviations on page 2.*        *NOTE: All dosage recommendations are for adults (unless otherwise indicated) and assume normal renal function. §Alternatives consider allergy, PK, compliance, local resistance, cost.

**TABLE 1 (20)**

| ANATOMIC SITE/DIAGNOSIS/ MODIFYING CIRCUMSTANCES | ETIOLOGIES (usual) | SUGGESTED REGIMENS* | | ADJUNCT DIAGNOSTIC OR THERAPEUTIC MEASURES AND COMMENTS |
|---|---|---|---|---|
| | | PRIMARY | ALTERNATIVE§ | |
| **GASTROINTESTINAL/Gastrointestinal Infections by Anatomic Site:** Esophagus to Rectum *(continued)* | | | | |
| Diverticulitis, perirectal abscess, peritonitis<br>*Also see Peritonitis, page 49*<br><br>*NEJM 2018;379:1635* | Enterobacteriaceae, occasionally P. aeruginosa, Bacteroides sp., enterococci | **Outpatient rx—mild diverticulitis, drained perirectal abscess:**<br>[(TMP-SMX-DS bid) or CIP 750 mg bid or Levo 750 mg q24h)] + Metro 500 mg q6h. All px x 7-10 days.<br>**Mild-moderate disease—Inpatient—Parenteral Rx: (e.g., focal periappendiceal peritonitis, peridiverticular abscess, endomyometritis)**<br>PIP-TZ 3.375 gm IV q6h or 4.5 gm IV q8h or Erta 1 gm IV q24h or Moxi 400 mg IV q24h<br>**Severe life-threatening disease, ICU patient:**<br>IMP 500 mg IV q6h or MER 1 gm IV q8h or Dori 500 mg q8h (1-hr infusion).<br>For Ceftolo-tazo & Ceftaz-avi dosing, see Table 10D, page 128] page 49. | **AM-CL-ER** 1000/62.5 mg 2 tabs po bid x 7-10 days **OR** Moxi 400 mg po q24h x 7-10 days.<br><br>[(CIP 400 mg IV q12h) or (Levo 750 mg IV q24h)] + [Metro 500 mg IV q6h or 1 gm IV q12h) **OR Moxi** 400 mg IV q24h<br><br>**AMP + Metro + (CIP** 400 mg IV q12h or **Levo** 750 mg IV q24h) **OR (AMP** 2 gm IV q4h) + **Metro** 500 mg IV q6h + **Aminoglycoside§**<br>*(see Table 10D, page 128)]*<br>**Severe penicillin/cephalosporin allergy: (Aztreonam** 2 gm IV q6h to q8h) + I**Metro** (500 mg IV q6h) or (1 gm IV q12h)] **OR** [(CIP 400 mg IV q12h) or **Levo) + Metro].** | Must "cover" both Gm-neg. aerobic & Gm-neg. anaerobic bacteria. **Drugs active only vs. anaerobic Gm-neg. bacilli:** clinda, metro. **Drugs active only vs. aerobic Gm-neg. bacilli:** APAG, P Ceph 2/3/4 *(see Table 10A, page 112)*, aztreonam, CIP, Levo. **Drugs active vs. both aerobic/anaerobic Gm-neg. bacteria:** cefoxitin, cefotetan, TC-CL, PIP-TZ, AM-SB, ERTA, DORI, IMP, MER, Moxi, & tigecycline.<br><br>**Increasing resistance of B. fragilis group**<br><br>| | Clinda | Moxi | Cefoxitin | Cefotetan |<br>|---|---|---|---|---|<br>| % Resistant: | 42-80 | 34-45 | 48-60 | 19-35 |<br><br>*Ref: Anaerobe 17:147, 2011; AAC 56:1247, 2012; Surg Infect 10:111, 2009.*<br>**Resistance (B. fragilis):** Metro, PIP-TZ rare. Resistance to FQ increased in enteric bacteria, particularly if any FQ used recently. **Ertapenem** poorly active vs. P. aeruginosa/Acinetobacter sp. **Concomitant surgical management important**, esp. with moderate-severe disease. Role of enterococci remains debatable. Probably need drugs active vs. enterococci in pts with infections of biliary tract. Probably pathogenic in infections of biliary tract. Concomitant surgical management essential to cure. Probably pathogenic in pts with valvular heart disease.<br>**Tigecycline: Black Box Warning:** All cause mortality higher in pts treated with tigecycline (2.5%) than comparators (1.8%) in meta-analysis of clinical trials. Cause of mortality risk difference of 0.6% (95% CI, 0.1, 1.2) not established. Tigecycline should be essential for use in situations when alternative treatments are not suitable *(FDA MedWatch Sep 27, 2013)*. AGA guidelines recommend antibiotics not be used selectively in acute, uncomplicated diverticulitis *(Gastro 149: 1944, 2015)*. |
| **GENITAL TRACT: Mixture of empiric & specific treatment. Divided by sex of the patient. For sexual assault (rape), see Table 15A, page 154.**<br>*See CDC Guidelines for Sexually Transmitted Diseases: MMWR 64(RR-3):1, 2015; Med Lett 2017;59:105.* | | | | |
| **Both Women & Men:** | | | | |
| Chancroid<br>*(Curr Op Inf Dis 29:52, 2016)*<br>Ulcer is painful. | H. ducreyi | **Ceftriaxone** 250 mg IM single dose **OR Azithro** 1 gm po single dose | **CIP** 500 mg bid po x 3 days **OR Erythro base** 500 mg po tid x 7 days. | In HIV+ pts, failures reported with single dose azithro *(CID 21:409, 1995)*. Evaluate after 7 days, ulcer should objectively improve. All patients treated for chancroid should be tested for HIV and syphilis. All sex partners of pts with chancroid should be examined and treated if they have evidence of disease or have had sex with index pt within the last 10 days. |
| Non-gonococcal or post-gonococcal urethritis, cervicitis<br>**NOTE: Assume concomitant N. gonorrhoeae** (Chlamydia conjunctivitis, see page 14) | Chlamydia 50%, Mycoplasma genitalium (30%). Other known etiologies (10-15%): trichomonas, herpes simplex virus, *see JID 206:357, 2012.* Ref: CID 61:S774, 2015 | **(Doxy** 100 mg bid po x 7 days) or **(Azithro** 1 gm po as single dose). **Evaluate & treat sex partner**<br>**Pregnancy: Azithro** 1 gm po single dose **OR Amox** 500 mg po tid x 7 days | **(Erythro base** 500 mg po qid po x 7 days) or **Ofloxo** 300 mg po x 7 days) or **(Levo** 500 mg q24h) x 7 days).<br>**In pregnancy: Erythro base** 500 mg po qid for 7 days<br>**Doxy & FQs contraindicated** | **Diagnosis:** NAAT for C. trachomatis & N. gonorrhoeae on urine or cervix or urethra specimens *(AnIM 142:914, 2005).* Test all urethritis/cervicitis pts for HIV & syphilis.<br>**Evaluate & treat sex partners.**<br>Azithromycin 1 gm was superior to doxycycline for M. genitalium male urethritis *(CID 48:1649, 2009)*, but may select resistance leading to failure of multi-dose azithromycin retreatment regimens *(CID 48:1655, 2009).* |

§ Aminoglycoside = antipseudomonal aminoglycosidic aminoglycoside, e.g., Amikacin, Gentamicin, Tobramycin, Plazomicin

*Abbreviations on page 2.* *NOTE: All dosage recommendations are for adults (unless otherwise indicated) and assume normal renal function. § Alternatives consider allergy, PK, compliance, local resistance, cost.*

**TABLE 1 (21)**

| ANATOMIC SITE/DIAGNOSIS/ MODIFYING CIRCUMSTANCES | ETIOLOGIES (usual) | SUGGESTED REGIMENS* PRIMARY | ALTERNATIVE§ | ADJUNCT DIAGNOSTIC OR THERAPEUTIC MEASURES AND COMMENTS |
|---|---|---|---|---|
| **GENITAL TRACT/Both Women & Men** (continued) - CDC Guidelines: *MMWR 64(RR-3):1, 2015* | | | | |
| Non-gonococcal urethritis: **Mycoplasma genitalium** Ref: *CID 61:S802, 2015.* | Mycoplasma genitalium. | **Azithro** 500 mg po x 1 then 250 mg po once daily x 4 days or **Azithro** 1 gm po x 1 dose | **Moxi** 400 mg once daily x 10-14 days | Diagnosis by NAAT, but usually not available. **Doxy** ineffective. No cell wall so beta-lactams ineffective. Cure with single dose Azithro only 67% (*CID 61:1389, 2015*). Emerging resistance with Moxi (*Em Inf Dis 23:809, 2017*). Pristinamycin may work (*CID 2015;60:1228*). |
| Recurrent/persistent urethritis | C. trachomatis (43%), **M. genitalium** (30%), **T. vaginalis** (13%) (*CID 52:163, 2011*) | **Metro** 2 gm po x 1 dose + **Azithro** 1 gm po x 1 dose | **Tinidazole** 2 gm po x 1 + **Azithro** 1 gm po x 1 | High failure rate of Azithro if M. genitalium (*CID 56:934, 2013*). Can try Moxi 400 mg po once daily x 10 days if Azithro failure (*PLoS One 3:e3618, 2008*). New FQ resistance in Japan (*JAC 69:2376, 2014*). |
| Rectal, proctitis MSM and increasingly in women | C. trachomatis, M. genitalium, N. gonorrhoeae, syphilis, HSV | Treat for GC and chlamydia; **Doxy** 100 bid x 7 days preferred over Azithro | If LGV suspected treat **Doxy** 100 bid x 21 days | **Proctitis:** prefer Doxy x 7 days (*Sex Trans Dis 41:79, 2014*). Higher failures with azithro (*JAC 70:961, 2015*). |
| **Gonorrhea  FQs no longer recommended for treatment of gonococcal infections** (*See CDC Guidelines MMWR 64(RR-3):1, 2015; CID 61:S785, 2015*). **Cephalosporin resistance:** *JAMA 309:163 & 185, 2013.* Case report of Azithro/Ceph resist strain treated with ERTA in UK (*Eurosurv 23:5 2018*). | | | | |
| Conjunctivitis (adult) | N. gonorrhoeae | **Ceftriaxone** 1 gm IM or IV single dose + **Azithro** | | Consider one-time saline lavage of eye. |
| Disseminated gonococcal infection (DGI, dermatitis-arthritis syndrome) | N. gonorrhoeae | **Ceftriaxone** 1 gm IV q24h + **Azithro** 1 gm po x 1 | (**Cefotaxime** 1 gm q8h IV or **Ceftizoxime** 1 gm q8h IV) + **Azithro** 1 gm po x 1 | **Treat for a minimum of 7 days.** Owing to high-level resistance to oral cephalosporins and fluoroquinolones in the community, "Step-down" therapy should be avoided unless susceptibilities are known and demonstrate full activity of cephalosporin or fluoroquinolone R/O meningitis/endocarditis. **Treat** presumptively for concomitant **C. trachomatis.** Azithro recommended to cover resistant GC (usually tetra resistant, too) and C. trachomatis. |
| Endocarditis | N. gonorrhoeae | **Ceftriaxone** 1-2 gm IV q12-24 hours x 4 weeks + **Azithro** 1 gm po x 1 | | GC endocarditis may occur in the absence of concomitant urogenital symptoms (*Infection 42: 425, 2014*). Severe valve destruction may occur. Ceftriaxone resistance in *N. gonorrhoeae* has been reported (*AAC 55: 3538, 2011*); determine susceptibility of any isolate recovered. |
| Pharyngitis Dx: NAAT | N. gonorrhoeae | **Ceftriaxone** 250 mg IM x 1 + (**Azithro** 1 gm po x 1). | Due to resistance concerns, **do not use FQs.** | Pharyngeal GC more difficult to eradicate. **Repeat NAAT 14 days post-rx. Spectinomycin**NUS, **cefixime, cefpodoxime & cefuroxime not effective** |
| Urethritis, cervicitis, proctitis (uncomplicated) For prostatitis, see page 29. **Diagnosis:** Nucleic acid amplification test (NAAT) on vaginal swab, urine or urethral swab *MMWR 64(RR-3):1, 2015* | N. gonorrhoeae (50% of pts with urethritis, cervicitis have concomitant C. trachomatis—treat for both even if NAAT indicates single pathogen). | **Ceftriaxone** 250 mg IM x 1 + **Azithro** 1 gm po x 1; **Rx failure:** Ceftriaxone 500 mg IM x 1 + Azithro 2 gm po x 1; treat partner; NAAT for test of cure 1 wk post-treatment **Severe Pen/Ceph allergy:** (Gent 240 mg IM x 1 + Azithro 2 gm po x 1 dose) OR (Gemi 320 mg + Azithro 2 gm po x 1 dose) (nausea in >20%) | | Screen for syphilis. **Other alternatives for GC (Test of Cure is no longer recommended one week after Rx for ALL of these approaches listed below):** • **Oral cephalosporin use is no longer recommended** as primary therapy due to emergence of resistance, *MMWR 67:590, 2012.* • Other single-dose cephalosporins; ceftizoxime 500 mg IM, cefoxitin 2 gm IM + probenecid 1 gm po, cefotaxime 500 mg IM. |
| Granuloma inguinale (Donovanosis) | Klebsiella (formerly Calymmatobacterium) granulomatis | **Azithro** 1 gm po q wk x 3 wks | **TMP-SMX** one DS tablet bid x 3 wks **OR Erythro** 500 mg po bid x 3 wks **OR CIP** 750 mg po bid x 3 wks **OR Doxy** 100 mg po bid x 3 wks. | Clinical response usually seen in 1 wk; **Rx until all lesions healed**, may take 4 wks. Treatment failures & recurrence seen with Doxy & TMP-SMX. Relapse can occur 6-18 months after apparently effective Rx. If improvement not evident in first few days, some experts add Gent 1 mg/kg IV q8h. |
| Herpes simplex virus Human papilloma virus (HPV) | *See Table 14A, page 181* *See Table 14A, page 186* | | | |

*Abbreviations on page 2.* *NOTE: All dosage recommendations are for adults (unless otherwise indicated) and assume normal renal function. §Alternatives consider allergy, PK, compliance, local resistance, cost.*

**TABLE 1 (22)**

| ANATOMIC SITE/DIAGNOSIS/ MODIFYING CIRCUMSTANCES | ETIOLOGIES (usual) | SUGGESTED REGIMENS* | | ADJUNCT DIAGNOSTIC OR THERAPEUTIC MEASURES AND COMMENTS |
|---|---|---|---|---|
| | | PRIMARY | ALTERNATIVE[b] | |
| **GENITAL TRACT/Both Women & Men** (continued) | | | | |
| **Lymphogranuloma venereum**<br><br>Ref: CID 61:S865, 2015 | Chlamydia trachomatis, serovars. L1, L2, L3 | Doxy 100 mg po bid x 21 days | Erythro 500 mg po qid x 21 days or Azithro 1000 mg po q wk x 3 wks (clinical data lacking). | Dx based on serology; biopsy contraindicated because sinus tracts develop. Nucleic acid ampli tests for C. trachomatis will be positive. In MSM, presents as fever, rectal ulcer, anal discharge (CID 39:996, 2004; Dis Colon Rectum 52:507, 2009). |
| **Phthirus pubis (pubic lice, "crabs")** & scabies | Phthirus pubis & Sarcoptes scabiei | See Table 13A, page 172 | | |
| **Syphilis** Diagnosis: JAMA 312:1922, 2014; treatment: JAMA 312:1905, 2014; management: CID 61:S818, 2015. Overview: Lancet 389: 1550, 2017. | | | | |
| **Early, primary, secondary, or latent <1 yr.** Defn: Screen with treponema-specific antibody of or RPR/VDRL, see JCM 50:2 & 148, 2012; CID 58:1116, 2014.<br><br>Chancre is painless. | T. pallidum | **Benzathine pen G (Bicillin L-A)** 2.4 million units IM x 1 (See Comment) | (Doxy 100 mg po bid x 14 days) or (Tetra 500 mg po qid x 14 days) or (Ceftriaxone 1 gm IV/IM q24h x 10–14 days). Follow-up mandatory.<br><br>Ceftriaxone efficacy (CID 2017;65:1683)<br><br>Doxy considered safe regardless of age for rx ≤21 days (AAP Redbook 2018) | If early or congenital syphilis, quantitative VDRL at 0, 3, 6, 12 & 24 mos after rx. If 1° or 2° syphilis, VDRL should ↓ 2 tubes at 6 mos, 3 tubes 12 mos, & 4 tubes 24 mos. Update on congenital syphilis (MMWR 64(RR-3):1, 2015). Early latent: 2 tubes ↓ at 12 mos. With 1°, 50% will be RPR seronegative at 12 mos., 24% neg. FT/ABS (2–3 yrs (AnlM 114:1005, 1991). If titers fail to fall, examine CSF. If CSF (+) treat as neurosyphilis; if CSF is negative, retreat with benzathine Pen G 2.4 mu IM weekly x 3 wks. **If no other options:** Azithro 2 gm po x 1 dose (equivalent to Benzathine pen 2.4 M x 1 dose in early syphilis (J Infect Dis 201:1729, 2010). Azithro-resistant syphilis documented in California, Ireland, & elsewhere.<br>**NOTE:** Use of benzathine procaine penicillin is inappropriate! |
| **More than 1 yr's duration (latent of indeterminate duration, cardiovascular, late benign gumma)** | | **Benzathine pen G (Bicillin L-A)** 2.4 million units IM x 1 week x 3 = 7.2 million units | Doxy 100 mg po bid x 28 days or Tetra 500 mg po qid x 28 days. Ceftriaxone 1 gm IV or IM daily for 10–14 days MAY be an alternative. (No clinical data; consult an ID specialist). | No published data on efficacy of alternatives. **Indications for LP (CDC):** neurologic symptoms, treatment failure, any eye or ear involvement, other evidence of active syphilis (aortitis, gumma, iritis). |
| **Neurosyphilis**—Very difficult to treat. Includes ocular (retro-bulbar neuritis) syphilis<br>**All need CSF exam.**<br><br>HIV infection (AIDS)<br>CDC STD guidelines:<br>MMWR 64 (3), June 5, 2015 | | **Pen G** 18–24 million units per day either as continuous infusion or as 3–4 million units IV q4h x 10–14 days. Treatment same as HIV uninfected. Treat early neurosyphilis regardless of CD4 count; MMWR 56:625, 2007. | **Procaine pen G** 2.4 million units IM q24h + **probenecid** 0.5 gm po qid) both x 10–14 days—See Comment. | **Ceftriaxone** 2 gm (IV or IM) q24h x 14 days. For penicillin allergy: either desensitize or obtain infectious diseases consultation. Serologic criteria for response to rx: 4-fold or greater ↓ in VDRL titer over 6–12 mos.<br><br>See Syphilis discussion in CDC Guidelines MMWR 64(RR-3):1, 2015. Doxy, tetracycline contraindicated. Erythro not recommended because of high risk of failure to cure fetus. |
| **Pregnancy and syphilis** | | Same as Non-pregnant, some recommend 2nd dose (2.4 million units) **Benzathine Pen G** 1 wk after initial dose esp. in 3rd trimester or with 2° syphilis | Skin test for penicillin allergy. Desensitize if necessary, as parenteral pen G is only therapy with documented efficacy. | Monthly quantitative VDRL or equivalent. If 4-fold ↑, re-treat. Doxy, tetracycline contraindicated. Erythro not recommended because of high risk of failure to cure fetus. |

NOTE: Screen MSM and/or HIV pts every 3–12 mos (JAMA 315:2321 & 2328, 2016). Pregnancy: screen all (JAMA 2018;320:911)

For penicillin desensitization method, see Table 7, page 91 and MMWR 64(RR-3):1, 2015

**NOTE:** Test all pts with syphilis for HIV; test all HIV patients for latent syphilis.

Abbreviations on page 2.

*NOTE: All dosage recommendations are for adults (unless otherwise indicated) and assume normal renal function. § Alternatives consider allergy, PK, compliance, local resistance, cost.

TABLE 1 (23)

| ANATOMIC SITE/DIAGNOSIS/ MODIFYING CIRCUMSTANCES | ETIOLOGIES (usual) | SUGGESTED REGIMENS* | | ADJUNCT DIAGNOSTIC OR THERAPEUTIC MEASURES AND COMMENTS |
|---|---|---|---|---|
| | | PRIMARY | ALTERNATIVE§ | |
| **GENITAL TRACT/Both Women & Men/Syphilis:** *(continued)* | | | | |
| Congenital syphilis (Update on Congenital Syphilis: MMWR 64(RR-3):1, 2015) | T. pallidum | **Aqueous crystalline Pen G** 50,000 units/kg per dose IV q12h x 7 days, then q8h for 10 days total. | **Procaine Pen G** 50,000 units/kg IM q24h for 10 days | Another alternative: **Ceftriaxone** ≤30 days old, 75 mg/kg IV/IM q24h (use with caution in infants with jaundice) or >30 days old 100 mg/kg IV/IM q24h. Treat 10-14 days. If symptomatic, ophthalmologic exam indicated. If more than 1 day of rx missed, restart entire course. **Need serologic follow-up!** |
| Warts, anogenital | *See Table 14A, page 186* | | | |
| **Women:** | | | | |
| Amnionitis, septic abortion | Bacteroides, esp. Prevotella bivia; Group B, A streptococci; Enterobacteriaceae; C. trachomatis. Rarely U. urealyticum. | [(Cefoxitin or Dori^NM or IMP or MER or AM-SB or Erta or PIP-TZ) + **Doxy**] OR [Clinda + (Aminoglycoside or Ceftriaxone)] *Dosage: see footnote9* NOTE: in US and Europe, 1/3 of Grp B Strep resistant to clindamycin. | | DoC of uterus. **In septic abortion,** Clostridium perfringens may cause fulminant intravascular hemolysis. **In postpartum patients with** enigmatic fever and/or pulmonary emboli, **consider septic pelvic vein thrombophlebitis** (see *Vascular septic pelvic vein thrombophlebitis, page 72*). After discharge: doxy or clinda for C. trachomatis. |
| Cervicitis, mucopurulent Treatment based on results of nucleic acid amplification test | N. gonorrhoeae Chlamydia trachomatis | Treat for Gonorrhea, *page 25* Treat for non-gonococcal urethritis, *page 25* if due to *Mycoplasma genitalium*, less likely to respond to doxy than azithro and emerging resistance to both azithro and FQ. | | Criteria for diagnosis: 1) (muco) purulent endocervical exudate and/or 2) sustained endocervical bleeding after passage of cotton swab. >10 WBC/ hpf of vaginal fluid is suggestive. Intracellular gram-neg diplococci are specific but insensitive. If in doubt, send swab or urine for culture, EIA or nucleic acid amplification test and treat for both. |
| **Endomyometritis/septic pelvic phlebitis** | | | | |
| Early postpartum (1st 48 hrs) (usually after C-section) | Bacteroides, esp. Prevotella bivia; Group B, A streptococci; Enterobacteriaceae; C. trachomatis; M. hominis | [(Cefoxitin or Erta or IMP or MER or AM-SB or Ceftriaxone) + **Doxy**] or [Clinda + (Aminoglycoside or Ceftriaxone)] *Dosage: see footnote9* | | See *Comments under Amnionitis, septic abortion, above* |
| Late postpartum (48 hrs to 6 wks) (usually after vaginal delivery) | C. trachomatis | **Doxy** 100 mg IV or po q12h times 14 days | | Tetracyclines not recommended in nursing mothers; discontinue nursing. M. hominis sensitive to tetra, clinda, not erythro. |
| Fitzhugh-Curtis syndrome | N. gonorrhoeae | Treat as for pelvic inflammatory disease immediately below. | | Perihepatitis (violin-string adhesions). Sudden onset of RUQ pain. Associated with salpingitis. Transaminases elevated in <30% of cases. |
| Pelvic actinomycosis: usually tubo-ovarian abscess | A. Israelii most common | **AMP** 200 mg/kg/day in 3-4 divided doses x 4-6 wks then **Pen VK** 2-4 gm/day in 4 divided doses x 6-12 mo | **Doxy** or **Ceftriaxone** or **Clinda** | Complication of intrauterine device (IUD). Remove IUD. Can use **Pen G** 10-20 million units/day IV instead of **AMP** x 4-6 wks. |

9 **P Ceph 2 (Cefoxitin** 2 gm IV q6-8h, **Cefotetan** 2 gm IV q12h, **Cefuroxime** 750 mg IV q12h; **AM-SB** 3 gm IV q6h; for nosocomial pneumonia; 4.5 gm IV q8h or 4-hr infusion of 3.375 gm q8h; **Doxy** 100 mg IV/po q12h; **Clinda** 450-900 mg IV/po q8h; **Aminoglycoside (Gent,** see *Table 10D, page 128*); **P Ceph 3 (Cefotaxime** 2 gm IV q8h, **Ceftriaxone** 2 gm IV q24h); **Dori** 500 mg IV q8h (1-hr infusion); **Erta** 1 gm IV q24h; **IMP** 0.5 gm IV q6h; **MER** 1 gm IV q8h; **Azithro** 1 gm IV q24h; **Linezolid** 600 mg IV/po q12h; **Vanco** 1 gm IV q12h

*Abbreviations on page 2.*     *\*NOTE: All dosage recommendations are for adults (unless otherwise indicated) and assume normal renal function. PK, compliance, local resistance, cost. § Alternatives consider allergy, PK, compliance, local resistance, cost.*

TABLE 1 (24)

| ANATOMIC SITE/DIAGNOSIS/ MODIFYING CIRCUMSTANCES | ETIOLOGIES (usual) | SUGGESTED REGIMENS* | | ADJUNCT DIAGNOSTIC OR THERAPEUTIC MEASURES AND COMMENTS |
|---|---|---|---|---|
| | | PRIMARY | ALTERNATIVE§ | |
| **GENITAL TRACT/Women** (continued) | | | | |
| **Pelvic Inflammatory Disease (PID), salpingitis, tubo-ovarian abscess** | | | | |
| Outpatient rx: limit to pts with temp <38°C, WBC <11,000 per mm³, minimal evidence of peritonitis, active bowel sounds & able to tolerate oral nourishment<br><br>*NEJM 372:2039, 2015;*<br>*CDC Guidelines MMWR 64(RR-3):1, 2015* | N. gonorrhoeae, chlamydia, bacteroides, Enterobacteriaceae, streptococci, especially G. agalactiae.<br>Less commonly:<br>G. vaginalis, Haemophilus influenzae, cytomegalovirus (CMV), M. genitalium, U. urealyticum | **Outpatient rx:** [(**Ceftriaxone** 250 mg IM or IV x 1) (± **Metro** 500 mg po bid x 14 days) + (**Doxy** 100 mg po bid x 14 days)]. **OR** (**Cefoxitin** 2 gm IM with **Probenecid** 1 gm po both as single dose) plus **Doxy** 100 mg po bid times 14 days) | **Inpatient regimens:**<br>[(**Cefotetan** 2 gm IV q12h or **Cefoxitin** 2 gm IV q6h) + (**Doxy** 100 mg IV/po q12h)]<br><br>(**Clinda** 900 mg IV q8h) + **Gent** 2 mg/kg loading dose, then 1.5 mg/kg q8h or 4.5 mg/kg once per day) + **Doxy** 100 mg po bid x 14 days | **Another alternative parenteral regimen:**<br>**AM-SB** 3 gm IV q6h + **Doxy** 100 mg IV/po q12h. Recommended treatments don't cover M. genitalium so if no response after 7-10 days consider M. genitalium NAAT and treat with **Moxi** 400 mg/day 14 days.<br><br>Remember: Evaluate and treat sex partner. FQs not recommended due to increasing resistance *(MMWR 64(RR-3):1, 2015 & cdc.gov/std/ treatment).*<br><br>Suggest initial inpatient evaluation/therapy for pts with tubo-ovarian abscess. For inpatient regimens, continue treatment until satisfactory response for ≥24-hr before switching to outpatient regimen. Improved routine testing for chlamydia and gonorrhea among outpatients resulted in reduced hospitalization and ectopic pregnancy rates *(J Adolescent Health 51:80, 2012)* |
| **Vaginitis—** *MMWR 64(RR-3):1, 2015* | | | | |
| **Candidiasis**<br>Pruritus, thick cheesy discharge.<br>See *Table 11A, page 134* | Candida albicans 80-90%.<br>C. glabrata, C. tropicalis may be increasing & are less susceptible to azoles | **Oral azoles: Fluconazole** 150 mg po x 1 dose. For milder cases, Topical Therapy with one of the over the counter preparations usually is successful (e.g., clotrimazole, butoconazole, miconazole, or tioconazole) as creams or vaginal suppositories. | **Butoconazole, Clotrimazole, Miconazole, Tioconazole, Terconazole** (all intravaginal): variety of strengths - from 1 dose to 7-14 days *(See Table 11A, page 134)* | Nystatin vag. tabs, times 14 days less effective. Other rx for azole-resistant strains: gentian violet, boric acid.<br>If recurrent candidiasis (4 or more episodes per yr): 6 mos. suppression with: fluconazole 150 mg po q week or itraconazole 100 mg po q24hr or clotrimazole vag. suppositories 500 mg q week. |
| **Trichomoniasis**<br>*(CID 61:S837, 2015)*<br>Copious foamy discharge, pH >4.5<br>Treat sexual partners—<br>see Comment | Trichomonas vaginalis<br>**Dx:** NAAT & PCR available<br>& most sensitive; wet mount not sensitive.<br>Ref: *JCM 54:7, 2016.* | **Metro** 500 mg po bid x 7 days OR 2 gm single dose. **Tinidazole** 2 gm po single dose more effective than Metro 2 gm; If HIV+ always give 7 day course OR **Tinidazole** 2 gm po single dose.<br>**Pregnancy:** See Comment. | **For rx failure:** Re-treat with metro 500 mg po bid x 7 days; If 2nd failure: metro 2 gm po q24h x 3-5 days. If 3rd failure: **Tinidazole** 2 gm po q24h x 5 days. **Clinda** 0.3 gm bid x 7 days or **Clinda ovules** 100 mg intravaginally at bedtime x 3 days. **Secnidazole** 2 gm packet intravaginally at bedtime x 7 days | **Treat male sexual partners: Metro** 2 gm x 1 dose Nearly 20% men with NGU are infected with trichomonas. For alternative option in refractory cases, see *CID 33:1341, 2001.*<br>**Pregnancy:** No data indicating metro teratogenic or mutagenic. For discussion of treating trichomonas, including issues in pregnancy, see *MMWR 64(RR-3):1, 2015; Curr Drug Safety 2015;10:170.* |
| **Bacterial vaginosis (BV)**<br>Malodorous vaginal discharge, pH >4.5 | Etiology unclear: associated with Gardnerella vaginalis, mobiluncus, Mycoplasma hominis, Prevotella sp., & Atopobium vaginae et al. | **Metro** 0.5 gm po bid x 7 days or **Metro vaginal gel¹⁰** (1 applicator intravaginally) 1x/day x 5 days<br>OR<br>2% **Clinda vaginal cream** 5 gm intravaginally at bedtime x 7 days | **Clinda** 0.3 gm po bid x 7 days or **Clinda ovules** 100 mg intravaginally at bedtime x 3 days. **Secnidazole** 2 gm packet (apple-sauce, yogurt, pudding) x 1 dose over 30 min. | **Treatment of male sex partner not indicated unless balanitis present.** Recurrence 50% ↑ in cure rate if abstain from sex or use condoms: *CID 44:213 & 220, 2007.* Oral Metro or oral Clinda 7-day regimens *(see CDC STD Guidelines: MMWR 64(RR-3):1, 2015).* If recurrent BV, can try adding **boric acid** to suppressive regimen: Metro 0.5 gm po bid x 7 days, then vaginal boric acid gelatin capsule 600 mg hs x 21 days, followed by Metro vaginal gel 2x/week x 16 weeks *(Sex Trans Dis 36:732, 2009).* |

¹⁰ 1 applicator contains 5 gm of gel with 37.5 mg metronidazole

*Abbreviations on page 2.*   \*NOTE: All dosage recommendations are for adults (unless otherwise indicated) and assume normal renal function. PK, compliance, local resistance, cost.

§ Alternatives consider allergy, PK, compliance, local resistance, cost.

**TABLE 1 (25)**

| ANATOMIC SITE/DIAGNOSIS/ MODIFYING CIRCUMSTANCES | ETIOLOGIES (usual) | SUGGESTED REGIMENS* | | ADJUNCT DIAGNOSTIC OR THERAPEUTIC MEASURES AND COMMENTS |
|---|---|---|---|---|
| | | PRIMARY | ALTERNATIVE§ | |
| **GENITAL TRACT** *(continued)* | | | | |
| **Men:** | | | | |
| **Balanitis** | Candida 40%, Group B strep, gardenella | **Metro** 2 gm po x 1 dose OR **Fluconazole** 150 mg po x 1 dose | OR **Itra** 200 mg po bid x 1 day. | Occurs in 1/4 of male sex partners of women infected with candida. Exclude circinate balanitis (Reiter's syndrome); (non-infectious) responds to hydrocortisone cream. |
| **Epididymo-orchitis** *(CID 61:S770, 2015)* | | | | |
| Age <35 years | N. gonorrhoeae, Chlamydia trachomatis | **[Ceftriaxone** 250 mg IM x 1 + **Doxy** 100 mg po bid x 10 days] + bed rest, scrotal elevation, analgesics. | | Enterobacteriaceae occasionally encountered. Test all pts age <35 yrs for HIV and syphilis. |
| Age >35 years or MSM (insertive partners in anal intercourse) | Enterobacteriaceae (coliforms) | **[Levo** 500-750 mg IV/po once daily] OR [**Oflox** 300 mg po bid] or (400 mg IV twice daily)] for 10-14 days AM-SB, P Ceph 3, PIP-TZ *(Dosage: see footnote* on page 27)* for MSM can be mixed GC/chlamydia with enterics so treat with FQ AND Ceftriaxone 250 mg IM x1) Also: bed rest, scrotal elevation, analgesics. | | Midstream pyuria and scrotal pain and edema. **NOTE:** Do urine NAAT (nucleic acid amplification test) to ensure absence of N. gonorrhoeae with concomitant risk of FQ-resistant gonorrhoeae or of chlamydia if using agents without reliable activity. Other causes include: mumps, brucella, TB, intravesicular BCG, B. pseudomallei, coccidioides, Behcet's. |
| **Non-gonococcal urethritis** | *See page 25 (CID 61:S763, 2015)* | | | |
| **Prostatitis**—Review: CID 50:1641, 2010. See Guidelines 2015 http://onlinelibrary.wiley.com/doi/10.1111/bju.13101/epdf | | | | |
| Acute | N. gonorrhoeae, C. trachomatis | **Ceftriaxone** 250 mg IM x 1 then **Doxy** 100 mg bid x 10 days. | | FQs no longer recommended for gonococcal infections. Test for HIV. In AIDS pts, prostate may be focus of Cryptococcus neoformans. |
| Uncomplicated (with risk of STD, age <35 yrs). | Enterobacteriaceae (coliforms) | **FQ** *(dosage: see Epididymo-orchitis, >35 yrs, above).* Some recommend 3-4 wks therapy. If uncertain, do NAAT for C. trachomatis and N. gonorrhoeae. If resistant enterobacteriaceae, use ERTA 1 gm IV qd. If resistant pseudomonas, use IMP or MER (500 mg IV q6 or q8 respectively). | | Treat as acute urinary infection, 14 days (not single dose regimen). Some |
| Uncomplicated with low risk of STD | Enterobacteriaceae (coliforms) | or **TMP-SMX** 1 DS tablet (160 mg TMP) po bid x 10-14 days (minimum). Some authorities recommend 4 weeks of therapy. | | |
| Chronic bacterial | Enterobacteriaceae 80%, enterococci 15%, P. aeruginosa | **CIP** 500 mg po bid x 4-6 wks OR **Levo** 750 mg po q24h x 4 wks. | **TMP-SMX-DS** 1 tab po bid x 1-3 mos (Fosfomycin: see Comment) | **With treatment failures** consider infected prostatic calculi. FDA approved dose of levo is 500 mg; editors prefer higher dose. Fosfomycin penetrates prostate; case report of success with 3 gm po q24h x 12-16 wks (CID 61:1141, 2015) or 3 gm q3d x 6 wks. (AAC 60:1854, 2016). |
| Chronic prostatitis/chronic pain syndrome | The most common prostatitis syndrome. Etiology is unknown. | α-adrenergic blocking agents are controversial *(AnIM 133:367, 2000).* | | Pt has six of prostatitis but negative cultures and no cells in prostatic secretions. Rev: TMP-SMX-DS (AnIM 141:581 & 639, 2004). 100 mg IV q6 or q8 respectively). AAC 46:157, 2000. In randomized double-blind study, CIP and an alpha-blocker of no benefit |
| **HAND** *(Bites: See Skin)* | | | | |
| **Paronychia** | | | | |
| Nail biting, manicuring | Staph. aureus (maybe MRSA) | Incision & drainage; culture | **TMP-SMX-DS** 1-2 tabs po bid while waiting for culture result. | *See Table 6 for alternatives.* Occasionally—candida, gram-negative rods. |
| Contact with saliva— dentists, anesthesiologists, wrestlers | Herpes simplex (Whitlow) | **Acyclovir** 400 mg tid po x 10 days | **Famciclovir** or **Valacyclovir,** see Comment | Gram stain and routine culture negative. Famciclovir/valacyclovir for primary genital herpes; see *Table 14A, page 181* |
| Dishwasher (prolonged water immersion) | Candida sp. | **Clotrimazole** (topical) | | Avoid immersion of hands in water as much as possible. |

29

*Abbreviations on page 2.*   \*NOTE: *All dosage recommendations are for adults (unless otherwise indicated) and assume normal renal function.* § *Alternatives consider allergy, PK, compliance, local resistance, cost.*

**TABLE 1 (26)**

| ANATOMIC SITE/DIAGNOSIS/ MODIFYING CIRCUMSTANCES | ETIOLOGIES (usual) | SUGGESTED REGIMENS* | | ADJUNCT DIAGNOSTIC OR THERAPEUTIC MEASURES AND COMMENTS |
|---|---|---|---|---|
| | | PRIMARY | ALTERNATIVE§ | |
| **HEART** | | | | |
| **Infective endocarditis—Native valve—empirical rx awaiting cultures—No IV illicit drugs** | Diagnostic criteria include evidence of continuous bacteremia (multiple positive blood cultures), new murmur (worsening of old murmur) of valvular insufficiency, definite emboli, and echocardiographic (transthoracic or transesophageal) evidence of valvular vegetations. Refs.: *Circulation 132:1435, 2015.* | | | |
| Valvular or congenital heart disease but no modifying circumstances See *Table 15C, page 222* for prophylaxis | Viridans strep 30-40%, "other" strep 15-25%, enterococci 5-18%, staphylococci 20-35% (including coag-neg staphylococci (*CID 46:232, 2008).* | Vanco 15-20 mg/kg q8-12h (target trough conc of 15-20 µg/mL) + Ceftriaxone 2 gm 24h OR Vanco 15-20 mg/kg q8-12h (target trough conc of 15-20 µg/mL) + Gent 1 mg/kg q8h IV/IM | Substitute **Dapto** 6 mg/kg IV q24h (or q48h for CrCl <30 mL/min) for **Vanco** | For antimicrobial prophylaxis, see *Table 15C, page 222.* If patient not acutely ill and not in heart failure, wait for blood culture results. If initial 3 blood cultures neg. after 24-48 hrs, obtain 2-3 more blood cultures before empiric therapy started. Gent dose is for CrCl of 80 mL/min or greater; even low-dose Gentamicin for only a few days carries risk of nephrotoxicity *(CID 48:713, 2009).* Gent is used for synergy; peak levels need not exceed 4 µg/mL and troughs should be <1 µg/mL. Coagulase-negative staphylococci can occasionally cause native valve endocarditis *(CID 46:232, 2008).* Modify therapy based on identification of specific pathogen as soon as possible to obtain best coverage and to avoid toxicities. **Surgery indications:** See *NEJM 368:1425, 2013.* Role of surgery in pts with left-sided endocarditis & large vegetation *(NEJM 366:2466, 2012).* No difference in 15 yr survival between bioprosthetic and mechanical valve *(JAMA 312:1323, 2014).* |
| **Infective endocarditis—Native valve—culture positive** Ref. *Circulation 132:1435, 2015.* | | | | |
| Viridans strep, S. bovis (*S. gallolyticus*) with **pen G MIC ≤0.12 mcg/mL** | Viridans strep, S. bovis (*S. gallolyticus subsp. gallolyticus*). | **(Pen G** 12-18 million units/day IV, divided q4h - q4h **OR (Ceftriaxone** 2 gm IV q24h) x 4 wks | [(**Pen G or Ceftriaxone** 2 gm IV q24h) + **Gent** 3 mg per kg IV q24h] x 2 wks. | 4-wks regimen preferred for most patients. Avoid 2-wks regimen for patients age >65 years, those with cardiac or extracardiac abscess, creatinine clearance of <50 mL/min, impaired eighth cranial nerve function, or Abiotrophia, Granulicatella, or Gemella spp infection. Vancomycin 15 mg/kg q12h x 4 weeks, dose adjusted to achieve trough concentrations of 10-15 µg/mL for patients allergic to or intolerant of Pen or Ceftriaxone. |
| Viridans strep, S. bovis (*S. gallolyticus*) with **pen G MIC >0.12 to <0.5 mcg/mL** | Viridans strep, S. bovis (*S. gallolyticus subsp. gallolyticus*). | **Pen G** 24 million units/day IV (divided q4h) x 4 wks) + **Gent** 3 mg/kg IV q24h x 2 wks | **Vanco** 15 mg/kg q12h x 4 wks, dose adjusted to achieve trough concentrations of 10-15 µg/mL | If the isolate is Ceftriaxone susceptible (MIC <0.5 µg/mL), then Ceftriaxone x 4 wks alone is an option. |
| Viridans strep, S. bovis, **nutritionally variant streptococci** (new names are: Abiotrophia sp. & Granulicatella sp.) | Viridans strep, S. bovis, **nutritionally variant streptococci** (new names are: Abiotrophia sp. & Granulicatella sp.) | **Pen G** 24 million units per 24h IV, divided q4h x 4 wks) + (**Gent** 3 mg/kg/d in 2-3 divided doses x 4 wks)] OR (**AMP** 12 gm/day IV, divided q4h + **Gent** as above x 4 wks) | **Vanco** 15 mg/kg q12h x 4 wks, dose adjusted to achieve trough concentrations of 10-15 µg/mL | If the isolate is Ceftriaxone susceptible (MIC <0.5 µg/mL), then Ceftriaxone x 4 wks alone is an option. |
| For viridans strep or S. bovis with **pen G MIC ≥0.5 mcg/mL** **NOTE:** Inf. Dis. consultation suggested | | | **Vanco** 15 mg/kg q12h x 4 wks, dose adjusted to achieve trough concentrations of 10-15 µg/mL | For streptococci with Ceftriaxone MIC ≤0.5 µg/mL, Ceftriaxone 2 gm q24h can be substituted for ampicillin. For gentamicin given 1 mg/kg q8h target peak serum concentration of 3-4 µg/mL and trough serum concentration of <1 µg/mL. |

*Abbreviations on page 2.*  *NOTE: All dosage recommendations are for adults (unless otherwise indicated) and assume normal renal function. § Alternatives consider allergy, PK, compliance, local resistance, cost.*

**TABLE 1 (27)**

**HEART/Infective endocarditis—Native valve—culture positive** (continued) Ref: *Circulation 132:1435, 2015.*

| ANATOMIC SITE/DIAGNOSIS/ MODIFYING CIRCUMSTANCES | ETIOLOGIES (usual) | SUGGESTED REGIMENS* | | ADJUNCT DIAGNOSTIC OR THERAPEUTIC MEASURES AND COMMENTS |
|---|---|---|---|---|
| | | **PRIMARY** | **ALTERNATIVE§** | |
| Enterococci, penicillin and aminoglycoside susceptible | E. faecalis E. faecium | [(AMP 2 gm IV q4h + Pen G 24 million units) + Gent 3 mg/kg/d IV in 2-3 divided doses] x 4–6 wks | [(AMP 2 gm IV q4h + Ceftriaxone 2 gm IV q12h) x 6 wks] Penicillin-intolerant patient only: (Vanco 30 mg/kg/d IV in 2-3 divided doses + Gent 1 mg/kg IV q8h) x 6 wks | **Native valve:** 4 ks Pen or AMP + Gent if symptoms <3 mo; 6 wks if symptoms >3 mo; **prosthetic valve:** 6 wks. Adjust dose of **Gent** to achieve peak serum conc. of 3-4 µg/mL and trough of <1 µg/mL. Target **Vanco** trough of 15-20 µg/mL. **AMP+Ceftriaxone** preferred for patients with creatinine clearance <50 mL/min or who develop such as on gent regimen. Vanco + Gent toxic; consider pen desensitization. |
| Enterococci, Penicillin susceptible, Gentamicin resistant (MIC >500 µg/mL), streptomycin susceptible (MIC <1500 µg/mL). | E. faecalis E. faecium | (AMP 2 gm IV q4h + Ceftriaxone 2 gm IV q12h) x 6 wks | [(AMP 2 gm IV q4h or Pen G 24 million units) + streptomycin 15 mg/kg IV q24h] x 4–6 wks. | May have to consider surgical removal of infected valve. Must confirm streptomycin MIC for synergy if strep combo used. **AMP + Ceftriaxone** regimen preferred, if creatinine clearance <50 mL/min, concern for impaired eighth nerve function. |
| Enterococci, Penicillin, aminoglycoside, Vancomycin resistant | E. faecalis E. faecium | Dapto 8-12 mg/kg IV q24h + AMP 2 gm IV q4h | Linezolid 600 mg IV/po q12h | **Quinupristin-Dalfopristin** 7.5 mg/kg IV q8h (via central line for E. faecium, not active vs E. faecalis). Duration of therapy ≥8 weeks, expert consultation strongly advised. Valve replacement often required for cure. |
| Infective endocarditis, Gram-negative bacilli | Enterobacteriaceae or P. aeruginosa | Optimal therapy unknown, infectious diseases consult recommended; an aminoglycoside (Tobra if P. aeruginosa) + (Cefepime or MER) is a reasonable option. | | Choice of agents based on in vitro susceptibilities, fluoroquinolone an option instead of aminoglycoside, but few data. |
| Infective endocarditis, fungal | Candida sp. Aspergillus | Optimal therapy unknown, infectious diseases consultation recommended; an azole or echinocandin is a reasonable empirical choice. High failure rate with medical therapy alone, consider early surgery. | | |
| **Staphylococcal endocarditis** **Aortic &/or mitral valve infection—MSSA** Surgery indications; see Comment page 30. | Staph. aureus, methicillin-sensitive | Nafcillin/Oxacillin 2 gm q4h x 4–6 wks | [(Cefazolin 2 gm IV q8h x 4–6 wks) OR Vanco 30-60 mg/kg/d in 2-3 divided doses to achieve trough of 15-20 mcg/mL x 4–6 wks. | If IgE-mediated penicillin allergy, 10% cross-reactivity to cephalosporins (AnIM 141:16, 2004). **Cefazolin** and **Nafcillin** probably similar in efficacy and Cefazolin better tolerated (CID 54:1700, 2012; Clin Micro Infect 24:152, 2018). Presence of cefazolin inoculum effect may limit efficacy (Open Forum Infect Dis. 2018 May 23;5(6):ofy123). |
| **Aortic and/or mitral valve— MRSA** | Staph. aureus, methicillin-resistant | Vanco 30-60 mg/kg per day in 2-3 divided doses to achieve target trough concentrations of 15-20 mcg/mL recommended for serious infections. | Dapto 8-12 mg/kg IV q24h (Not FDA approved for this indication or dose) | For other indications, see Table 6, page 90. Daptomycin references: JAC 69:926 & 2921, 2013. Case reports of success with Telavancin (JAC 65:1315, 2010; AAC 54:5376, 2010; JAC 66: 2186, 2011) and ceftaroline (JAC 67:1267, 2012; J Infect Chemother 19: 42, 2013). |
| **Tricuspid valve infection (usually IVDUs); MSSA, uncomplicated** | Staph. aureus, methicillin-sensitive | Nafcillin/Oxacillin 2 gm IV q4h x 2 wks (uncomplicated) | If penicillin allergy: Vanco 30-60 mg/kg/d in 2-3 divided doses to achieve trough of 15-20 mcg/mL x 4 wks OR Dapto 8-12 mg/kg IV q24h x 4 wks OR Cefazolin 2 gm IV q8h x 4 wks | **2-week regimen not long enough** if metastatic infection (e.g., osteo) or left-sided endocarditis. **Dapto** resistance can occur de novo, after or during vanco, or after/during dapto therapy. See Comments on MSSA above. |

Abbreviations on page 2.     *NOTE: All dosage recommendations are for adults (unless otherwise indicated) and assume normal renal function. §Alternatives consider allergy; PK, compliance, local resistance, cost.

TABLE 1 (28)

| ANATOMIC SITE/DIAGNOSIS/ MODIFYING CIRCUMSTANCES | ETIOLOGIES (usual) | SUGGESTED REGIMENS* PRIMARY | ALTERNATIVE§ | ADJUNCT DIAGNOSTIC OR THERAPEUTIC MEASURES AND COMMENTS |
|---|---|---|---|---|
| **HEART/Infective endocarditis—Native valve—culture positive** *(continued)* | | | | |
| Tricuspid valve—MRSA | Staph. aureus, methicillin-resistant | Vanco 15-20 mg/kg q8-12h IV to achieve target trough concentrations of 15-20 mcg/mL recommended for serious infections x 4-6 wks. | Dapto 8-12 mg/kg IV q24h x 4-6 wks (*NEJM 355: 653, 2006*). (*See Comments & table 6, page 90*) | Dapto 8-12 mg/kg IV q24h not FDA-approved dose. |
| Slow-growing fastidious Gm-neg. bacilli—any valve | HACEK group (*See Comments*). | Ceftriaxone 2 gm IV q24h x 4 wks OR **Moxi** 400 mg po/IV q12h x 4 wks | AM-SB 3 gm IV q6h x 4 wks OR **Levo** 750 mg po/IV q24h x 4 wks OR **Moxi** 400 mg po/IV q24h x 4 wks | HACEK (acronym for Haemophilus parainfluenza, Aggregatibacter, Actinobacillus, Cardiobacterium, Eikenella, Kingella). AMP 2 gm IV q4h an option if growth of isolate in vitro is sufficient for reliable determination of ampicillin susceptibility. |
| Bartonella species—any valve | B. henselae, B. quintana | Doxy 100 mg IV/po bid x 6 weeks + **Gent** 3 mg/kg/day IV divided in 3 equal doses x 2 wks | If can't use gentamicin: Doxy 100 mg IV/po bid x 6 wks + RIF 300 mg IV/po bid x 2 wks | Dx: Immunofluorescent antibody titer ≥1:800; blood cultures only occ. positive, or PCR of tissue from surgery. B. quintana transmitted by body lice among homeless. Doxy considered safe regardless of age for rx ≤21 days (*AAP Redbook 2018*). |
| **Infective endocarditis— "culture negative"** Fever, valvular disease, and ECHO vegetations ± emboli and neg. cultures. | | Etiology in 348 cases studied by serology, culture, histopath, & molecular detection: C. burnetii 48%, Bartonella sp. 28%, and rarely (Abiotrophia elegans (nutritionally variant strep), Mycoplasma hominis, Tropheryma whipplei—together 1%), & rest without etiology identified (most on antibiotic). See *CID 51:131, 2010* for approach to work-up. Chronic Q fever: *CID 2017;65:1872.* AHA treatment guidelines *Circulation 132:1435, 2015.* Study from Germany suggests T. whipplei is 4th most common cause (*J Clin Micro 50:216, 2012*). | | |
| **Infective endocarditis— empiric therapy (cultures pending)** | | Etiology as above. S. aureus now most common cause (*JAMA 297:1354, 2007*). | | |
| Early (<2 mos post-op) | S. epidermidis, S. aureus. Rarely, Enterobacteriaceae, diphtheroids, fungi. | Vanco 15-20 mg/kg q8-12h + **Gent** 1 mg/kg IV q8h + **RIF** 600 mg po q24h | | Early surgical consultation advised especially if etiology S. aureus, evidence of heart failure, presence of diabetes and/or renal failure, or concern for valve ring abscess. Early valve surgery not associated with improved 1 year survival in patients with S. aureus prosthetic valve infection (*CID 60:741, 2015*). |
| Late (>2 mos post-op) | S. epidermidis, viridans strep, enterococci, S. aureus | Vanco 15-20 mg/kg IV q8-12h + **Gent** 1 mg/kg/kg IV q8h + **RIF** 300 mg po q8h x 14 days. | | |
| **Infective endocarditis— Prosthetic valve—positive blood cultures** Surgical consultation advised: | Staph. epidermidis | (Vanco 15-20 mg/kg IV q8-12h + **RIF** 300 mg po q8h) x 6 wks + **Gent** 1 mg/kg IV q8h x 2 wks. | | If S. epidermidis is susceptible to nafcillin/oxacillin in vitro (not common), then substitute nafcillin (or oxacillin) for vanco. Target vanco trough concentrations 15-20 mcg/mL. |
| Indications for surgery: severe heart failure, S. aureus infection, prosthetic dehiscence, resistant organism, emboli due to large vegetation (See AHA guidelines; *Circulation 132:1435, 2015*). | Staph. aureus | Methicillin sensitive: (**Nafcillin/Oxacillin** 2 gm IV q8-12h + **RIF** 300 mg po q8h) x 6 wks + **Gent** 1 mg per kg IV q8h x 2 wks. Methicillin resistant: (**Vanco** 15-20 mg/kg IV q8-12h (to achieve a target trough of 15-20 mcg/mL) + **RIF** 300 mg po q8h) x 6 wks + **Gent** 1 mg per kg IV q8h x 2 wks. | | Some clinicians prefer to wait 2-3 days after starting vanco/gent before starting RIF, to decrease bacterial density and thus minimize risk of selecting rifampin-resistant subpopulations. |
| | Viridans strep, enterococci | See *Infective endocarditis, native valve, culture positive, page 30.* Treat for 6 weeks. | | |
| | Enterobacteriaceae or P. aeruginosa | [(**Cefepime** 2 gm IV q8h or **MER** 2 gm IV q8h) or (**PIP-TZ** 4.5 gm IV q6h) + **Tobra** 1.5-2 mg/kg IV q8h] | | In theory, could substitute CIP for aminoglycoside, but no clinical data and resistance is common. Select definitive regimen based on susceptibility results. Can occur with native valves also. |
| | Candida, aspergillus | *Table 11, page 132* | | High mortality. Valve replacement plus antifungal therapy standard therapy but some success with antifungal therapy alone. |

TABLE 1 (29)

| ANATOMIC SITE/DIAGNOSIS/ MODIFYING CIRCUMSTANCES | ETIOLOGIES (usual) | SUGGESTED REGIMENS* | | ADJUNCT DIAGNOSTIC OR THERAPEUTIC MEASURES AND COMMENTS |
|---|---|---|---|---|
| | | PRIMARY | ALTERNATIVE§ | |
| **HEART** (continued) | | | | |
| **Infective endocarditis—Q fever** Emerg Infect Dis 21:1183, 2015 JCM 52:1637, 2014 | Coxiella burnetii | **Doxy** 100 mg bid + **hydroxychloroquine** 600 mg/day for at least 18 mos (Mayo Clin Proc 83:574, 2008). Pregnancy: Need long term **TMP-SMX** (see CID 45:548, 2007). | | **Dx:** IFA > 800 phase I IgG plus evidence of endocarditis or vasculopathy or signs of chronic Q fever **OR** positive Coxiella burnetii PCR of blood or tissue. Possible chronic Q fever = IFA > 800 phase I IgG. Treatment duration: 18 mos for native valve, 24 mos for prosthetic valve. Monitor serologically for 5 yrs. |
| **Pacemaker/defibrillator infections** | S. aureus (40%), S. epidermidis (40%), Gram-negative bacilli (5%), fungi (5%). | Device removal + **Vanco** 15-20 mg/kg IV q8-12h (methicillin-resistant strain). If methicillin-susceptible staphylococci: **Nafcillin/Oxacillin** 2 gm IV q4h OR **Cefazolin** 2 gm IV q8h | Device removal + **Dapto** 8-10 mg per kg IV q24h[NAI] | **Duration of rx after device removal:** For "pocket" or subcutaneous infection, 10-14 days; if lead-assoc. endocarditis, 4-6 wks depending on organism. Device removal and absence of valvular vegetation assoc. with significantly higher survival at 1 yr (JAMA 307:1727, 2012). British guidelines: JAC 70:325, 2015. |
| **Pericarditis, bacterial** | Staph. aureus, Strep. pneumoniae, Group A strep, Enterobacteriaceae | [**Vanco** 15-20 mg/kg q8-12h + (**Ceftriaxone** 2 gm q24h OR **Cefepime** 2 gm IV q8h)] (Dosage, see footnote[11]) | **Vanco + CIP** 400 mg q12h (see footnote[11]) | Drainage required if signs of tamponade. Adjust regimen based on results of organism ID and susceptibility. Use Nafcillin, Oxacillin, or Cefazolin for confirmed MSSA infection. |
| **Rheumatic fever** with carditis Ref.: Ln 366:155, 2005 | Post-infectious sequelae of Group A strep infection (usually pharyngitis) | ASA, and usually prednisone 2 mg/kg po q24h for symptomatic treatment of fever, arthritis, arthralgia. May not influence carditis. | | Clinical Features: Carditis, polyarthritis, chorea, subcutaneous nodules, erythema marginatum. Prophylaxis: see page 65. ASA dose: 80-100 mg/kg/day (pediatric), 4-8 gm/day (adult). Eradication of group A streptococcus also recommended: Child, Penicillin V, 250 mg po tid x 10 days; adult, Penicillin V 500 mg po tid x 10 days. |
| **Ventricular assist device-related infection** Manifest & mgmt: CID 57:1438, 2013 Prevent & mgmt: CID 64: 222, 2017 | S. aureus, S. epidermidis, aerobic gm-neg bacilli, Candida sp | After culture of blood, wounds, drive line, device pocket and maybe pump: **Vanco** 15-20 mg/kg IV q8-12h + **Cefepime** 2 gm IV q12h) + **Fluconazole** 800 mg IV q24h. | | Can substitute **Daptomycin** 10 mg/kg/d[NAI] for **Vanco**, (**CIP** 400 mg IV q12h or **Levo** 750 mg IV q24h) for cefepime, and (**Vori, Caspo, Micafungin** or **Anidulafungin**) for **fluconazole**. Modify regimen based on results of culture and susceptibility tests. Higher than FDA-approved Dapto dose because of potential emergence of resistance. |
| **JOINT**—Also see Lyme Disease, page 62 | | | | |
| **Reactive arthritis** | | | | |
| **Reiter's syndrome** (See Comment for definition) | Occurs wks after infection with chlamydia trachomatis, Campylobacter jejuni, Yersinia enterocolitica, Shigella/Salmonella sp. | Only treatment is non-steroidal anti-inflammatory drugs | | **Definition:** Urethritis, conjunctivitis, arthritis, and sometimes uveitis and rash. An asymmetrical oligoarthritis of ankles, knees, feet, sacroilitis. **Rash:** palms and soles—keratoderma blennorrhagica; circinate balanitis of glans penis. HLA-B27 positive predisposes to Reiter's. |
| **Poststreptococcal reactive arthritis** (See Rheumatic fever, above) | Immune reaction after strep pharyngitis: (1) arthritis onset in <10 days, (2) lasts months, (3) unresponsive to ASA | Treat strep pharyngitis and then NSAIDs (prednisone needed in some pts) | | A reactive arthritis after a B-hemolytic strep infection in absence of sufficient Jones criteria for acute rheumatic fever. Ref.: Pediatr Emerg Care 28:1185, 2012. |

[11] **Aminoglycosides** (See Table 10D, page 128), **IMP** 0.5 gm IV q6h, **MER** 1 gm IV q8h, **Nafcillin** or **Oxacillin** 2 gm IV q4h, **PIP-TZ** 3.375 gm IV q6h or 4.5 gm IV q8h, **AM-SB** 3 gm IV q6h, **P Ceph** 1 (**cephalothin** 2 gm IV q4h or **cefazolin** 2 gm IV q8h), **CIP** 750 mg po bid or 400 mg IV q8h, **Vanco** 1 gm IV q12h, **RIF** 600 mg IV q8h, **Aztreonam** 2 gm IV q8h, **Cefepime** 2 gm IV q12h

Abbreviations on page 2.     *NOTE: All dosage recommendations are for adults (unless otherwise indicated) and assume normal renal function. § Alternatives consider allergy, PK, compliance, local resistance, cost.

**TABLE 1 (30)**

| ANATOMIC SITE/DIAGNOSIS/ MODIFYING CIRCUMSTANCES | ETIOLOGIES (usual) | SUGGESTED REGIMENS* | | ADJUNCT DIAGNOSTIC OR THERAPEUTIC MEASURES AND COMMENTS |
|---|---|---|---|---|
| | | PRIMARY | ALTERNATIVE§ | |
| **JOINT** (continued) | | | | |
| **Septic arthritis:** Treatment requires both adequate drainage of purulent joint fluid and appropriate antimicrobial therapy. **There is no need to inject antimicrobials into joints.** Empiric therapy after collection of blood and joint fluid for culture; review Gram stain of joint fluid. | | | | |
| **Infants <3 mos (neonate)** | Staph. aureus, Enterobacteriaceae, Group B strep. | **If MRSA not a concern:** (Nafcillin OR Cefazolin) + Cefotaxime | **If MRSA a concern:** Vanco + Cefotaxime | Blood cultures frequently positive. Adjacent bone involved in 2/3 pts. Group B strep and gonococcal most common community-acquired etiologies. Kingella kingae suscept. to ceftriaxone (Ped Infect Dis J 2016, 35:340). |
| **Children (3 mos–14 yrs)** | S. aureus 27%, S. pyogenes & S. pneumo 14%, H. influ 3%, Gm-neg. bacilli 6%, other (GC, N. mening) 14%; unk 36% | **MRSA prevalence high: Vanco + Cefotaxime** MRSA prevalence low: **Cefazolin** | | Marked ↓ in H. influenzae since use of conjugate vaccine. **NOTE:** Septic arthritis due to salmonella has no association with sickle cell disease, unlike salmonella osteomyelitis. 10 days of treatment as effective as a 30-day treatment course if there is a good clinical response and CRP levels normalize quickly (CID 48(1201, 2009). |
| **Adults** (review Gram stain): See page 62 for Lyme Disease and page 62 for gonococcal arthritis | | | | |
| **Acute monoarticular** **At risk for sexually-transmitted disease** | **N. gonorrhoeae** (See page 25), S. aureus, streptococci, rarely aerobic Gm-neg. bacilli | **Gram stain negative: Ceftriaxone** 1 gm IV q24h or **Cefotaxime** 1 gm IV q8h or **Ceftizoxime** 1 gm IV q8h | If Gram stain shows Gm+ cocci in clusters: **Vanco** 15-20 mg/kg IV q8-12h. | Suspected gonococcal infections (GC): culture urethra, cervix, anal canal, throat, blood, joint fluid. For treatment comments, see *Disseminated GC, page 25.* **Add Azithromycin 1 gm po or Doxycycline 100 mg twice daily for 7 days if GC proven or suspected.** |
| **Not at risk for sexually-transmitted disease** | S. aureus, streptococci, Gm-neg. bacilli | Gram stain shows Gram-pos. cocci: **Vanco** 15-20 mg/kg IV q8-12h. Gram stain shows Gram-neg bacilli: **Cefepime** 2 gm q8h IV OR **Meropenem** 1 gm q8h IV. Gram stain neg: **Vanco** 15-20 mg/kg IV q8-12h + (**Ceftriaxone** 1 gm IV q24h OR **Cefepime** 2 gm q8h IV (preferred for possible healthcare-associated infection)) | | Differential includes gout and chondrocalcinosis (pseudogout). **Look for crystals in joint fluid.** Adjust regimen based on culture and susceptibility. **NOTE:** See *Table 6* for MRSA treatment. |
| **Chronic monoarticular** | Brucella, nocardia, mycobacteria, fungi | *For treatment duration, see Table 3, page 77.* See specific bacterial organism (Table 2) and/or mycobacteria (Table 12) | | |
| **Polyarticular, usually acute** | **Gonococci,** B. burgdorferi (Lyme), acute rheumatic fever; viruses, e.g., hepatitis B, rubella vaccine, parvo B19, staph and strep may also cause polyarticular infections | Gram stain usually negative for GC. If sexually active, culture urethra, cervix, anal canal, throat, blood, joint fluid, and then: **Ceftriaxone** 1 gm IV q24h. No STD risk, Gram stain negative: **Vanco + Ceftriaxone** OR **Cefepime.** | | GC may be associated with pustular/hemorrhagic skin lesions and tenosynovitis; treat with **Ceftriaxone** for 7 days and with **Azithromycin** 1 gm po x1 OR **Doxycycline** 100 mg twice daily for 7 days if GC proven or suspected. Consider Lyme disease if exposure areas known to harbor infected ticks (see page 62); usually large joint. Vanco+ CIP or Levo also an option if low STD risk. Expanded differential includes gout, pseudogout, reactive arthritis (HLA-B27 pos.). |
| **Septic arthritis, post intra-articular injection** | MSSE/MRSE 40% MSSA/MRSA 20%, P. aeruginosa, Propionibacteria, AFB | **NO empiric therapy.** Arthroscopy for culture/sensitivity, crystals, washout | | Treat based on culture results x 14 days (assumes no foreign body present). |

*NOTE: All dosage recommendations are for adults (unless otherwise indicated) and assume normal renal function. § Alternatives consider allergy, PK, compliance, local resistance, cost.

Abbreviations on page 2.

**TABLE 1 (31)**

| ANATOMIC SITE/DIAGNOSIS/ MODIFYING CIRCUMSTANCES | ETIOLOGIES (usual) | SUGGESTED REGIMENS* | | ADJUNCT DIAGNOSTIC OR THERAPEUTIC MEASURES AND COMMENTS |
|---|---|---|---|---|
| | | PRIMARY | ALTERNATIVE§ | |
| **JOINT** (continued) | | | | |
| **Infected prosthetic joint (PJI)**<br>• Suspect infection if sinus tract or wound drainage; acutely/chronically painful prosthesis; or high ESR/CRP assoc. w/painful prosthesis.<br>• **Empiric therapy is NOT recommended.** Treat based on culture and sensitivity results.<br>• **3 surgical options:**<br>1) Debridement and prosthesis retention (if sx <3 wks or of implantation <30 days);<br>2) 1 stage, direct exchange;<br>3) 2 stage: debridement, removal, reimplantation<br>• **IDSA Guidelines:** CID 56:e1, 2013.<br>• Data do not allow assessment of value of adding antibacterial cement to temporary joint spacers (CID 55:474, 2012).<br>• Evidence of systemic absorption of Tobra from antibiotic-impregnated cement spacers (CID 58:1783, 2014).<br><br>(Continued on next page) | MSSA/MSSE | **Debridement/Retention:**<br>(**Nafcillin/Oxacillin** 2 gm IV q4h **+ RIF** 300 mg po bid) OR (**Cefazolin** 2 gm IV q8h **+ RIF** 300 mg po bid) OR **RIF** 300 mg po bid q 2-6 wks followed by [(**CIP** 750 mg po bid OR **Levo** 750 mg po bid) **+ RIF** 300 mg po q24h) for 3-6 months (shorter duration for total hip arthroplasty)<br>**1-stage exchange:** IV/po regimen as above for 3 mos<br>**2-stage exchange:** regimen as above for 4-6 wks | (**Dapto** 8-10 mg/kg IV q24h OR **Linezolid** 600 mg po/IV bid) **± RIF** 300 mg po bid | • **Confirm isolate susceptibility to fluoroquinolone and rifampin:** for fluoroquinolone-resistant isolate consider using other active highly bioavailable agent, e.g., TMP-SMX, Doxy, Minocycline, Amoxicillin-Clavulanate, Cephalexin, or Linezolid.<br>• Enterococcal infection: addition of aminoglycoside optional.<br>• *P. aeruginosa* infection: consider adding aminoglycoside if isolate is susceptible. (but if this improves outcome unclear.)<br>• Prosthesis retention most important risk factor for treatment failure (Clin Microbiol Infect 16:1789, 2010). (Linezolid 600 mg + Rifampin 300 mg) may be effective as salvage therapy if device removal not possible (Antimicrob Agents Chemother 55-4308, 2011).<br>• If prosthesis is retained, consider long-term, suppressive therapy, particularly for staphylococcal infections: depending on in vitro susceptibility options include TMP-SMX, Doxycycline, Minocycline, Amoxicillin, Ciprofloxacin, Cephalexin. |
| | MRSA/MRSE | **Debridement/Retention:**<br>(**Vanco** 15-20 mg/kg IV q8-12h **+ RIF** 300 mg po bid) q 2-6 weeks followed by [(**CIP** 750 mg po bid OR **Levo** 750 mg po q24h) **+ RIF** 300 mg po bid] for 3-6 months (shorter duration for total hip arthroplasty)<br>**1-stage exchange:** IV/po regimen as above for 3 mos<br>**2-stage exchange:** regimen as above for 4-6 wks | (**Dapto** 8-10 mg/kg IV q24h OR **Linezolid** 600 mg po/IV bid) **± RIF** 300 mg po bid | • Culture yield may be increased by sonication of prosthesis (N Engl J Med 357:654, 2007).<br>• Other treatment consideration: Rifampin is bactericidal vs. biofilm-producing bacteria. Never use Rifampin alone due to rapid development of resistance. Rifampin 300 mg po/IV bid + Fusidic acid[ns] 500 mg po/IV tid is another option (Clin Micro Inf 12(S3):93, 2006).<br>• Watch for toxicity if Linezolid is used for more than 2 weeks of therapy.<br>• Role of longer durations of therapy or chronic suppressive therapy in Gram-negative or Pseudomonas PJI not established. |
| (Continued on next page) | Streptococci (Grps A, B, C, D, viridans, other) | **Debridement/Retention:**<br>(Poorer outcomes with retention compared with removal and exchange, CID 64:1742, 2017). **Pen G** 20 million units IV continuous infusion q24h or in 6 divided doses OR **Ceftriaxone** 2 gm IV q24h x 4-6 wks<br>**1 or 2 stage exchange:** regimen as above for 4-6 wks | **Vanco** 15 mg/kg IV q12h | |

Abbreviations on page 2. *NOTE: All dosage recommendations are for adults (unless otherwise indicated) and assume normal renal function. § Alternatives consider allergy, PK, compliance, local resistance, cost.

**TABLE 1 (32)**

| ANATOMIC SITE/DIAGNOSIS/ MODIFYING CIRCUMSTANCES | ETIOLOGIES (usual) | SUGGESTED REGIMENS* | | ADJUNCT DIAGNOSTIC OR THERAPEUTIC MEASURES AND COMMENTS |
|---|---|---|---|---|
| | | PRIMARY | ALTERNATIVE§ | |
| JOINT/Infected prosthetic joint (PJI) *(continued)* | | | | |
| *(Continued from previous page)* | Enterococci | **Debridement/Retention: Pen-susceptible: (AMP:** 200 mg/kg/day IV in divided doses q6h or **Pen G** 20 million units/day IV by continuous infusion or in 6 divided doses) x 4-6 wks **Pen-resistant: Vanco** 15 mg/kg IV q12h x 4-6 wks **1 or 2 stage exchange:** regimen as above for 4-6 wks | **Dapto** 8-10 mg/kg IV q24h OR **Linezolid** 600 mg po/IV bid | *(Continued from previous page)* |
| | Cutibacterium acnes (Hold broth cultures, especially in infections of the shoulder, for 10 days with blind subculture to maximize recovery of C. acnes (*J Clin Microbiol 54:3043, 2016*). | **Debridement/Retention: Pen G** 20 million units IV continuous infusion or in 6 divided doses OR **Ceftriaxone** 2 gm IV q24h x 4-6 wks **1 or 2 stage exchange:** regimen as above for 4-6 wks | **Vanco** 15 mg/kg IV q12h OR **Clinda** 300-450 mg po qid | |
| | Gm-neg enteric bacilli | **Debridement/Retention: Erta** 1 gm q24h IV OR other beta-lactam (e.g., **Ceftriaxone** 2 gm IV q24h OR **Cefepime** 2 gm IV q12h, based on susceptibility) x 4-6 wks **1 or 2 stage exchange:** regimen as above for 4-6 wks | **CIP** 750 po bid | |
| | P. aeruginosa | **Debridement/Retention: Cefepime** 2 gm IV q12h OR **MER** 1 gm IV q8h + **Tobra** 5.1 mg/kg once daily IV x 4-6 wks **1 or 2 stage exchange:** regimen as above for 4-6 wks | **CIP** 750 po bid or 400 mg IV q8h | |
| **Rheumatoid arthritis** | **TNF inhibitors** (adalimumab, certolizumab, etanercept, golimumab, infliximab) and other anti-inflammatory biologics (tofacitinib, rituximab, tocilizumab, abatacept) † risk of TBc, fungal infection, legionella, listeria, and malignancy. Hep B flare may be fatal. *See Med Lett 55:1, 2013 for full listing.* | | | Empiric MRSA coverage recommended if risk factors are present and in high prevalence areas. Immunosuppression, not duration of therapy, is a risk factor for recurrence; 7 days of therapy may be sufficient for immuno-competent patients undergoing one-stage bursectomy (*JAC 65:1008, 2010*). |
| **Septic bursitis:** **Olecranon bursitis;** **prepatellar bursitis** | Staph. aureus >80%, M. tuberculosis (rare), M. marinum (rare) | **(Nafcillin/Oxacillin** 2 gm IV q4h OR **Cefazolin** 2 gm IV q8h if MSSA. Oral step-down: **Diclox** 500 mg po qid | **(Vanco** 15-20 mg/kg IV q8-12h or **Linezolid** 600 mg po bid) if MRSA. Another option: **Dapto** 6 mg/kg IV q24h. | |

Abbreviations on page 2.     *NOTE: All dosage recommendations are for adults (unless otherwise indicated) and assume normal renal function. § Alternatives consider allergy, PK, compliance, local resistance, cost.

**TABLE 1 (33)**

| ANATOMIC SITE/DIAGNOSIS/ MODIFYING CIRCUMSTANCES | ETIOLOGIES (usual) | SUGGESTED REGIMENS* | | ADJUNCT DIAGNOSTIC OR THERAPEUTIC MEASURES AND COMMENTS |
|---|---|---|---|---|
| | | **PRIMARY** | **ALTERNATIVE§** | |
| **KIDNEY & BLADDER** (Reviewed in *Nature Rev 13:269, 2015; IDSA Guidelines CID 52: e103, 2011*) | | | | |
| **Acute Uncomplicated Cystitis & Pyelonephritis in Women** | | | | |
| **Cystitis** Diagnosis: dysuria, frequency, urgency, suprapubic pain & no vaginal symptoms *See AAC 60:2860, 7535 & 7536, 2016* | E. coli (75–95%) P. mirabilis K. pneumoniae S. saprophyticus Presence of enterococci, Grp B Streptococcus, S. epidermidis suggests contamination Often no need for culture if uncomplicated | **Nitrofurantoin (Macrobid)** 100 mg po bid x 5 OR **TMP-SMX DS** 1 tab po bid x 3 days (Avoid TMP-SMX if 20% or more local E. coli are resistant) OR **Fosfomycin** 3 gm po x 1 dose (less effective than nitrofurantoin in RCT, *JAMA 2018,319:1771 & 1781*) | **CIP** 250 mg bid or extended release 500 mg q24h x 3 days **Levo** 250 mg q24h x 3 days **AM-CL** 875/125 mg bid x 5-7 days **Cephalexin** 500 mg bid x 5-7 days **Cefdinir** 300 mg bid x 3-7 days **Pivmecillinam (NUS)** 400 mg bid for 3-7 days | • **Pyridium** (phenazopyridine) may hasten resolution of dysuria. • Beta-lactams are less effective. • Nitrofurantoin & Fosfomycin active vs. ESBLs; however, if early pyelonephritis avoid these drugs due to low renal concentrations. • Vaginitis can mimic symptoms of cystitis. • Outpatient therapy of UTIs due to MDR bacteria: - Fosfomycin & nitrofurantoin usually active. - Increasing TMP-SMX & FQ resistance (*AAC 2016,60:2680*). - Beta-lactams least efficacious. - Ref: *CID 2016,63:960.* • In prospective comparative study, no benefit to replacement of needed chronic Foley catheter (*J Am Geriatric Soc 2018,66:1779*). |
| **Pyelonephritis** Diagnosis: Fever, CVA, pain, nausea/vomiting | Same as for Cystitis, above. Need urine culture & sensitivity testing | *LOW RISK for resistant bacteria:* **CIP** 500 mg po bid OR **CIP-ER** 1000 mg po once daily OR **Levo** 750 mg po once daily x 5-7 days OR **Ceftriaxone** 1 gm IV qd x 10 days (can transition to po FQ or TMP-SMX 1 DS bid if suscept) *HIGH RISK for MDR bacteria:* consider **Erta** 1 gm IV qd or, if critically ill and/or had recent Pseudomonas infection, **MER** 1 gm IV q8h | *Low risk for resistant bacteria:* **Erta** 1 gm IV q24 OR **Gent** 5mg/kg IV qd. When transitioning to po, if FQ or TMP-SMX not an option, consider oral B-lactams to complete 14 days (may be less effective): **Cefixime** 400 mg po qd (*Emerg Med J 2002; 19:19*) **AM-CL** 875 mg/125 mg po bid | • When tolerating po fluids, can transition to oral therapy; drug choice based on culture/sens results. • Consider imaging (US / CT) if critical illness, new renal failure, history of nephrolithiasis, ureteral colic, obstructive uropathy, urine pH ≥ 7.0, or failure to respond to appropriate therapy. • **HIGH-RISK for resistant bacteria include prior highly-resistant bacteria in urine, recent inpatient health- care facility stay, obstructive uropathy, recent fluoroquinolone or B-lactam exposure, recent travel to Asia, Middle East or Africa in past 3 months)** |
| **Pregnancy: Asymptomatic bacteriuria & cystitis** Drug choice based on culture / sensitivity results; do follow-up culture one week after last dose of antibiotic. | E. coli (70%) Klebsiella sp. Enterobacter sp. Grp B Streptococcus | **Nitrofurantoin (Macrobid)** (but not in 3rd trimester) 100 mg po q12h x 5-7 days OR **AM-CL** 875 mg po bid x 5-7 days OR **Cephalexin** 500 mg po q6h x 3-7 days | **TMP-SMX DS** (but not in 1st trimester or at term) 1 tab po q12h x 3 days OR **AM-CL** 500 mg/125 mg 100 mg po q12h x 7 days | • Treatment recommended to avoid progression to cystitis or pyelonephritis. • Untreated bacteriuria associated with increased risk of low birth wt, preterm birth & increased perinatal mortality. • If post-treatment culture positive, re-treat with different drug of longer course of same drug. • Avoid nitrofurantoin in 3rd trimester due to risk of hemolytic anemia in newborn. |
| **Pregnancy: Acute pyelonephritis** Diagnosis: CVA pain, fever, nausea/vomiting in 2nd/3rd trimester. *See Comment* | Same as for Cystitis, above Regimens are empiric therapy (*See Comment*) | **Moderately ill: Ceftriaxone** 1 gm IV q24h OR **Cefepime** 1 gm IV q12h. If Pen-allergic, **Aztreonam** 1 gm IV q8h (no activity vs. Gram-pos cocci) **Severely ill: Pip-Tazo** 3.375 gm IV q6h OR **MER** 500 mg IV q8h OR **Erta** 1 gm IV q24h | | • Differential dx includes: placental abruption & infection of amniotic fluid. • Try to avoid FQs and AGs during pregnancy. • Switch to po therapy after afebrile x 48 hrs. • **Treat for 10-14 days.** • If pyelo recurs, re-treat. Once asymptomatic continue suppressive therapy for duration of pregnancy: Nitrofurantoin 50-100 mg qhs OR Cephalexin 250-500 mg po qhs. |

*Abbreviations on page 2.*    *NOTE: All dosage recommendations are for adults (unless otherwise indicated) and assume normal renal function. § Alternatives consider allergy, PK, compliance, local resistance, cost.*

**TABLE 1 (34)**

| ANATOMIC SITE/DIAGNOSIS/ MODIFYING CIRCUMSTANCES | ETIOLOGIES (usual) | SUGGESTED REGIMENS* PRIMARY | SUGGESTED REGIMENS* ALTERNATIVE§ | ADJUNCT DIAGNOSTIC OR THERAPEUTIC MEASURES AND COMMENTS |
|---|---|---|---|---|
| **KIDNEY & BLADDER/Acute Uncomplicated Cystitis & Pyelonephritis in Women** (continued) | | | | |
| **Recurrent UTIs in Women** (2 or more infections in 6 mos/ 3 or more infections in 1 yr) Risk factors: family history, spermicide use, presence of cystocele, elevated post-void residual urine volume | Same as for Cystitis, above Regimens are options for antimicrobial prophylaxis | Preventive strategies include avoid spermicide, increase fluid intake (additional 1.5L/ day) (JAMA Intern Med 2018; 178:1509), Methenamine hippurate 1gm PO BID (Cochrane Database Syst Rev 2012), post-coital antibiotics (**Nitrofurantoin** 100 mg OR TMP-SMX 80 mg/400 mg OR TMP 100 mg OR **Cephalexin** 250 mg immediately after intercourse (JAMA 1993; 264: 703). In post-menopausal women use intravaginal estrogen: 0.5 mg Estriol cream intravaginal daily x 2 weeks and then twice weekly as maintenance (N Engl J Med 1993; 329: 753) | When primary options fail, consider daily abx prophylaxis based on susceptibility of pathogen. Can include **TMP-SMX SS, cephalexin** 250 mg, or **nitrofurantoin** 50-100 mg daily) | • No strong evidence to support use of cranberry juice. • Probiotics need more study. • In DBRPCT of women age >65 yrs in nursing home, cranberry capsules resulted in no difference in bacteriuria/pyuria (JAMA 2016;316:1873 & 1879). |
| **Asymptomatic Bacteriuria in Women** Defined: 2 consecutive clean catch urine cultures with ≥10⁵ CFU/mL of same organism | Same as for Cystitis, above | **Treatment indicated:** pregnancy, urologic procedure causing bleeding from mucosa | **No treatment indicated:** non-pregnant premenopausal women, spinal cord injury pts, elderly women in/out of nursing home, prosthetic joint surgery | • Asymptomatic bacteriuria & pyuria are discordant; 60% of pts with pyuria have no bacteriuria and pyuria commonly accompanies asymptomatic bacteriuria. • In DBRPCT of women in nursing homes, compared cranberry capsules vs. placebo; no difference in bacteriuria/pyuria (JAMA 2016;316:1873 & 1879). |
| **Acute Uncomplicated Cystitis & Pyelonephritis in Men.** Risk of uncomplicated UTI increased with history of insertive anal sex & lack of circumcision. See also, Complicated UTIs in Men & Women, below | | | | |
| **Cystitis** | E. coli (75-95%) Rarely other enterobacteriaceae | **TMP-SMX DS** 1 tab po bid x 7 days OR **CIP** 500 mg po bid OR **CIP-ER** 1000 mg po once daily OR **Levo** 750 mg po once daily x 5 days | | • If recurrent, evaluate for prostatitis. • Cystitis plus symptoms of bladder outlet obstruction suggests concomitant acute bacterial prostatitis. • Consider presence of STDs. Recommend NAAT for C. trachomatis & N. gonorrhoeae. • Avoid Nitrofurantoin due to low renal concentration in prostate. |
| **Pyelonephritis** | Pockets of FQ-resistant ESBL producing E. coli (EID 2016;22:1594) | Low risk of MDR-GNB: **CIP** 400 mg IV q12h OR **Levo** 750 mg IV once daily x 7-14 days | High risk of MDR-GNB: **MER** 0.5-1 gm IV q8h x 7-14 days OR **Erta** 1gm IV q12. If critically illness or recent Pseudomonas infection use **MER** 1 gm IV q8h. | • If any hint of obstructive uropathy, image collecting system asap. • Case report: Fosfomycin 3 gm daily used for MDR gm-neg bacilli (CID 61:1141, 2015). |

Abbreviations on page 2.        *NOTE: All dosage recommendations are for adults (unless otherwise indicated) and assume normal renal function. § Alternatives consider allergy, PK, compliance, local resistance, cost.

TABLE 1 (35)

39

| ANATOMIC SITE/DIAGNOSIS/ MODIFYING CIRCUMSTANCES | ETIOLOGIES (usual) | SUGGESTED REGIMENS* | | ADJUNCT DIAGNOSTIC OR THERAPEUTIC MEASURES AND COMMENTS |
|---|---|---|---|---|
| | | PRIMARY | ALTERNATIVE§ | |
| **KIDNEY & BLADDER** *(continued)* | | | | |
| **Acute Complicated UTIs in Men & Women** | | | | |
| **Defined:** UTI plus co-morbid condition that increases infection severity & risk of failure, e.g., diabetes, pregnancy, late diagnosis, chronic Foley catheter, suprapubic tube, obstruction secondary to stone, anatomic abnormalities, immunosuppression | E. coli or Other enterobacteriaceae plus: P. aeruginosa Enterococci S. aureus Candida sp. | Prior to empiric therapy, urine culture & sensitivity. If hypotensive blood cultures. If obstructive uropathy suspected, need imaging of urinary tract asap. *See Comments* **Low risk of MDR GNB:** **Levo** 750 mg IV once daily OR **Ceftriaxone** 1 gm IV once daily OR **Cefepime** 1 gm IV q12h OR **PIP-TZ** 3.375 gm IV q6h OR **Gent** 5 mg/kg IV Once daily. **If Pen-allergic:** **Aztreonam** 2 gm IV q8h | **Risk of MDR GNB ≥20%:** **MER** 0.5-1 gm IV q8h OR **Ceftolo-tazo** 1.5 gm IV q8h OR **Ceftaz-avi** 2.5 gm IV q8h OR **MER-vabor** 4 gm IV q8h, *See Comment* | • **Uncontrolled infection**, esp. if obstruction, can result in emphysematous pyelonephritis, renal abscess, carbuncle, papillary necrosis or perinephric abscess. • Due to co-morbidities & frequent infections, increased risk of drug-resistance pathogens. • Due to high incidence of resistance and infection severity, Nitrofurantoin, Fosfomycin & TMP-SMX should not be used for empiric therapy. • If enterococci cultured, need to adjust therapy based on in vitro susceptibility. • Duration of treatment varies with status of co-morbid conditions, need for urologic procedures & individualized pt clinical response. • Pip-Tazo inferior to MER vs. ceftriaxone-resistant E. coli/K. pneumo *(JAMA 2018;320:979 & 984).* |
| **LIVER** *(for Primary (Spontaneous) Bacterial Peritonitis (SBP), see page 49)* | | | | |
| **Cholangitis** | Esophageal flora | *See Gallbladder, page 18* | | Short term prophylactic antibiotics in cirrhotics with G-I hemorr, with or without ascites, decreases rate of bacterial infection & ↑ survival *(J Hepatol 60:1310, 2014).* |
| **Cirrhosis & variceal bleeding** | | **CIP** 400 mg IV q12h x. max. of 7 days | **Ceftriaxone** 1 gm IV once daily for max. of 7 days | |
| **Hepatic abscess** Klebsiella liver abscess ref.: *Ln ID 12:881, 2012* | Enterobacteriaceae (esp. Klebsiella sp.), bacteroides, enterococci, Entamoeba histolytica, Yersinia entero-colitica (rare), Fusobacterium necrophorum *(Lemierre's).* For echinococcus, see Table 13, page 171. For cat-scratch disease (CSD), see pages 48 & 61 | **Metro + Ceftriaxone** OR **Cefoxitin** OR **PIP-TZ** OR **AM-SB** OR **CIP** or **Levo** | **Metro** (for amoeba) + either **IMP, MER** OR **Dori** | **Serological tests for amebiasis should be done on all patients;** if neg, surgical drainage or percutaneous aspiration. In pyogenic abscess, ½ have identifiable GI source or underlying biliary tract disease. If amoeba serology positive, treat with **Metro** alone without surgery. Empiric **Metro** included for both E. histolytica & bacteroides. **Hemochromatosis** associated with Yersinia enterocolitica liver abscess; regimens listed are effective for yersinia. Klebsiella pneumonia genotype K1 associated ocular & CNS Klebsiella infections. |
| **Hepatic encephalopathy** | Urease-producing gut bacteria | Rifaximin 550 mg po bid (take with lactulose) | | Ref. *NEJM 375:1660, 2016.* |
| **Leptospirosis** | Leptospirosis, see page 64 | *See page 61* | | |
| **Peliosis hepatis in AIDS pts** | Bartonella henselae and B. quintana | | | |
| **Post-transplant infected "biloma"** | Enterococci (incl. VRE), candida, Gm-neg. bacilli (P. aeruginosa 8%), anaerobes 5% | **Linezolid** 600 mg IV bid + **PIP-TZ** 4.5 gm IV q6h + **Fluconazole** 400 mg IV q24h | **Dapto** 6 mg/kg per day + **Levo** 750 mg IV q24h + **Fluconazole** 400 mg IV q24h | Suspect if fever & abdominal pain post-transplant. Exclude hepatic artery thrombosis. Presence of candida and/or VRE bad prognosticators. |
| **Viral hepatitis** | Hepatitis A, B, C, D, E, G | *See Table 14E and Table 14F* | | |

*Abbreviations on page 2.      *NOTE: All dosage recommendations are for adults (unless otherwise indicated) and assume normal renal function. § Alternatives consider allergy, PK, compliance, local resistance, cost.*

**TABLE 1 (36)**

| ANATOMIC SITE/DIAGNOSIS/ MODIFYING CIRCUMSTANCES | ETIOLOGIES (usual) | SUGGESTED REGIMENS* | | ADJUNCT DIAGNOSTIC OR THERAPEUTIC MEASURES AND COMMENTS |
|---|---|---|---|---|
| | | PRIMARY | ALTERNATIVE§ | |
| **LUNG/Bronchi** | | | | |
| **Bronchiolitis/wheezy bronchitis (expiratory wheezing)** | | | | |
| Infants/children (≤ age 5) See RSV, Table 14A page 187 Ref.: Ln 368-312, 2006 | Respiratory syncytial virus (RSV) 50% during paraifluenza 25%, human metapneumovirus | Antibiotics not useful, mainstay of therapy is oxygen and hydration. Ribavirin not recommended for bronchiolitis except HSCT and perhaps other transplant pts | | RSV most important. Rapid diagnosis with antigen detection methods. For prevention of a humanized mouse monoclonal antibody, **palivizumab**. See Table 14A, page 187. RSV immune globulin is no longer available. Guidance from the American Academy of Pediatrics recommends use of Palivizumab only in newborn infants born at 29 weeks gestation (or earlier) and in special populations (e.g., those infants with significant heart disease). (Pediatrics 2014;134:415–420) |
| **Bronchitis** | | | | |
| Infants/children (≤ age 5) Ref.: JAMA 312:2678, 2014 | <Age 2: Adenovirus; age 2-5: parainfluenza 3 virus, human metapneumovirus Usually viral. M. pneumoniae 5%, C. pneumoniae 5%. See Persistent cough (Pertussis). | Antibiotics not indicated. Antitussive ± inhaled bronchodilators. Throat swab PCR available for Dx of mycoplasma or chlamydia. | Antibiotics indicated only with associated sinusitis or heavy growth on throat culture for S. pneumo., Group A strep, H. influenzae or M. pneumoniae | Purulent sputum alone not an indication for antibiotic therapy. Expect cough to last 2 weeks. If fever/rigors, get chest x-ray. **If mycoplasma documented, prefer doxy over macrolides due to increasing macrolide resistance** (JAC 68:506, 2013). |
| Adolescents and adults with acute tracheobronchitis (Acute bronchitis) | Bordetella pertussis & occ. Bordetella parapertussis. Also consider asthma, gastro-esophageal reflux, post-nasal drip, mycoplasma and also chlamydia. | **Peds doses: Azithro / Clarithro** po OR **Erythro estolate**[14] OR **TMP-SMX** (doses in footnote) | **Adult doses: Azithro** po 500 mg day 1, 250 mg days 2-5 OR **Clarithro** 500 mg bid x 7 days OR **Erythro** 500 mg po qid x 14 days OR **TMP-SMX-DS** 1 tab bid times 14 days OR (**Clarithro** 500 mg po bid or 1 gm extended release q24h x 7 days) | **3 stages of illness:** catarrhal (1-2 wks), paroxysmal coughing (2-4 wks), and convalescence (1-2 wks). Treatment may abort or eliminate pertussis in catarrhal stage, but does not shorten the paroxysmal stage. Diagnosis: PCR on nasopharyngeal secretions or ↑ pertussis-toxin antibody. **Rx aimed at eradication of NP carriage.** In non-outbreak setting, likelihood of pertussis increased if post-tussive emesis or inspiratory whoop present. |
| **Persistent cough (>14 days), afebrile during paroxysms of cough. Pertussis (whooping cough)** 10–20% adults with cough >14 days have pertussis (Review: Chest 146:205, 2014) | | | | |
| Pertussis: Prophylaxis of household contacts | Drugs and doses as per treatment immediately above. Vaccination of newborn contacts: | | | Recommended by Am. Acad. Ped. Red Book 2006 for all household or close contacts; community-wide prophylaxis not recommended. |
| Acute bacterial exacerbation of chronic bronchitis (ABECB), adults (almost always smokers with COPD) Ref.: NEJM 359:2355, 2008. | Viruses 20–50%, C. pneumo-niae 5%, M. pneumoniae <1%, role of S. pneumo, H. influenzae & M. catarrhalis controversial. Tobacco use, air pollution contribute. | **Severe ABECB** = ↑ dyspnea, ↑ sputum viscosity/purulence, ↑ low O₂ sat, (2) inhaled anticholinergic bronchodilator; (3) non-invasive positive pressure ventilation. | Severe volume. For severe ABECB: (1) consider chest x-ray, esp. if febrile 6/ oral corticosteroid for just 5 days (JAMA 309:2223, 2013); (4) D/C tobacco use; (5) | Role of antimicrobial therapy is debated even for severe disease, but study of >80,000 patients shows value of antimicrobial therapy in patients hospitalized with severe disease (JAMA 303(20):2035, 2010). **For mild or moderate disease, no antimicrobial treatment** vs. drug-resistant S. pneumo. Limit **Gemi** to 5 days to decrease risk of rash. **Azithro** 250 mg daily x 1 yr modestly reduced frequency of acute exacerbations in pts with milder disease (NEJM 365:689, 2011). |

**TABLE 1 (37)**

| ANATOMIC SITE/DIAGNOSIS/ MODIFYING CIRCUMSTANCES | ETIOLOGIES (usual) | SUGGESTED REGIMENS* | | ADJUNCT DIAGNOSTIC OR THERAPEUTIC MEASURES AND COMMENTS |
|---|---|---|---|---|
| | | PRIMARY | ALTERNATIVE§ | |
| **LUNG/Bronchi** (continued) | | | | |
| **Bronchiectasis**<br>*Thorax 65 (Suppl 1): i1, 2010; Am J Respir Crit Care Med 188:647, 2013.* | H. influ., P. aeruginosa, and rarely S. pneumo. | **Gemi, Levo,** or **Moxi** x 7–10 days. *Dosage in footnote[12].* | | Many potential etiologies: obstruction, ↓ immune globulins, cystic fibrosis, dyskinetic cilia, tobacco, prior severe or recurrent necrotizing bronchitis; e.g. pertussis. |
| *Acute exacerbation*<br>*Prevention of exacerbation* | Not applicable | Two randomized trials of **Erythro** 250 mg bid (*JAMA 309:1260, 2013*) or **Azithro** 250 mg od (*JAMA 309:1251, 2013*) x 1 year showed significant reduction in the rate of acute exacerbations, better preservation of lung function, and better quality of life versus placebo in adults with non-cystic fibrosis bronchiectasis. | | **Caveats:** higher rates of macrolide resistance in oropharyngeal flora, potential for increased risk of a) cardiovascular deaths from macrolide-induced QTc prolongation, b) liver toxicity, or c) hearing loss (*see JAMA 309:1295, 2013*).<br>**Pre-treatment screening:** baseline liver function tests, electrocardiogram; assess hearing; sputum culture to exclude mycobacterial disease. |
| *Specific organisms* | Aspergillus (*see Table 11*) and MAi (*Table 12*) and P. aeruginosa (*Table 5B*). | | | |
| **Pneumonia: CONSIDER TUBERCULOSIS IN ALL PATIENTS; ISOLATE ALL SUSPECT PATIENTS** | | | | |
| **Neonatal: Birth to 1 month** | Viruses: CMV, rubella, H. simplex<br>**Bacteria:** Group B strep, listeria, coliforms, S. aureus, P. aeruginosa<br>**Other:** Chlamydia trachomatis, syphilis | **AMP + Gent ± Cefotaxime.** Add **Vanco** if MRSA a concern. For chlamydia therapy, **Erythro** 12.5 mg per kg po or IV qid times 14 days. | | Blood cultures indicated. Consider C. trachomatis if afebrile pneumonia, staccato cough, IgM >18; therapy with erythro or sulfisoxazole.<br>If MRSA documented, **Vanco, Clinda, & Linezolid** alternatives. **Linezolid** dosage from birth to age 11 yrs is 10 mg per kg q8h. |
| **Age 1–3 months**<br>Pneumonitis syndrome.<br>Usually afebrile | C. trachomatis, RSV, parainfluenza virus 3, human metapneumovirus, Bordetella, S. pneumoniae, S. aureus (rare) | **Outpatient: po**<br>**Amox** 90–100 mg/kg/d x 10–14 days OR **Azithro** 10 mg/kg x 1 dose then 5 mg/kg once daily x 4 days | **Inpatient:**<br>• **If febrile: Erythro** 10 mg/kg IV q6h or **Azithro** 2.5 mg/kg IV q12h (see **Comment**)<br>• **If febrile: Cefotaxime** 200 mg/kg per day div q8h OR **Ceftriaxone** 75–100 mg/kg q24h | Pneumonitis syndrome: Cough, tachypnea, dyspnea, diffuse infiltrates, afebrile. Usually requires hospital care. Reports of hypertrophic pyloric stenosis after erythro under age 6 wks; not sure about azithro, bid azithro dosing theoretically might ↓ risk of hypertrophic pyloric stenosis. If lobar pneumonia, give AMP 200–300 mg per kg per day for S. pneumoniae. No empiric coverage for S. aureus, as it is rare etiology. |
| | | For **RSV**, see Bronchiolitis, page 40 | | |
| **Infants and Children, age >3 months to 18 yrs** (IDSA Treatment Guidelines: *CID 53:617, 2011*). | | | | |
| **Outpatient** | RSV, human metapneumovirus, rhinovirus, influenza virus, adenovirus, parainfluenza virus, Mycoplasma, H. influenzae, S. pneumoniae, S. aureus (rare) | **Amox** 90 mg/kg in 2 divided doses x 5 days | **Azithro** 10 mg/kg x 1 dose (max 500 mg), then 5 mg/kg (max 250 mg) x 4 days OR **AM-CL** 90 mg/kg (Amox comp) in 2 divided doses x 5 days | Antimicrobial therapy not routinely required for preschool-aged children with CAP as most infections are viral etiologies. |

*Abbreviations on page 2.*   *NOTE: All dosage recommendations are for adults (unless otherwise indicated) and assume normal renal function. §Alternatives consider allergy, PK, compliance, local resistance, cost.*

**TABLE 1 (38B)**

| ANATOMIC SITE/DIAGNOSIS/ MODIFYING CIRCUMSTANCES | ETIOLOGIES (usual) | SUGGESTED REGIMENS* | | ADJUNCT DIAGNOSTIC OR THERAPEUTIC MEASURES AND COMMENTS |
|---|---|---|---|---|
| | | PRIMARY | ALTERNATIVE§ | |
| **LUNG/Bronchi/Pneumonia** *(continued)* | | | | |
| **Inpatient** | As above | Fully immunized: **AMP** 50 mg/kg IV q6h; Not fully immunized: **Cefotaxime** 150 mg/kg IV divided q8h | Fully immunized: **Cefotaxime** 150 mg/kg IV divided q8h | If atypical infection suspected, add **Azithro** 10 mg/kg × 1 dose (max 500 mg), then 5 mg/kg (max 250 mg) × 4 days. If community MRSA suspected, add **Vanco** 15-20 mg/kg/day divided q6-8h OR **Clinda** 40 mg/kg/day divided q6-8h. Depending on clinical response, may switch to orals or oral agents as early as 2-3 days. |
| **Adults (over age 18) — IDSA/ATS Guideline for CAP in adults:** *CID 44 (Suppl 2): S27-S72, 2007; NEJM 370-543, 2014; NEJM 371:1679, 2014.* | | | | |
| **Community-acquired, empiric therapy for outpatient** Prognosis prediction: CURB-65 *(Thorax 58:377, 2003)* C: confusion = 1 pt U: BUN >19 mg/dl = 1 pt R: RR >30/min = 1 pt B: BP <90/60 = 1 pt Age >65 yr = 1 pt Total = 1, ok to treat as out-patient, ≥2 hospitalization recommended | S. pneumo, atypicals and mycoplasma in particular, Hemophilus, Moraxella, viral pathogens: up to 30% of cases *(BMC Infect Dis 15:89, 2015)* and co-infection, often viral, in ~20% of cases *(BMC Infect Dis 15:64, 2015.)* | **Azithro** 500 mg po day 1 then 250 mg daily day 2-5 OR **Clarithro** 500 mg po bid or **Clarithro-ER** 1 gm po q24h 5 days OR **Doxy** 100 mg po bid × 5-7 days OR if Doxy unavailable **Minocycline** 200 mg po/IV × 1, then 100 mg po/IV q12h | **Levo** 750 mg po q24h × 5 days OR **Moxi** 400 mg po q24h × 5 days OR **AM-CL (1000/62.5)** (extended rel.) 2 tabs po bid or **Amox** 1 gm po tid) + [**Azithro** or **Clarithro** × 7 days] | **Azithro/clarithro:** active against atypical pneumonia agents, but S. pneumo resistance as high as 20-30%; **alternative regimen (Levo** or **Moxi)** recommended if high local prevalence of macrolide resistance or co-morbidities (e.g., COPD, alcoholism, CHF). **Moxi** has anaerobic activity and may be preferred over levo for post-obstructive pneumonia or aspiration. **Amox-CL or Amox + Azithro or Clarithro** another alternative for patients with comorbidities, in setting of high prevalence of S. pneumo macrolide resistance, or if prior antibiotic in last 3 mo. Oral cephalosporins (cefdinir 300 mg q12h, cefpodoxime 200 mg q12h or cefprozil 500 mg q12h) can be substituted for Amox-Clav or Amox. |
| **Community-acquired, empiric therapy for patient admitted to hospital, non-ICU** *(See NEJM 370-543, 2014)* | As above + legionella, Gram-negative bacilli IVDU: S. aureus Post-influenza: S. aureus, S. pneumo. No pathogen detected in majority of patients, viruses more common than bacteria *(NEJM 373-415, 2015.)* | (**Ceftriaxone** 1 g IV q24h or **Cefotaxime** 600 mg q12h IV) + **Azithro** 500 mg IV/po q24h | **Levo** 750 mg IV/po q24h OR **Moxi** 400 mg IV/po q24h OR **Gati** 400 mg IV q24h (not available in US) (**Ceftriaxone** OR **Ceftaroline**) + **Doxy** 100 mg IV/po q12h. | Administration of antibiotic within 6h associated with improved survival in pneumonia with severe sepsis *(Eur Respir J 39:156, 2012).* Duration of therapy 5-7 days. Better outcome with ceftaroline than Ceftriaxone in one RCT *(Lancet ID 15:161, 2015).* Improved outcome with β-lactam/macrolide combo vs β-lactam alone in hospitalized CAP of moderate- or high- severity *(Thorax 68:493, 2013).* Blood and sputum cultures recommended. Test for influenza during influenza season. Consider urinary pneumococcal antigen and urinary legionella for sicker patients. |
| **Community-acquired, empiric therapy for patient admitted to ICU** | As above | As above + [**Vanco** 15-20 mg/kg IV q8-12h OR **Linezolid** 600 mg IV/po q12h] **Procalcitonin:** Several clinical trials and meta-analyses indicate that normalization of procalcitonin levels can be used to guide duration of antibiotic therapy. Safe to discontinue antibiotics when procalcitonin level has decreased to 0.1-0.2 mcg/mL. *(CID 55:651, 2012; JAMA 309:717, 2013).* | As above +[**Vanco** 15-20 mg/kg IV q8-12h OR **Linezolid** 600 mg IV/po q12h] | Add **Vanco** 15-20 mg/kg IV q8-12h for pneumonia with concomitant or precedent influenza or for pneumonia in an IVDU. **Do nasal PCR for S. aureus; if neg, safe to dc vanco** *(AJCM 2015;24:8; AAC 2017;61:e02071-16).* **Legionella:** Most all legionella species detected by urine antigen; if suspicious perform culture or do PCR on airway secretions *(CID 57:1275, 2013).* |

Abbreviations on page 2.     *NOTE: All dosage recommendations are for adults (unless otherwise indicated) and assume normal renal function. § Alternatives consider allergy, PK, compliance, local resistance, cost.*

**TABLE 1 (39)**

| ANATOMIC SITE/DIAGNOSIS/ MODIFYING CIRCUMSTANCES | ETIOLOGIES (usual) | SUGGESTED REGIMENS* PRIMARY | SUGGESTED REGIMENS* ALTERNATIVE§ | ADJUNCT DIAGNOSTIC OR THERAPEUTIC MEASURES AND COMMENTS |
|---|---|---|---|---|
| **LUNG/Bronchi/Pneumonia** (continued) | | | | |
| **Hospital-acquired or Ventilator-associated pneumonia** IDSA guidelines: CID 63:e61, 2016 | As above + MDR Gram-negatives. In 39 of 174 pts with non-ventilator HAP, respiratory virus detected (Resp Med 2017;122:76) | **Cefepime** 2 gm IV q12h OR **PIP-TZ** 4.5 gm q6h. Per Guidelines, suggest use of adjunctive inhaled antibiotic if etiologic bacteria are susceptible to only polymyxins or AG. Suggest: testing may identify other active agents, e.g., **Ceftaz-avi**, **MER-vabor**. | **MER** 1 gm IV q8h OR **Levo** 750 mg IV/po q24h. Proposed regimens in Table 10F. | Add **Vanco** or **Linezolid** if unit or hospital MRSA prevalence >10-20%, prior MRSA use within 90 days, acute renal replacement therapy prior to VAP onset, septic shock or high risk of mortality, ARDS preceding VAP, unknown MRSA prevalence or presence of MRSA risk factors (e.g., IVDU, prior MRSA infection or colonization). For suspected pseudomonas or high risk of mortality add **CIP** 400 mg IV q8h or **Levo** 750 mg IV q24h or **Tobra** 5 mg/kg IV q24h or **AMK** 15 mg/kg IV q24h. **Aztreonam** 2 gm IV q8h can substitute for other beta-lactams if there is beta-lactam hypersensitivity, but lacks coverage for S. aureus. Consider addition of Colistin if carbapenem-resistant Gram-negative is suspected. |
| **Pneumonia —Selected specific therapy after culture results (sputum, blood, pleural fluid, etc.) available.** Also see Table 2, page 73 | | | | |
| **Acinetobacter baumannii** (See also Table 5B); CID 2018;67:1455; AAC 2017;61:e01268-16 | Patients with VAP; long ICU stay with repeated antibiotic exposure | **Empiric rx:** positive culture, no in vitro suscept results, prevalence of resistance < 20%: **Cefepime. Ceftazidime.** **AM-SB** (Doses in footnote[13]). If prevalence of resistance > 20%: (**AM-SB** + **MER** + **Polymyxin B**) (See Comments for dosing) | **Specific rx:** culture & suscept results known, susceptible organism: **Cefepime.** **Ceftazidime. AM-SB or FQ.** If MDR organism & critically ill: **MER** + **AM-SB** + **Polymyxin B** | Combination rx for XDR strains in critically ill pts. Based on in vitro hollow-fiber data (AAC 2017;61:e01268-16) High dose Amp-sulb safe & effective in prospective observational clin studies (J Infect 2008;56:432; Scand J Inf Dis 2007;39:38). Regimen details: **AM-SB** 8/4 gm IV over 4 hr q8h + **MER** 2 gm IV q8h + **Polymyxin B** 2.5 mg/kg IV over 2 hr (loading dose), then 12 hr later start 1.43 mg/kg IV q12h (maint dose). |
| **Actinomycosis** | A. Israelii and rarely others | **AMP** 200 mg/kg/day in 3-4 divided doses x 4-6 wks then **Pen VK** 2-4 gm/day in 4 divided doses x 6-12 mo. | **Doxy** or **Ceftriaxone** OR **Clinda** IV x 4-6 wks, then po x 6-12 mo | Can use **Pen G** instead of AMP: 10-20 million units/day IV x 4-6 wks, then Pen VK po 6-12 mo. |

[13] Doses of antibiotics used to treat pneumonia due to Acinetobacter sp., Klebsiella sp, and Pseudomonas sp. Penicillins: **Pip-Tazo** loading dose 4.5 gm IV over 30 min, then, 4 hrs later, start 3.375 gm IV over 4 hrs & repeat q8h; **AM-SB** 3 gm IV q6h. Cephalosporins: **Ceftazidime** 2 gm IV q8h; **Ceftaz-avi** 2.5 gm IV q8h; **Ceftolo-tazo** 1.5 gm IV q8h; FQs: **CIP** 400 mg IV q8h; **Levo** 750 mg IV q24h. Carbapenems: **MER** 1-2 gm IV q8h; **MER-vabor** 4 gm IV over 3 hrs q8h; **MER** 0.5-1 gm q8h. Aminoglycosides: **Gent/Tobra** 7 mg/kg IV x 1, then 5 mg/kg IV q8h. **Polymyxin B** 2.5 mg/kg IV over 2 hrs, then 12 hrs later, 1.5 mg/kg over 1 hr & repeat q12h. **Minocycline** 200 mg IV x 1, then 100 mg IV q12h

Abbreviations on page 2.      *NOTE: All dosage recommendations are for adults (unless otherwise indicated) and assume normal renal function. § Alternatives consider allergy, PK, compliance, local resistance, cost.

**TABLE 1 (40)**

**LUNG/Bronchi/Pneumonia/Selected specific therapy after culture results (sputum, blood, pleural fluid, etc.) available.** *(continued)*

| ANATOMIC SITE/DIAGNOSIS/MODIFYING CIRCUMSTANCES | ETIOLOGIES (usual) | SUGGESTED REGIMENS* PRIMARY | ALTERNATIVE* *(continued)* | ADJUNCT DIAGNOSTIC OR THERAPEUTIC MEASURES AND COMMENTS |
|---|---|---|---|---|
| **Anthrax** (applies to oropharyngeal & gastrointestinal forms) **Inhalation** **To report possible bioterrorism event: 770-488-7100** Ref: www.bt.cdc.gov; CDC panel recommendations for adults: *Emerg Infect Dis* 20(2). Doi: 10.3201/eid2002.130687. AAP recommendations for children: *Pediatrics* 133:e1411, 2014. | Bacillus anthracis Plague, tularemia: See page 46. Chest x-ray: mediastinal widening & pleural effusion | **Adults (including pregnancy):** CIP 400 mg IV q8h + (Linezolid 600 mg IV q12h or Clinda 900 mg IV q8h) + **Meropenem** 2 gm IV q8h (see comments) + **raxibacumab** 40 mg/kg IV (over 2 hrs). Switch to po after 2 wks if stable. **CIP** 500 mg po q12h or **Doxy** 100 mg q12h to complete 60-day regimen. | **Children (including pregnancy):** CIP 10 mg/kg IV q8h (max 400 mg per dose) + [Linezolid 10 mg/kg IV q8h (age <12 yr) or Linezolid 15 mg/kg q12h (age >12 yr) (max 600 mg per dose)] + MER 40 mg/kg IV q8h (max 600 mg per dose) + raxibacumab 40-80 mg/kg IV over 2 hrs. Switch to po after 2 wks if stable: CIP 15 mg/kg q12h or 100 mg q12h (>45 kg) q12h to complete 60-day regimen for oral dosage. | 1. Meropenem or Doxy preferred over Clinda for meningitis.<br>2. Pen G 4 million units IV q4h (children, max 4 million units per dose) IV q4h can be substituted for Meropenem for pen-susceptible strain.<br>3. For children <8 years of age tooth staining likely with Doxy for 60 days. Alternatives for oral switch include Clinda 10 mg/kg q8h (max dose 600 mg) or Levo 8 mg/kg q12h (max dose 250 mg) q12h for <50 kg, 500 mg q24h ≥50 kg or for pen-susceptible strains Amox 25 mg/kg (max dose 1 gm) q8h or Pen VK 25 mg/kg (max dose 1 gm) q8h.<br>4. Levo and Moxi are alternatives to CIP<br>5. Anthrax immune globulin (**Anthrasil**). FDA approved for emergency use (U.S. national stockpile).<br>6. Obiltoxaximab 16 mg/kg is an alternative to Raxibacumab. |
| **Anthrax, prophylaxis:** See: *Emerg Infect Dis* 20(2), doi: 10.3201/eid2002.130687. 60 days of **antimicrobial prophylaxis** + 3-dose series of Biothrax (Anthrax Vaccine Adsorbed | | **Adults (including pregnancy):** CIP 500 mg po q12h or **Doxy** 100 mg po q12h x 60 days +3-dose series of Biothrax Anthrax Vaccine Adsorbed | **Children: CIP** or **Doxy** (see above for dosing) x 60 days (not FDA approved, to be made available on investigational basis) | 1. Consider alternatives to Doxy for use in pregnancy.<br>2. Alternatives include Clinda, Levo, Moxi, and for pen-susceptible strains Amox or Pen VK. |
| **Burkholderia (Pseudomonas) pseudomallei** (etiology of melioidosis) Can cause primary or secondary skin infection See *NEJM* 367:1035, 2012 | Gram-negative | **Initial parenteral rx:** Ceftaz 30–50 mg per kg IV q8h or IMP 20 mg per kg IV q8h. Rx minimum 10 days and improving, then no therapy | **Post-parenteral po rx Adults** (see Comment for children): TMP-SMX 5 mg/kg (TMP component) bid + **Doxy** 2 mg/kg bid x 3 mos. | Children age ≤8 yrs & pregnancy: AM-CL-ER 1000/62.5, 2 tabs po bid times 20 wks.<br>Even with compliance, relapse rate is 10%.<br>Max. daily ceftazidime dose: 6 gm.<br>For treatment of MDR strains: *Expert Rev Anti-infect Ther* 2018;16:87. |
| **Chlamydia pneumoniae** | Chlamydophila pneumoniae | **Azithro** 500 mg IV once then 250 mg x 4 days OR **Levo** 750 mg x 5 days | **Doxy** 100 mg q12h x 5 days OR **Clarithro** 500 mg bid x 5 days | Clinical diagnosis, rarely confirmed microbiologically. |
| **Haemophilus influenzae** | β-lactamase negative β-lactamase positive | AMP IV, **Amox** po. **TMP-SMX** **AM-CL, O Ceph 2/3, P Ceph 3, FQ** Dosage: Table 10A. | **TMP-SMX**, Azithro/Clarithro, Doxy, FQ | 25–35% strains β-lactamase positive. ↑ resistance to both TMP-SMX and Azithro. See Table 10A, page 112 for dosages |
| **Klebsiella sp.—ESBL pos. & other coliforms**[14] | β-lactamase positive | IMP or MER; if resistant: **Ceftolo-tazo, Ceftaz-avi** or **MER-vabor** (See footnote[13] for dosing) | **Ceftolo-tazo, Ceftaz-avi, Ceftaz-avi** or **Aztho** 500 mg x1 on day 1 then 250 mg x4 for total of 7-10 days. | ESBL inactivates all cephalosporins, β-lactams/β-lactamase inhibitor drug activity not predictable; co-resistance to all FQs & often aminoglycosides. Failure of Pip-tazo vs. ESBLs (*JAMA* 2018;320:979-989).<br>Consider longer courses of therapy for immunocompromised hosts, severe illness. |
| **Legionella pneumonia** | Legionella pneumophila, other legionella species | **Levo** 750 mg po/IV or **Moxi** 400 mg po/IV x 7-10 days | **Azithro** 500 mg x1 on day 1 then 250 mg x4 for total of 7-10 days. | Trend for better outcomes with FQ over macrolide (*CAC* 69:2354, 2014).<br>Alternatives consider allergy, PK, compliance, local resistance, cost. |

[14] Dogma on duration of therapy not possible with so many variables: i.e. certainty of diagnosis, infecting organism, severity of infection & co-morbidities. Agree with efforts to de-escalate & shorten course. Treat at least 7-8 days. Need clinical evidence of response: fever resolution, improved oxygenation, falling WBC. Refs: *AJRCCM* 171:388, 2005; *CID* 43:S75, 2006; *COID* 19:185, 2006.

*Abbreviations on page 2.* *NOTE: All dosage recommendations are for adults (unless otherwise indicated) and assume normal renal function. See Abbreviations on page 2.*

**TABLE 1 (41)**

LUNG/Bronchi/Pneumonia/Selected specific therapy after culture results (sputum, blood, pleural fluid, etc.) available. *(continued)*

| ANATOMIC SITE/DIAGNOSIS/ MODIFYING CIRCUMSTANCES | ETIOLOGIES (usual) | SUGGESTED REGIMENS* PRIMARY | ALTERNATIVE§ | ADJUNCT DIAGNOSTIC OR THERAPEUTIC MEASURES AND COMMENTS |
|---|---|---|---|---|
| Moraxella catarrhalis | 93% β-lactamase positive | **AM-CL, O Ceph 2/3, P Ceph 2/3, Macrolides[15], FQ, TMP-SMX.** See Table 10A, page 112 for dosages | | |
| **Mycoplasma pneumoniae** | M. pneumoniae | **Doxy** 100 mg q12h x 7-10 days; Peds: Doxy safe regardless of age for rx ≤ 21 days *(AAP Redbook 2018).* | **Azithro** 500 mg po on day 1 and then 250 mg po once daily for 4 days *(See Comments)* **OR** **Levo** 750 mg po/IV x 5 days | **Doxy** another option. *See Table 10A, page 112 for dosages.* If Doxy not available, Mino 200 mg po/IV x 1 dose, then 100 mg po/IV bid. Increasing prevalence of macrolide resistance so Doxy then Levo are preferred agents for documented mycoplasma infection. Cold agglutinin ass. complications *(JAMA 2018;319:1377).* |
| **Nocardia pneumonia** Expert Help: Wallace Lab, UT-Tyler 903-877-7680; Dr. (+1) 404-639-3158 Ref: *Medicine 88:250, 2009.* | N. asteroides, N. brasiliensis | **TMP-SMX** 15 mg/kg/day IV po in 2-4 divided doses + **Imipenem** 500 mg IV q6h for ≥ 3-4 wks, **then** **TMP-SMX** 10 mg/kg/day in 2-4 divided doses x 3-6 mos. | **IMP-TMP** IV q6h + **Amikacin** 7.5 mg/kg IV q12h x 3-4 wks & then po **TMP-SMX** | **Duration:** 3 mos. if immunocompetent; 6 mos. if immunocompromised. **Measure peak sulfonamide levels:** Target is 100-150 mcg/mL 2 hrs post po dose. **Linezolid** active in vitro. In vitro resistance to TMP-SMX may be increasing *(Clin Infect Dis 51:1445, 2010),* but whether this is associated with worse outcomes is unknown. |
| **Pseudomonas aeruginosa** Adjunctive Colistin inhalation rx for severe pneumonia, see Table 10F *(Virulence 8:403, 2017).* | Risk factors: cystic fibrosis, neutropenia, mechanical ventilation, tracheostomy | Mild, low risk of MDR GNB: Monotherapy: **[PIP-TZ Ceftazidime, Cefepime, IMP, MER or Aztreonam] or [CIP or Levo]** *(Dosing in footnote[a])* | Septic; ± high risk for MDR GNB: Combination rx: **[PIP-TZ, Ceftaz or Cefepime] + (Tobra) or CIP or [Tobra IV) + (CIP or Levo)] or [CIP or Levo]** *(Dosing in footnote[a])* | Known ESBL producer: MER or **Cefolo-tazo*** or **Ceftaz-avi*** or **MER-vabor***. Known KPC producer: **Ceftaz-avi*** or **MER-vabor**. Known metallo-type (NDM) carbapenemase producer: (**Ceftaz-avi*** + **Aztreonam**). *Dosing in footnote[14]* * not FDA-approved indication |
| **Q Fever** Acute atypical pneumonia. See *MMWR 62 (3):1, 2013.* | Coxiella burnetii | **Doxy** 100 mg bid x 14 days Doxy safe regardless of age for rx ≤ 21 days *(AAP Redbook 2018)* | Valvular heart disease: (**Doxy** 100 mg po bid + **hydroxychloroquine** 200 mg po). See Comment | In pregnancy: **TMP-SMX DS** 1 tab po bid throughout pregnancy. Even in absence of valvular heart disease, 1% of pts develop endocarditis *(CID 62:537, 2016).* If hydroxychloroquine intolerant, Doxy + FQ is alternative *(CID 2018;66:719).* |
| **Staphylococcus aureus** Duration of treatment: 2-3 wks if just pneumonia; 6-8 wks if concomitant endocarditis and/or osteomyelitis. IDSA Guidelines, *CID 52 [Feb 1]:1, 2011.* | Nafcillin/oxacillin susceptible | **Nafcillin/oxacillin** 2 gm IV q4h | **Vanco** 30-60 mg/kg/d IV in 2-3 divided doses or **Linezolid** 600 mg IV/po q12h. | Adjust dose of vancomycin to achieve target trough concentrations of 15-20 mcg/mL. Some authorities recommend a 25-30 mg/kg loading dose (actual body weight) for MRSA pneumonia *(CID 49:325, 2009).* |
| | MRSA | **Vanco** 15-20 mg/kg q8-12h IV in 2-3 divided doses, or **Linezolid** 600 mg IV/po q12h | **Dapto** not an option; if pneumonia developed during dapto rx *(CID 49:1286, 2009).* **Ceftaroline** 600 mg IV q8h | Prospective trial for MRSA pneumonia: cure rate with Linezolid (58%), Vanco (47%), p = 0.042; no difference in mortality *(CID 54:621, 2012).* **Televancin** 10 mg/kg IV x 60 min q24h another option. Perhaps lower efficacy if CrCl <50mL/min *(AAC 56:2030, 2014).* |
| **Stenotrophomonas maltophilia** | | **TMP-SMX** 15-20 mg/kg/day div q8h (TMP component) | **Mino** 200 mg IV qd *(AAC 2016;71:1071).* | FQ is an alternative if susceptible. Rarely may need to use polymyxin combination therapy. |
| **Streptococcus pneumoniae** | Pen-susceptible | **AMP** 2 gm IV q6h, **Amox** 1 gm po tid, **Pen G IV[16], Doxy, O Ceph 2/3;** may add **Azithro** 500 mg IV q12h *(AAC 69:1441, 2014).* See Table 10A, page 112 for dosages. Treat until afebrile, (min. of 5 days) and/or until serum procalcitonin normal. | | In CAP trial, **Ceftaroline** 600 mg IV q12h superior to Ceftriaxone *(CID 51:641, 2010).* |
| | Pen-resistant, high level | **FQs** with enhanced activity: **Gemi, Levo, Moxi.** See Table 10A, page 112 for dosages. If all options not possible (e.g., allergy), **Linezolid** active: 600 mg IV or q12h. *Dosages Table 10A, page 88 for more data.* **Vanco** IV—see Table 5, page 88 3-5 days (min. of 5 days). In CAP trial, **Ceftaroline** 600 mg IV q12h superior to Ceftriaxone *(CID 51:641, 2010).* | | |

[15] **Macrolide** = Azithromycin, Clarithromycin and Erythromycin.

[16] **IV Pen G dosage:** no meningitis, 2 million units IV q4h. If concomitant meningitis, 4 million units IV q4h.

Abbreviations on page 2.     *NOTE: All dosage recommendations are for adults (unless otherwise indicated) and assume normal renal function. § Alternatives consider allergy, PK, compliance, local resistance, cost.*

**TABLE 1 (42)**

| ANATOMIC SITE/DIAGNOSIS/ MODIFYING CIRCUMSTANCES | ETIOLOGIES (usual) | SUGGESTED REGIMENS[*] PRIMARY | ALTERNATIVE[§] | ADJUNCT DIAGNOSTIC OR THERAPEUTIC MEASURES AND COMMENTS |
|---|---|---|---|---|
| **LUNG/Bronchi/Pneumonia/Selected specific therapy after culture results (sputum, blood, pleural fluid, etc.) available.** *(continued)* | | | | |
| **Tuberemia** Inhalational tularemia **Treatment** Ref.: *JAMA 285:2763, 2001 & www.bt.cdc.gov* | Francisella tularemia | (Streptomycin 15 mg per kg IV bid) or (Gent 5 mg per kg IV qd) times 10 days | Doxy 100 mg IV or po bid times 14–21 days or CIP 400 mg IV (or 750 mg po) bid times 14–21 days. | Pregnancy: *as for non-pregnant adults.* Tobramycin should work. |
| **Postexposure prophylaxis** | | Doxy 100 mg po bid times 14 days | CIP 500 mg po bid times 14 days | Pregnancy: As for non-pregnant adults |
| **Viral (interstitial) pneumonia suspected** *See Influenza, Table 14A, page 185.* Ref.: *Chest 133:1221, 2008.* | Consider: **Influenza**, adenovirus, coronavirus (MERS/SARS), hantavirus, metapneumovirus, parainfluenza virus, respiratory syncytial virus. | Oseltamivir 75 mg po bid for 5 days or Zanamivir two 5 mg inhalations twice a day for 5 days. | | No known efficacious drugs for adenovirus, coronavirus, hantavirus, metapneumovirus, parainfluenza or RSV. Need travel (MERS/SARS) & exposure (Hanta) history. RSV and human metapneumovirus as serious as influenza in the elderly (*NEJM 352:1749 & 1810, 2005; CID 44:1152 & 1159, 2007*). |
| **Yersinia pestis (Plague)** *EID 2017;23:553; MMWR 64:918, 2015* | Y. pestis if aerosolized, suspect bioterror. | (Gent 5 mg/kg IV q24h or Streptomycin 30 mg/kg/day in 2 div doses) x 10 days | CIP 500 mg po bid or 400 mg IV q12h | Doxy 200 mg IV q12h x 1 day, then 100 mg po bid x 7–10 days. Chloro also effective but potentially toxic. Consider if evidence of plague meningitis. |
| **LUNG—Other Specific Infections** | | | | |
| **Aspiration pneumonia/anaerobic lung infection/lung abscess** | Anaerobes and viridans group streptococci predominate. | Clinda 300–450 mg po tid OR AM-SB 3 g IV q6h OR Ceftriaxone 1 gm IV q24h + Metro 500 mg IV q6h OR 1 gm IV q12h | Moxi 400 mg po q24h OR Erta 1 gm IV q24h. | Typically anaerobic infection of the lung: aspiration pneumonitis, necrotizing pneumonia, lung abscess and empyema (*REF. Anaerobe 18:235, 2012*). Other treatment options: PIP-TZ 3.375 g IV q6h or Moxi 400 mg IV/po q24h or AM-CL 875/125 mg bid. Note: Different from chemical pneumonitis after aspiration of sterile gastric acid (*CID 2018;67:513*). |
| **Chronic pneumonia with fever, night sweats and weight loss** | M. tuberculosis, coccidioidomycosis, histoplasmosis | *See Table 11 and Table 12.* For risk associated with TNF inhibitors, see *CID 41(Suppl 3):S187, 2005.* | | Risk factors: HIV+, foreign-born, alcoholism, contact with TB, travel into developing countries. |
| **Cystic fibrosis** **Acute exacerbation of pulmonary symptoms** Choice of therapy should be based on results of respiratory cultures. | S. aureus or H. influenzae early in disease. P. aeruginosa later in disease. Nontuberculous mycobacteria emerging as an important pathogen (*Semin Respir Crit Care Med 34:124, 2013*) | For **P. aeruginosa**: (Peds doses) Tobra 3.3 mg/kg q8h or 12 mg/kg IV q24h. Combine tobra with PIP-TZ 4.5 gm IV q6h or Ceftaz 50 mg/kg IV q8h to max of 6 gm per day. If resistant to above, CIP/Levo used if P. aeruginosa susceptible. *See footnote[§] & Comment* | For **S. aureus: (1)** MSSA—Oxacillin/Nafcillin 2 gm IV q4h. **(2)** MRSA–Vanco 15–20 mg/kg (actual wt) IV q8–12h (to achieve target trough concentration of 15–20 µg/mL. | **Cystic Fibrosis Foundation Guidelines:** 1. Combination therapy for P. aeruginosa infection. 2. Once-daily dosing for aminoglycosides. 3. Need more data on continuous infusion beta-lactam therapy. 4. Routine use of steroid not recommended. **Inhalation options** (P. aeruginosa suppression): 1) Nebulized tobra 300 mg bid x 28 days, no rx for 28 days, repeat; 2) Inhaled tobra powder-hand held: 4-28 mg cap bid x 28 days, no rx for 28 days, repeat; Nebulized aztreonam (Cayston): 75 mg tid after pre-dose bronchodilator. Ref. *Med Lett 56:51, 2014.* |
| **Burkholderia (Pseudomonas) cepacia.** Mechanisms of resistance. (*Semin Respir Crit Care Med 36:99, 2015*) | | TMP-SMX 5 mg per kg (TMP) IV q6h. Need culture & sens results to guide rx. | Chloro 15–20 mg per kg IV/po q6h | B. cepacia has become a major pathogen. Patients develop progressive respiratory failure; 62% mortality at 1 yr. **Fail to respond to aminoglycosides,** anti-pseudomonal beta-lactams. Patients with B. cepacia should be isolated from other CF patients. |

[*] Other options: (Tobra + Aztreonam 50 mg per kg IV q8h); (IMP 15–25 mg per kg IV q6h + Tobra); CIP commonly used in children, e.g., CIP IV/po + Ceftaz IV (*LnID 3-537, 2003*).

Abbreviations on page 2.    [*]*NOTE: All dosage recommendations are for adults (unless otherwise indicated) and assume normal renal function. §Alternatives consider allergy, PK, compliance, local resistance, cost.*

# TABLE 1 (43)

| ANATOMIC SITE/DIAGNOSIS/ MODIFYING CIRCUMSTANCES | ETIOLOGIES (usual) | SUGGESTED REGIMENS* | | ADJUNCT DIAGNOSTIC OR THERAPEUTIC MEASURES AND COMMENTS |
|---|---|---|---|---|
| | | PRIMARY | ALTERNATIVE§ | |
| **LUNG—Other Specific Infections** *(continued)* | | | | |
| **Empyema.** *IDSA Treatment Guidelines for Children, CID 53:617, 2011; exudative pleural effusion criteria (JAMA 311:2422, 2014).* | | | | |
| Neonatal | Staph. aureus. | See *Pneumonia, neonatal, page 41* | | Drainage indicated. |
| Infants/children (1 month-5 yrs) | Staph. aureus, Strep. pneumoniae, H. influenzae | See *Pneumonia, age 1 month-5 years, page 41* | | Drainage indicated. |
| Child >5 yrs to Adult—Diagnostic thoracentesis; chest tube for empyemas | | | | |
| Acute, usually parapneumonic. *For dosage, see Table 10B or footnote page 27* | Strep. pneumoniae, Group A strep | Cefotaxime or Ceftriaxone (Dosage, see footnote* page 27) | Vanco | Tissue Plasminogen Activator (10 mg) + DNase (5 mg) bid x 3 days via chest tube improves outcome (NEJM 365:518, 2011). |
| | Staph. aureus. Check for MRSA | Nafcillin/Oxacillin if MSSA | Vanco or Linezolid if MRSA. | Usually complication of S. aureus pneumonia &/or bacteremia. |
| | H influenzae | Ceftriaxone | | |
| Subacute/chronic | Anaerobic strep., Strep. milleri; Bacteroides sp., Enterobacteriaceae, M. tuberculosis | Clinda 450-900 mg IV q8h + Ceftriaxone | TMP-SMX or AM-SB Cefoxitin or IMP or PIP-TZ or AM-SB (Dosage, see footnote* page 27) | Pleuropnic Gm-neg. bacilli, ↑ resistance to TMP-SMX. Intrapleural tissue plasminogen activator (t-PA) 10 mg + DNase 5 mg via chest tube twice daily for 3 days improved fluid drainage, reduced frequency of surgery, and reduced duration of the hospital stay; neither agent effective alone (N Engl J Med 365:518, 2011). Pro/con debate: Chest 145:14, 17, 20, 2014. Pleural biopsy with culture for mycobacteria and histology if TBc suspected. |
| **Human immunodeficiency virus infection (HIV+):** | | | | |
| CD4 T-lymphocytes <200 per mm³ or clinical AIDS Dry cough, progressive dyspnea, & diffuse infiltrate Prednisone first if suspect pneumocystis (see Comment) | Pneumocystis jirovecii (PJP or PCP) most likely; also MTB, fungi, Kaposi's sarcoma, & lymphoma NOTE: AIDS pts may develop pneumonia due to DRSP or other pathogens—see below | *Rx listed here is for severe pneumocystis; see Table 11A, page 141 for regimens for mild disease.* Prednisone 1° (see Comment), then: TMP-SMX [IV: 15 mg per kg per day q8h (TMP component) or po: 2 DS tabs q8h], total of 21 days | (Clinda 600 mg IV q8h + Primaquine 30 mg po q24h) or (pentamidine isethionate 21 mg per kg per day IV) times 21 days See Comment | Diagnosis (induced sputum or bronchial wash) for histology or monoclonal antibody strains or PCR. Prednisone 40 mg bid po times 5 days then 40 mg q24h times 5 days then 20 mg q24h po times 11 days is indicated with PCP should be given at initiation of anti-PCP rx; don't wait until pt's condition deteriorates. If PCP studies negative, consider bacterial pneumonia, TBc, cocci, histo, crypto, Kaposi's sarcoma or lymphoma. Pentamidine not active vs. bacterial pathogens. |
| CD4 T-lymphocytes normal Acute onset, purulent sputum & pulmonary infiltrates ± pleuritic pain. Isolate pt and TBc excluded: Adults | Strep. pneumoniae, H. influenzae, aerobic Gm-neg. bacilli (including P. aeruginosa), Legionella rare, MTB. | Ceftriaxone 1 gm IV q24h (over age 65 1 gm IV q24h) + Azithro. Could use Levo, or Moxi IV as alternative (see Comment) | | For suspected bacterial pneumonia, other regimens for CAP also are options. |
| **LYMPH NODES** (approaches below apply to lymphadenitis without an obvious primary source) | | | | |
| **Lymphadenitis, acute** | | | | |
| Generalized | Etiologies: EBV, early HIV infection, syphilis, toxoplasma, tularemia, lymphoma, others. For differential diagnosis of fever and lymphadenopathy see NEJM 369:2333, 2013. | | | |
| **By Region:** | | | | |
| Cervical—see cat-scratch disease (CSD) | CSD (B. henselae), Grp A strep, Staph. aureus, anaerobes, MTB (scrofula), M. avium, M. scrofulaceum, M. malmoense, toxo, tularemia | History & physical exam directs evaluation. If nodes fluctuant, aspirate and base rx on Gram & acid-fast stains. **Kikuchi-Fujimoto** disease causes fever and benign self-limited adenopathy; the etiology is unknown (Blood 122:917, 2012). | | |

*Abbreviations on page 2.*

*NOTE: All dosage recommendations are for adults (unless otherwise indicated) and assume normal renal function. PK, compliance, local resistance, cost.*
§ *Alternatives consider allergy, PK, compliance, local resistance, cost.*

**TABLE 1 (44)**

| ANATOMIC SITE/DIAGNOSIS/ MODIFYING CIRCUMSTANCES | ETIOLOGIES (usual) | SUGGESTED REGIMENS* | | ADJUNCT DIAGNOSTIC OR THERAPEUTIC MEASURES AND COMMENTS |
|---|---|---|---|---|
| | | **PRIMARY** | **ALTERNATIVE§** | |
| **LYMPH NODES/Lymphadenitis, acute/By Region** *(continued)* | | | | |
| Inguinal | | | | |
|   Sexually transmitted | HSV, chancroid, syphilis, LGV | | | |
|   Not sexually transmitted | GAS, SA, tularemia, CSD, Y. pestis (plague) | | Consider bubonic plague & glandular tularemia. | |
| Axillary | GAS, SA, CSD, tularemia, Y. pestis, sporotrichosis. | | Consider bubonic plague & glandular tularemia. | |
| **Extremity, with associated nodular lymphangitis** | Sporotrichosis, leishmania, Nocardia brasiliensis, Mycobacterium marinum, Mycobacterium chelonae, tularemia. | | Treatment varies with specific etiology. | A distinctive form of lymphangitis characterized by subcutaneous swellings along inflamed lymphatic channels. Primary site of skin invasion usually present; regional adenopathy variable. |
| **Nocardia lymphadenitis & skin abscesses** | N. asteroides, N. brasiliensis | TMP-SMX 5-10 mg/kg/day based on TMP IV/po div in 2-4 doses | **Sulfisoxazole** 2 gm po qid or **Minocycline** 100-200 mg po bid. | **Duration:** 3 mos. if immunocompetent; 6 mos. if immunocompromised. (Ann Pharmacother 41:1694, 2007). Linezolid 600 mg po bid reported effective. |
| **By Pathogen:** | | | | |
| **Cat-scratch disease— immunocompetent patient** Axillary/epitrochlear nodes 46%, neck 26%, inguinal 17% (Int J Antimicrob Agts 44:16, 2014) | Bartonella henselae | **Adult: Azithro** 500 mg po x 1, then 250 mg/day x 4 days. **Peds** (<45.5 kg): **Azithro** soln/n 10 mg/kg x 1, then 5 mg/kg per day x 4 days. | Adult: **Clarithro** 500 mg po bid or **RIF** 300 mg po bid or **TMP-SMX DS** 1 tab po bid or **CIP** 500 mg po bid (duration at least 10 days) | **Dx:** Antibody titer, PCR increasingly available. **Hepatosplenic, CNS or Retinal infection: Doxy** 100 mg po bid + **RIF** 300 mg po bid) x 4-6 wks. Needle drainage of suppurative node(s) provides patient comfort. |
| **Bubonic plague** (see also, plague pneumonia) Ref: MMWR 64:918, 2015 | Yersinia pestis | (**Streptomycin** 30 mg/kg/day IV in 2 div doses or **Gentamicin** 5 mg/kg/day IV single dose) x 10 days | (**Levo** 500 mg IV/po once daily or **CIP** 500 mg po (or 400 mg IV) q12h) x 10 days or **Moxi** 400 mg IV/po q24h x 10-14 days | **Doxy** 200 mg IV/po bid x 1 day, then 100 mg IV/po bid x 10 days another option. FQs effective in animals & small case series (EID 2017;23:553). Peds dose 4.4 mg/kg/day div bid safe regardless of age for rx ≤21 days (AAP Redbook 2018). |
| **MOUTH** | | | | |
| **Aphthous stomatitis, recurrent** | Etiology unknown | Topical steroids (Kenalog in Orabase) may ↓ pain and swelling | | |
| **Actinomycosis: "Lumpy jaw" after dental or jaw trauma** | Actinomyces israelii | **AMP** 200 mg/kg/day IV in 3-4 divided doses x 2-6 wks then **Pen VK** 2-4 gm/day in 4 divided doses x 6-12 mo | (**Ceftriaxone** 2 gm IV q24h or **Clinda** 600-900 mg IV q8h) x 4-6 wks, then **Pen VK** 2-4 gm/day x 6-12 mos | **NOTE:** Metro not active vs. actinomyces. Recommendations for a 2-6 week run-in IV therapy prior to long oral therapy are traditional and empirical. There are case reports of successful treatment with oral therapy preceded by much shorter durations of IV therapy, as little as 3 days, or no IV therapy at all (Chest 126:2211, 2005), particularly for less severe disease. Durations shorter than 3 months may also be effective in less bulky disease. |
| **Buccal cellulitis** Children <5 yrs | H. influenzae | **Ceftriaxone** 50 mg/kg IV q24h | **AM-CL** 45-90 mg/kg po div bid or **TMP-SMX** 8-12 mg/kg (TMP comp) IV/po div q6h | With Hib immunization, invasive H. influenzae infections have ↓ by 95%. Now occurring in infants prior to immunization. |
| **Candida Stomatitis ("Thrush")** | C. albicans | **Fluconazole** | Echinocandin | See Table 11, page 132. |
| **Dental (Tooth) abscess** | Aerobic & anaerobic Strep sp. | Mild: **AM-CL** 875/125 mg po bid | Severe: **PIP-TZ** 3.375 gm IV q6h | Surgical drainage / debridement. If Pen-allergic: **Clinda** 600 mg IV q6-8h |
| **Herpetic stomatitis** | Herpes simplex virus 1 & 2 | See Table 14A | | |
| **Submandibular space infection, bilateral (Ludwig's angina)** | Oral anaerobes, facultative streptococci, S. aureus (rare) | **PIP-TZ** or **Pen G** (+ **Metro** IV) | **Clinda** 600 mg IV q6-8h (For Pen-allergic) | Ensure adequate airway and early surgical debridement. Add Vanco IV if gram-positive cocci on gram stain. Look for dental infection. |
| **Ulcerative gingivitis (Vincent's angina or Trench mouth)** | Oral anaerobes + vitamin deficiency | **Pen G** 4 million units IV q4h or **Metro** 500 mg IV q8h | **Clinda** 600 mg IV q8h | Replete vitamins (A-D). Can mimic scurvy. Severe form is NOMA (Cancrum oris) (Ln 368:147, 2006) |

*NOTE: All dosage recommendations are for adults (unless otherwise indicated) and assume normal renal function. § Alternatives consider allergy, PK, compliance, local resistance, cost.*

*Abbreviations on page 2.*

**TABLE 1 (45)**

| ANATOMIC SITE/DIAGNOSIS/ MODIFYING CIRCUMSTANCES | ETIOLOGIES (usual) | SUGGESTED REGIMENS* — PRIMARY | SUGGESTED REGIMENS* — ALTERNATIVE§ | ADJUNCT DIAGNOSTIC OR THERAPEUTIC MEASURES AND COMMENTS |
|---|---|---|---|---|
| **MUSCLE** | | | | |
| "Gas gangrene" Contaminated traumatic wound. Can be spontaneous without trauma. | C. perfringens, other histotoxic Clostridium sp. | (Clinda 900 mg IV q8h) + (Pen G 24 million units/day div. q4–6h IV) | | Susceptibility of C. tertium to penicillins and metronidazole is variable; resistance to clindamycin and 3GCs is common, so vanco or metro (500 mg q8h) recommended. IMP or MER expected to have activity in vitro against Clostridium spp. |
| Pyomyositis | Staph. aureus, Group A strep, (rarely Gm-neg. bacilli), variety of anaerobic organisms | (Nafcillin or Oxacillin 2 gm IV q4h) or Cefazolin 2 gm IV q8h if MSSA | Vanco 15–20 mg/kg q8-12h if MRSA | In immunocompromised or if otherwise suspected, add gram-negative and/ or anaerobic coverage. Evaluate for drainage of abscesses. |
| **PANCREAS** | | | | |
| Acute alcoholic (without necrosis or pancreatitis) (idiopathic) pancreatitis | Not bacterial | None No necrosis on CT | | 1–9% become infected but prospective studies show no advantage of prophylactic antimicrobials. Observe for pancreatic abscesses or necrosis which require therapy. |
| Post-necrotizing pancreatitis; infected pseudocyst; pancreatic abscess | Enterobacteriaceae, enterococci, S. aureus, S. epidermidis, anaerobes, candida | Need culture of abscess/infected pseudocyst to direct therapy; PIP-TZ is reasonable empiric therapy. | | Can often get specimen by fine-needle aspiration. Moxi, MER, IMP, ERTA are all options (AAC 56:6434, 2012). |
| Antimicrobial prophylaxis, necrotizing pancreatitis | As above | Patients with necrotizing pancreatitis who develop gas in the area of necrosis, rising inflammatory markers or persistent fever may be suspected of having infected pancreatic necrosis and would be candidates for antibiotic therapy. Meta-analysis: initiation of antibiotics within 72 hrs of sx onset reduced infected pancreatic necrosis (J Hepatobil Pancreat Sci 2015;22:316). | | |
| **PAROTID GLAND** | | | | |
| "Hot" tender parotid swelling | S. aureus, S. pyogenes, oral flora, & aerobic Gm-neg. bacilli (rare), mumps, rarely enterovirus/influenza; parainfluenza | (Nafcillin/Oxacillin 2 gm IV q4h or cefazolin 2 gm IV q8h if MSSA. Vanco if MRSA. Metro or Clinda for anaerobes | Metro or Clinda 2 gm IV q8h if MSSA. Metro or Clinda for anaerobes | Predisposing factors: stone(s) in Stensen's duct, dehydration. Therapy depends on ID of specific etiologic agent. |
| "Cold" non-tender parotid swelling | Granulomatous disease (e.g. mycobacteria, fungi, sarcoidosis, Sjögren's syndrome, drugs (iodides, et al.), diabetes, cirrhosis, tumors | | | History/lab results may narrow differential; may need biopsy for diagnosis. |
| **PERITONEUM/PERITONITIS:** | | | | |
| Primary (Spontaneous) Bacterial Peritonitis (SBP) Dx: Pos culture & ≥250 PMN/mcL of ascites fluid Ref: Aliment Pharmacol Ther 2015;41:1116 | E. coli 33% Other enterobacteriaceae 11% P. aeruginosa 1% Gm+ cocci 40% Strept sp 15% Staph sp 18% Enterococci 9% | **Community-acquired: low risk of MDR GNB, VRE:** PIP-TZ 3.375 gm IV q6h or Ceftriaxone 2 gm IV q24h or (if beta lactam allergy) CIP 400 mg IV q12h (J Hepatol 60:1310, 2014) | **Nosocomial: high risk of MDR GNB, VRE:** MER 1 gm IV q8h + Dapto 6 mg/kg IV q24h **Note:** In random trial, combination superior to Ceftaz alone (Hepatology 63:1299, 2016) | **Diagnosis of SBP:** For microbiologic dx: inoculate 10mL of ascitic fluid into one aerobic and one anaerobic blood culture bottles; yield better if inoculate 2 aerobic and 2 anaerobic bottles. Comment: for VRE, random higher doses of Dapto, eg 8-10 mg/kg per day. Secondary prophylaxis: Norfloxacin 400 mg po daily or CIP 500 mg po daily until transplantation or liver function improves to compensated. In RCT, CIP 750 mg po once weekly as effective as Norflox 400 mg po daily (Am J Gastroenterol 2018;113:1167). |
| | | • Average duration of rx 5 days (not based on severity of infection) | | |
| | | • To protect renal function: on day 1 & day 3 give IV albumin 1.5 gm/kg | | |
| Prophylaxis after UGI (Variceal) bleeding | | Hospitalized pts: Ceftriaxone 1 gm, IV once daily x 7 days or Norfloxacin 400 mg po bid x 7 days or CIP 500 mg po bid x 7 days | | |
| **Prevention of SBP** (Amer. J Gastro 104:993, 2009): Cirrhosis & ascites (Aliment Pharmacol Ther 2015;41:1116) For prevention after UGI bleeding, see Liver, page 39 | | CIP 500 mg/day (J Hepatol 2008;48:774) | | TMP-SMX 1 peritonitis or spontaneous bacteremia from 27% to 3% (ANM 122:595, 1995). Ref for CIP: Hepatology 22:1171, 1995. |

Abbreviations on page 2.    *NOTE: All dosage recommendations are for adults (unless otherwise indicated) and assume normal renal function. § Alternatives consider allergy, PK, compliance, local resistance, cost.

**TABLE 1 (46)**

| ANATOMIC SITE/DIAGNOSIS/ MODIFYING CIRCUMSTANCES | ETIOLOGIES (usual) | SUGGESTED REGIMENS* | | ADJUNCT DIAGNOSTIC OR THERAPEUTIC MEASURES AND COMMENTS |
|---|---|---|---|---|
| | | PRIMARY | ALTERNATIVE§ | |
| **PERITONEUM/PERITONITIS** *(continued)* | | | | |
| **Secondary (bowel perforation, ruptured appendix, ruptured diverticuli)** Ref: *CID 50:133, 2010 (IDSA Guidelines)* **Antifungal rx?** No need if successful uncomplicated 1st surgery for viscus perforation. Treat for candida if: pure culture from abdomen or blood, in controlled study, no benefit from preemptive rx to prevent invasive candidiasis *(CID 61:1671, 2015).* | Enterobacteriaceae, Bacteroides sp, enterococci, P. aeruginosa (3-15%). C. albicans (see Comment) If VRE documented, dapto may work *(Int J Antimicrob Agents 32:369, 2008).* See *Table 5A* for other options for treatment of VRE. | **Mild-moderate disease—Inpatient—parenteral rx:** (e.g., focal peritonitis/perforated appendicitis, peridiverticular abscess). Usually **need source control** PIP-TZ 3.375 gm IV q6h or 4.5 gm IV q8h or 4-hr infusion of 3.375 gm q8h **OR Erta** 1 gm IV q24h **OR Moxi** 400 mg IV q24h | [(**CIP** 400 mg IV q12h or **Levo** 750 mg IV q24h) + (**Metro** 1 gm IV q12h)] or (**CFP** 2 gm q12h + **Metro**) **NOTE:** avoid tigecycline unless no other alternative due to increased mortality risk (FDA warning). | Must "cover" both Gm-neg, aerobic & Gm-neg, anaerobic bacteria. Empiric coverage of MRSA, enterococci and candida not necessary unless culture indicates infection. Cover enterococci if valvular heart disease. **Drugs active only vs. anaerobic Gm-neg. bacilli:** Metro. **Drugs active only vs. aerobic Gm-neg. bacilli:** aminoglycosides, P Ceph 2/3/4, Aztreonam, AP Pen, CIP, Levo, Ceftolozane-tazo, Ceftaz-avibactam. **Drugs active vs. both aerobic/anaerobic Gm-neg. bacteria:** PIP-TZ, DORI, IMP, MER, tigecycline, eravacycline. Increasing resistance of Bacteroides species *(Anaerobe 17:147, 2013; AAC 56:1247, 2012)* to: |
| | | | | | Metro | Cefotetan | Cefoxitin | Clindamycin |
| | | | | | **% Resistant** | 5-30 | 17-87 | 19-35 |
| | | | | | Essentially no resistance of Bacteroides to: Metro, PIP-TZ, Carbapenems. Case report of B. fragilis resistant to all drugs except minocycline, tigecycline & linezolid *(MMWR 62:694, 2013).* Ertapenem not active vs. P. aeruginosa/Acinetobacter species. |
| **Pediatric appendicitis.** In retrospective review, **Ceftriaxone** 50 mg/kg (max 2 gm) once daily + **Metro** 30 mg/kg (max 1500 mg) once daily as effective as **Erta** *(JPIDS 2017:5:57)* | | **Severe life-threatening disease—ICU patient:** **Surgery for source control** IMP 500 mg IV q6h or **MER** 1 gm IV q8h or **Dori** 500 mg IV q8h (1-hr infusion) or **Ceftolozane-tazobactam** 1.5 gm IV q8h + **Metro** 500 mg q8h) or (**Ceftaz-avi** 2.5 gm IV over 2 hrs q8h + **Metro** 500 mg q8h) **Concomitant surgical management important.** | [**AMP + Metro + (CIP** 400 mg IV q8h or **Levo** 750 mg IV q24h) **OR** [**AMP** 2 gm IV q6h + **Metro** 500 mg IV q6h + **aminoglycoside** (see *Table 10D, page 128*)] | If absence of ongoing fecal contamination, aerobic/anaerobic culture of peritoneal exudate/abscess may be of help in guiding specific therapy. Less need for aminoglycosides. **With severe pen allergy, can "cover"** Gm-neg aerobes with CIP or Aztreonam. Remember **Dori/IMP/MER are β-lactams.** IMP dose increased to 1 gm q6h if suspect P. aeruginosa and pt. is critically ill. Resistance to Moxi increasing. See *CID 59:698, 2014* (suscept. of anaerobic bacteria). Recent data suggest that short course antibiotic Rx (approx 4 days) may be sufficient where there is adequate source control of complicated intra-abdominal infections *(NEJM 372:21, 2015).* |
| **Abdominal actinomycosis** | A. Israelii and rarely others | **AMP** 200 mg/kg/day in 3-4 divided doses x 4-6 wks then **Pen VK** 2-4 gm/day in 4 divided doses x 6-12 mo | **Doxy** or **Ceftriaxone** or **Clinda** | Presents as mass +/- fistula tract after abdominal surgery, e.g., for ruptured appendix. Can use IV Pen G instead of AMP: 10-20 million units/day IV x 4-6 wks. |
| **Associated with chronic ambulatory peritoneal dialysis** (Abdominal pain, cloudy dialysate, dialysate WBC >100 cell/μL with >50% neutrophils, normal = <8 cells/μL; Ref: *Perit Dial Int 30-393, 2010*.) | Gm+ 45%, Gm- 15%, Multiple 1%, Fungi 2%, MTB 3% *(Perit Dial Int 24:424, 2004).* | **Empiric therapy:** Need activity vs. MRSA (**Vanco**) and gram-negative bacilli (**Ceftaz, Carbapenem, CIP, Aztreonam, Gent**). Add **Fluconazole** if gram stain shows yeast, For bacteremia, IV dosing. For dosing detail, see *Table 19, page 252.* | | **For diagnosis:** concentrate several hundred mL of removed dialysis fluid by centrifugation. Gram stain concentrate and then inject into aerobic/anaerobic blood culture bottles. A positive Gram stain will guide initial therapy. If culture shows Staph. epidermidis and no S. aureus, good chance of "saving" dialysis catheter. If multiple organisms cultured, consider catheter removal and for **bowel perforation and for catheter removal.** See *Perit Dialysis Int 29:5, 2009.* Other indications for catheter removal: relapsing/refractory peritonitis, fungal peritonitis, catheter tunnel infection. |

*NOTE: All dosage recommendations are for adults (unless otherwise indicated) and assume normal renal function. PK, pharmacokinetics; §Alternatives consider allergy, PK, compliance, local resistance, cost.*

## TABLE 1 (47)

| ANATOMIC SITE/DIAGNOSIS/ MODIFYING CIRCUMSTANCES | ETIOLOGIES (usual) | SUGGESTED REGIMENS* | | ADJUNCT DIAGNOSTIC OR THERAPEUTIC MEASURES AND COMMENTS |
|---|---|---|---|---|
| | | PRIMARY | ALTERNATIVE§ | |
| **PHARYNX** **Pharyngitis/Tonsillitis:** "Strep throat" **Exudative or Diffuse Erythema** Associated cough, rhinorrhea, hoarseness and/or oral ulcers suggest viral etiology. Student health clinic pts: Gp A Strep in 10% (AnIM 162:241, 2002). 37% & 8%, respectively, in another study. F. necrophorum in 13.5% (age 14-20 yrs) (JCM 2017;55:1147). IDSA Guidelines on Group A Strep: CID 55:1279, 2012. Pros & cons of diagnostics (JCM 2016;54:2413). Even with rapid detection of S. pyogenes, probably still need back-up culture if rapid test is negative (AJM 2016;54:2413). 2 PCR (NAAT) assays for GpA strep FDA approved: Cobas & Xpert Xpress Strep A: Superior to antigen detection (JCM 2018;56:e01310). | Group A, C, G Strep; EBV; Primary HIV; N. gonorrhea; Respiratory viruses. F. necrophorum found in 20%, Gp A Strep in 10% (AnIM 162:241, 2002). | For Strep pharyngitis (adult): (Pen V OR Benzathine Pen) OR Cefdinir OR Cefpodoxime. If suspect F. necrophorum: AM-CL OR Amox Peds: Pen V OR Amox Doses in footnote[18]. | For Strep pharyngitis: Clinda OR Azithro OR Clarithro. If suspect F. necrophorum: Metro; Resistant to macrolides Doses in footnote[18]. | **Dx: Rapid Strep test.** If rapid test neg, do culture (CID 59:643, 2014). No need for post-treatment rapid strep test or culture. **Complications of Strep pharyngitis:** 1. Acute rheumatic fever - follows Grp A S. pyogenes infection, rare after Grp C/G infection. See footnote*. For prevention, start treatment within 9 days of onset of symptoms. 2. Children age <7 yrs at risk for post-streptococcal glomerulonephritis. 3. Pediatric autoimmune neuropsychiatric disorder associated with Grp A Strep (PANDAS) infection. 4. Peritonsillar abscess: Suppurative phlebitis are potential complications. |
| Gonococcal pharyngitis | | Ceftriaxone 250 mg IM x 1 dose + Azithro 1 gm po x 1 dose | FQs not recommended due to resistance | Not effective for pharyngeal GC: spectinomycin, cefixime, cefpodoxime and cefuroxime. Ref: MMWR 61:590, 2012. See most recent CDC STD guidelines. |
| Proven S. pyogenes recurrence or documented relapse | Gp A Strep | Cefdinir OR Cefpodoxime | AM-CL OR Clinda | Doses in footnote[18]. Prospective study favors AM-CL (JAC 1999;24:227). |
| | Gp A infections: 6 in 1 yr; 4 in 2 consecutive yrs | Benefit of tonsillectomy unclear (Peds 2017;139:e20163490) | | Hard to distinguish Grp A Strep infection from chronic Grp A Strep carriage and/or repeat viral infections. |
| Peritonsillar abscess - Sometimes a serious complication of exudative pharyngitis ("Quinsy") (JAC 66:1941, 2013). Other complications | F. necrophorum (44%) (JCM 2018;56:e00487-18) Gp A Strep (33%) Grp C/G Strep (9%) S. anginosus grp | Surgical drainage plus: PIP-TZ 3.375 gm IV q6h or (Metro 500 mg IV/po q6-8h + Ceftriaxone 2 gm IV q24h) | Pen allergic: Clinda 600-900 mg IV q6-8h | Avoid macrolides: Fusobacterium is resistant. Reports of beta-lactamase production by oral anaerobes (Anaerobe 9:105, 2003). See jugular vein suppurative phlebitis, page 52. Etiologies ref: Eur J Clin Micro Infect Dis 2015;34:549. Culture results may allow de-escalation to AM-SB 3 gm IV q6h. |
| See parapharyngeal space infection and jugular vein suppurative phlebitis (see next page) | | | | |

[18] **Treatment of Group A, C & G strep:** Treatment durations are from approved package inserts. Subsequent studies indicate efficacy of shorter treatment courses. **All po unless otherwise indicated.**

**PEDS DOSAGE: Benzathine penicillin** 25,000 units per kg IM to max. 1.2 million units; **Pen V** 250 mg bid or tid x 10d (wt <27kg); **Amox** 50 mg/kg once daily (max 1000 mg) x 10 days; **AM-CL** 45 mg per kg per day div q12h x 10 days; **Cephalexin** 20 mg/kg/dose bid (max 500 mg/dose) x 10 days; **Cefuroxime axetil** 20 mg per kg per day div. bid x 5 days; **Cefprozil** 7.5 mg per kg q12h x 10 days; **Cefpodoxime** 10 mg per kg per day div q12h x 5 days; **Cefdinir** 7 mg per kg q12h x 5 days or 14 mg per kg q24h x 10 days; **Cefadroxil** 30 mg/kg once daily (max 1 gm/day) x 10 days; **Clarithro** 15 mg per kg per day div bid or 250 mg qid x 10 days; **Azithro** 12 mg per kg once daily x 5 days; clinda 20-30 mg per kg per day div. q8h x 10 days.

**ADULT DOSAGE: Benzathine penicillin** 1.2 million units IM x 1; **Pen V** 500 mg qid or 250 mg qid x 10 days; **Cefditoren** 200 mg tid x 10 days; **Cefuroxime axetil** 250 mg bid x 4 days; **Cefpodoxime proxetil** 100 mg bid x 5 days; **Cefdinir** 300 mg q12h x 5 days or 600 mg q24h x 5 days; **Cefditoren** 200 mg bid; **Cefprozil** 500 mg q12h x 10 days; **NOTE: All: O Ceph 2** drugs approved for 10-day rx of strep pharyngitis; increasing number of studies show efficacy of shorter courses. **Clarithro** 250 mg bid x 10 days; **Clarithro** 500 mg q24h x 4 days or 500 mg q24h x 3 days; Clinda 300 mg tid x 10 days.

[19] Primary rationale for therapy is eradication of Group A Strep (GAS) and prevention of acute rheumatic fever (ARF). Benzathine penicillin G has been shown in clinical trials to a rate of ARF from 2.8 to 0.2%. This was associated with clearance of GAS on pharyngeal cultures (CID 19:1110, 1994). Subsequent studies have been based on cultures, not actual prevention of symptoms.

*NOTE: All dosage recommendations are for adults (unless otherwise indicated) and assume normal renal function. § Alternatives consider allergy, PK, compliance, local resistance, cost.

Abbreviations on page 2.

**TABLE 1 (48)**

| ANATOMIC SITE/DIAGNOSIS/ MODIFYING CIRCUMSTANCES | ETIOLOGIES (usual) | SUGGESTED REGIMENS* | | ADJUNCT DIAGNOSTIC OR THERAPEUTIC MEASURES AND COMMENTS |
|---|---|---|---|---|
| | | **PRIMARY** | **ALTERNATIVE§** | |
| **PHARYNX/Pharyngitis/Tonsillitis/Exudative or Diffuse Erythema** *(continued)* | | | | |
| **Membranous pharyngitis due to Diphtheria**<br><br>Respiratory isolation, nasal & pharyngeal cultures (special media), obtain antitoxin. **Place pt in respiratory droplet isolation.** | C. *diphtheriae* (human to human), C. *ulcerans* (animal to human), C. *pseudotuberculosis* (animal to human) (rare) | **Treatment: antibiotics + antitoxin**<br>**Antibiotic therapy: Erythro** 500 mg IV qid OR/OR **Pen G** 50,000 units/kg/day (max 1.2 million units/kg. Can switch to **Pen VK** 250 mg po qid when able. Treat for 14 days | **Diphtheria antitoxin:** Horse serum. Obtain from CDC, +1 404-639-2889. Do scratch test before IV therapy. Dose depends on stage of illness: <48hrs: 20,000-40,000 units; if NP membranes: 40,000-60,000 units; >3 days & bull neck: 80,000-120,000 units | **Ensure adequate airway.** EKG & cardiac enzymes. F/U cultures 2 wks post-treatment to document cure. Then, diphtheria toxoid immunization. Culture contacts; treat contacts with either single dose of **Pen G** IM: 600,000 units if age <6 yrs, 1.2 million units if age ≥6 yrs. If Pen-allergic, **Erythro** 500 mg po qid x 7-10 days. Assess immunization status of close contacts: toxoid vaccine as indicated. In vitro, C. diphtheriae suscept. to clarithro, azithro, clinda, FQs, TMP/SMX. |
| **Vesicular, ulcerative pharyngitis** (viral) | Coxsackie A9, B1-5, ECHO (multiple types), Enterovirus 71, Herpes simplex 1,2 | Antibacterial agents not indicated. For HSV-1,2: **acyclovir** 400 mg tid po x 10 days. | HIV: **Famciclovir** 250 mg po tid x 7 days or **Valacyclovir** 1000 mg po bid x 7-10 days | Small vesicles posterior pharynx suggests enterovirus. Viruses are most common etiology of acute pharyngitis. **Suspect viral if concurrent conjunctivitis, coryza, cough, skin rash, hoarseness.** |
| **Epiglottitis (Supraglottis): Concern in life-threatening obstruction of the airway** | | | | |
| Children | H. influenzae (rare), S. pyogenes, S. pneumoniae, S. aureus (includes MRSA), viruses | **Peds dosage: Cefotaxime** 50 mg per kg IV q8h or **Ceftriaxone** 50 mg per kg IV q24h) + **Vanco** | **Peds dosage: Levo** 10 mg/kg IV q24h + **Clinda** 7.5 mg/kg/day IV q6h | Have tracheostomy set "at bedside". **Levo** use in children is justified as emergency empiric therapy in pts with severe beta-lactam allergy. Ref: *Ped Clin N Amer 53:215, 2006.* Use of steroids is controversial; do not recommend. |
| Adults | Group A strep, H. influenzae (rare) & many others | Same regimens as for children. See footnote20 | **Adult dosage:**<br>**PIP-TZ** 3.375 gm IV q6h or **AM-SB** 3 gm IV q6h | |
| **Parapharyngeal space infection** [Spaces include: sublingual, submandibular (Ludwig's angina) (*see page 48*) lateral pharyngeal, retropharyngeal, pretracheal & descending mediastinitis] | | | | |
| Poor dental hygiene, dental extractions, foreign bodies (e.g., toothpicks, fish bones). Refs: *Infection 2016;44:77, Otol Head Neck Surg 2016;155:155* | Polymicrobic: S. aureus, Strep sp., anaerobes, Eikenella corrodens. Anaerobes outnumber aerobes 10:1. | [(**Clinda** 600-900 mg IV q8h or (**Pen G** 24 million units/day by cont. infusion or div q4-6h IV) + **Metro** 1 gm IV load and then 0.5 gm IV q6h] | **Clinda** 600-900 mg IV q8h.<br>**Avoid macrolides:**<br>fusobacterium is resistant | Close observation of airway, 1/3 require intubation. MRI or CT to identify abscess; **surgical drainage. Metro** may be given 1 gm IV q12h. Complications: infection of carotid (rupture possible) & jugular vein phlebitis. |
| **Jugular vein suppurative phlebitis (Lemierre's syndrome)** *LnID 12:808, 2012.* | Fusobacterium necrophorum in vast majority (*CCM 2018;56:e00487-18*) | **PIP-TZ** 4.5 gm IV q8h or **IMP** 500 mg IV q6h or **Metro** 500 mg po/IV q8h + **Ceftriaxone** 2 gm IV once daily | **Clinda** 600-900 mg IV q8h. **Avoid macrolides:** fusobacterium is resistant | Emboli: pulmonary and systemic common. Erosion into carotid artery can occur. Lemierre described F. necrophorum in 1936; other anaerobes & Gm-positive cocci are less common etiologies of suppurative phlebitis post-pharyngitis. |
| **Laryngitis** (hoarseness) | Viral (90%) | Not indicated | | |

[20] Parapharyngeal space infection: **Ceftriaxone** 2 gm IV q24h; **Cefotaxime** 2 gm IV q4-8h; **PIP-TZ** 3.375 gm IV q6h or 4-hr infusion of 3.375 gm q8h; **TMP-SMX** 8-10 mg per kg per day (based on TMP component) div q6h, q8h, or q12h; **Clinda** 600-900 mg IV q6-8h; **Levo** 750 mg IV q24h; **Vanco** 15 mg/kg IV q12h.

*NOTE: All dosage recommendations are for adults (unless otherwise indicated) and assume normal renal function. § Alternatives consider allergy; PK, compliance, local resistance, cost.*

Abbreviations on page 2.

## TABLE 1 (49)

| ANATOMIC SITE/DIAGNOSIS/ MODIFYING CIRCUMSTANCES | ETIOLOGIES (usual) | SUGGESTED REGIMENS* | | ADJUNCT DIAGNOSTIC OR THERAPEUTIC MEASURES AND COMMENTS |
|---|---|---|---|---|
| | | PRIMARY | ALTERNATIVE§ | |
| **SINUSES, PARANASAL** | | | | |
| **Sinusitis, acute** Guidelines: *Pediatrics 132:e262 & 284, 2013* (American Academy of Pediatrics); *Otolaryngol Head Neck Surg 2015;152 (Suppl 2):S1* | | | | |
| **Treatment goals:** • Speed resolution • Prevent bacterial complications (*see Comment*) • Prevent chronic sinusitis • Avoid unnecessary use of antibiotics  Discussion of when to start antibacterial rx *(AnIM 2017;166:201)* | S. pneumonia 33% H. influenza 32% M. catarrhalis 9% Anaerobes 6% Grp A strep 2% Viruses 15-18% S. aureus 10% (*See Comment*) | Most common: obstruction of sinus ostia from virus or allergy. Treatment: Saline irrigation. **Antibiotics for bacterial sinusitis if:** 1) fever, pain, purulent nasal discharge; 2) still symptomatic after 10 days with no antibiotic; 3) clinical failure despite antibiotic therapy.  *No penicillin allergy:* **Peds** or **Adult: Amox** 90 mg/kg/day divided q12h or **AM-CL** suspension 90 mg/kg/day (Amox comp) divided q12h. Treat for 10-14 days **Adult: AM-CL** 1000/62.5-2 tabs po bid x 5-7 days | *Penicillin allergy* **Peds (if anaphylaxis): Clinda** 30-40 mg/kg/day divided tid or qid x 10-14 days (see Comment) **Peds (no anaphylaxis): Cefpodoxime** 10 mg/kg/day po div q12h. **Adult (if anaphylaxis):** Levo or Doxy **Adult (no anaphylaxis):** Cefpodoxime 200 mg po bid | **Treatment:** Panda: Haemophilus & Moraxella sp. are resistant; may need 2nd drug • Duration of rx: 5-7 days (*IDSA Guidelines*), 10-14 days (*Amer Acad Ped Guidelines*) • Adjunctive rx: 1) do not use topical decongestant for >3 days; 2) no definite benefit from nasal steroids or antihistamines; 3) saline irrigation may help • Avoid macrolides & TMP-SMX due to resistance • Empiric rx does not target S. aureus: incidence same in pts & controls (*CID 45:e121, 2007*) Potential complications: transient hyposmia, orbital infection, epidural abscess, brain abscess, meningitis, cavernous sinus thrombosis. For other adult drugs and doses, see footnote[21] |
| **Clinical failure after 3 days** | As above; consider diagnostic tap/aspirate | **Mild/Mod. Disease: AM-CL-ER** OR (**Cefpodoxime, Cefprozil,** or **Cefdinir**) *Treat 5-10 days. Adult doses in footnote[21]* | **Severe Disease:** Gati[NUS], Gemi, Levo, Moxi | Severe/hospitalized: **AM-SB** 3 gm IV q6h or **Ceftriaxone** 1-2 gm IV q24h or **Levo** 750 mg IV/po q24h. If no response in 48 hrs, CT sinus & surgical consult. |
| **Diabetes mellitus with acute ketoacidosis; neutropenia; deferoxamine rx: Mucormycosis** | Rhizopus sp. (mucor), aspergillus | See Table 11, pages 131 & 140 | | |
| **Hospitalized + nasotracheal or nasogastric intubation** | Gm-neg. bacilli 47% (pseudomonas, acinetobacter, E. coli common), Gm+ (S. aureus) 35%, yeasts 18%. Polymicrobial in 80% | Remove nasotracheal tube: if fever persists and ENT available, recommend sinus aspiration for C/S & S. aureus PCR prior to empiric therapy **IMP** 0.5 gm IV q6h or **MER** 1 gm IV q8h. Add **Vanco** for MRSA if Gram stain suggestive. | (**Ceftaz** 2 gm IV q8h + **vanco**) or **CFP** 2 gm IV q12h + **Vanco**). | After 7 days of nasotracheal or nasogastric tubes, 95% have x-ray "sinusitis" (fluid in sinuses), but on transnasal puncture only 38% culture + (*AJRCCM 150:776, 1994*). For pts requiring mechanical ventilation with nosocomial sinusitis, bacterial sinusitis occurs in <10% (*CID 27:851, 1998*). May feed fluconazole if yeast on Gram stain of sinus aspirate. |
| **Sinusitis, chronic Adults** **Defined:** (drainage, blockage, facial pain, ↓ sense of smell) + (Polyps, purulence and/or abnormal endoscopy or sinus CT scan: *JAMA 314:926, 2015*) | Multifactorial inflammation of upper airways | Standard maintenance therapy: Saline irrigation + topical corticosteroids | Intermittent/Rescue therapy: For symptomatic exacerbation: oral steroid x 4 wks; for polyps + purulence: **Doxy** 200 mg po x 1 dose, then 100 mg po once daily x 20 days | Leukotriene antagonists considered only for pts with nasal polyps. No antihistamines unless clearly allergic sinusitis. Some suggest >12 wks of macrolide rx; data only supportive; worry about AEs. |

[21] **Adult doses for sinusitis (all oral): AM-CL-ER** 2000/125 mg bid, **amox high-dose (HD)** 1 gm bid, **Clarithro** 500 mg bid or **Clarithro ext. release** 1 gm q24h, **Doxy** 100 mg bid, **respiratory FQs** (**Gati** 400 mg q24h[NUS] due to hypo/hyperglycemia, **Gemi** 320 mg q24h (*not FDA indication but should work*), **Levo** 750 mg q24h x 5 days, **Moxi** 400 mg q24h), **O Ceph** (**Cefdinir** 300 mg q12h or 600 mg q24h, **Cefprozil** 250–500 mg bid, **Cefuroxime** 500 mg bid), **TMP-SMX** 1 double-strength (TMP 160 mg) bid (results after 3- and 10-day rx similar).

Abbreviations on page 2.     *NOTE: All dosage recommendations are for adults (unless otherwise indicated) and assume normal renal function. PK: compliance, local resistance, cost

§ Alternatives consider allergy, PK, compliance, local resistance, cost

**TABLE 1 (50)**

| ANATOMIC SITE/DIAGNOSIS/ MODIFYING CIRCUMSTANCES | ETIOLOGIES (usual) | SUGGESTED REGIMENS* PRIMARY | SUGGESTED REGIMENS* ALTERNATIVE§ | ADJUNCT DIAGNOSTIC OR THERAPEUTIC MEASURES AND COMMENTS |
|---|---|---|---|---|
| **SKIN** See IDSA Guideline: CID 59:147, 2014. | | | | |
| **Acne vulgaris** See IDSA Guideline (Med Lett 2016,58:13; JAMA 2016,316:1402; J Am AcadDerm 2016,74-945). **Dermatology consult recommended.** **BP = benzoyl peroxide; TR = topical retinoid; AB = antibiotic** | | | | |
| **Mild** (all topical therapy). | | BP or TR or (BP + TR) or topical (BP + AB) | Add TR or BP if not used. Consider topical **Dapsone**. | • TR as monotherapy for comedonal acne or with topical AB for mixed or inflammatory acne • **Clinda** & **Erythro** are recommended topical AB • Only use systemic AB if moderate or severe acne that is resistant to topical therapy • Try to limit systemic AB use to 3 mos • Oral isotretinoin should be restricted to severe nodular acne, recalcitrant acne or acne that causes psychosocial distress and/or scarring |
| **Moderate** (topical or combined topical + oral therapy) | | Topical combination therapy: (BP + AB + TR) OR (BP + AB) or (BP + TR) OR Oral/topical combination therapy: (Oral AB + TR + BP + topical AB) | Change combination as in Primary or (if female) add oral contraceptive or oral combination to | |
| **Severe** (oral antibiotic + topical therapy and maybe oral retinoid) | | (Oral AB + topical combination therapy: BP + AB + retinoid) OR (Oral AB + oral isotretinoin) | Consider different oral AB or (if female) add oral contraceptive or oral spironolactone. | |
| **Acne rosacea** Ref: NEJM 2017;377:1754 | Skin mite: Demodex folliculorum (Arch Derm 146:896, 2010) | For Erythema stage: generic **Metro** gel or cream bid x 8-12 weeks | Papulopustular: **Ivermectin (Soolantra)** 1% cream once daily x 8-12 weeks (Expensive) | Systemic oral therapy reserved for severe disease, e.g., **Doxy** 40 mg (low dose) once daily +/- **isotretinoin** 0.1-0.5 mg/kg/d (low dose) x 6-8 mos. Many other therapy options, see NEJM 2017;377:1754. |
| **Anthrax, cutaneous** **To report bioterrorism event:** 770-488-7100; **For info:** www.bt.cdc.gov Treat as inhalation anthrax if systemic illness. Refs: JAMA 2002,287:2236 Refs: ARCC4 18;41333, 2011 (Review): CID 59:147, 2014 (Clinical Prac. Guideline); Pediatrics 133:e1411, 2014. | B. anthracis Spores are introduced into/ under the skin by contact with infected animals/animal products. See Lung, page 44. | **Adults:** CIP 500 mg po q12h or **Doxy** 10 mg po q12h. **Peds:** CIP 15 mg/kg (max dose 500 mg) po q12h or for pen-susceptible strain **Amox** 25 mg/kg (max dose 1 gm) po q8h For bioterrorism exposure, 3-dose series of Biothrax Anthrax Vaccine Adsorbed is indicated. | | 1. Duration of therapy 60 days for bioterrorism event because of potential inhalational exposure and 7-10 days for naturally acquired disease. 2. Consider alternative to Doxy for pregnancy: 3. Alternatives for adults: Levo 750 mg q24h or Moxi 400 mg q24h or Clinda 600 mg q8h or for pen-susceptible strains Amox 1 gm q8h or Pen VK 500 mg q6h. 4. Alternatives for children: Doxy 2.2 mg/kg (max dose 100 mg) q12h (tooth staining likely with 60-day regimen age <8 years) or Clindamycin 10 mg/kg (max dose 600 mg) q8h or Levo 8 mg/kg q12h (max dose 250 mg) if <50 kg and 500 mg q24h if >50 kg |
| **Bacillary angiomatosis:** For other Bartonella infections, see Cat-scratch disease lymphadenitis, page 48, and Bartonella systemic infections, page 61 | | | | |
| In immunocompromised (HIV-1, bone marrow transplant) patients | Bartonella henselae and quintana | **Clarithro** 500 mg po bid or ext. release 1 gm po q24h or **Azithro** 250 mg po q24h (see Comment) | **Erythro** 500 mg po bid or **Doxy** 100 mg po bid or (**Doxy** 100 mg po bid + **RIF** 300 mg po bid) | For AIDS pts, continue suppressive therapy until HIV treated and CD4 >200 cells/μL for 6 mos. **Drugs to avoid:** TMP-SMX, CIP, Pen, cephalosporins. |

*NOTE: All dosage recommendations are for adults (unless otherwise indicated) and assume normal/renal function. § Alternatives consider allergy, PK, compliance, local resistance, cost.

TABLE 1 (51)

| ANATOMIC SITE/DIAGNOSIS/ MODIFYING CIRCUMSTANCES | ETIOLOGIES (usual) | SUGGESTED REGIMENS* | | ADJUNCT DIAGNOSTIC OR THERAPEUTIC MEASURES AND COMMENTS |
|---|---|---|---|---|
| | | PRIMARY | ALTERNATIVE§ | |
| **SKIN** *(continued)* | | | | |
| **Bite: Remember tetanus prophylaxis**— *See Table 20B, page 254 for rabies prophylaxis.* Review: *CMR 24:231, 2011.* **Avoid primary wound closure.** | | | | |
| **Alligator** *(Alligator mississipiensis)* | Gram negatives including Aeromonas hydrophila, Clostridium sp. | Severe wound: Surgical debridement + **CIP 400 mg IV q12h** (or **Levo 750 mg po bid or** IV/750 mg po bid or **AM-SB** 3 gm IV q6h; **OR Pip-Tazo** 4.5 g m IV q8h) | Severe wound: Surgical debridement + (**TMP-SMX** 8-10 mg/kg/day IV div q6h or q8h + **AM-CL** 875/125 mg po bid or 500/125 mg po bid | Oral flora of American alligator isolated: Aeromonas hydrophila and other gram-negatives, and anaerobes including Clostridium spp (*S Med J 82:262, 1989*). |
| | | | **Cefepime 2 gm IV q8h + Metro 500 mg q8h**) | |
| | | **AM-CL** 875/125 mg po bid or 500/125 mg po bid | **Doxy** 100 mg po bid | |
| **Bat, raccoon, skunk** | Strep & staph from skin; rabies | | | In Americas, **anti-rabies rx indicated:** rabies immune globulin + vaccine. (*See Table 20B, page 254*). |
| **Bear** | S. aureus, coagulase-negative staph, viridans streptococci, Enterobacteriaceae, Aeromonas, B. cereus, Neisseria spp, L. durans (*Clin Microbiol Rev 24: 231, 2011*) | **PIP-TZ** 4.5 gm IV q8h | **Vanco** IV (trough 15-20 mcg/mL) + (**Cefepime** 2 gm IV OR **CIP** 400 mg IV q8-12h) + **Metro** 500 mg q8h **OR AM-CL** 875 mg po bid + **CIP** 500-750 mg po bid. | Injuries often result in hospital level care. Infection with Mycobacterium fortuitum reported (*J Clin Micro 43: 1009, 2005*). Rabies occurs in bears (*MMWR 48: 761, 1999*). |
| **Camel** | S. aureus, Streptococcus spp, P. aeruginosa, Other Gm-neg bacilli | **PIP-TZ** 4.5 gm q8h | **Cephalexin** 500 mg po bid + **CIP** 750 mg bid | See *EJCMID 18:918, 1999.* Rabies can occur in camels (*PLoS Negl Trop Dis. 2016; 10(9): e00048900*). |
| **Cat:** 80% get infected, culture & treat empirically. | **Pasteurella multocida**, Streptococci, Staph. aureus, Neisseria, Moraxella. | **AM-CL** 875/125 mg po bid 1000/62.5 mg 2 tabs po bid | **Cefuroxime axetil** 0.5 gm po q12h or **Doxy** 100 mg po bid. **Do not use cephalexin.** Sens. to FQs in vitro. | **P. multocida resistant to dicloxacillin, cephalexin, clinda; many strains resistant to erythro** (most sensitive to azithro but no clinical data). P. multocida infection develops within 24 hrs. Observe for osteomyelitis. If culture + for only P. multocida, can switch to pen G IV or pen VK po, *See Dog Bite.* |
| Cat-scratch disease: *page 48* | | | | |
| **Catfish sting** | Toxins (pain may respond to immersion in hot water as tolerated) Evaluate for retained foreign body (spine) May become secondarily infected | **Doxy** 100 mg po bid + **AM-CL** 875/125 mg po bid | **Doxy** 100 mg po bid | Toxin injury presents as immediate pain, erythema, edema; resembles strep cellulitis. May become infected with marine organisms or staphylococci (*CID 14: 689, 1992*). |
| **Dog:** Only 5% get infected; treat only if bite severe or bad co-morbidity (e.g. diabetes). | **Pasteurella canis**, S. aureus, Fusobacterium sp, Capnocytophaga canimorsus. | **AM-CL** 875/125 mg po bid 1000/62.5 mg 2 tabs po bid | Adult: **Clinda** 300 mg po q6h Child: **Clinda + TMP-SMX** | Consider anti-rabies prophylaxis: rabies immune globulin + vaccine (*see Table 20B*). Capnocytophaga in splenectomized pts may cause local eschar, sepsis with DIC. **P. canis resistant to diclox, cephalexin, clinda and erythro;** sensitive to Ceftriaxone, cefuroxime, cefpodoxime and FQs. |
| **Horse** | Actinobacillus, Pasteurella, Enteric Gram negative bacilli, S. aureus, streptococci, anaerobes | **AM-CL** 875/125 mg po bid | **Doxy** 100 mg po bid | Debridement often needed. IV antibiotics may be needed for severe wounds. Strep. equi meningitis and brain abscess reported (*Lancet 376: 1194, 2010*) |

*Abbreviations on page 2.   *NOTE: All dosage recommendations are for adults (unless otherwise indicated) and assume normal renal function. § Alternatives consider allergy, PK, compliance, local resistance, cost.*

**TABLE 1 (52)**

| ANATOMIC SITE/DIAGNOSIS/ MODIFYING CIRCUMSTANCES | ETIOLOGIES (usual) | SUGGESTED REGIMENS* | | ADJUNCT DIAGNOSTIC OR THERAPEUTIC MEASURES AND COMMENTS |
|---|---|---|---|---|
| | | PRIMARY | ALTERNATIVE§ | |
| **SKIN/Bite (continued)** | | | | |
| **Human** For bacteriology, see CID 37:1481, 2003 | Viridans strep 100%, Staph epidermidis 53%, corynebacterium 41%, **eikenella 29%**, bacteroides 82%, peptostrep 26% | **Early** (not yet infected): **AM-CL** 875/125 mg po bid times 5 days. **Later:** Signs of infection (usually in 3-24 hrs): (**AM-SB** 1.5 gm IV q6h or **Cefoxitin** 2 gm IV q8h or (**PIP-TZ** 3.375 gm IV q6h or 4.5 gm q8h or 4-hr infusion of 3.375 gm q8h). Pen allergy: **Clinda** + (either **CIP** or **TMP-SMX**) | **PIP-TZ** 4.5 gm IV q8h | **Cleaning, irrigation and debridement most important.** For clenched fist injuries, x-rays should be obtained. Bites inflicted by hospitalized pts, consider aerobic Gm-neg. bacilli. **Eikenella resistant to clinda, nafcillin/ oxacillin, metro, P Ceph 1, and erythro; susceptible to FQs and TMP-SMX.** |
| **Komodo dragon** | Staphylococcus spp, Bacillus spp, Aeromonas, Pseudomonas spp, Enterobacteriaceae, Burkholderia, anaerobes | **AM-CL** 875 mg po bid plus **CIP** 750 mg po bid | | Microbiology: see CMR 24: 231, 2011. Also have toxic venom (PNAS 106: 8969, 2009). |
| **Leech (Medicinal)** (Ln 381:1686, 2013) | Aeromonas hydrophila | **CIP** (400 mg IV or 750 mg po) bid + **Doxy** 100 mg IV/po bid | **TMP-SMX DS** 1 tab po bid | Aeromonas in GI tract of leeches. Some use prophylactic antibiotics when leeches used medicinally. |
| **Pig** (swine) | Polymicrobic Gm+ cocci, Gm-neg. bacilli, anaerobes, Pasteurella sp, Actinobacillus suis. | **AM-CL** 875/125 mg po bid | **P Ceph 3** or **AM-SB** or **IMP** | Information limited but infection is common and serious (Ln 348:888, 1996). Pigs may be colonized with MRSA (Clin Microbiol Rev 24: 231, 2011). Potential pathogens include Streptococcus suis leading to meningitis (NEJM 354: 1325, 2006; Rinsho Shinkeigaku 53:732, 2013) |
| **Prairie dog** | Monkeypox | See Table 14A, page 186. No rx recommended | | Tularemia and bubonic plague reported after prairie dog bites. |
| **Primate, Monkey, non-human** See Table 14A, Herpes simiae. | Herpesvirus simiae | **Valacyclovir** (PEP) or **Acyclovir** or **Ganciclovir** | | From macaques, risk of infection with herpes B virus; rare but potentially fatal encephalitis/myelitis (CID 35: 1191, 2002). Potential risk of rabies. Bacteria similar to human bites (CID 24: 231, 2011); for deep bites, can use antibiotics as for human bites. |
| **Rat** | Spirillum minus & Streptobacillus moniliformis | **AM-CL** 875/125 mg po bid | **Doxy** 100 mg po bid | Anti-rabies rx not indicated. Causes rat bite fever (Streptobacillus moniliformis): Pen G or doxy, alternatively erythro or clinda. |
| **Seal** | Marine mycoplasma | **Tetracycline** or **Doxy** for 2-4 wks | | Can take weeks to appear after bite. Disseminated disease reported (CID 62:491, 2016). Differential includes sealpox, resembling Orf (Br J Derm 152: 791, 2005) and other bacteria: Bisgaardia hudsonensis (J Infect 63: 86, 2011) and Streptococcus halichoeri (J Clin Microbiol 54: 739, 2016). |
| **Snake: pit viper** (Ref.: NEJM 347:347, 2002) | Pseudomonas sp, Enterobacteriaceae, Staph. aureus and epidermidis, Clostridium sp. | **Primary therapy is antivenom.** (Am J Med 2018;131:1367). **PIP/Tazo** (Emerg Clin N Amer 35: 339, 2017). | | Tetanus prophylaxis indicated. No need for antibiotic prophylaxis (J Clin Microbiol 54: 739, 2016). Adjust per culture results |
| **Spider bite:** Most necrotic ulcers attributed to spiders are probably due to another cause, e.g., cutaneous anthrax (Ln 364:549, 2004) or **MRSA infection** (spider bite painful; anthrax not painful.) | | | | |
| **Widow** (Latrodectus) | Not infectious | None | | May be confused with "acute abdomen". Diazepam or calcium gluconate helpful to control pain, muscle spasm. Tetanus prophylaxis. |
| **Brown recluse** (Loxosceles) NEJM 352:700, 2005 | Not infectious. Overdiagnosed! Spider distribution limited to Central & desert SW of US. | Bite usually self-limited & self-healing. Rx of proven efficacy. **Dapsone** 50 mg po q24h often used despite marginal supportive data | | Dapsone causes hemolysis (check for G6PD deficiency). Can cause hepatitis; baseline & weekly liver panels suggested. |
| **Swan** | P aeruginosa | **CIP** 750 mg po bid | | Case report of P aeruginosa infection (Lancet 350: 340, 1997). However, other aquatic organisms or host skin organisms have potential to cause infection. |
| **Tasmanian devil** | Pasteurella multocida (CID 14: 1266, 1992) | Treat as cat bite | | 15% of P multocida from devils were TMP-SMX resistant (Lett Appl Microbiol 62: 237, 2016) |

Abbreviations on page 2.    *NOTE: All dosage recommendations are for adults (unless otherwise indicated) and assume normal renal function. § Alternatives consider allergy, PK, compliance, local resistance, cost.

TABLE 1 (53)

| ANATOMIC SITE/DIAGNOSIS/ MODIFYING CIRCUMSTANCES | ETIOLOGIES (usual) | SUGGESTED REGIMENS* PRIMARY | SUGGESTED REGIMENS* ALTERNATIVE§ | ADJUNCT DIAGNOSTIC OR THERAPEUTIC MEASURES AND COMMENTS |
|---|---|---|---|---|
| **SKIN** (continued) | | | | |
| **Boils—Furunculosis** | | | | |
| Active lesions *See Table 6, page 90* | Staph. aureus, both MSSA & MRSA. *IDSA Guidelines: CID 59:147, 2014* | **Boils and abscesses** uncomplicated (e.g., no immunosuppression) **I&D + TMP/SMX 1 DS** (if BMI >40) bid or **I&D + Clinda** 300 mg bid equally efficacious (see *NEJM 372:1093, 2015, NEJM 2016, 374-823; and NEJM 375:2545, 2017*). **Incision and Drainage mainstay of therapy!** | | Other options: **Doxy** 100 mg po bid for 5–10 days; **Fusidic acid**ⁿᵘˢ 250–500 mg po q8–12h ± **RIF**. **Cephalexin** 500 mg po tid-qid or **Dicloxacillin** 500 mg po tid-qid, only in low prevalence setting for MRSA. Also: **Dalbavancin** 1.5 gm IV x 1 or **Oritavancin** 1200 mg IV x 1. If dx uncertainty or assessing adequacy of I&D, ultrasound is helpful (*NEJM 370:1039, 2014*). **NOTE: needle aspiration is inadequate.** |
| To lessen number of furuncle recurrences —decolonization *For surgical prophylaxis, see Table 15B, page 219.* | MSSA & MRSA. *IDSA Guidelines: CID 59:e10, 2014* | 7-day therapy: **Chlorhexidine** (2%) washes daily; 2% **Mupirocin ointment** anterior nares 2x daily | **Mupirocin ointment** in anterior nares bid x 7 days + **Chlorhexidine** (2%) washes daily x 7 days + (**TMP-SMX DS** 1 tab po bid + **Doxy** 100 mg po bid) x 7 days | Optimal regimen uncertain. Can substitute bleach baths for chlorhexidine (*Inf Control Hosp Epidemiol 32:872, 2011*) but only modest effect (*CID 58:679, 2014*). In vitro resistance of mupirocin & retapamulin roughly 10% (*AAC 56:2878, 2014*). One review found mupirocin resistance ranging from 1–81% (*JAC 70:2681, 2015*). |
| **Burns.** Overall management: ISBI Practice Guideline (Burns): *Burns 2016;42:953.* | | | | |
| Initial wound care Use burn unit, if available Topical rx options (*NEJM 359:1037, 2008; Clin Plastic Surg 36:597, 2009*) | **Not infected** Prophylaxis for potential pathogens: Gm-pos cocci Gm-neg bacilli Candida | Early excision & wound closure. Variety of skin grafts/substitutes. Shower hydrotherapy. Topical antimicrobials | Silver sulfadiazine cream 1% applied 1-2 x daily. Minimal pain. Transient reversible neutropenia due to margination in burn – not marrow toxicity | Mafenide acetate cream is an alternative but painful to apply. Anti-tetanus prophylaxis indicated. **Severe burn rx on ventilator:** prophylactic AM-SB or Cefazolin may reduce mortality (*CID 62:60 & 67, 2016*). |
| Burn wound sepsis | Strep. pyogenes, Enterobacter sp., S. aureus, S. epidermidis, E. faecalis, E. coli, P. aeruginosa Fungi (rare). Herpesvirus (rare). | **Vanco** high dose to rapidly achieve trough concentration of 15-20 μg/mL + (**MER** 1 gm IV q8h or **Cefepime** 2 gm IV q8h) + **Fluconazole** 6 mg/kg IV qd *See Comments for alternatives* | **Vanco** 15 mg/kg (actual wt) IV q8-12h (to achieve target trough concentration of 15-20 μg/mL x 7-10 days | Vanco allergic/intolerant: **Dapto** 6-10 mg/kg IV qd IgE mediated allergy to beta lactams: **Aztreonam** 2 gm IV q8h ESBL: use a carbapenem; carbapenemase-producer: **Ceftaz-avi or MER-vabor** (*See Table 5B*) |
| **Cellulitis, erysipelas: NOTE:** Consider diseases that masquerade as cellulitis; e.g. stasis dermatitis (*Clev Clin J Med 79:547, 2012*) | | | | |
| Extremities, non-diabetic. *For diabetes, see below.* Practice guidelines: *CID 59:147, 2014.* **NOTE:** stasis dermatitis can masquerade as erysipelas (*J Am Acad Derm 2015;73-70*) | Streptococcus sp., Groups A, B, C & G, Staph. aureus, including MRSA (but rare). Strep sp: No purulence. Staph sp: Purulence. Etiologic study (*OFID, doi 10.1093 OFID/OFV18T*) | **Inpatient:** Elevate legs. **Pen G** 1-2 million units IV q6h or **Cefazolin** 1 gm IV q8h. If Pen allergic (not IgE mediated): **Cefazolin.** If IgE mediated: **Vanco.** | **Outpatient: Elevate legs. Pen VK** 500 mg po qid, & hs or **Cephalexin** 500 mg qid x 7-10 days. **Pen-allergic: Azithro** 500 mg x 1 dose, then 250 mg once daily x 4 days (total 5 days). Rarely, **Linezolid** 600 mg po bid or **Tedizolid** 200 mg po q24h or **Dalba** 1000 mg po q12h x 5-14 days. | • Erysipelas: Elevate legs, treat T. pedis if present, if no purulence, no need for culture • If unsure as to presence of deep abscess, bedside ultrasound can help. • If present: (furunculosis (boils) • **TMP-SMX 1 DS** bid OR **Clinda** 300 mg for uncomplicated cellulitis in non-diabetic outpatients (*NEJM 372:2460, 2015*) • **Oritavancin** 1200 mg IV x1 OR **Dalbavancin** 1.5 gm IV x 1 also effective for outpatient therapy of more severe infections in patients who might otherwise be admitted to the hospital. (see *NEJM 370:2180, 2014, NEJM 370:2169, 2014*) • No benefit of adding **TMP-SMX** to Cephalexin for MRSA coverage (*JAMA 317:2088, 2017*). |
| Facial, adult (erysipelas) | Strep. sp. (Grp A, B, C & G), Staph. aureus (to include MRSA), S. pneumo | **Vanco** 15 mg/kg (actual wt) IV q8-12h (to achieve target trough concentration of 15-20 μg/mL x 7-10 days | **Dapto** 4 mg/kg IV q 24h or **Linezolid** 600 mg IV q 12h. Treat 7-10 days if not bacteremic | **Choice of empiric therapy** must have activity vs. **S. aureus.** S. aureus can mimic streptococcal erysipelas of an extremity. Forced to treat empirically for MRSA until in vitro susceptibilities available. |

*Abbreviations on page 2.* *NOTE: All dosage recommendations are for adults (unless otherwise indicated) and assume normal renal function. §Alternatives consider allergy, PK, compliance, local resistance, cost.*

**TABLE 1 (54)**

| ANATOMIC SITE/DIAGNOSIS/ MODIFYING CIRCUMSTANCES | ETIOLOGIES (usual) | SUGGESTED REGIMENS* | | ADJUNCT DIAGNOSTIC OR THERAPEUTIC MEASURES AND COMMENTS |
|---|---|---|---|---|
| | | PRIMARY | ALTERNATIVE§ | |
| **SKIN** (continued) | | | | |
| **Diabetes mellitus and erysipelas** (See Foot, "Diabetic", page 18) | Strep. sp. (Grp A, B, C & G), Staph. aureus, Enterobacteriaceae; Anaerobes | **Early mild: TMP-SMX** 1-2 tabs po bid + (**Pen VK** 500 mg po qid or **Cephalexin** 500 mg po qid). **For severe disease: IMP, MER, Erta** or **Dori IV + (Linezolid** 600 mg IV/po bid or **vanco** IV or **dapto** 4 mg/kg IV q 24h). *Dosage, page 18, Diabetic foot* | **(Pen VK** 500 mg po bid + | Prompt surgical debridement indicated to rule out necrotizing fasciitis and to obtain cultures. If septic, obtain x-ray of extremity to demonstrate gas. **Prognosis dependent on blood supply: assess arteries.** See *diabetic foot, page 18.* For severe disease, use regimen that targets both aerobic gram-neg bacilli & MRSA. Caution re hyperaremia with TMP-SMX in those with reduced renal function or concomitant drugs causing hyperkalemia. |
| **Erysipelas 2° to lymphedema** (congenital = Milroy's disease); post-breast surgery with lymph node dissection | Streptococcus sp. Groups A, C, G | **Benzathine pen G** 1.2 million units IM q4 wks or **Pen VK** 500 mg po bid or **Azithro** 250 mg po qd | | Indicated only if pt is having frequent episodes of cellulitis. Benefit in controlled clinical trial *(NEJM 368:1695, 2013).* |
| **Erythema multiforme** | H. simplex type 1, mycoplasma, Strep. pyogenes, drugs (sulfonamides, phenytoin, penicillins) | | | Treat underlying disorder / Remove offending drug; symptomatic. Rx. |
| **Erythema nodosum** | Sarcoidosis, inflammatory bowel disease, MTB, coccidioidomycosis, yersinia, sulfonamides, Whipple's disease. | | | **Rx: NSAIDs; glucocorticoids** if refractory. Identify and treat precipitant disease if possible. |
| **Erythrasma** | Corynebacterium minutissimum | **Localized infection: Topical Clinda** 2-3 x daily x 7-14 days | **Widespread infection: Clarithro** 500 mg po bid or **Erythro** 250 mg po bid) x 14 days | Dx: Coral red fluorescence with Wood's lamp. If infection recurs, prophylactic bathing with anti-bacterial soap or wash with benzyl peroxide. One-time dose of Clari 1 gm po reported to be effective *(Intl J Derm 52:576, 2013).* **Clarithro** 1 gm po x 1 reported to be effective x 2-4 weeks reported to be effective. |
| **Folliculitis** | S. aureus, candida, P. aeruginosa common | Usually self-limited; no Rx needed. Could use topical mupirocin for Staph and topical antifungal for Candida. | | |
| **Furunculosis** | Staph. aureus | See Boils, page 57 | | |
| **Hemorrhagic bullous lesions** Hx of sea water-contaminated abrasion or eating raw seafood in cirrhotic pt. | Vibrio vulnificus | **Ceftriaxone** 2 gm IV q24h + (**Doxy** or **Minocycline**) 100 mg po/IV bid. Peds: Doxy 4.4 mg/kg/day div bid (safe regardless of age for rx ≤21 days) *(AAP Redbook 2018)* | **CIP** 750 mg po bid or 400 mg IV bid OR **Levo** 750 mg IV q24h | Wound infection in healthy hosts, but bacteremia mostly in cirrhotics or use of TNF-inhibitors. Pathogenesis: Exposure to contaminated seawater. Can cause necrotizing fasciitis. Surgical debridement needed. Ref: *NEJM 2016,375:1780.* |
| **Herpes zoster** (shingles): See Table 14A | | | | |

*NOTE: All dosage recommendations are for adults (unless otherwise indicated) and assume normal renal function. § Alternatives consider allergy, PK compliance, local resistance, cost.

**TABLE 1 (55)**

| ANATOMIC SITE/DIAGNOSIS/ MODIFYING CIRCUMSTANCES | ETIOLOGIES (usual) | SUGGESTED REGIMENS* PRIMARY | ALTERNATIVE§ | ADJUNCT DIAGNOSTIC OR THERAPEUTIC MEASURES AND COMMENTS |
|---|---|---|---|---|
| **SKIN** (continued) | | | | |
| **Impetigo**—See CID 59-147, 2014. | | | | |
| "Honey-crust" lesions (non-bullous). Ecthyma is closely related. Causes "punched out" skin lesions. | **Group A strep** impetigo (rarely Strept. sp. Groups B, C or G); crusted lesions can be Staph. aureus + streptococci. Staph. aureus may be secondary colonizer. | **Few lesions: (Mupirocin** ointment 2% tid or **fusidic acid cream**[NUS] [EU] 2%, OR **retapamulin** ointment, 1% bid. Treat for 5 days | **Numerous lesions: Pen VK** 250-500 mg po q6h x 5 days or **Benzathine Pen** 600,000 units IM x 1 or **TMP-SMX** po x 3-5 days (Lancet 384:2132, 2014) | **Topical rx:** OTC ointments (bacitracin, neomycin, polymyxin B) not as effective as prescription ointments. For mild disease, topical rx as good as po antibiotics (Cochrane Database Syst Rev C0003261, 2012). **Ecthyma:** Infection deeper into epidermis than impetigo. May need parenteral penicillin. Military outbreaks reported: CID 48: 1213 & 1220, 2009 (good images). |
| Bullous (if ruptured), thin "varnish-like" crust | Staph. aureus MSSA & MRSA: strains that produce exfoliative toxin A. | **For MSSA:** po therapy with Diclox, Oxacillin, Cephalexin, AM-CL, Clinda, TMP-SMX-DS, OR Mupirocin ointment OR Retapamulin ointment | **For MRSA: Mupirocin** ointment OR po therapy with, TMP-SMX-DS, Minocycline, Doxy, Clinda. Treat for 7 days | |
| | | For dosages, see Table 10A | | |
| **Infected wound, extremity—Post-trauma** (for bites, see page 55; for post-operative, see below)—Gram stain negative | | | | |
| Mild to moderate; uncomplicated. Debride wound, if necessary. | Polymicrobic: S. aureus (MSSA & MRSA), aerobic & anaerobic strep. | **Clinda** 300-450 mg po tid | **Minocycline** 100 mg po bid or **linezolid** 600 mg po bid | **Culture & sensitivity, check Gram stain. Tetanus toxoid if indicated. Mild infection:** Suggested drugs focus on S. aureus & Strep species. If suspect Gm-neg. bacilli, add **AM-CL-ER** 1000/62.5 two tabs po bid. |
| Febrile with sepsis—hospitalized Debride wound, if necessary. | Enterobacteriaceae, C. perfringens, C. tetani; if water exposure, Pseudomonas sp., Aeromonas sp. | **[PIP-TZ** or **Dori**[NUS] OR **IMP** or **MER** or **Erta** (Dosage, page 27)] + **Vanco** 15-20 mg/kg q8-12h | **(Vanco** 15-20 mg/kg IV q8-12h OR **Dapto** 6 mg/kg IV q 24h OR **Ceftaroline 600 mg IV q12h OR Televancin** 10 mg/kg IV q24h) + **CIP** 400 mg IV q12h (q8h if P. aeruginosa) OR **Levo** 750 mg IV q24h) | If MRSA is erythro-resistant, may have inducible resistance to clinda. **Fever—sepsis:** Another alternative is **Linezolid** 600 mg IV/po q12h. If Gm-neg. bacilli & severe pen allergy, **CIP** or **Levo** |
| **Infected wound, post-operative—Gram stain positive cocci - see below** | | | | |
| **Surgery not involving GI or female genital tract** | | | | |
| Without sepsis (mild, afebrile) | Staph. aureus, Group A, B, C or G strep sp. | **Clinda** 300-450 mg po tid | **Dapto** 4 mg per kg IV q24h or **televancin** 10 mg/kg IV q24h | **Check Gram stain of exudate.** If Gm-neg. bacilli, **add** β-lactam/β-lactamase inhibitor: **AM-CL-ER** po or (**ERTA** or **PIP-TZ**) IV. Dosage on page 27. |
| With sepsis (severe, febrile) | | **Vanco** 15-20 mg/kg IV q8-12h (to achieve target trough concentration of 15-20 µg/mL) | | |
| **Surgery involving GI tract** (includes oropharynx, esophagus) or female genital tract—fever, neutrophilia | MSSA/MRSA, coliforms, bacteroides & other anaerobes | **[PIP-TZ** (**P. Ceph 3 + Metro**) or **Dori** or **IMP** or **MER**] + (**Vanco** 1 gm IV q12h or **Dapto** 6 mg/kg IV q 24h) if severely ill. **Mild infection: AM-CL-ER** 1000/62.5 mg 2 tabs po bid + TMP-SMX-DS 1-2 tabs po bid if Gm+ cocci on Gram stain. Dosages Table 10A & footnote 23, page 66. | | **For all treatment options, see Peritonitis, page 49.** Most important: Drain wound & get cultures. Can sub **Linezolid** for vanco. Can sub **CIP** or **Levo** if local susceptibility permits. |
| **Meleney's synergistic gangrene** | See Necrotizing Fasciitis, page 60 | | | |

Abbreviations on page 2.     *NOTE: All dosage recommendations are for adults (unless otherwise indicated) and assume normal renal function. §Alternatives consider allergy, PK, compliance, local resistance, cost.

**TABLE 1 (56)**

| ANATOMIC SITE/DIAGNOSIS/ MODIFYING CIRCUMSTANCES | ETIOLOGIES (usual) | SUGGESTED REGIMENS* | | ADJUNCT DIAGNOSTIC OR THERAPEUTIC MEASURES AND COMMENTS |
|---|---|---|---|---|
| | | PRIMARY | ALTERNATIVE$ | |
| **SKIN/Infected wound, post-operative—Gram stain negative** *(continued)* | | | | |
| **Infected wound, post-op, febrile patient— Positive gram stain: Gram-positive cocci in clusters** | S. aureus, possibly MRSA | **Do culture & sensitivity: open & drain wound**<br><br>**Oral:** TMP-SMX-DS 1 tab bid or **Clinda** 300–450 mg po tid *(see Comment)* | **IV:** Vanco 15-20 mg/kg q8-12h or **Dapto** 4-6 mg/kg IV q24h or **Ceftaroline** 600 mg IV q12h or **Telavancin** 10 mg/kg IV q24h | Need culture & sensitivity to verify MRSA. Other po options for CA-MRSA include **minocycline** 100 mg po q12h or **Doxy** 100 mg po q12h or **linezolid** 600 mg po q12h. If MRSA clinda-sensitive but erythro-resistant, watch out for inducible clinda resistance. Dalbavancin and oritavancin recently FDA approved for treatment of acute bacterial skin and skin structure infections are single-dose options for parenteral out-patient therapy. |
| **Necrotizing fasciitis ("flesh-eating bacteria")** Reviews: *Infect Dis Clin N Amer 2017;31:497; NEJM 2017;377:2253.* | | | | |
| Post-surgery, trauma, or strepto-coccal skin infections<br><br>*See Gas gangrene, page 49, & Toxic shock, page 68.*<br>*Refs: NEJM 2017;377:2253;*<br>*IDSA Guidelines: CID 2014;59:e10* | **5 types:** (1) Strep sp., Grp A; (2) Clostridia sp.; (3) polymicrobic: aerobic + anaerobic (if S. aureus + anaerobic strep = Meleney's synergistic gangrene); (4) MRSA; (5) V. vulnificus; (6) Klebsiella sp; (7) Aeromonas sp. | *For treatment of clostridia, see Muscle, gas gangrene, page 49.*<br>Meleney's synergistic gangrene, Fournier's gangrene, necrotizing fasciitis have common pathophysiology. **All require prompt surgical debridement + antibiotics.** Dx of necrotizing fasciitis req incision & probing of fascial plane. **Need Gram stain/culture** to determine if etiology is strep, clostridia, polymicrobial, or S. aureus.<br>**Treatment: Pen G** if strep or clostridia, **IMP** or **MER** if polymicrobial, add **Vanco OR Dapto** if MRSA suspected.<br>**NOTE: If strep necrotizing fasciitis,** treat with **penicillin & clinda** (900 mg IV q6h). **if clostridia ± gas gangrene,** add **clinda**, *page 68.* IVIG not recommended.<br>*(see page 49).* **See toxic shock syndrome, streptococcal, page 68.** | | |
| **Puncture wound—nail, toothpick** | Through tennis shoe: P. aeruginosa | Local debridement to remove foreign body & tetanus prophylaxis; no antibiotic therapy. | | Osteomyelitis evolves in only 1–2% of plantar puncture wounds. Consider x-ray if chance of radio-opaque foreign body. |
| **Staphylococcal scalded skin syndrome**<br>Ref: *PIDJ 19:819, 2000* | Toxin-producing S. aureus | **Nafcillin/Oxacillin** 2 gm IV q4h (children: 150 mg/kg / day div. q6h) x 5–7 days for MSSA. **Vanco** 15-20 mg/kg q8-12h (children 40–60 mg/kg/day div. q6h) for MRSA | | Toxin causes **intraepidermal split** and positive Nikolsky sign. Biopsy differentiates: drugs cause epidermal/dermal split, **called toxic epidermal necrolysis**—more serious. |
| **Ulcerated skin lesions:** | Consider: anthrax, tularemia, P. aeruginosa (ecthyma gangrenosum), plague, blastomycosis, spider (rarely), mucormycosis, mycobacteria, leishmania, YAWS; arterial insufficiency, venous stasis, and others. | | | |
| Ulcerated skin: venous/arterial insufficiency; pressure (infected decubiti)<br>Care of non-healing, non-infected ulcers (AnIM 159:532, 2013; AnIM 162:S39, 2015). | Polymicrobic: Streptococcus sp. (Groups A, C, G), enterococci; anaerobic strep, Enterobacteriaceae, Pseudomonas sp., Bacteroides sp., Staph. aureus | Severe local or possible bacteremia: **IMP** or **MER** or **Dori** or **PIP-TZ**.<br>If Gm-pos cocci on gram stain, add **Vanco.** | [**CIP** (or **Levo**) + **Metro**] or<br>[**CFP** (or **Ceftaz**) + **Metro**].<br>If Gm-pos cocci on gram stain, add **Vanco.**<br>*Dosages, see footnotes 4, 5, 6, 9, 11, 24* | • If ulcer clinically inflamed, treat IV with no topical rx. If not clinically inflamed, consider debridement, removal of foreign body, lessening direct pressure for weight-bearing limbs & leg elevation (if no arterial insufficiency).<br>• Society of Vascular Surgery guidelines recommend against routine use of topical antimicrobials (*J Vasc Surg 60 (2 Suppl): 3S, 2014*).<br>Silver sulfadiazine 1% cream: insufficient evidence.<br>**Chlorhexidine & povidone iodine may harm "granulation tissue"—Avoid.** If not inflamed, healing improved on air bed, protein supplement, radiant heat, electrical stimulation (*AnIM 159:39, 2013*). |
| **Whirlpool: (Hot Tub) folliculitis** | Pseudomonas aeruginosa | Usually self-limited, treatment not indicated | | Decontaminate hot tub: drain and chlorinate. Also associated with exfoliative beauty aids (loofah sponges). |
| **Whirlpool: Nail Salon, soft tissue infection** | Mycobacterium (fortuitum or chelonae) | Minocycline, **Doxy** or **CIP** | | For more serious or progressive infection see recommendations for M. fortuitum. |
| **SPLEEN. For post-splenectomy prophylaxis,** see Table 15A, page 217; for Septic Shock Post-Splenectomy, see Table 1, page 68. Vaccines: CID 58:309, 2014. | | | | |
| **Splenic abscess** | Staph. aureus, streptococci | **Nafcillin/Oxacillin** 2 gm IV q4h or **Cefazolin** 2 gm IV q8h if MSSA | **Vanco** 15-20 mg/kg IV q8-12h (target trough concentration of 15-20 μg/mL). | Burkholderia (Pseudomonas) pseudomallei is common cause of splenic abscess in SE Asia. Presents with fever and LUQ pain. Usual treatment is antimicrobial therapy and splenectomy. |
| **Endocarditis, bacteremia** | | | | |

*Abbreviations on page 2.*    *NOTE: All dosage recommendations are for adults (unless otherwise indicated) and assume normal renal function. § Alternatives consider allergy, PK, compliance, local resistance, cost.*

TABLE 1 (57)

| ANATOMIC SITE/DIAGNOSIS/ MODIFYING CIRCUMSTANCES | ETIOLOGIES (usual) | SUGGESTED REGIMENS* | | ADJUNCT DIAGNOSTIC OR THERAPEUTIC MEASURES AND COMMENTS |
|---|---|---|---|---|
| | | PRIMARY | ALTERNATIVE§ | |
| **SPLEEN/Splenic abscess** (continued) | | | | |
| Contiguous from intra-abdominal site | Polymicrobic | *Treat as Peritonitis, secondary, page 49* | | |
| Immunocompromised | Candida sp. | Amphotericin B | Fluconazole, caspofungin | *See Candida, Table 11* |
| **SYSTEMIC SYNDROMES (FEBRILE/NON-FEBRILE) Spread by infected TICK, FLEA, or LICE** | | | | |
| Epidemiologic history crucial. **Babesiosis, Lyme disease, & Anaplasma (Ehrlichiosis)** have same reservoir & tick vector. | | | | |
| **Babesiosis:** see *JAMA 315:1767, 2016.* Do not treat if asymptomatic, young, has spleen, and immunocompetent; can be fatal in lymphoma pts. | Etiol.: B. microti et al. Vector: Usually Ixodes ticks Host: White-footed mouse & others | [(Atovaquone 750 mg po q12h) + (Azithro 600 mg po day 1, then 500–1000 mg per day) times 7–10 days]. If severe infection [Clinda 1.2 gm IV bid or 600 mg po bid times 7 days + Quinine 650 mg po tid times 7 days. **Ped. dosage:** Clinda 20–40 mg per kg per day and quinine 25 mg per kg per day]. **Exchange transfusion**–See Comment | | **Seven diseases where pathogen visible in peripheral blood smear:** African/ American trypanosomiasis; babesia; bartonellosis; filariasis; malaria; relapsing fever. **Dx:** Giemsa-stained blood smear; antibody test available. PCR if available. **Rx: Exchange transfusions successful adjunct if used early, in severe disease.** May need treatment for 6 or more wks if immunocompromised. Look for Lyme and/or Anaplasma co-infection. |
| **Bartonella infections:** Treatment review: *Int J Antimicrob Agts 44:16, 2014.* | | | | |
| Bacteremia, asymptomatic | B. quintana, B. henselae | Doxy 100 mg po/IV bid x 4 wks + Gent 1 mg/kg qhs x 1st 2 wks | | Rule out endocarditis. Found in homeless, alcoholics, esp. if lice/leg pain. Often missed since asymptomatic. |
| Cat-scratch disease | B. henselae | Azithro 500 mg po x 1 dose, then 250 mg/day x 4 days. For symptomatic only–*see Lymphadenitis, page 48:* usually lymphadenitis, hepatitis, splenitis, FUO, neuroretinitis, transverse myelitis, oculoglandular disease. | | |
| Bacillary angiomatosis; Peliosis hepatis—AIDS | B. henselae, B. quintana | **Uncomplicated:** Erythro 500 mg po qid x 3 months or longer OR Doxy 100 mg po bid x 3 months or longer | **Complicated (CNS involvement):** Doxy 100 mg IV/po bid + RIF 300 mg po bid | **Do not use:** TMP-SMX, CIP, Pen, Ceph. **Manifestations of Bartonella infections:** **Immunocompetent:** Bacteremia/endocarditis/FUO/ encephalitis Cat scratch osteo Vertebral osteo Trench fever Parinaud's oculoglandular syndrome |
| | | Regardless of CD4 count, DC therapy after 3-4 mos. & observe. If no relapse, no suppressive rx. If relapse, **Doxy, Azithro** or **Erythro** x 3 mos. Stop when CD4 >200 x 6 mos. | | **HIV/AIDS:** Bacillary angiomatosis Bacillary peliosis Bacteremia/endocarditis/FUO |
| **Endocarditis** (see page 30) *Int J Antimicrob Agts 44:16, 2014* | B. henselae, B. quintana | **Surgical removal of infected valve.** If suspect endocarditis: Ceftriaxone 2 gm IV once daily x 6 weeks + Gent 1 mg/ kg IV q8h x 14 days + Doxy 100 mg IV q8h x 14 days | **If proven endocarditis: Doxy 100 mg IV/po bid x 6 wks + Gent 1 mg/kg IV q8h x 11 days** | **Gentamicin toxicity:** If Gent toxicity, substitute Rifampin 300 mg IV/po bid x 14 days. Role of valve removal surgery to cure unclear. Presents as SBE. Diagnosis: ECHO, serology & PCR of resected heart valve. **Note:** Empiric treatment for possible endocarditis due to Strept. sp. while awaiting blood culture results. |
| **Oroya fever (acute)** & **Verruga peruana (chronic) (South American Bartonellosis)** | B. bacilliformis; *AAC 48:192, 2014; Pediatrics 128:e1034, 2011* | Oroya fever: (Adult)/CIP 500 mg po bid + Ceftriaxone 1 gm IV once daily) x 14 days OR (Chloro 50-75 mg/kg/day IV po in 4 div doses + Ceftriaxone 1 gm IV once daily) x 14 days. | **Verruga peruana:** (Adult) Azithro 500 mg po once daily x 7 days OR CIP 500 mg po bid x 7-10 days | **Oroya fever (Pregnancy): AM-CL** 1000/62.5 mg po bid. Oroya fever, severe infection (Child): (**CIP** or **Chloro**) + **Ceftriaxone** **Verruga peruana (Child):** Azithro 10 mg/kg po once daily x 7 days OR **CIP** 20 mg/kg po in 2 div doses x 14 days |
| **Trench fever (FUO)** | B. quintana | No endocarditis: Doxy 100 mg po bid x 4 wks + Gent 3 mg/kg once daily for 1st 2 wks of therapy (AAC 48:1921, 2004). | | Vector is body louse. Do not use: TMP-SMX, FQs, cefazolin or Pen. If endocarditis, need longer rx. See *Emerg ID 2:217, 2006).* |

Abbreviations on page 2.  **\*NOTE:** All dosage recommendations are for adults (unless otherwise indicated) and assume normal renal function. § Alternatives consider allergy, PK, compliance, local resistance, cost.

TABLE 1 (58)

| ANATOMIC SITE/DIAGNOSIS/ MODIFYING CIRCUMSTANCES | ETIOLOGIES (usual) | SUGGESTED REGIMENS* PRIMARY | SUGGESTED REGIMENS* ALTERNATIVE§ | ADJUNCT DIAGNOSTIC OR THERAPEUTIC MEASURES AND COMMENTS |
|---|---|---|---|---|
| **SYSTEMIC SYNDROMES (FEBRILE/NON-FEBRILE)/Spread by infected TICK, FLEA, or LICE** *(continued)* | | | | |
| **Ehrlichiosis²**, CDC def. is one of: (1) 4x ↑ IFA antibody, (2) detection of Ehrlichia DNA in blood or CSF by PCR, (3) visible morulae in WBC and IFA ≥1:64. New species in WI, MN *(NEJM 365:422, 2011)*. | | | | |
| **Human monocytic ehrlichiosis (HME)** *CID 45(Suppl 1):S1, 2007* | Ehrlichia chaffeensis (Lone Star tick is vector) | Doxy 100 mg po/IV bid x 7–10 days *(Peds, see footnote²³)* | Tetracycline 500 mg po qid x 7–10 days. No current tx. for children or pregnancy | 30 states: mostly SE of line from NJ to Ill. to Missouri to Oklahoma to Texas. History of outdoor activity and tick exposure. Lymph node. Fever, rash (36%), leukopenia and thrombocytopenia. Blood smears no help. PCR for early dx. |
| **Human Anaplasmosis** (formerly known as Human granulocytic ehrlichiosis) *MMWR 65:1, 2016; JAMA 315:1767, 2016.* | Anaplasma (Ehrlichia) phagocytophilum (Ixodes sp. ticks also vector). Dog variant is Ehrlichia ewingii | Doxy 100 mg po or IV x 7–14 days *(Peds, see footnote²³)* | Tetracycline 500 mg po qid x 7–14 days. Not in children or pregnancy. Chloro is an alternative. | Upper Midwest, NE, West Coast & Europe. H/O tick exposure. April–Sept. Febrile flu-like illness after outdoor activity. No rash. Leukopenia/ thrombocytopenia common. **Dx:** PCR best; blood smear insensitive *(Am J Trop Med Hyg 93:66, 2015)*. **Rx:** RIF active in vitro *(DCNA 22:433, 2008)* but worry about resistance developing. Minocycline should work if doxy not available. |
| **Lyme Disease   NOTE:** Think about concomitant tick-borne disease—e.g., babesiosis, anaplasmosis and ehrlichiosis. **Guidelines:** *CID 51:1, 2010; NEJM 370:1724, 2014; JAMA 315:1767, 2016.* | | | | |
| Bite by ixodes-infected tick in an endemic area — **Postexposure prophylaxis** | Borrelia burgdorferi **IDSA guidelines:** *CID 51:1, 2010* Rarely, Borrelia mayonii *(Int J Syst Evol Microbiol 2016; 66:4878)* | If endemic area, if nymphal partially engorged deer tick: Doxy 200 mg po x 1 dose with food *(Peds, see footnote²³)* | If not endemic area, not engorged, not deer tick: No treatment | Prophylaxis study in endemic area: erythema migrans developed in 3% of the control group and 0.4% doxy group *(NEJM 345:79 & 133, 2001)*. Can substitute **Minocycline** for Doxy. Doxy is unavailable. |
| **Early** (erythema migrans) Serologic tests negative | | Doxy 100 mg po bid or **Amoxicillin** 500 mg po tid or **cefuroxime axetil** 500 mg po bid All regimens x 14–21 days. *(Peds, see footnote²³)* | **Amoxicillin** 500 mg po tid or cefuroxime axetil 500 mg po bid x 14–21 days. **Azithro** 500 mg po q24h x 7–10 days. | High rate of clinical failure with azithro & erythro *(Drugs 57:157, 1999)*. **Peds** (all po for 14–21 days): **Amox** 50 mg per kg per day in 3 div. doses or Cefuroxime axetil 30 mg per kg per day in 2 div. doses or **Azithro** 10 mg/kg (max 500 mg) per day for 7–10 days. |
| **Carditis** *See Comment* | IgM—Need 2 of 3 positive of kilodaltons (kD): 23, 39, 41, 45, 58, 66, 93 IgG—Need 5 of 10 positive of kilodaltons (kD): 18, 21, 28, 30, 39, 41, 45, 58, 66, 93 *(AnIM 138:697, 2003)*. Azithro 500 mg (Peds dosing, see Comments and footnote²³) | (**Ceftriaxone** 2 gm IV q24h) or (**Cefotaxime** 2 gm IV q8h) or (**Pen G** 3 million units IV q4h) x 14–21 days | **Doxy** (see Comments) 100 mg po bid x footnote²³) 14–21 days or **Amoxicillin** 500 mg po bid x 14–21 days | Lesions usually homogenous—not target-like. *(AnIM 136:423, 2002)*. First degree AV block: Oral regimen. Generally High degree AV block (PR >0.3 sec.): IV therapy—permanent pacemaker not necessary, but temporary pacing in 39% *(CID 59:996, 2014)*. |
| **Facial nerve paralysis** (isolated finding, early) | Interest in 2 tier diagnostic approach: 1) standard Lyme ELISA & if positive; 2) C6 peptide ELISA. Better sensitivity/specificity. | (Doxy 100 mg po bid) or (**Amoxicillin** 500 mg po) tid x 14–21 days *(Peds, see footnote²³)* | **Ceftriaxone** 2 gm IV q24h x 14–21 days | LP suggested excluding central neurologic disease. If LP neg., oral regimen OK. If abnormal or not done, suggest parenteral Ceftriaxone. |
| **Meningitis, encephalitis** *For encephalopathy, see Comment* | Guidance on diagnostics: *ED 22:2169, 2016; JAMA 2018;320:636; CID 2018;67:1133.* | **Ceftriaxone** 2 gm IV q24h x 14–28 days | (**Pen G** 20 million units IV q24h in div doses) or (**Cefotaxime** 2 gm IV q8h) x 14–28 days | Encephalopathy: memory difficulty, depression, somnolence, or headache, CSF abnormalities. 89% had objective CSF abnormalities. No compelling evidence that prolonged treatment has any benefit in post-Lyme syndrome *(NEJM 374:1209, 2016)*. |
| **Arthritis** | | (Doxy 100 mg po bid) *(Peds, see footnote²³)* or (**Amoxicillin** 500 mg po tid) x 28 days | (**Ceftriaxone** 2 gm IV q24h) or (**Pen G** 20–24 million units per day IV) x 14–28 days | Start with 1 mo of therapy; if only partial response, treat for a second mo. |
| **Pregnancy** | | **Amoxicillin** 500 mg po tid x 21 days | If pen. allergic: (**Azithro** 500 mg po q24h x 7–10 days) or (**Erythro** 500 mg po qid x 14–21 days). Choice should not include doxy. | |

²² In endemic area (New York), high % of both adult ticks and nymphs were jointly infected with Anaplasma (HGE) and B. burgdorferi *(NEJM 337:49, 1997)*.
²³ **Important Note:** Use of **Doxycycline** in children is considered safe regardless of age for treatment duration of ≤21 days. Pediatric dose: 4.4 mg/kg/day divided bid *(AAP Redbook 2018)*.

*NOTE: All dosage recommendations are for adults (unless otherwise indicated) and assume normal renal function. § Alternatives consider allergy, PK, compliance, local resistance, cost.*

Abbreviations on page 2.

**TABLE 1 (59)**

| ANATOMIC SITE/DIAGNOSIS/ MODIFYING CIRCUMSTANCES | ETIOLOGIES (usual) | SUGGESTED REGIMENS* | | ADJUNCT DIAGNOSTIC OR THERAPEUTIC MEASURES AND COMMENTS |
|---|---|---|---|---|
| | | PRIMARY | ALTERNATIVE§ | |
| **SYSTEMIC SYNDROMES (FEBRILE/NON-FEBRILE)/Spread by infected TICK, FLEA, or LICE/Lyme Disease** *(continued)* | | | | |
| **Post-Lyme Disease Syndromes** | | None indicated | | No benefit from rx (AJM 126:665, 2013; CID 5:1, 2010; AAC 58:6701, 2014; NEJM 345:85, 2001). Constructive review: CID 58:1267, 2014. |
| **Plague, bacteremic** (see also Bubonic plague and plague pneumonia) | Yersinia pestis | (**Streptomycin** 30 mg/kg/day IV in 2 div doses OR **Gentamicin** 5 mg/kg/day IV single dose) x 10 days | [**Levo** 500 mg IV/po once daily or **CIP** 500 mg po or 400 mg IV q12h] x 10 days another option. FQs effective in animals & small case series (EID 20:1,23-553). | **Doxy** 200 mg IV/po bid x 1 day, then 100 mg IV/po bid x 7-10 days |
| **Relapsing fever** | | | | |
| Louse-borne (LBRF) | Borrelia recurrentis Reservoir is human Vector: Louse pediculus humanus | **Tetracycline** 500 mg IV/po x 1 dose or **Doxy** 100 mg IV/po x 1 dose (Peds, see footnote²³) | **Erytho** 500 mg IV/po x 1 dose | Jarisch-Herxheimer (fever, ↑ pulse, ↑ resp., ↓ blood pressure) in most patients (occurs in ~2 hrs.) Not prevented by prior steroids. **Dx: Examine peripheral blood smear during fever for spirochetes.** Can relapse up to 10 times. |
| Tick-borne (TBRF) | No Amer: B. hermsii, B. turicata; Africa: B. hispanica, B. crocidurae, B. duttonii; Russia: B. miyamoto (see Comment) | **Doxy** 100 mg po bid x 7-10 days (Peds, see footnote²³) | **Erytho** 500 mg po qid x 7-10 days | Jarisch-Herxheimer reaction may occur. Postexposure **Doxy** pre-emptive therapy highly effective (NEJM 355:148, 2006). B. miyamoto: Dx by ref lab serum PCR. Fever, headache, thrombocytopenia & tick exposure (NE USA). Seems to respond to Doxy, Azithro, Ceftriaxone (AnIM 163:91 & 141, 2015; NEJM 373-468, 2015). Resistant to Amox (AAC 2018:52:e00419). |
| **Rickettsial diseases** (MMWR 65:(RR-2):1, 2016). | | | | |
| **Spotted fevers (NOTE: Rickettsial pox not included)** | | | | |
| Rocky Mountain spotted fever (RMSF) (LnID 8:143, 2008 and MMWR 55 (RR-4), 2007) | R. rickettsii (Dermacentor tick vector) | **Doxy** 100 mg po/IV bid x 7 days or x 2 days after temp. normal. Some suggest loading dose: **Doxy** 200 mg IV/po q12h x 3 days, then 100 mg po bid | Pregnancy: **Chloro** 50 mg/kg/ day in 4 div doses. If cannot obtain Chloro, alternative is **Doxy** | Fever, rash (88%), petechiae 40-50%. **Rash spreads from distal extremities to trunk.** Rash in ~50% pts in first 72 hrs. Dx: Immunohistology on skin biopsy; confirmation with antibody titers. Highest incidence in SE and South Central states; also seen in Oklahoma, S. Dakota, Montana. Cases reported from 42 U.S. states. **NOTE: Only 3-18% of pts present with fever, rash, and hx of tick exposure; many early deaths in children & empiric doxy reasonable (MMWR 49:885, 2000).** |
| **NOTE:** Can mimic ehrlichiosis. Pattern of rash important—see Comment | | | | |
| Other spotted fevers, e.g., Rickettsial pox, African tick bite fever, R. parkeri | At least 8 species on 6 continents. (CID 45 (Supl 1) S39, 2007). | **Doxy** 100 mg po bid x 7 days (Peds, see footnote²³) | **Chloro** 500 mg IV/po qid x 7 days Children age < 8 yrs: **Azithro** or **Clarithro** (if mild disease) | Clinical diagnosis suggested by: 1) Fever, intense myalgia, headache; 2) exposure to tick; 3) localized eschar (black necrotic) or rash. Definitive Dx: PCR of blood, skin biopsy or sequential antibody tests. |
| **Typhus group—**Consider in returning travelers with fever | | | | |
| Louse-borne: epidemic typhus Ref: LnID 8:417, 2008 | R. prowazekii (vector is body or head louse) | **Doxy** 100 mg IV/po bid x 7 days; single 200 mg dose 95% effective. (Peds, see footnote²³) | **Chloro** 500 mg IV/po qid x 5 days | **Brill-Zinsser disease** (Ln 357:1198, 2007) is a relapse of typhus acquired during WWII. Truncal rash (64%) spreads centrifugally—opposite of RMSF. Louse borne typhus is a winter disease. Diagnosis by serology. R. prowazekii found in flying squirrels in SE US. Delouse clothing of infected pt. |

Abbreviations on page 2.          *NOTE: All dosage recommendations are for adults (unless otherwise indicated) and assume normal renal function. § Alternatives consider allergy, PK, compliance, local resistance, cost.

**TABLE 1 (60)**

| ANATOMIC SITE/DIAGNOSIS/ MODIFYING CIRCUMSTANCES | ETIOLOGIES (usual) | SUGGESTED REGIMENS* PRIMARY | ALTERNATIVE§ | ADJUNCT DIAGNOSTIC OR THERAPEUTIC MEASURES AND COMMENTS |
|---|---|---|---|---|
| **SYSTEMIC SYNDROMES (FEBRILE/NON-FEBRILE)/Spread by infected TICK, FLEA, or LICE/Rickettsial diseases** *(continued)* | | | | |
| Murine typhus (aka flea typhus): *EID 14:1019, 2008* Scrub typhus (*World J Crit Care 4:244, 2015*) | R. typhi (rat reservoir and flea vector): O. tsutsugamushi [rodent reservoir; vector is larval stage of mites (chiggers)] | **Doxy** 100 mg IV/po bid x 5 days **Doxy** 100 mg po/IV bid x 7 days. In pregnancy: **Azithro** 500 mg po x one dose | **Chloro** 500 mg IV/po qid x 5 days *(Peds, see footnote23)* **Chloro** 500 mg po/IV qid x 7 days | Rash in 20-54%, not diagnostic. Without treatment most pts recover in 2 wks. Faster recovery with treatment. Dx based on suspicion; confirmed serologically. Asian rim of Pacific. Confirm with serology. If Doxy resistance suspected, (**RIF** 600 mg po qd or **Azithro** 500 mg po qd x 5 days *(CID 20:867600)*. |
| Tularemia, typhoidal type Ref. **bioterrorism:** see *JAMA 285:2763, 2001; ID Clin No Amer 22:489, 2008; CID 58:744, 2009.* | Francisella tularensis. (Vector depends on geography; ticks, biting flies, mosquitoes identified). Direct inoculation of wounds. | Moderate/severe: [(**Gent** or **Tobra** 5 mg per kg per day div. q8h IV) or **Streptomycin** 10 mg/kg IV/IM q12h)] x 10 days | Mild: (**CIP** 400 mg IV (or 750 mg po) bid or **Doxy** 100 mg IV/po bid] x 14-21 days *(Peds, see footnote23)* | Diagnosis: Culture on cysteine-enriched media & serology. Dangerous in the lab. Hematogenous meningitis is a complication: treatment is **Streptomycin** + **Chloro** 50-100 mg/kg/day IV in 4 divided doses *(Arch Neuro) 66:523, 2009).* |
| **Other Zoonotic Systemic Bacterial Febrile Illnesses (not spread by fleas, lice or ticks): Obtain careful epidemiologic history** | | | | |
| **Brucellosis** Refs: *NEJM 352:2325, 2005; CID 46:426, 2008; MMWR 57:603, 2008; BMJ 336:701, 2008; PLoS One 7:e32090, 2012.* | B. abortus–cattle B. suis–swine B. melitensis–goats B. canis–dogs | **Non focal disease:** [**Doxy** 100 mg po bid x 6 wks + **Gent** 5 mg/kg once daily for 1-2 wks] **Spondylitis, Sacroiliitis:** [**Doxy** + **Gent** (as above) + **RIF**] x min 3 mos **Neurobrucellosis:** [**Doxy** + **RIF** + TMP-SMX] x 45 days to 6 mos **Endocarditis:** Surgery + [(**RIF** + **Doxy** + TMP-SMX) x 2-4 wks *(CID 56:1407, 2013)* + **Gent** for 2-4 wks] x 6 wks **Pregnancy:** Not much data. **RIF** 900 mg po once daily x 6 wks | [**Doxy** 100 mg po bid + **RIF** 600-900 mg po once daily] x 6 wks. Less optimal: **CIP** 500 mg po bid + (**Doxy** or **RIF**) x 6 wks. [**CIP** 750 mg po bid + **RIF** 600-900 mg po once daily] x min 3 mos [**Doxy** + **RIF** (as above) + **Ceftriaxone** 2 gm IV q12h until CSF returned to normal *(AAC 56:1523, 2012)* **RIF** 900 mg po once daily. + **TMP-SMX** 5 mg/kg (TMP comp) po bid x 4 wks | Bone involvement, esp. sacroiliitis in 20-30%. **Neurobrucellosis:** Usually meningitis. 1% of all pts with brucellosis. Role of corticosteroids unclear, not recommended. **Endocarditis:** Rare but most common cause of death. Need surgery + antimicrobials. **Pregnancy:** TMP-SMX may cause kernicterus if given during last week of pregnancy. |
| **Leptospirosis** *(Curr Topics Micro Immunol 387:65, 2015)* | Leptospira—in urine of domestic livestock, dogs, small rodents | **Severe illness:** Pen G 1.5 million units IV q6h or **Ceftriaxone** 2 gm q24h. Duration: 7 days | **Mild illness: Doxy** 100 mg IV/po q12h *(Peds, see footnote23)* or **Amox** 500 mg po tid x 7 days or **Azithro** 1 gm po x 1, then 500 mg po once daily x 2 days | Severity varies. Varies from mild anicteric illness to severe icteric disease (Weil's disease) with renal failure and myocarditis. AST/ALT do not exceed 5x normal. Jarisch-Herxheimer reaction can occur post-Pen therapy. |

Abbreviations on page 2.   *NOTE: All dosage recommendations are for adults (unless otherwise indicated) and assume normal renal function. § Alternatives consider allergy, PK, compliance, local resistance, cost.

TABLE 1 (61)

65

| ANATOMIC SITE/DIAGNOSIS/ MODIFYING CIRCUMSTANCES | ETIOLOGIES* (usual) | SUGGESTED REGIMENS* | | ADJUNCT DIAGNOSTIC OR THERAPEUTIC MEASURES AND COMMENTS |
|---|---|---|---|---|
| | | PRIMARY | ALTERNATIVE§ | |
| **SYSTEMIC SYNDROMES (FEBRILE/NON-FEBRILE)/Other Zoonotic Systemic Bacterial Febrile Illnesses** *(continued)* | | | | |
| **Salmonella bacteremia** other than S. typhi-non-typhoidal) | Salmonella enteritidis—a variety of serotypes from animal sources | If NOT acquired in Asia: **CIP** 400 mg IV q12h or **Levo** 750 mg po once daily) x 14 days *(See Comment)* | If acquired in Asia: **Ceftriaxone** 2 gm IV q24h or **Azithro** 1 gm po x 1 dose, then 500 mg po once daily x 5-7 days. Do NOT use FQs until susceptibility is determined. *(See Comment)* | In vitro resistance to nalidixic acid indicates relative resistance to FQs. Bacteremia can infect any organ/tissue: look for infection of atherosclerotic aorta, osteomyelitis in sickle cell pts. Rx duration range 14 days (immunocompetent) to 26 wks if mycotic aneurism or endocarditis. Alternative, if susceptible: **TMP-SMX** 8-10 mg/kg/day (TMP comp) divided q8h. CLSI has established new interpretive breakpoints for susceptibility to Ciprofloxacin: susceptible strains, MIC <0.06 μg/mL *(CID 55:1107, 2012)*. |
| **Miscellaneous Systemic Febrile Syndromes** | | | | |
| **Fever in Returning Travelers** Etiology by geographic exposure & clinical syndrome *(AnnIM 158:456, 2013).* | Dengue (Flavivirus) Malaria (Plasmodia sp) Typhoid (Salmonella sp) | Supportive care; *see Table 14A, page 178* Diagnosis: peripheral blood smear *See Table 1, page 65* | | Average incubation period 4 days; serodiagnosis. *See Table 13A, page 163* Average incubation 7-14 days; diarrhea in 45%. |
| **Kawasaki syndrome** 6 weeks to 12 yrs of age, peak at 1 yr of age; 85% below age 5. *Pediatrics 1247, 2009.* Tongue image *(NEJM 373:467, 2015)* | Self-limited vasculitis with ↑ temp, rash, conjunctivitis, strawberry tongue, cervical adenitis, arthritis, & coronary artery aneurysms | **IVIG** 2 gm per kg over 8-12 hrs x 1 + **ASA** 20-25 mg per kg qid THEN **ASA** 3-5 mg per kg per day x q24h times 6-8 wks | If still febrile after 1st dose of IVIG, some give a 2nd dose. In Japan **IVIG** + prednisolone 2 mg/kg/d Continue steroid until CRP normal for 15 days *(Lancet 379:1571, 2012).* | Iv gamma globulin (2 gm per kg over 10 hrs) in pts rx before 10th day of illness ↓ incidence of coronary artery lesions. *See Table 14A, page 187* for IVIG adverse effects. In children, wait until 11+ months after IVIG before giving live virus vaccines. |
| **Rheumatic Fever, acute** Ref.: *Ln 366:155, 2005* | Post-Group A strep pharyngitis (not Group B, C, or G) | (1) Symptom relief: **ASA** 80-100 mg per kg per day in children; 4-8 gm per day in adults. (2) Eradicate Group A strep: **Pen** times 10 days *(see Pharyngitis, page 51).* (3) Start prophylaxis: *see below* | | |
| **Prophylaxis** | | | | |
| Primary prophylaxis: Treat S. pyogenes pharyngitis | | **Benzathine pen G** 1.2 million units IM *(see Pharyngitis, page 51)* | **Penicillin** for 10 days prevents rheumatic fever even when started 7-9 days after onset of illness *(see page 51).* **Alternative: Penicillin V** 250 mg po bid or **Sulfadiazine (sulfisoxazole)** 1 gm po q24h or **Erythro** 250 mg po bid. | |
| Secondary prophylaxis (previous documented rheumatic fever) | | **Benzathine pen G** 1.2 million units IM q3-4 wks *(AAC 58:6735, 2014).* | **Duration?** No carditis: 5 yrs or until age 21, whichever is longer. Carditis without residual heart disease: 10 since last attack; carditis with residual valvular disease: 10 yrs since last episode or until age 40 whichever is longer *(J Am Coll Cardiol 63 e57, 2014).* | |
| **Typhoidal syndrome** (typhoid fever, enteric fever) FQ resistance increasing in infected travelers *(BMC Infect Dis 15:212, 2015)* | Salmonella typhi, S. paratyphi A, B, C & S. cholerasuis. **NOTE: In vitro resistance to nalidixic acid predicts clinical failure of CIP (FQs).** Do not use empiric FQs if Asia-acquired infection. Need susceptibility results. | If NOT acquired in Asia: **CIP** 400 mg IV q12h or **Levo** 750 mg po/IV q24h) x 7-14 days. *(See Comment)* **Peds:** **Azithro** 10 mg/kg once daily x 7 days *(AAC 51:819, 2007)* | If acquired in Asia: (**Ceftriaxone** 2 gm IV daily x 7-14 d) or (**Azithro** 1 gm x 1 dose, then 500 mg po daily x 7 days) or (**Chloro** 500 mg po/IV q6h x 14 d) *(See Comment)* | **Dexamethasone:** Use in severely ill pts: 1st dose just prior to antibiotic, **3 mg/kg IV, then 1 mg/kg q6h x 8 doses.** **Complications:** perforation of terminal ileum &/or cecum, osteo, septic arthritis, **mycotic aneurysm,** meningitis, hematogenous pneumonia. Failure of MER in pt with S. enterica strain producing ESBLs and resistant to FQs & azithro responded to addition of fosfomycin *(CID 2017:65:1754).* |

TABLE 1 (62)

| ANATOMIC SITE/DIAGNOSIS/ MODIFYING CIRCUMSTANCES | ETIOLOGIES (usual) | SUGGESTED REGIMENS* | | ADJUNCT DIAGNOSTIC OR THERAPEUTIC MEASURES AND COMMENTS |
|---|---|---|---|---|
| | | PRIMARY | ALTERNATIVE§ | |
| **SYSTEMIC SYNDROMES (FEBRILE/NON-FEBRILE)** (continued) | | | | |
| **Sepsis:** Following suggested empiric therapy assumes pt is bacteremic; mimicked by viral, fungal, rickettsial infections and pancreatitis (Intensive Care Med. 2017;43:304). | | | | |
| **Neonatal—early onset** Age <7 days | Group B strep, E. coli, klebsiella, enterobacter, Staph. aureus (uncommon), listeria (rare in U.S.) | **AMP** 150 mg/kg/day IV div q6h + **Cefotaxime** 100 mg/kg/day div q12h ± **Gent** 5 mg/kg q 24 or 2.5 mg/kg q8h IV or IM (if meningitis, consider increasing to **AMP** 200 mg/kg/day IV q6h and **Cefotaxime** 150 mg/kg/day q8h) | | Blood cultures are key but only 5-10% of febrile infants have bacterial infection. Discontinue antibiotics after 72 hrs if cultures and course do not support diagnosis. In Spain, listeria predominates; in S. America, salmonella. In Grp B Strep infection + severe beta-lactam allergy, alternatives include: erythro & clinda; report of clinda resistance at 38% & erythro resistance at 38% (AAC 56:739, 2012). |
| **Neonatal—late onset** Age >7 days | As above + H. influenzae & S. epidermidis | **AMP** 200-300 mg/kg/day IV q6h + **Cefotaxime** 75 mg/kg IV q12h or **AMP** 200 mg/kg/day IV div q6h + **Gent** 5 mg/kg q8h IV or IM | (**AMP** 200 mg/kg/day IV q6h + **Cefotaxime** 100 mg/kg q12h div or **AMP** 200 mg/kg/day IV q6h + **Gent** 5 mg/kg/day IV div q8h) or **Gent** 5 mg/kg/day once daily or q8h IV or IM. | **If MRSA is a concern, add Vanco** 15 mg/kg IV q12h (Wt < 2000 gm). See also Comment (early onset). |
| **Child; not neutropenic** | Strep, pneumoniae, meningococci, Staph. aureus (MSSA & MRSA), H. influenzae now rare. | (**Cefotaxime** 50 mg/kg IV q8h or **Ceftriaxone** 100 mg/kg IV q24h) + **Vanco** 15 mg/kg IV q6h | Aztreonam 7.5 mg/kg q6h + Linezolid | Major concerns are S. pneumoniae & community-associated MRSA. Coverage for Gm-neg. bacilli included but H. influenzae infection now rare. Meningococcemia mortality remains high (Ln 356:961, 2000). |
| **Adult; not neutropenic NO HYPOTENSION but LIFE-THREATENING**[24]—**For Septic shock, see page 68** | | | | **Sepsis:** life-threatening organ dysfunction (identified by an acute change in SOFA [Sequential (Sepsis-Related) Organ Failure Assessment] score ≥2 points) caused by a dysregulated host response to infection. |
| **Source unclear**—consider primary bacteremia, intra-abdominal or skin source. May be **Life-threatening.** Survival greater with quicker, effective empiric antibiotic Rx (NEJM 2017; 376:2235). | Aerobic Gm-neg. bacilli; S. aureus; streptococci; others | [**IMP** or **MER** + **Vanco**] OR (**PIP-TZ** + **Vanco**) If ESBL and/or carbapenemase-producing GNB, Empiric options pending clarification of clinical syndrome and culture results: **Low prevalence of resistance: Vanco + PIP-TZ If high prevalence of resistance,** see Table 5B, page 89 for treatment options Dosages in footnote[24] | [**Dapto** 6 mg/kg IV q24h) + (**Cefepime** or **PIP-TZ**). | **Septic shock** sepsis accompanied by circulatory and cellular/metabolic abnormalities sufficient to substantially increase mortality (see JAMA 2017; 317:847; JAMA 2017; 317:267). For patients in septic shock, unresponsive to volume resuscitation requiring on-going vasopressor therapy to maintain systolic BP > 90 mm Hg or MAP > 65 mm Hg consider hydrocortisone 50 mg IV q6h + fludrocortisone 50 mcg once daily via NG tube (NEJM 2018; 378:797; 809; 860 [editorial]). Note: Pip-tazo inferior to MER vs. ceftriaxone-resistant E. coli/K. pneumo (JAMA 2018;320:979 & 984). |
| **If suspect biliary source** (see Gallbladder page 18) | Enterococci + aerobic Gm-neg. bacilli | PIP-TZ (Do not use if ESBL producer) | Ceftriaxone + Metro or (CIP or Levo) + Metro Dosages–footnote[24] | If enterococci a concern, add ampicillin or vanco to metro regimens |
| **If community-acquired pneumonia** with severe sepsis or septic shock (see page 42 and following pages) | S. pneumoniae; MRSA; Legionella; Gm-neg. bacillus, others | (**Levo** or **Moxi**) + (**PIP-TZ**) + Vanco | Aztreonam + (**Levo** or **Moxi**) + Linezolid | Many categories of CAP, see material beginning at page 42. Suggestions based on most severe CAP, e.g., MRSA after influenza or Klebsiella pneumonia in an alcoholic. |
| **If illicit use IV drugs.** | S. aureus | Include **Vanco** to cover MRSA. | | |

[24] P Ceph 3 [**Cefotaxime** 2 gm IV q8h, use q4h if life-threatening; **Ceftriaxone** 2 gm IV q24h; **Cefepime** 2 gm IV q12h], **PIP-TZ** 3.375 gm IV q4h or 4-hr infusion of 3.375 gm q8h, **Aminoglycosides** (see Table 10D, page 128), **AMP** 200 mg/kg/day divided q6h, **Clinda** 900 mg IV q8h, **IMP** 0.5 gm IV q6h, **MER** 1 gm IV q8h, **Erta** 1 gm IV q24h, **Dori** 500 mg q8h (1-hr infusion), **Nafcillin/Oxacillin** 2 gm IV q4h; **Aztreonam** 2 gm IV q8h; **Metro** 1 gm loading dose then 0.5 gm q6h or 1 gm IV q12h, **Vanco** loading dose 25-30 mg/kg IV, then 15-20 mg/kg IV q8-12h (dose in obese pt, see Table 17C, page 250), **Ceftazidime** 2 gm IV q8h, **Ciprofloxacin** 400 mg IV q12h (q8h if neutropenic), **Cefpirome**[AMB] 2 gm IV q12h (q8h if neutropenic), **Levo** 750 mg IV q24h, **Linezolid** 600 mg IV q12h.

Abbreviations on page 2.      *NOTE: All dosage recommendations are for adults (unless otherwise indicated) and assume normal renal function. § Alternatives consider allergy, PK, compliance, local resistance, cost.

# TABLE 1 (63)

| ANATOMIC SITE/DIAGNOSIS/ MODIFYING CIRCUMSTANCES | ETIOLOGIES (usual) | SUGGESTED REGIMENS* | | ADJUNCT DIAGNOSTIC OR THERAPEUTIC MEASURES AND COMMENTS |
|---|---|---|---|---|
| | | PRIMARY | ALTERNATIVE§ | |
| **SYSTEMIC SYNDROMES (FEBRILE/NON-FEBRILE)/Sepsis/Adult/not neutropenic** *(continued)* | | | | |
| If suspect intra-abdominal source | Mixture aerobic & anaerobic Gm-neg. bacilli | See secondary peritonitis, page 50. | | |
| If petechial rash | Meningococcemia | Ceftriaxone 2 gm IV q12h (until sure, no meningitis); consider Rocky Mountain spotted fever—see page 63. | | |
| If suspect urinary source, e.g. pyelonephritis | Aerobic Gm-neg. bacilli & enterococci | See pyelonephritis, page 37. Prefer a carbapenem for patients with severe sepsis or septic shock to cover ESBL producers. | | |
| **Neutropenia: Child or Adult (absolute PMN count <500 per mm³) in cancer and transplant patients.** Guidelines (inpatient): CID 2011;52:427, (outpatient): J Clin Oncol 31:794, 2013) | | | | |
| **Prophylaxis** (J Clin Oncol 31:794, 2013) | | | | |
| Post-chemotherapy— impending neutropenia | Pneumocystis (PCP), Viridans strep | In patients expected to have PMN <100 for >7 days consider Levo 500-750 mg po q24h. Acute leukemias undergoing intensive induction consider addition of Fluc 400 mg q24h. In patients with AML or MDS who have prolonged neutropenia, consider Posa instead at 200 mg TID (N Engl J Med 356:348, 2007). Safe & effective during induction Rx for acute lymphoblastic leukemia (ALL) (CID 2017;65:1790). | | |
| Post allogeneic stem cell transplant | Aerobic Gm-neg. bacilli, ↑ risk pneumocystis, herpes viruses, candida aspergillus | TMP-SMX (vs. PCP) + Acyclovir (vs. HSV/VZV)+ pre-emptive monitoring for CMV + Posaconazole (vs. mold) | | In autologous HCT, not active prophylaxis nor CMV screening is recommended. Fluc OK with TMP-SMX and acyclovir. |
| **Empiric therapy—febrile neutropenia (≥38.3°C for >1 hr or sustained >38°C and absolute neutrophil count <500 cells/µL)** (IDSA Guidelines: CID 52:427, 2012). (Outpatients: J Clin Oncol doi:10.1200/JCO 2017;77:6211.) | | | | |
| Low-risk adults Anticipate <7 days neutropenia, no co-morb., can take po meds | Aerobic Gm-neg bacilli, Viridans strep | CIP 750 mg po bid + AM-CL 875 /125 mg po bid. Treat until absolute neutrophil count >1000 cells/µL | Treat as outpatients with 24/7 access to inpatient care if: no focal findings, no hypotension, no COPD, no fungal infection, no dehydration, age range 16-60 yrs; reliable and compliant pts & family. If pen allergy: can substitute Clinda 300 mg po qid for AM-CL | |
| High-risk adults and children (Anticipate >7 days profound neutropenia, active co-morbidities) | Aerobic Gm. bacilli; to include P. aeruginosa; cephalosporin-resistant viridans strep; MRSA | **Empiric therapy:** CFP, IMP, MER, Dori, or PIP-TZ. Consider addition of Vanco as below.<br>Dosages: See footnote on page 66 and Table 10B.<br>Include empiric Vanco if: Suspected CLABSI; severe mucositis; SSTI, PNA, or hypotension | **Combination therapy:** If pt has severe sepsis/shock, consider add Tobra + Vanco + Echinocandin | Increasing resistance of viridans streptococci to penicillins, cephalosporins & FQs (CID 34:1469 & 1524, 2002). **What if severe IgE-mediated β-lactam allergy?** Aztreonam plus Tobra. Work-up should include blood, urine, CXR with additional testing based on symptoms. Low threshold for CT scan. If cultures remain neg. but pt afebrile, treat until absolute neutrophil count ≥500 cells/µL. **Note:** Pip-tazo inferior to MER vs. ceftriaxone-resistant E. coli/K. pneumo (JAMA 2018;320:979 & 984). |
| **Persistent fever and neutropenia after 5 days of empiric antibacterial therapy—see CID 52:427, 2011.** | | | | |
| | Candida species, aspergillus, VRE, resistant GNB | Add either (**Caspofungin** 70 mg IV day 1, then 50 mg IV q24h or **Micafungin** 100 mg IV q24h or **Anidulafungin** 200 mg IV x 1 dose, then 100 mg IV q24h) **OR Voriconazole** 6 mg per kg IV q12h times 2 doses, then 4 mg per kg IV q12h | | Conventional **Ampho B** causes more fever & nephrotoxicity & lower efficacy than lipid-based ampho B; both **Caspofungin** & **Voriconazole** better tolerated & perhaps more efficacious than lipid-based Ampho B (NEJM 346:225, 2002 & 351:1391 & 1445, 2005). |

Abbreviations on page 2.

*NOTE: All dosage recommendations are for adults (unless otherwise indicated) and assume normal renal function. § Alternatives consider allergy, PK, compliance, local resistance, cost.

**TABLE 1 (64)**

| ANATOMIC SITE/DIAGNOSIS/ MODIFYING CIRCUMSTANCES | ETIOLOGIES (usual) | SUGGESTED REGIMENS* | | ADJUNCT DIAGNOSTIC OR THERAPEUTIC MEASURES AND COMMENTS |
|---|---|---|---|---|
| | | PRIMARY | ALTERNATIVE§ | |
| **SYSTEMIC SYNDROMES (FEBRILE/NON-FEBRILE)/Sepsis** *(continued)* | | | | |
| **Shock syndromes** | | | | |
| **Septic shock: Fever & hypotension**<br>**Bacteremic shock, endotoxin shock**<br><br>*Goals:*<br>*1. Effective antibiotics*<br>*2. Fluid resuscitation*<br>*3. Vasoactive drugs, if needed*<br>*4. Source control*<br>*(Intensive Care Med 2017;43:304; JAMA 2017;317:267 & 347)* | Bacteremia with aerobic Gm-neg. bacteria or Gm+ cocci | • Lower mortality with **sepsis treatment "bundle"** *(NEJM 2017;376:2235, 2223)*<br>• Blood cultures & serum lactate<br>• Initiate effective antibiotic therapy:<br>  o No clear source & MDR GNB are rare: **PIP-TZ + Vanco**<br>  o No clear source but high prevalence of MDR GNB: if suspect, **MER or IMP**<br>• IV crystalloid: 20-40 mL/kg for hypotension or elevated lactate *(NEJM 2018;378:829 & 862)*<br>• If hypotensive after fluids, **nor-epinephrine**<br>• Attempt to identify & correct source of bacteremia<br>• Monitor lactate & central venous O$_2$ sat (target ≥70%)<br>• Transfuse if hematocrit <30% *(NEJM 371:1381, 2014)*<br>• See **Comment** for continuation. | | • For septic shock unresponsive to volume resuscitation and requiring on-going vasopressor therapy to maintain systolic BP > 90 mm Hg or MAP > 65 mm Hg consider hydrocortisone 50 mg IV q6h + fludrocortisone 50 mcg once daily via NG tube *(N Engl J Med 2018; 378:797, 809; and 860 [editorial]).*<br>• Insulin Rx: Current target is glucose level of 140-180 mg/dL. Attempts at tight control (80-110 mg/dL) resulted in excessive hypoglycemia.<br>• Impact of early effective antibiotic therapy *(NEJM 2017;376:2235)*<br>• Bacteremia due to carbapenemase-producing K. pneumoniae: **Ceftaz-avi** or **MER-vabor**.<br>• Shock associated with leaky capillaries which results in increased volume of drug distribution. Hence, need loading dose of antibiotics and, early in treatment, larger maintenance doses *(AAC 59:2995, 2015)* |
| **Septic shock: post-splenectomy or functional asplenia.** Asplenic pt care: *Chest 2016, 150:1994* | S. pneumoniae, N. meningitidis, H. influenzae, Capnocytophaga (DF-2) | No dog bite: **Ceftriaxone** 2 gm IV q24h (1 to 2 gm q12h if meningitis).<br>Post-dog bite: (**PIP-TZ** 3.375 gm IV q6h OR **MER** 1 gm IV q8h) + **Clinda** 900 mg IV q8h | No dog bite: (**Levo** 750 mg or **Moxi** 400 mg) once IV q24h | Howell-Jolly bodies in peripheral blood smear confirm absence of functional spleen.<br>Often results in **symmetrical peripheral gangrene of digits** due to severe DIC. For prophylaxis, see *Table 15A, page 217.* Vaccines: *CID 56:309, 2014.* |
| **Toxic shock syndrome, Clostridium sordellii**<br>Clinical picture: vascular leak, hemoconcentration, leukemoid reaction, afebrile | Clostridium sordellii-hemorrhagic & lethal toxins | Fluids, aq. **Pen G** 18-20 million units per day div. q4-6h • **Clinda** 900 mg IV q8h. **Surgical debridement is key.** | | Occurs in variety of settings that produce anaerobic tissue, e.g., illicit drug use, post-partum. Several deaths reported after use of abortifacient regimen of mifepristone (RU486) & misoprostol. *(NEJM 363:2540, 2010).* |
| **Toxic shock syndrome, staphylococcal**<br>**Colonization** by toxin-producing Staph. aureus of: vagina (tampon-assoc.), surgical/traumatic wounds, endometrium, burns | Staph. aureus (toxic shock toxin-mediated) | (**Nafcillin/Oxacillin** 2 gm IV q4h) or (if MRSA, **Vanco** 15-20 mg/kg q8-12h) + **Clinda** 600-900 mg IV q8h | **Cefazolin** 1-2 gm IV q8h) or (if MRSA, **Vanco** 15-20 mg/kg q8-12h OR **Dapto** 6 mg/kg IV q24h) **Clinda** 600-900 mg IV q8h | Benefit of adjunctive IVIG unclear but may be reasonable for patients with persistent hypotension. Rationale for Clinda is inhibition of toxin production; Linezolid also an option to inhibit toxin production. |

*Abbreviations on page 2.* *NOTE: All dosage recommendations are for adults (unless otherwise indicated) and assume normal renal function. §Alternatives consider allergy, PK, compliance, local resistance, cost.

**TABLE 1 (65)**

| ANATOMIC SITE/DIAGNOSIS/ MODIFYING CIRCUMSTANCES | ETIOLOGIES (usual) | SUGGESTED REGIMENS* | | ADJUNCT DIAGNOSTIC OR THERAPEUTIC MEASURES AND COMMENTS |
|---|---|---|---|---|
| | | PRIMARY | ALTERNATIVE§ | |
| **Systemic Syndromes (Febrile/Non-Febrile)/Sepsis/Shock syndromes** *(continued)* | | | | |
| **Toxic shock syndrome, streptococcal. NOTE:** For Necrotizing fasciitis without toxic shock, *see page 60.* Ref: *NEJM 2017;377:2253.* | | | | |
| Associated with invasive disease, i.e., erysipelas, necrotizing fasciitis; secondary strep infection of varicella. Secondary household contact TSS cases reported. | Group A, B, C, & G Strep. pyogenes, Group B Strep ref: *EID 15:223, 2009.* | (**Pen G** 24 million units per day IV in div. doses) + **Clinda** 900 mg IV q8h | **Ceftriaxone** 2 gm IV q24h + **Clinda** 900 mg IV q8h | **Definition:** Isolation of Group A strep, hypotension and ≥2 of: renal impairment, coagulopathy, liver involvement, ARDS, generalized rash, soft tissue necrosis. Associated with invasive disease. **Surgery usually required.** |
| | | Prospective observational study *(CID 59:358, 366 & 851, 2014)* indicates:<br>• Clinda decreases mortality<br>• High incidence of secondary cases in household contacts | | Clinda added to decrease toxin production.<br>**Adjunctive IVIG** (1 gm/kg on day 1, 0.5 gm/kg on days 2 and 3) may be of benefit *(CID 2018;67:1434)(meta-analysis).* |
| **Toxin-Mediated Syndromes—no fever unless complicated** | | | | |
| **Botulism** *(CID 2017;66(suppl.1):S11. As biologic weapon: JAMA 285:1059, 2001).* As biologic weapon: *https://www.cdc.gov/botulism/index.html)* | Clostridium botulinum | For all types: Follow vital capacity; other supportive care | Equine antitoxin: Contact the local or state health department (1-800-222-1222) or CDC (1-770-488-7100) or for infant botulism (1-510-231-7600. | |
| **Food-borne**<br>Dyspnea at presentation bad sign. *(CID 43:1247, 2006).* | Less common: C. barati, C. butyricum | If no ileus, purge GI tract | Heptavalent equine serum antitoxin—CDC<br>(See Comment.) | **Antimicrobials:** May make infant botulism worse. Untested in wound botulism. When used, pen G 10–20 million units per day usual dose. If complications (pneumonia, UTI) occur, avoid antimicrobials with assoc. neuromuscular blockade, i.e., aminoglycosides, tetracycline, polymyxins. |
| **Infant**<br>(Adult intestinal botulism is rare variant: *EJN 18:1, 2012).* | Submit blood, wound tissue, and/or implicated food (as pertinent) for mouse toxin bioassay. | Age < 1 year: Human botulinum immunoglobulin. Age > 1 year: Equine serum heptavalent antitoxin.<br>DO NOT WAIT FOR LAB CONFIRMATION TO TREAT SUSPECTED CASES | No antibiotics: may lyse C. botulinum in gut and ↑ load of toxin | **Differential dx:** Guillain-Barré, myasthenia gravis, tick paralysis, organophosphate toxicity, West Nile virus. EMG can help. |
| **Wound** | | Debridement & anaerobic cultures. No proven value of local antitoxin. Role of antibiotics untested. | Trivalent equine antitoxin | Wound botulism associated with injection drug use. Mouse bioassay failed to detect toxin in 1/3 of patients *(CID 48:1669, 2009).* |
| **Tetanus:** Trismus, generalized muscle rigidity, muscle spasm Ref: *AnIM 154:329, 2011.* | C. tetani–production of tetanospasmin toxin | **Six treatment steps:**<br>1. Urgent endotracheal intubation to protect the airway. Laryngeal spasm is common. Early tracheostomy.<br>2. Eliminate reflex spasms with diazepam, 20 mg/kg/day IV or midazolam. Reports of benefit combining diazepam with magnesium sulfate *(Ln 368:1436, 2006).* Worst cases: need neuromuscular blockade with vecuronium.<br>3. Neutralize toxin: Human hyperimmune globulin IM, start tetanus immunization—no immunity from clinical tetanus.<br>4. Surgically debride infected source tissue. Start antibiotic: **Pen G** 3 million units IV q4h or **Doxy** 100 mg IV q12h or **Metro** 1000 mg IV q12h) x 7–10 days.<br>5. Avoid light as may precipitate muscle spasms.<br>6. Use beta blockers, e.g., short acting esmolol, to control sympathetic hyperactivity. | | |

*Abbreviations on page 2.*   *NOTE: All dosage recommendations are for adults (unless otherwise indicated) and assume normal renal function. § Alternatives consider allergy, PK, compliance, local resistance, cost.*

TABLE 1 (66)

| ANATOMIC SITE/DIAGNOSIS/ MODIFYING CIRCUMSTANCES | ETIOLOGIES (usual) | SUGGESTED REGIMENS* | | ADJUNCT DIAGNOSTIC OR THERAPEUTIC MEASURES AND COMMENTS |
|---|---|---|---|---|
| | | PRIMARY | ALTERNATIVE§ | |
| **VASCULAR** | | | | |
| **Catheter Related Blood Stream Infections (CRBSI).** Ref: *Infect Dis Clin No Amer 2018 Dec;32(4):765-787* | | | | |
| Tunneled & non-tunneled central venous catheters (CVC), including peripherally-inserted central catheters (PICC). For management of peripheral IV, midline, arterial & hemodialysis catheters, see *Infect Dis Clin No Amer 2018 Dec;32(4):765-787.* **Diagnosis:** concomitant blood cultures from CVC & peripheral vein. A differential time to positive (DTP) of ≥2 hr favors infection of the CVC. | If suspect Gm+ bacteria: empiric rx for MSSA, MRSA, MRSE | Vanco | Dapto | Recommend in all clinical settings due to high prevalence of MSSA, MRSA & MRSE |
| | If suspect Gm-neg bacteria: e.g., femoral line, neutropenic. Empiric rx if high risk of candidemia, e.g., prolonged antibiotic therapy, post-transplant neutropenia, hyperalimentation. | Not critically ill: **Cefepime** or **PIP-TZ** Critically ill: **MER** or **IMP** | | |
| | S. epidermidis in blood: MSSE or MRSE (most often) | Micafungin or Caspofungin | Isavuconazole | |
| | | IF no attempt to salvage catheter; remove catheter. For MSSE: **Vanco** or **Dapto** For MSSE: **Cefazolin** IF attempt to salvage catheter. Antibiotic as above + antibiotic lock therapy (ALT) x 10-14 days. (See Comment.) | | Antibiotic lock therapy (ALT) not FDA approved, Several options, but prefer sol'n of Minocycline 5 mg + EDTA 30 mg/mL in 25% alcohol. See *AAC 2016;60:3426.* Catheter "dwell" time of a minimum 2-4 hrs/day. |
| | S. aureus or S. lugdunensis in blood; attempts at salvage therapy not recommended | Remove catheter. For MSSA: (**Nafcillin/Oxacillin**) or **Cefazolin** x 2-6 wks For MRSA: **Vanco** or **Dapto** x 2-6 wks | | If bacteremia for >72 hrs after catheter removal, TEE 5-7 days after diagnosis of bacteremia. New CVC after removal of infected CVC, new blood cultures for 48-72 hrs. TEE if bacteremia persists longer than 72 hrs after the start of antibiotic therapy or patient has a prosthetic heart valve. |
| | Enterococcus sp. in blood. | Specific antibiotic rx based on culture iD & susceptibility testing If short term CVC: remove & treat for 7-14 days. If long term CVC: can attempt salvage with combination IV antibiotic + ALT x 10-14 days | | If GNB in blood, maybe Leuconostoc sp. or Lactobacillus sp. Both are Vanco resistant but sensitive to **Pen G**, **AMP** or **Clinda**. |
| | Aerobic Gm-neg bacilli (GNB) in blood (See Comment) | Mono- or combination therapy for *P. aeruginosa* (or other MDR bacteria). Remove catheter. Can attempt to salvage catheter with systemic antibiotic + ALT x 10-14 days. | | |
| | Candida sp. in blood | Remove CVC. **Micafungin** | Remove CVC. **Fluconazole** unless *C. krusei*, then **Isavuconazole** | |
| **Prevention of Catheter-Related Blood Stream Infection** | | | | |
| At Time of Catheter Insertion | 1. Maximum sterile barrier precaution 2. Skin prep with 0.5% chlorhexidine and alcohol 3. Use subclavian vein if possible; try to avoid femoral vein/artery | | | |
| Post Catheter Insertion | 1. Remove CVC as soon as possible 2. Scrub the hub of the catheter with alcohol or alcoholic chlorhexidine 3. Patient bathing with chlorhexidine 4. Change site dressing weekly if transparent or semi-transparent; every 2 days if gauze dressing | | | |
| Emerging Prevention Methods | 1. Antimicrobial-coated catheters 2. Chlorhexidine impregnated dressings 3. Antibiotic impregnated needles and connectors 4. Catheter lock solutions (CID 2014;59:1741) | | | |

*Abbreviations on page 2.*   *NOTE: All dosage recommendations are for adults (unless otherwise indicated) and assume normal renal function. §Alternatives consider allergy, PK, compliance, local resistance, cost.*

TABLE 1 (67)

| ANATOMIC SITE/DIAGNOSIS/ MODIFYING CIRCUMSTANCES | ETIOLOGIES (usual) | SUGGESTED REGIMENS* | | ADJUNCT DIAGNOSTIC OR THERAPEUTIC MEASURES AND COMMENTS |
|---|---|---|---|---|
| | | PRIMARY | ALTERNATIVE§ | |
| **VASCULAR/CATHETER Related Blood Stream Infections (CRBSI)** *(continued)* | | | | |
| Mycotic aneurysm | S. aureus (28-71%), S. epidermidis, Salmonella sp. (15-24%), M.TBc, S. pneumonia, many others | **Vanco** (dose sufficient to achieve trough level of 15-20 μg/mL) + (**Ceftriaxone** or **PIP-TZ** or **CIP**) **Treatment is combination of antibiotic + surgical resection with revascularization.** | **Dapto** could be substituted for Vanco. For GNB: **Cefepime** or **Carbapenems** | Report of success with Ceftaroline with surgery for mycotic aneurysm due to VISA S. aureus resistant to daptomycin *(BMJ Case Rep 2015; PMID 25833910)*. Best diagnostic imaging: CT angiogram. Blood cultures positive in 50-85%. **De-escalate to specific therapy when culture results known.** Treatment duration varies but usually 6 wks from date of definitive surgery. |
| **Suppurative (Septic) Thrombophlebitis** | | | | |
| **Cranial dural sinus:** | | | | |
| **Cavernous Sinus:** CN III, IV, V (branches V1/V2), VI at risk (Note: V1 and V2, numbers are subscript) | S. aureus (70%) Streptococcus sp. Anaerobes (rare) Mucormycosis (diabetes) | [**Vanco** (dose for trough conc of 15-20 μg/mL) + **Ceftriaxone** 2 gm IV q12h], add **Metro** 500 mg IV q8h if dental/sinus source | [**Dapto** 8-12 mg/kg IV q24h OR **Linezolid** 600 mg IV q12h), add **Metro** 500 mg IV q8h if dental/sinus source | • Diagnosis: CT or MRI • Treatment: 1) obtain specimen for culture; 2) empiric antibiotics; 3) may need adjunctive surgery; 4) heparin until afebrile, then coumadin for several weeks |
| **Lateral Sinus:** Complication of otitis media/mastoiditis (pathogens similar to otitis media) | Polymicrobial (often) Aerobes, e.g., Proteus sp. E. coli P. aeruginosa S. aureus B. fragilis Other GNB | **Cefepime** 2 gm IV q8h + **Metro** 500 mg IV q8h + **Vanco** (dose for trough conc of 15-20 μg/mL) | **MER** 2 gm IV q8h + **Linezolid** 600 mg IV q12h | • Diagnosis: CT or MRI • Treatment: 1) consider radical mastoidectomy; 2) obtain cultures; 3) antibiotics; 4) anticoagulation controversial • Prognosis: favorable |
| **Superior Sagittal Sinus:** Complication of bacterial meningitis or bacterial frontal sinusitis. Treat as for meningitis | S. pneumoniae N. meningitidis H. influenzae (rare) S. aureus (very rare) | **Ceftriaxone** 2 gm IV q12h + **Vanco** (trough conc of 15-20 μg/mL) + **Dexamethasone** | **MER** 2 gm IV q8h + **Vanco** (trough conc of 15-20 μg/mL) + **Dexamethasone** | • Diagnosis: MRI • Pathology: MRI; causes cortical vein thrombosis, hemorrhagic infarcts and brainstem herniation • Anticoagulants not recommended |

*Abbreviations on page 2.* *NOTE: All dosage recommendations are for adults (unless otherwise indicated) and assume normal renal function. §Alternatives consider allergy, PK, compliance, local resistance, cost.*

TABLE 1 (68)

| ANATOMIC SITE/DIAGNOSIS/ MODIFYING CIRCUMSTANCES | ETIOLOGIES (usual) | SUGGESTED REGIMENS* | | ADJUNCT DIAGNOSTIC OR THERAPEUTIC MEASURES AND COMMENTS |
|---|---|---|---|---|
| | | PRIMARY | ALTERNATIVE§ | |
| **VASCULAR/Suppurative (Septic) Thrombophlebitis** *(continued)* | | | | |
| **Jugular Vein, Lemierre's Syndrome:** Complication of pharyngitis, tonsillitis, dental infection, EBV. Ref: *NEJM 371:2018, 2015.* | Fusobacterium necrophorum (anaerobe) Less often: Other Fusobacterium S. pyogenes Bacteroides sp. | (**PIP-TZ** 3.375 gm IV q6h OR **AM-SB** 3 gm IV q6h) x 4 weeks | **IMP** 500 mg IV q6h OR (**Metro** 500 mg IV q6h + **Ceftriaxone** 2 gm IV once daily) x 4 weeks. Another option: **Clinda** 600-900 mg IV q8h | • Diagnosis: Preceding pharyngitis and antibiotics therapy, persistent fever and pulmonary emboli<br>• Imaging: Hi-res CT scan<br>• Role of anticoagulants unclear |
| **Pelvic Vein:** Includes ovarian vein and deep pelvic vein phlebitis | Aerobic gram-neg bacilli Streptococcus sp. Anaerobes | Antibiotics + anticoagulation (heparin, then coumadin) *Low prevalence of MDR GNB:* **PIP-TZ** 3.375 gm IV q6h or 4.5 gm IV q8h OR (**Ceftriaxone** 2 gm IV once daily + **Metro** 500 mg IV q8h) | *High prevalence of MDR GNB:* **MER** 1 gm IV q8h. If severe beta-lactam allergy: (**CIP** 400 mg IV q12h + **Metro** 500 mg IV q8h) | • Diagnosis: ovarian vein infection presents 1 week post-partum with fever & local pain; deep pelvic vein presents 3-5 days post-delivery with fever but no local pain. CT or MRI may help.<br>• Treat until afebrile for 48 hrs & WBC normal<br>• Coumadin for 6 weeks |
| **Portal Vein (Pylephlebitis):** Complication of diverticulitis, appendicitis and (rarely) other intra-abdominal infection | Aerobic gram-neg bacilli: E.coli, Klebsiella & Proteus most common Other: aerobic/anaerobic streptococci, B. fragilis, Clostridia | *Low prevalence of MDR GNB (<20%):* **PIP-TZ** 4.5 gm IV q8h OR (**CIP** 400 mg IV q12h + **Metro** 500 mg IV q8h) | *High prevalence of MDR GNB (≥20%):* If ESBL producer: **Meropenem** 1 gm IV q8h. If carbapenemase producer: (**Polymyxin B** (preferred) or **Colistin**) + **MER** | • Diagnosis: Pain, fever, neutrophilia in pt with intra-abdominal infection.<br>• Abdominal CT scan<br>• Pyogenic liver abscess is a complication<br>• No anticoagulants unless hypercoagulable disease (neoplasm) indicated<br>• Surgery on vein not indicated |

*Abbreviations on page 2.   *NOTE: All dosage recommendations are for adults (unless otherwise indicated) and assume normal renal function. § Alternatives consider allergy, PK, compliance, local resistance, cost.*

**TABLE 2 – RECOMMENDED ANTIMICROBIAL AGENTS AGAINST SELECTED BACTERIA**

| BACTERIAL SPECIES | ANTIMICROBIAL AGENT (See page 2 for abbreviations) | | |
|---|---|---|---|
| | **RECOMMENDED** | **ALTERNATIVE** | **ALSO EFFECTIVE[1] (COMMENTS)** |
| Achromobacter xylosoxidans spp xylosoxidans (formerly Alcaligenes) | IMP, MER, DORI (no DORI for pneumonia) | TMP-SMX. Some strains susc. to ceftaz, PIP-TZ | Resistant to aminoglycosides, most cephalosporins & FQs. Ref: Ann Amer Thor Soc 12:252, 2015 |
| Acinetobacter calcoaceticus— baumannii complex | If suscept: IMP or MER. For MDR strains: Polymyxin B + (IMP or MER) + AM-SB | AM-SB used for activity of sulbactam | Resistant to aminoglycosides, FQs. Minocycline, effective against many strains (CID 51:79, 2010) |
| Actinomyces israelii | AMP or Pen G | Doxy, Ceftriaxone | Clindamycin, Erythro |
| Aerococcus urinae (cystitis) | Amox or Nitrofurantoin | Fosfomycin (A. urinae only); CIP (if susceptible) | Susceptible to Pen G. Frequently resistant to FQs. Increased Ceftriaxone MICs. Generally resistant to TMP-SMX |
| Aeromonas hydrophila & other sp. | CIP or Levo | TMP-SMX or (P Ceph 3, 4) | See AAC 56:1110, 2012. |
| Arcanobacterium haemolyticum | Azithro | Pen G, Ceftriaxone, Vancomycin, and many other agents | Resistance to TMP-SMX (AAC 38: 142, 1994). Resistance to Levofloxacin, Clindamycin reported (J Med Microbiol 64: 369, 2015) |
| **Bacillus anthracis (anthrax): inhalation** | See Table 1, page 44. | | |
| Bacillus cereus, B. subtilis | Vancomycin, Clinda | FQ, IMP | |
| Bacteroides sp., B. fragilis & others | Metronidazole or PIP-TZ | DORI, ERTA, IMP, MER, AM-CL | Increasing resistance to: Clinda, Cefoxitin, Cefotetan, Moxi. Ref: CID 59:698, 2014. |
| **Bartonella henselae, quintana** See Table 1, pages 32, 48, 54, 61 | Varies with disease entity & immune status. Active: Azithro, Clarithro, Erythro, Doxy & in combination: RIF, Gent, Ceftriaxone. Not active: CIP, TMP-SMX, Pen, most cephalosporins, Aztreonam. | | |
| Bordetella pertussis | Azithro or clarithro | TMP-SMX | See PIDJ 31:78, 2012. |
| **Borrelia burgdorferi, B. afzelii, B. garinii** (Lyme & relapsing fever) | See specific disease entity | | |
| Brucella sp. | Drugs & duration vary with localization or non-localization. See specific disease entities. PLoS One 7:e32090, 2012. | | |
| Burkholderia cepacia | TMP-SMX or MER or CIP | Minocycline or chloramphenicol | Multiple mechanisms of resistance. Need culture & sensitivity to guide therapy (Sem Resp Crit Care Med 36:99, 2015) |
| Burkholderia pseudomallei Curr Opin Infect Dis 23:554, 2010; CID 41:1105, 2005 | Initially, IV Ceftaz or IMP or MER, then po (TMP-SMX + Doxy x 3 mos) (AAC 49:4010, 2005). One study showed TMP-SMX alone was non-inferior to combination with Doxy (Lancet 383: 807, 2014) | | (Thai, 12–80% strains resist to TMP-SMX). FQ not very active in vitro. AM-CL possible alternative to TMP-SMX (Int J Antimicrob Agents 43: 310, 2014). |
| Campylobacter jejuni | Azithro | Erythro or CIP | TMP-SMX, Pen & cephalosporins not active. |
| Campylobacter fetus | Gentamicin | IMP or Ceftriaxone | AMP, Chloramphenicol |
| Capnocytophaga ochracea (DF-1) | Dog bite: Clinda or AM-CL | Septic shock, post-splenectomy: PIP-TZ, Clinda, IMP, DORI, MER | FQ activity variable; aminoglycosides, TMP-SMX & Polymyxins have limited activity. |
| Capnocytophaga canimorsus (DF-2) | Dog bite: AM-CL, PIP-TZ, CFP | | LN ID 9:439, 2009. |
| Chlamydophila pneumoniae | Doxy | Azithro, FQ | Clarithro |
| Chlamydia trachomatis | Doxy or Azithro | Erythro | |
| Citrobacter diversus (koseri), C. freundii | Life threatening illness: IMP, MER, DORI | Non-life threatening illness: CIP or Gent | Emergence of resistance: AAC 52:995, 2007. |
| **Clostridium (Clostridioides) difficile** | Mild illness: Vanco (po) | Moderate/severe illness: Vanco (po) or Fidaxomicin (CID 51:1306, 2010). | See also Table 1, page 20 re severity of disease. |
| Clostridium perfringens | Pen G ± clindamycin | Doxy | Erythro, Chloramphenicol, Cefazolin, Cefoxitin, PIP-TZ, Carbapenems |
| Clostridium tetani | Metronidazole | Doxy | Role of antibiotics unclear. |
| Corynebacterium diphtheriae | Erythro + antitoxin | Pen G + antitoxin | RIF reported effective (CID 27:845, 1998) |
| Corynebacterium jeikeium | Vancomycin | Daptomycin (Resistance reported, JCM 47: 2328, 2009) | Most strains are resistant to pen and Erythro (Clin Microbiol Inf 2: 209, 1996) |
| Corynebacterium minutissimum | Clinda 1% lotion | Clarithro or Erythro | Causes erythrasma |
| Coxiella burnetii (Q fever) acute disease (CID 52:1431, 2011). | Doxy, FQ (see Table 1, page 33) | Erythro, Azithro, Clarithro | Endocarditis: Doxy + hydroxychloroquine (JID 188:1322, 2003; LnID 3:709, 2003; LnID 10:527, 2010). |
| chronic disease, e.g., endocarditis | Doxy + hydroxy chloroquine | TMP-SMX, Chloro | |

# TABLE 2A (2)

| BACTERIAL SPECIES | ANTIMICROBIAL AGENT (See page 2 for abbreviations) | | |
|---|---|---|---|
| | RECOMMENDED | ALTERNATIVE | ALSO EFFECTIVE[1] (COMMENTS) |
| Ehrlichia chaffeensis Ehrlichia ewingii Anaplasma phagocytophilum | Doxy | Rifampin (no large studies) | Chloro not effective. In severe infections, consider doxycycline desensitization if allergic (MMWR 65(2): 1, 2016). |
| Eikenella corrodens | AM-CL, IV Pen G | TMP-SMX, FQ | Resistant to Clinda, Cephalexin, Erythro, Metro, Diclox |
| Elizabethkingia meningoseptica (formerly Chryseobacterium) | Levo or TMP-SMX | CIP, Minocycline | Resistant to Pen, cephalosporins, carbapenems, aminoglycosides, Vanco (JCM 44:1181, 2006) |
| Enterobacter species | Recommended agents vary with clinical setting and degree and mechanism of resistance. | | |
| **Enterococcus faecalis** | Highly resistant. See Table 5A, page 88 | | |
| **Enterococcus faecium** | Highly resistant. See Table 5A, page 88 | | |
| Erysipelothrix rhusiopathiae | Penicillin G or amox | P Ceph 3, FQ | IMP, PIP-TZ (vancomycin, APAG, TMP-SMX resistant) |
| Escherichia coli | Can be highly resistant. Treatment varies with degree and mechanism of resistance, see Table 5B. | | |
| **Francisella tularensis (tularemia)** See Table 1, page 46 | Gentamicin, Tobramycin, or Streptomycin | Mild infection: Doxy or CIP | Chloramphenicol, RIF. Doxy/chloro bacteriostatic → relapses CID 53:e133, 2011. |
| Fusobacterium necrophorum | Metro, Ceftriaxone, PIP-TZ | IMP, MER, Clinda | Resistant to macrolides |
| Gardnerella vaginalis (bacterial vaginosis) | Metronidazole or Tinidazole | Clindamycin | See Table 1, page 28 for dosage |
| Helicobacter pylori | See Table 1, page 23 | | Drugs effective in vitro often fail in vivo. |
| Haemophilus aphrophilus (Aggregatibacter aphrophilus) | Ceftriaxone | CIP or Levo | Resistant to Vanco, Clinda, Methicillin |
| Haemophilus ducreyi (chancroid) | Azithro or Ceftriaxone | Erythro, CIP | Most strains resistant to Tetracycline, Amox, TMP-SMX |
| **Haemophilus influenzae** Meningitis, epiglottitis & other life-threatening illness | Cefotaxime, Ceftriaxone | AMP if susceptible and β-lactamase neg, FQs | Chloramphenicol rarely used due to hematotoxicity. |
|   non-life threatening illness | AM-CL, O Ceph 2/3 | | Azithro, Clarithro, Telithro |
| Klebsiella ozaenae/ rhinoscleromatis | CIP | Levo | Acta Otolaryngol 131:440, 2010. |
| Klebsiella species | Treatment varies with degree and mechanism of resistance, see Table 5B. | | |
| Lactobacillus species | Pen G or AMP | Clindamycin | **May be resistant to vancomycin** |
| Legionella sp. | Levo or Moxi | Azithro, Doxy | |
| Leptospira interrogans | Mild: Doxy or Amox | Severe: Pen G or ceftriaxone | |
| Leuconostoc | Pen G or AMP | Clinda | **NOTE: Resistant to vancomycin** |
| **Listeria monocytogenes** | AMP ± Gent for synergy | TMP-SMX | Erythro, penicillin G (high dose); APAG may be synergistic with ß-lactams. **Cephalosporin-resistant!** |
| Moraxella (Branhamella) catarrhalis | AM-CL or O Ceph 2/3, TMP-SMX | Azithro, Clarithro, Dirithromycin, Telithro | Erythro, Doxy, FQs |
| Morganella sp. (need in vitro susceptibility) | Recommendations vary with clinical syndrome, frequency & mechanism of resistance | | |
| **Mycoplasma pneumoniae** | Doxy | Azithro, Minocycline | Clindamycin & ß lactams NOT effective. Increasing macrolide resistance (JAC 68:506, 2013; AAC 58:1034, 2014). |
| **Neisseria gonorrhoeae** (gonococcus) | Ceftriaxone, | Azithro (high dose) | FQs and oral cephalosporins no longer recommended: high levels of resistance. |
| **Neisseria meningitidis** (meningococcus) | Ceftriaxone | Pen G, MER, Chloro | (Chloro less effective than other alternatives: see JAC 70:979, 2015) |
| **Nocardia asteroides** or **Nocardia brasiliensis** | TMP-SMX + IMP | Linezolid | Amikacin + (IMP or ceftriaxone or Cefotaxime) (AAC 58:795, 2014). |
| **Pasteurella multocida** | Pen G, AMP, Amox, AM-CL, Cefuroxime, Cefpodoxime | Doxy, Levo, Moxi, TMP-SMX | Resistant to Cephalexin, Oxacillin, Clindamycin, Erythro, Vanco. Rare beta-lactamase-producing isolates have been reported (EJCMID 20: 210, 2001). |
| Peptoniphilus sp. (Peptostreptococcus) | Pen G | Metronidazole | Some clinda resistance (Clin Micro Infect 2014;20:0857) |
| Plesiomonas shigelloides | CIP | TMP-SMX | AM-CL, Ceftriaxone & Chloro active. Resistant to: Amp, Tetra, aminoglycosides |
| Propionibacterium (now Cutibacterium) acnes (not acne) | Penicillin, Ceftriaxone | Vanco, Dapto, Linezolid | May be resistant to Metro. |
| Proteus sp, **Providencia sp**, (Need in vitro susceptibility) | Recommended drugs vary with clinical setting and frequency & mechanism of resistance. | | |

| BACTERIAL SPECIES | ANTIMICROBIAL AGENT *(See page 2 for abbreviations)* | | |
|---|---|---|---|
| | **RECOMMENDED** | **ALTERNATIVE** | **ALSO EFFECTIVE[1] (COMMENTS)** |
| **Pseudomonas aeruginosa** | No in vitro resistance: PIP-TZ, AP Ceph 3, DORI, IMP, MER, Tobra, CIP, Aztreonam. For serious inf., use AP β-lactam + (Tobra or CIP) | For UTI, if no in vitro resistance, single drugs effective: PIP-TZ, AP Ceph 3, Cefepime, IMP, MER, aminoglycoside, CIP, Aztreonam | If resistant to all beta lactams, FQs, aminoglycosides: Polymyxin B + MER or IMP. Do not use DORI for pneumonia. Suggest consult for extensively resistant strains. |
| **Rhodococcus (C. equi)** | Customary to use combination Rx. Choose 2 from: Azithro, Levo, or Rif *(Lancet ID 10:350, 2010)*. | (Vanco or IMP) + (Azithro, Levo or RIF) | Vancomycin active in vitro; intracellular location may impair efficacy *(CID 34:1379, 2002)*. Avoid Pen, Cephalosporins, Clinda, Tetra, TMP-SMX. |
| Rickettsia species (includes spotted fevers) | Doxy | Chloramphenicol (in pregnancy) | *See specific infections (Table 1). (MMWR 65(RR-2):1, 2016)* |
| **Salmonella typhi** *(CID 50:241, 2010; AAC 54:5201, 2010; BMC ID 51:37, 2005)* | If FQ & nalidixic acid susceptible: CIP | Ceftriaxone, Cefixime, Azithro, Chloro | Concomitant steroids in severely ill. Watch for relapse (1-6%) & ileal perforation. Chloro less effective than other alternatives: see *JAC 70:979, 2015)*. |
| Serratia marcescens | If no in vitro resistance: PIP-TZ, CIP, LEVO, Gent | If in vitro resistance due to ESBL: Carbapenem | Avoid extended spectrum Ceph if possible See specific syndrome if MDR documented. |
| **Shigella sp.** | FQ or azithro | Ceftriaxone is alternative; TMP-SMX depends on susceptibility. | |
| **Staph. aureus, methicillin-susceptible** | Oxacillin/Nafcillin | P Ceph 1, Vanco, Teicoplanin[NUS], Clinda, Ceftaroline | ERTA, IMP, MER, AM-CL, FQ, PIP-TZ, Linezolid, Dapto, Telavancin. |
| **Staph. aureus, methicillin-resistant (health-care associated)** IDSA Guidelines: CID 52 (Feb 1):1, 2011. | Vancomycin | Teicoplanin[NUS], Linezolid, Daptomycin, Telavancin, Ceftaroline | Fusidic acid[NUS]. >60% CIP-resistant in U.S. (Fosfomycin + RIF). See Table 6, page 90. |
| **Staph. aureus, methicillin-resistant [community- associated (CA-MRSA)]** | | | |
| | (TMP-SMX or Doxy or Mino) | Clinda (if D-test neg— see Table 5A & 6). | CA-MRSA usually not multiply-resistant. Oft resist. to Erythro & Variably to FQ. Vanco, Teico[NUS], Telavancin, Dapto, Ceftaroline can be used in pts requiring hospitalization (see Table 6, page 90). |
| | Vanco or Teico[NUS] | Linezolid or Dapto | |
| **Staph. epidermidis** | MSSE: oxacillin, nafcillin, cefazolin MRSE: Vancomycin | Dapto, linezolid | Rifampin (if Susceptible) often used with (FQ or TMP-SMX) for infections assoc with prostheses. |
| Staph. haemolyticus | If Oxa-susceptible: oxacillin, nafcillin, cefazolin If Oxa-resistant: Vancomycin | Dapto, linezolid | For UTI: TMP-SMX, nitrofurantoin, oral ceph, FQ may be active. |
| Staph. lugdunensis | If Oxa-susceptible: oxacillin, nafcillin, cefazolin If Oxa-susc: oral ceph or AM-CL. | Pen G if pen-susceptible. Daptomycin, linezolid. If Oxa-susc: oral ceph or AM-CL. | Approx 52% susceptible to Pen G and 95% to oxacillin; high rates of susc to doxy or TMP-SMX *(JCM 55: 585, 2017)*. |
| Staph. saprophyticus (UTI) | Oral cephalosporin or AM-CL | FQ | Almost always methicillin-susceptible |
| Stenotrophomonas (Xanthomonas, Pseudo-monas) maltophilia | TMP-SMX | Minocycline *(Diag Micro Infect Dis 85:352, 2016; JAC 2016,71:1071)* | FQ (if in vitro suscept)*(AAC 2014,58:176)* |
| Streptobacillus moniliformis | Penicillin G | Doxy | Maybe Erythro, Clinda, Ceftriaxone |
| Streptococcus anginosus group | Penicillin | Vanco or Ceftriaxone | Avoid FQs; macrolide resistance emerging |
| **Streptococcus pneumoniae** penicillin-susceptible | Penicillin G, Amox | Multiple agents effective, e.g., Ceph 2/3, Clinda | If meningitis, higher dose, see *Table 1, page 11*. |
| penicillin resistant (MIC ≥2.0) | Vanco, Levo, Ceftriaxone, Ceftaroline, Amox (HD), Linezolid | | |
| **Streptococcus pyogenes,** (Grp A), **Streptococcus sp** (Grp B, C, G). Erysipelas, bacteremia, TSS | Penicillin G, cephalosporin | Clinda, vanco, dapto, linezolid | For TSS, necrotizing fasciitis: Pen G+Clinda. Avoid FQ, TMP-SMX, tetracyclines. Pockets of macrolide/clinda resistance *(JCM 49: 439, 2011)*. |
| **Tropheryma whipplei** | Doxy + Hydroxychloroquine | Ceftriaxone or Mero, then TMP-SMX | Clinical failures with TMP-SMX |
| Vibrio cholerae | Azithro | CIP, Doxy | Rehydration salts primary therapy. Vaccine available. |
| Vibrio parahaemolyticus | Doxy | Azithro, CIP | If bacteremic, treat as for V. vulnificus |

[1] Agents are more variable in effectiveness than "Recommended" or "Alternative". Selection of "Alternative" or "Also Effective" based on in vitro susceptibility testing, pharmacokinetics, host factors such as auditory, renal, hepatic function, & cost.

**TABLE 2A (4)**

| BACTERIAL SPECIES | ANTIMICROBIAL AGENT *(See page 2 for abbreviations)* | | |
| --- | --- | --- | --- |
| | **RECOMMENDED** | **ALTERNATIVE** | **ALSO EFFECTIVE[1] (COMMENTS)** |
| Vibrio vulnificus, alginolyticus, damsela | Doxy + Ceftriaxone | Levo | *CID 52:788, 2011* |
| **Yersinia enterocolitica** | Ceftriaxone if bacteremic, CIP otherwise | TMP-SMX | CIP resistance (*JAC 53: 1068, 2004*); also resistance to Pen, Amp, 1st gen Cephs, Erythro. |
| **Yersinia pestis** (plague) | Streptomycin or Gent | Doxy or (CIP, Levo, Moxi) | Levo, Moxi. CDC advice for treatment and prevention (https://www.cdc.gov/plague/healthcare/clinicians.html). |

**TABLE 3 – SUGGESTED DURATION OF ANTIBIOTIC THERAPY FOR SELECTED
CLINICAL SYNDROMES IN IMMUNOCOMPETENT PATIENTS**

**Overview of variables affecting duration of therapy**

Variables involved in duration of therapy are summarized in Curr Opin Infect Dis 2015;28:170 and include:

- PK/PD of antibiotic used, e.g., long tissue half-life of Azithro
- Identified pathogen (etiology)
- Host factors, e.g., neutropenic, HIV
- Severity of infection, e.g., cystitis vs. bacteremia
- Severity of host inflammatory response as measured by biomarkers, e.g., serum procalcitonin

Due to these many variables, it is usually not possible to recommend a definite duration except where there is a single pathogen in a healthy person, e.g., E. coli cystitis or Legionella pneumonia. For most situations, need to individualize duration until the patient is clinically stable and biomarkers have normalized.

| CLINICAL SITUATION | | DURATION OF THERAPY |
|---|---|---|
| **SITE** | **CLINICAL DIAGNOSIS** | **(Days)** |
| **Bacteremia** | Bacteremia with removable focus (no endocarditis) | **10–14** *(See Table 1)* |
| **Bone** | Osteomyelitis, adult; acute | **42** *(Ln 385:875, 2015)* |
| | adult; chronic | Until ESR normal (often >3 months) |
| | child; acute; staph. and enterobacteriaceae | **21** |
| | child; acute; strep, meningococci, haemophilus | **14** |
| | | Can shorten **14/21** to **7** days if resolution of S&S and biomarkers normalize |
| **Ear** | Otitis media with effusion | <2 yrs: **10**; ≥2 yrs: **5–7** |
| **Endocardium** | Infective endocarditis, native valve: Viridans strep | **14 or 28** *(See Table 1, page 30)* |
| | Enterococci | **28 or 42** *(See Table 1, page 31)* |
| | Staph. aureus | **14** (R-sided only) or **28** *(See Table 1, page 31)* |
| **GI** | Bacillary dysentery (shigellosis)/traveler's diarrhea | single dose, up to **3** days if no response |
| *Also see* | Typhoid fever (S. typhi): Azithro | **5–7** (children/adolescents) |
| *Table 1* | Ceftriaxone | **7–14** [Short course ↑ effective *(AAC 44:450, 2000)*] |
| | FQ | **7–10** |
| | Chloramphenicol | **14** |
| | Helicobacter pylori | **14** days now preferred |
| | Pseudomembranous enterocolitis (C. difficile) | **10** |
| **Genital** | Non-gonococcal urethritis or mucopurulent cervicitis | **7** days doxy or single dose azithro |
| | Pelvic inflammatory disease | **14** |
| **Heart** | Pericarditis (purulent) | **28** or until resolution of S&S and biomarkers normalize |
| **Joint** | Septic arthritis (non-gonococcal): Adult | **14–28** |
| | Infant/child | **10–14** (Response varies, stop when resolution of S&S and biomarkers normalize). |
| | Gonococcal arthritis/disseminated GC infection | **7** *(See Table 1, page 25)* |
| **Kidney** | Cystitis, acute | **3** |
| | Pyelonephritis *(Ln 380:484, 2012)* | **7** (7 days if CIP used; 5 days if levo 750 mg) |
| **Lung** | Pneumonia, pneumococcal | 5-7 days or fall of serum procalcitonin by 80% |
| *(Curr Op ID* | Community-acquired pneumonia | or ≤ 0.25 ng/mL |
| *28:177, 2015)* | Pneumonia, enterobacteriaceae or pseudomonal | **14-21, often up to 42** (variable, until biomarkers normalize) |
| | Pneumonia, staphylococcal | **21–28** (variable, until biomarkers normalize) |
| | Pneumocystis pneumonia (PCP) in AIDS | **21** |
| | Other immunocompromised | **14** |
| | Legionella, mycoplasma, chlamydia | **5-14** days depending on severity of illness, up to 21 in immunocompromised |
| | Lung abscess | Usually **28–42**, but variable |
| **Meninges** | N. meningitidis | **7** |
| | H. influenzae | **7** |
| | S. pneumoniae | **10–14** |
| | Listeria meningoencephalitis, gp B strep, coliforms | **21** (longer in immunocompromised) |
| | *Child: relapses seldom occur until 3 or more days post-rx.* | |
| **Multiple systems** | Brucellosis *(See Table 1, page 64)* | **42** (depends on site of infection) |
| | Tularemia *(See Table 1, pages 48, 64)* | **7–21** depending on severity |
| **Muscle** | Gas gangrene (clostridial) | **10** but depends on severity |
| **Pharynx** | Group A strep pharyngitis | **10** (Pen VK), **5** (O Ceph 2/3, Azithro) *(PIDJ 36:507, 2017)* |
| | *Also see Pharyngitis, Table 1, page 51* | |
| | Diphtheria (membranous) | **14** (Pen G, Erythro) |
| | Carrier | **1** dose (Pen G), **7–10** (Erythro) |
| **Prostate** | Chronic prostatitis | **30–90** (TMP-SMX), **28–42** (FQ) |
| **Sinuses** | Acute bacterial sinusitis (usually viral etiology) | **5** |
| **Skin** | Cellulitis, erysipelas | **Until 3 days after acute inflamm disappears** |
| **Systemic** | Lyme disease | *See Table 1, page 62.* |
| | Rocky Mountain spotted fever *(See Table 1, page 63)* | **Until afebrile 2 days** |

# TABLE 4A – ANTIBACTERIAL ACTIVITY SPECTRA

The data provided are intended to serve as a general guide to antibacterial usefulness based on treatment guidelines and recommendations, in-vitro activity, predominant patterns of susceptibility or resistance, and/or demonstrated clinical effectiveness. **Variability in resistance patterns as a consequence of clinical differences (e.g., community-onset vs. ICU-acquired infection) should be taken into account when using this table because activities of certain agents can differ significantly from what is shown in the table,** which are by necessity based on aggregate information. We have revised and expanded the color / symbol key to provide a more descriptive categorization of the table data.

**++ = Recommended:** Agent is a first line therapy; reliably active in vitro, clinically effective, guideline recommended, recommended as a first-line agent or acceptable alternative agent in the Sanford Guide

**+ = Active:** Agent is a potential alternative agent (active in vitro, possesses class activity comparable to known effective agents or a therapeutically interchangeable agents and hence likely to be clinically effective, but second line due to overly broad spectrum, toxicity, limited clinical experience, or paucity of direct evidence of effectiveness)

**± = Variable:** Variable activity such that the agent, although clinically effective in some settings or types of infections is not reliably effective in others, or should be used in combination with another agent, and/or its efficacy is limited by resistance which has been associated with treatment failure

**0 = Not recommended:** Agent is a poor alternative to other agents because resistance to likely to be present or occur, due to poor drug penetration to site of infection or an unfavorable toxicity profile, or limited or anecdotal clinical data to support effectiveness

**? = Insufficient Data** to recommend use

**NA = No activity:** Agent has no activity against this pathogen

| | Penicillins | | | | | | | | | | | | Carbapenems | | | | | Aztreonam | Fluoroquinolone | | | | | | | | | Parenteral Cephalosporins | | | | | | | | | | | | |
|---|---|---|---|---|---|---|---|---|---|---|---|---|---|---|---|---|---|---|---|---|---|---|---|---|---|---|---|---|---|---|---|---|---|---|---|---|---|---|---|---|
| | Penicillin G | Penicillin VK | Nafcillin | Oxacillin | Cloxacillin | Flucloxacillin | Dicloxacillin | Ampicillin | Amoxicillin | Amox-Clav | Amp-Sulb | Pip-Tazo | Doripenem | Ertapenem | Imipenem | Meropenem | Mero-Vabor | Aztreonam | Ciprofloxacin | Delafloxacin | Ofloxacin | Levofloxacin | Moxifloxacin | Norfloxacin | Prulifloxacin | Gemifloxacin | Gatifloxacin | Cefazolin | Cefotetan | Cefoxitin | Cefuroxime | Cefotaxime | Ceftizoxime | Ceftriaxone | Ceftazidime | Cefepime | Ceftaz-Avibac | Ceftaroline | Ceftobiprole | Ceftol-Tazo |
| **Aerobic gram-pos cocci** | | | | | | | | | | | | | | | | | | | | | | | | | | | | | | | | | | | | | | | | |
| E. faecalis (S) | ++ | ± | 0 | 0 | 0 | 0 | 0 | ++ | ++ | + | + | + | 0 | 0 | + | ± | ± | 0 | ± | + | ± | + | + | + | 0 | + | + | 0 | 0 | 0 | 0 | 0 | 0 | 0 | 0 | 0 | 0 | ++ | + | 0 |
| E. faecium (S) | ± | 0 | 0 | 0 | 0 | 0 | 0 | ± | ± | ± | ± | ± | 0 | 0 | 0 | 0 | 0 | 0 | 0 | + | 0 | 0 | 0 | + | 0 | + | + | 0 | 0 | 0 | 0 | 0 | 0 | 0 | 0 | 0 | 0 | + | 0 | 0 |
| E. faecalis (VRE) | ± | 0 | 0 | 0 | 0 | 0 | 0 | ± | ± | ± | ± | ± | 0 | 0 | ± | 0 | 0 | 0 | 0 | + | 0 | 0 | 0 | 0 | 0 | 0 | 0 | 0 | 0 | 0 | 0 | 0 | 0 | 0 | 0 | 0 | 0 | + | + | 0 |
| E. faecium (VRE) | 0 | 0 | 0 | 0 | 0 | 0 | 0 | 0 | 0 | 0 | 0 | 0 | 0 | 0 | 0 | 0 | 0 | 0 | 0 | + | 0 | 0 | 0 | 0 | 0 | 0 | 0 | 0 | 0 | 0 | 0 | 0 | 0 | 0 | 0 | 0 | 0 | 0 | 0 | ? |
| S. aureus MSSA | ± | ± | ++ | ++ | ++ | ++ | ++ | 0 | 0 | + | + | + | + | + | + | + | + | 0 | + | + | + | + | + | ± | ± | + | + | ++ | + | + | + | + | + | +± | ± | + | + | + | + | + |
| S. aureus HA-MRSA | 0 | 0 | 0 | 0 | 0 | 0 | 0 | 0 | 0 | 0 | 0 | 0 | 0 | 0 | 0 | 0 | 0 | 0 | 0 | + | 0 | 0 | 0 | 0 | 0 | 0 | 0 | 0 | 0 | 0 | 0 | 0 | 0 | 0 | 0 | 0 | 0 | + | + | 0 |
| S. aureus CA-MRSA | 0 | 0 | 0 | 0 | 0 | 0 | 0 | 0 | 0 | 0 | 0 | 0 | 0 | 0 | 0 | 0 | 0 | 0 | ± | + | 0 | ± | ± | 0 | 0 | ± | ± | 0 | 0 | 0 | 0 | 0 | 0 | 0 | 0 | 0 | 0 | + | + | 0 |
| Staph coag-neg (S) | ± | ± | ++ | ++ | ++ | ++ | ++ | ± | ± | + | + | + | + | + | + | + | + | 0 | ± | + | ± | + | + | ± | ± | + | + | + | + | + | + | + | + | + | ± | + | + | + | + | + |
| Staph coag-neg (R) | 0 | 0 | 0 | 0 | 0 | 0 | 0 | 0 | 0 | 0 | 0 | 0 | 0 | 0 | 0 | 0 | 0 | 0 | 0 | + | 0 | 0 | 0 | 0 | 0 | 0 | 0 | 0 | 0 | 0 | 0 | 0 | 0 | 0 | 0 | 0 | 0 | + | + | 0 |
| S. epidermidis (S) | ± | ± | ++ | ++ | ++ | ++ | ++ | ± | ± | + | + | + | + | + | + | + | + | 0 | ± | + | ± | + | +± | ± | ± | + | + | + | + | + | + | + | + | + | ± | + | + | + | + | ? |
| S. epidermidis (R) | 0 | 0 | 0 | 0 | 0 | 0 | 0 | 0 | 0 | 0 | 0 | 0 | 0 | 0 | 0 | 0 | 0 | 0 | 0 | + | 0 | 0 | 0 | 0 | 0 | ± | ± | 0 | 0 | 0 | 0 | 0 | 0 | 0 | 0 | 0 | 0 | + | + | 0 |
| S. lugdunensis | ± | ± | ++ | ++ | ++ | ++ | ++ | + | + | + | + | + | + | + | + | + | + | 0 | + | + | + | + | + | ± | + | + | + | + | + | + | + | + | + | + | ± | + | + | + | + | ? |
| S. saprophyticus | + | + | ++ | ++ | ++ | ++ | ++ | + | + | + | ++ | ++ | + | + | + | + | + | ± | ± | + | ± | ± | ± | + | + | + | + | + | + | + | + | + | + | + | + | + | + | + | + | ? |
| S. anginosus grp | ++ | ± | + | + | + | + | + | + | + | + | + | + | + | + | + | + | + | 0 | ± | + | ± | ± | +± | 0 | 0 | ± | ± | + | + | + | + | + | + | + | + | + | + | + | + | + |
| Strep. pyogenes (A) | ++ | ++ | + | + | + | + | + | ++ | ++ | + | + | + | + | + | + | + | + | 0 | ± | + | ± | + | + | 0 | 0 | + | + | + | + | + | + | + | + | + | + | + | + | + | + | + |
| Strep. agalactiae (B) | ++ | ++ | + | + | + | + | + | ++ | ++ | + | + | + | + | + | + | + | + | 0 | ± | + | ± | +± | +± | 0 | 0 | +± | +± | + | + | + | + | + | + | + | + | + | + | + | + | + |

TABLE 4A (2)

| | | Penicillins | | | | | | | | | | | | Carbapenems | | | | | | Fluoroquinolone | | | | | | | | | Parenteral Cephalosporins | | | | | | | | | | | | |
|---|---|---|---|---|---|---|---|---|---|---|---|---|---|---|---|---|---|---|---|---|---|---|---|---|---|---|---|---|---|---|---|---|---|---|---|---|---|---|---|---|---|---|
| | | Penicillin G | Penicillin VK | Nafcillin | Oxacillin | Cloxacillin | Flucloxacillin | Dicloxacillin | Ampicillin | Amoxicillin | Amox-Clav | Amp-Sulb | Pip-Tazo | Doripenem | Ertapenem | Imipenem | Meropenem | Mero-Vabor | Aztreonam | Ciprofloxacin | Delafloxacin | Ofloxacin | Levofloxacin | Moxifloxacin | Norfloxacin | Prulifloxacin | Gemifloxacin | Gatifloxacin | Cefazolin | Cefotetan | Cefoxitin | Cefuroxime | Cefotaxime | Ceftizoxime | Ceftriaxone | Ceftazidime | Cefepime | Ceftaz-Avibac | Ceftaroline | Ceftobiprole | Ceftol-Tazo |
| **Aerobic gram-pos cocci** *(continued)* | | | | | | | | | | | | | | | | | | | | | | | | | | | | | | | | | | | | | | | | | |
| | Strep. gp C, F, G | ++ | ++ | + | + | + | + | + | + | + | + | + | + | + | + | + | + | + | O | +! | + | +! | +! | +! | O | +! | +! | +! | + | + | + | + | + | + | + | + | + | + | + | + | + |
| | Strep. pneumoniae | ++ | ++ | + | + | + | + | + | + | + | + | + | + | + | + | + | + | + | O | +! | + | +! | + | + | O | +! | + | + | + | + | + | + | + | + | + | + | + | + | + | + | + |
| | Viridans Strep. | +! | +! | +! | +! | +! | +! | +! | +! | +! | +! | +! | +! | + | + | + | + | + | O | +! | + | +! | +! | +! | O | +! | +! | + | + | + | + | + | +‡ | + | +‡ | +! | +! | + | + | +! | +! |
| **Aerobic gram-pos bacilli** | | | | | | | | | | | | | | | | | | | | | | | | | | | | | | | | | | | | | | | | | | |
| | Arcanobacter. sp | + | ? | ? | ? | ? | ? | ? | + | + | + | + | + | + | + | + | + | + | O | ? | ? | ? | + | + | O | ? | ? | + | + | + | + | + | + | + | + | + | + | + | + | + | ? |
| | C. diphtheriae | ++ | ++ | O | O | O | O | O | + | + | + | + | + | ? | ? | ? | ? | + | O | ? | ? | ? | ? | ? | O | ? | ? | ? | + | + | + | + | + | + | + | + | + | ? | + | + | ? |
| | C. jeikeium | O | O | O | O | O | O | O | O | O | O | O | O | O | O | O | O | +! | O | O | + | O | O | +! | O | +! | +! | ? | O | O | O | O | O | O | O | O | O | O | O | O | O |
| | L. monocytogenes | + | + | O | O | O | O | O | ++ | ++ | +! | +! | O | ? | ? | ? | +! | + | O | O | + | O | O | O | O | O | O | ? | O | O | O | O | O | O | O | O | O | O | O | O | O |
| | Nocardia sp. | O | O | O | O | O | O | O | O | O | +! | ? | ? | ? | ? | ++ | +! | + | O | O | + | O | O | O | O | O | O | O | O | + | O | O | O | O | O | O | O | O | O | O | O |
| **Aerobic GNB - Enteric** | | | | | | | | | | | | | | | | | | | | | | | | | | | | | | | | | | | | | | | | | | |
| | Aeromonas sp. | O | O | O | O | O | O | O | O | O | +! | +! | + | + | + | + | + | + | + | + | + | + | + | + | + | + | + | + | O | O | O | ? | + | + | + | + | + | + | ? | ? | ? |
| | C. jejuni | O | O | O | O | O | O | O | + | + | + | + | O | + | + | + | + | + | ? | + | + | + | + | + | +! | + | + | + | O | O | O | O | ? | ? | ? | ? | O | ? | O | O | O |
| | Citrobacter sp. | O | O | O | O | O | O | O | O | O | O | O | ++ | + | +! | +! | + | + | +! | + | + | + | + | + | +! | + | + | + | O | O | O | O | +! | +! | +! | +! | +! | + | ? | + | + |
| | C. koseri | O | O | O | O | O | O | O | O | O | O | O | ++ | + | +! | ++ | + | ? | +! | + | + | + | + | + | +! | + | +! | + | O | O | O | O | +! | +! | +! | +! | ++ | + | O | + | + |
| | E. aerogenes | O | O | O | O | O | O | O | O | O | O | O | + | + | + | + | + | + | + | + | + | + | + | + | + | + | + | + | O | O | O | O | + | + | + | + | + | + | + | + | O |
| | E. cloacae | O | O | O | O | O | O | O | O | O | O | O | + | + | + | + | + | +‡ | + | + | + | + | + | + | + | + | + | + | O | O | O | O | + | + | + | + | + | + | + | + | + |
| | E. coli (S) | O | O | O | O | O | O | O | +! | +! | + | + | + | + | + | + | + | + | + | + | + | + | + | + | +! | + | + | + | + | + | +! | O | O | O | O | O | O | + | + | + | O |
| | E. coli, Klebs ESBL | O | O | O | O | O | O | O | O | O | O | O | O | + | ++ | ++ | +‡ | ++ | O | O | +! | O | O | O | +! | O | O | O | O | O | +! | O | O | O | O | O | O | + | O | O | O |
| | E. coli, Klebs KPC | O | O | O | O | O | O | O | O | O | O | O | O | O | O | O | O | O | O | O | + | O | O | O | O | O | O | O | O | O | O | O | O | O | O | +! | O | ‡ | O | O | O |
| | E. coli, Klebs MBL | O | O | O | O | O | O | O | O | O | O | O | O | O | O | O | O | O | O | +! | + | O | +! | O | +! | +! | +! | +! | O | O | O | O | O | O | O | +! | +! | O | O | O | O |
| | Enterics CRE, NOS | O | O | O | O | O | O | O | O | O | O | O | O | O | O | O | O | + | O | + | + | + | + | + | + | + | + | + | O | + | + | O | O | O | O | O | O | +! | O | O | O |
| | K. oxytoca | O | O | O | O | O | O | O | O | O | + | + | + | + | + | + | + | + | + | + | + | + | + | + | +! | + | + | + | + | + | + | O | + | + | + | + | + | + | + | + | + |
| | K. pneumoniae (S) | O | O | O | O | O | O | O | O | O | + | + | + | +! | + | + | + | + | O | + | + | + | + | + | +! | + | + | + | + | + | + | O | + | + | + | + | ++ | ‡ | + | + | + |
| | Morganella sp. | O | O | O | O | O | O | O | O | O | O | + | + | +! | +! | +! | + | + | +! | + | + | + | + | ? | +! | + | + | + | O | + | + | O | + | + | + | + | ++ | +! | + | + | ? |
| | P. mirabilis | O | O | O | O | O | O | O | + | + | + | + | + | +! | + | +! | + | + | + | + | + | + | + | ? | +! | +! | + | + | + | + | + | O | + | + | + | + | + | + | + | + | + |
| | P. vulgaris | O | O | O | O | O | O | O | O | O | + | + | + | ? | ? | ? | + | + | + | + | + | + | + | ? | +! | +! | ? | ? | O | + | + | O | + | + | + | + | + | + | + | ? | + |
| | Providencia sp. | O | O | O | O | O | O | O | O | O | O | + | ? | +! | +! | +! | + | + | O | + | + | + | + | ? | +! | + | ? | ? | O | + | + | O | + | + | + | + | + | + | + | ? | + |

TABLE 4A (3)

| | Penicillins | | | | | | | | | | | | Carbapenems | | | | | | Fluoroquinolone | | | | | | | | | Parenteral Cephalosporins | | | | | | | | | | | | |
|---|---|---|---|---|---|---|---|---|---|---|---|---|---|---|---|---|---|---|---|---|---|---|---|---|---|---|---|---|---|---|---|---|---|---|---|---|---|---|---|---|
| | Penicillin G | Penicillin VK | Nafcillin | Oxacillin | Cloxacillin | Flucloxacillin | Dicloxacillin | Ampicillin | Amoxicillin | Amox-Clav | Amp-Sulb | Pip-Tazo | Doripenem | Ertapenem | Imipenem | Meropenem | Mero-Vabor | Aztreonam | Ciprofloxacin | Delafloxacin | Ofloxacin | Levofloxacin | Moxifloxacin | Norfloxacin | Prulifloxacin | Gemifloxacin | Gatifloxacin | Cefazolin | Cefotetan | Cefoxitin | Cefuroxime | Cefotaxime | Ceftizoxime | Ceftriaxone | Ceftazidime | Cefepime | Ceftaz-Avibac | Ceftaroline | Ceftobiprole | Ceftol-Tazo |
| **Aerobic GNB - Enteric** *(continued)* | | | | | | | | | | | | | | | | | | | | | | | | | | | | | | | | | | | | | | | | |
| Salmonella sp. | o | o | o | o | o | o | o | +\| | +\| | + | + | + | + | + | + | + | + | + | + | + | + | + | + | o | + | + | + | o | + | ? | ? | + | + | + | + | + | + | ? | ? | ? |
| Serratia sp. | o | o | o | o | o | o | o | o | o | o | + | + | + | + | + | + | + | + | + | + | + | + | + | o | + | + | + | o | + | o | o | o | o | + | + | + | + | ? | ? | ? |
| Shigella sp. | o | o | o | o | o | o | o | o | o | + | + | + | + | + | + | + | + | + | ‡ | + | ‡ | ‡ | + | o | ‡ | ++ | + | o | o | ? | o | o | o | + | o | + | o | ? | ? | ? |
| Y. enterocolitica | o | o | o | o | o | o | o | o | o | +\| | +\| | + | ? | + | + | + | + | + | ‡ | + | + | ‡ | + | o | ‡ | ? | + | o | +\| | +\| | +\| | ‡ | +\| | ‡ | +\| | ‡ | ? | ? | ? | ? |
| **Aerobic GNB - Non-enteric** | | | | | | | | | | | | | | | | | | | | | | | | | | | | | | | | | | | | | | | | |
| Bartonella sp. | o | o | o | o | o | o | o | o | o | o | o | o | o | ? | o | o | o | o | o | o | o | +\| | o | o | o | o | o | o | o | o | o | o | o | o | o | o | o | o | o | o |
| B. pertussis | o | +\| | o | o | o | o | o | o | o | o | o | o | o | ? | o | o | o | o | o | o | o | ? | ? | ? | o | ? | ? | o | o | o | o | o | o | ‡ | o | + | o | o | o | o |
| B. burgdorferi | + | o | o | o | o | o | o | ++ | ++ | + | + | + | + | + | + | + | + | o | o | o | o | + | ? | o | ? | ? | ? | o | o | o | + | + | ++ | ++ | o | ? | o | ? | ? | ? |
| Brucella sp. | o | o | o | o | o | o | o | o | o | o | o | o | ? | ? | ? | ? | ? | o | + | o | +\| | + | + | ? | + | + | + | o | o | o | o | + | + | +\| | o | o | ? | ? | o | ? |
| Capnocytophaga | +\| | +\| | o | o | o | o | o | +\| | +\| | + | + | ‡ | + | + | ‡ | + | + | ? | +\| | + | + | + | + | ? | + | + | + | o | ? | ? | + | + | + | + | o | o | ? | ? | ? | ? |
| C. burnetii | o | o | o | o | o | o | o | o | o | o | o | o | o | ? | o | o | o | o | +\| | ? | +\| | +\| | +\| | ? | +\| | +\| | +\| | o | o | o | o | o | o | o | o | o | o | o | o | o |
| Ehrlichia, Anaplas | o | o | o | o | o | o | o | o | o | o | o | o | o | o | o | o | o | o | o | o | o | o | o | o | o | o | o | o | o | o | o | o | o | o | o | o | o | o | o | o |
| Eikenella sp | o | +\| | o | o | o | o | o | +\| | +\| | + | + | + | + | + | + | + | + | o | ‡ | + | ‡ | + | + | ++ | ‡ | + | + | o | o | o | + | + | ‡ | + | o | o | ? | ? | ? | ? |
| F. tularensis | o | o | o | o | o | o | o | o | o | o | o | o | ? | ? | ? | ? | ? | ? | ++ | ? | + | + | ? | ? | + | + | + | o | o | o | o | o | o | o | o | o | o | ? | o | ? |
| H. ducreyi | o | o | o | o | o | o | o | o | o | + | + | + | + | + | + | + | + | + | ‡ | + | ‡ | + | + | ++ | ‡ | + | + | o | ? | ? | + | + | ‡ | + | o | o | ? | ? | ? | ? |
| H. influenzae | o | +\| | o | o | o | o | o | +\| | +\| | + | + | + | + | + | + | + | + | + | + | + | + | + | ++ | + | + | + | + | o | ? | ? | + | + | ‡ | + | + | + | + | + | + | + |
| Kingella sp | + | + | o | o | o | o | o | + | + | + | + | + | + | + | + | + | + | + | + | + | + | + | + | ‡ | + | + | + | o | o | ? | + | + | + | + | o | o | ? | ? | ? | ? |
| K. granulomatis | o | o | o | o | o | o | o | o | o | ‡ | ‡ | + | + | + | + | + | + | o | ++ | + | ++ | ++ | + | + | ++ | + | + | o | o | o | o | ‡ | o | o | o | o | o | ? | ? | ? |
| Legionella sp. | o | o | o | o | o | o | o | o | o | o | o | o | o | o | o | o | o | o | ++ | + | ++ | ++ | + | + | ++ | ++ | + | o | o | o | o | o | o | o | o | o | o | o | o | o |
| Leptospira sp. | ++ | ++ | o | o | o | o | o | ++ | ++ | ‡ | ‡ | + | + | + | + | + | + | o | + | + | + | + | + | o | + | + | + | o | o | o | o | ‡ | o | +\| | o | o | o | o | o | o |
| M. catarrhalis | o | o | o | o | o | o | o | o | o | + | + | o | + | + | + | + | + | + | + | + | + | + | + | +\| | + | + | + | o | o | ? | +\| | + | +\| | + | + | + | + | ++ | + | + |
| N. gonorrhoeae | o | o | o | o | o | o | o | o | o | o | o | o | + | + | + | + | + | o | ? | +\| | ? | + | ? | o | ? | o | +\| | o | o | o | o | ++ | o | +\| | + | + | o | + | ? | ? |
| N. meningitidis | + | + | o | o | o | o | o | ‡ | ‡ | ‡ | ‡ | + | + | + | + | + | + | o | +\| | + | +\| | + | + | o | + | + | + | o | o | o | o | +\| | + | ++ | + | o | + | + | ? | ? |
| P. multocida | + | +\| | o | o | o | o | o | ‡ | ‡ | ‡ | ‡ | + | + | + | + | + | + | + | +\| | + | +\| | + | + | +\| | + | + | + | o | ? | +\| | + | +\| | +\| | + | o | o | ? | ? | ? | ? |
| R. rickettsii | o | o | o | o | o | o | o | o | o | o | o | o | o | o | o | o | o | o | o | o | o | o | o | o | o | o | o | o | o | o | o | o | o | o | o | o | o | o | o | o |
| T. pallidum | ++ | ++ | o | o | o | o | o | o | o | o | o | o | ? | ? | ? | ? | ? | ? | o | o | o | o | o | o | o | o | o | o | o | o | o | + | + | ++ | o | ? | o | ? | ? | ? |
| V. cholera | o | o | o | o | o | o | o | o | o | + | + | + | + | + | + | + | + | o | + | o | + | + | + | + | + | + | + | o | o | o | o | o | o | + | o | + | o | ? | o | ? |
| V. parahaemolyticus | o | o | o | o | o | o | o | o | o | o | o | ? | + | + | + | + | ? | ? | + | ? | + | + | ? | ? | ? | ? | ? | o | ? | o | o | o | o | + | o | + | ? | ? | ? | ? |

TABLE 4A (4)

| | Penicillins | | | | | | | | | | | | Carbapenems | | | | | | Fluoroquinolone | | | | | | | | | Parenteral Cephalosporins | | | | | | | | | | | | |
|---|---|---|---|---|---|---|---|---|---|---|---|---|---|---|---|---|---|---|---|---|---|---|---|---|---|---|---|---|---|---|---|---|---|---|---|---|---|---|---|---|
| | Penicillin G | Penicillin VK | Nafcillin | Oxacillin | Cloxacillin | Flucloxacillin | Dicloxacillin | Ampicillin | Amoxicillin | Amox-Clav | Amp-Sulb | Pip-Tazo | Doripenem | Ertapenem | Imipenem | Meropenem | Mero-Vabor | Aztreonam | Ciprofloxacin | Delafloxacin | Ofloxacin | Levofloxacin | Moxifloxacin | Norfloxacin | Prulifloxacin | Gemifloxacin | Gatifloxacin | Cefazolin | Cefotetan | Cefoxitin | Cefuroxime | Cefotaxime | Ceftizoxime | Ceftriaxone | Ceftazidime | Cefepime | Ceftaz-Avibac | Ceftaroline | Ceftobiprole | Ceftol-Tazo |
| **Aerobic GNB - Non-enteric** *(continued)* | | | | | | | | | | | | | | | | | | | | | | | | | | | | | | | | | | | | | | | | |
| V. vulnificus | 0 | 0 | 0 | 0 | 0 | 0 | 0 | 0 | 0 | 0 | 0 | 0 | ? | ? | ? | ? | ? | ? | + | ? | + | + | ? | 0 | + | ? | ? | 0 | 0 | 0 | 0 | + | + | + | + | + | + | ? | ? | ? |
| Y. pestis | 0 | 0 | 0 | 0 | 0 | 0 | 0 | 0 | 0 | 0 | 0 | 0 | 0 | 0 | 0 | 0 | 0 | 0 | + | ? | + | + | ? | 0 | + | ? | ? | 0 | 0 | 0 | 0 | 0 | 0 | 0 | 0 | 0 | ? | 0 | ? | 0 |
| **Aerobic GNB non-fermenter** | | | | | | | | | | | | | | | | | | | | | | | | | | | | | | | | | | | | | | | | |
| A. baumannii | 0 | 0 | 0 | 0 | 0 | 0 | 0 | 0 | 0 | 0 | +± | +± | + | 0 | +± | +± | +± | 0 | +± | ? | +± | + | +± | +± | +± | ? | ? | 0 | 0 | 0 | 0 | 0 | 0 | +± | +± | +± | ? | ? | ? | +± |
| B. cepacia | 0 | 0 | 0 | 0 | 0 | 0 | 0 | 0 | 0 | 0 | 0 | 0 | 0 | 0 | +± | +± | +± | 0 | 0 | ? | 0 | + | 0 | 0 | 0 | 0 | 0 | 0 | 0 | 0 | 0 | 0 | 0 | 0 | + | +± | ? | 0 | 0 | + |
| P. aeruginosa | 0 | 0 | 0 | 0 | 0 | 0 | 0 | 0 | 0 | 0 | 0 | + | + | 0 | + | + | + | + | + | + | 0 | + | 0 | + | + | 0 | ? | 0 | 0 | 0 | 0 | 0 | 0 | 0 | + | + | + | 0 | ? | + |
| S. maltophilia | 0 | 0 | 0 | 0 | 0 | 0 | 0 | 0 | 0 | 0 | 0 | +± | 0 | 0 | 0 | 0 | 0 | 0 | + | ? | 0 | +± | +± | 0 | + | ? | ? | 0 | 0 | 0 | 0 | 0 | 0 | 0 | +± | 0 | +± | 0 | 0 | + |
| **Aerobic - cell wall-deficient** | | | | | | | | | | | | | | | | | | | | | | | | | | | | | | | | | | | | | | | | |
| C. trachomatis | 0 | 0 | 0 | 0 | 0 | 0 | 0 | 0 | 0 | 0 | 0 | 0 | 0 | 0 | 0 | 0 | 0 | 0 | 0 | ? | ++ | ++ | ? | 0 | + | + | ? | 0 | 0 | 0 | 0 | 0 | 0 | 0 | 0 | 0 | 0 | 0 | 0 | 0 |
| Chlamydophila sp. | 0 | 0 | 0 | 0 | 0 | 0 | 0 | 0 | 0 | 0 | 0 | 0 | 0 | 0 | 0 | 0 | 0 | 0 | 0 | ? | + | + | + | + | ? | + | + | 0 | 0 | 0 | 0 | 0 | 0 | 0 | 0 | 0 | 0 | 0 | 0 | 0 |
| M. genitalium | 0 | 0 | 0 | 0 | 0 | 0 | 0 | 0 | 0 | 0 | 0 | 0 | 0 | 0 | 0 | 0 | 0 | 0 | + | ? | ? | +± | ++ | ? | ? | ? | ? | 0 | 0 | 0 | 0 | 0 | 0 | 0 | 0 | 0 | 0 | 0 | 0 | 0 |
| M. pneumoniae | 0 | 0 | 0 | 0 | 0 | 0 | 0 | 0 | 0 | 0 | 0 | 0 | 0 | 0 | 0 | 0 | 0 | 0 | + | ? | +± | ++ | ++ | 0 | + | + | + | 0 | 0 | 0 | 0 | 0 | 0 | 0 | 0 | 0 | 0 | 0 | + | + |
| U. urealyticum | 0 | 0 | 0 | 0 | 0 | 0 | 0 | 0 | 0 | 0 | 0 | 0 | 0 | 0 | 0 | 0 | 0 | 0 | + | ? | + | + | + | 0 | + | + | ? | 0 | 0 | 0 | 0 | 0 | 0 | 0 | 0 | 0 | 0 | 0 | + | + |
| **Anaerobic GNB** | | | | | | | | | | | | | | | | | | | | | | | | | | | | | | | | | | | | | | | | |
| B. fragilis | 0 | 0 | 0 | 0 | 0 | 0 | 0 | 0 | 0 | ++ | + | ++ | + | + | ++ | ++ | ++ | 0 | 0 | ? | ++ | + | +± | 0 | 0 | ? | 0 | 0 | +± | ++ | 0 | 0 | 0 | 0 | 0 | 0 | 0 | 0 | + | + |
| F. necrophorum | ± | ± | 0 | 0 | 0 | 0 | 0 | +± | +± | + | + | + | + | + | + | + | + | 0 | 0 | ? | + | 0 | + | 0 | 0 | ? | 0 | + | + | +± | + | + | + | + | ? | ? | ? | ? | ? | + |
| P. melaninogenica | ± | ± | 0 | 0 | 0 | 0 | 0 | +± | +± | + | + | + | + | + | + | + | + | 0 | 0 | ? | + | +± | + | 0 | 0 | ? | 0 | + | + | + | + | + | + | + | ? | ? | ? | ? | ? | + |
| **Anaerobic gram-positive** | | | | | | | | | | | | | | | | | | | | | | | | | | | | | | | | | | | | | | | | |
| Actinomyces sp. | ++ | ++ | 0 | 0 | 0 | 0 | 0 | ++ | ++ | ++ | + | + | + | + | + | + | + | 0 | 0 | ? | 0 | 0 | ? | 0 | 0 | ? | 0 | + | + | + | + | + | + | + | ? | ? | ? | ? | ? | ? |
| C. difficile | 0 | 0 | 0 | 0 | 0 | 0 | 0 | + | + | + | + | + | + | + | + | + | + | 0 | 0 | ? | 0 | 0 | 0 | 0 | 0 | 0 | 0 | 0 | + | + | 0 | 0 | 0 | 0 | 0 | 0 | 0 | 0 | 0 |
| Clostridium sp. | ++ | + | 0 | 0 | 0 | 0 | 0 | + | + | + | + | + | + | + | + | + | + | 0 | 0 | ? | 0 | 0 | +± | 0 | 0 | ? | 0 | + | + | + | + | + | + | + | ? | 0 | ? | + | ? | +± |
| P. acnes | ++ | + | ? | ? | ? | ? | ? | + | + | + | + | + | + | + | + | + | + | 0 | 0 | ? | + | + | +± | 0 | +± | ? | +± | + | + | + | + | + | + | ++ | ? | ? | + | ? | + | + |
| Peptostreptococci | ++ | ++ | 0 | ? | ? | ? | ++ | ++ | + | + | + | + | + | + | + | + | + | 0 | 0 | + | + | + | + | 0 | 0 | ? | + | + | + | + | + | + | + | + | ‡ | + | + | + | + | + |

**TABLE 4A (5)**

| | E. faecalis (S) | E. faecium (S) | E. faecalis (VRE) | E. faecium (VRE) | S. aureus MSSA | S. aureus HA-MRSA | S. aureus CA-MRSA | Staph coag-neg (S) | Staph coag-neg (R) | S. epidermidis (S) | S. epidermidis (R) | S. lugdunensis | S. saprophyticus | S. anginosus grp | Strep. pyogenes (A) | Strep. agalactiae (B) | Strep. gp C, F, G | Strep. pneumoniae | Viridans Strep. | Arcanobacter. sp | C. diphtheriae | C. jeikeium | L. monocytogenes | Nocardia sp. |
|---|---|---|---|---|---|---|---|---|---|---|---|---|---|---|---|---|---|---|---|---|---|---|---|---|
| **Other — Quinu-Dalfo** | o | + | o | + | + | + | + | + | + | + | + | + | o | + | + | + | + | o | + | + | o | o | ? | o |
| **Metronidazole** | o | o | o | o | o | o | o | o | o | o | o | o | o | o | o | o | o | o | o | o | o | o | o | o |
| **Fosfomycin (po)** | ± | ± | ± | ± | o | o | o | o | o | o | o | ± | o | o | o | o | o | o | o | o | o | o | o | o |
| **Fosfomycin (IV)** | ± | ± | ± | ± | + | + | + | + | ± | ± | + | o | ± | o | + | + | + | o | o | o | o | o | o | o |
| **Nitrofurantoin** | + | + | + | + | o | o | o | o | o | o | o | + | o | o | o | o | o | o | o | o | o | o | o | o |
| **TMP-SMX** | o | o | o | o | + | + | + | + | + | + | + | + | o | + | ± | + | + | ± | ± | o | o | o | o | ++ |
| **Rif (comb)** | ± | ± | ± | ± | ± | ± | ± | ± | ± | ± | ± | + | o | + | + | + | + | + | ? | o | o | o | o | o |
| **Fusidic Acid** | ± | ± | o | o | + | + | + | + | + | + | + | o | ? | ? | ? | ? | ? | ? | ? | o | o | o | o | o |
| **Poly — Colistin** | o | o | o | o | o | o | o | o | o | o | o | o | o | o | o | o | o | o | o | o | o | o | o | o |
| **Polymyxin B** | o | o | o | o | o | o | o | o | o | o | o | o | o | o | o | o | o | o | o | o | o | o | o | o |
| **Ox-lid — Tedizolid** | + | + | + | + | + | + | + | + | + | + | + | o | + | + | + | + | + | + | + | ? | o | ? | o | ? |
| **Linezolid** | + | + | ± | + | + | ±± | + | + | ±± | + | + | o | + | + | + | + | + | + | + | + | o | + | + | ? |
| **Glyco/Lipo — Dalbavancin** | + | + | o | o | + | + | + | + | + | + | + | ? | + | + | + | + | + | ? | + | ? | o | o | o | o |
| **Oritavancin** | + | + | + | + | + | + | + | + | + | + | + | ? | + | + | + | + | + | ? | + | ? | o | o | o | o |
| **Telavancin** | + | ± | ± | ± | + | + | + | + | + | + | + | + | + | + | + | + | + | + | + | + | o | + | o | o |
| **Teicoplanin** | ±± | ± | o | o | + | + | ±± | + | ±± | + | ±± | + | + | + | + | + | + | + | ±± | + | o | + | o | o |
| **Vancomycin** | ±± | ± | o | o | + | + | ±± | + | ±± | + | ±± | + | + | + | + | + | + | + | ±± | ±± | + | ±± | + | o |
| **Daptomycin** | + | + | + | + | ±± | ±± | + | + | ±± | ±± | + | + | + | o | + | + | + | + | ±± | + | o | + | o | o |
| **Tetracyclines — Tigecycline** | + | + | ± | + | + | + | + | + | + | + | + | + | + | + | + | + | + | + | + | + | o | + | o | ? |
| **Tetracycline** | ± | ± | ± | ± | + | + | ± | + | ± | + | ± | + | + | ± | ? | ? | ± | ± | ±± | + | o | ? | o | ? |
| **Omadacycline** | + | + | ± | ± | + | + | + | + | + | + | + | + | + | + | + | + | + | + | + | + | o | o | o | ? |
| **Minocycline** | ± | ± | ± | ± | + | + | + | + | + | + | + | + | + | ? | ? | ? | + | ± | + | + | ? | o | o | ± |
| **Eravacycline** | + | + | ± | + | + | + | + | + | + | + | + | + | + | + | + | + | + | + | + | + | + | o | o | ? |
| **Doxycycline** | ± | ± | ± | ± | + | + | + | + | + | + | + | + | ± | ? | ? | ± | ? | ± | ± | ±± | ? | ? | o | ? |
| **Macrolides — Telithromycin** | o | o | o | o | + | ± | + | + | o | + | o | + | + | + | + | + | + | + | + | + | + | o | o | ? |
| **Clarithromycin** | o | o | o | o | ± | o | ± | + | o | + | o | + | ± | ± | ± | ± | ± | ± | ± | ++ | ± | o | o | ? |
| **Azithromycin** | o | o | o | o | ± | o | ± | + | o | + | o | + | ± | ± | ± | ± | ± | ± | ± | ± | ± | o | o | ? |
| **Erythromycin** | o | o | o | o | ± | o | ± | + | o | + | o | + | ± | ± | ± | ± | ± | ± | ± | o | o | o | o | o |
| **Clindamycin** | o | o | o | o | + | + | + | + | ± | + | + | + | + | + | + | + | + | + | ± | ++ | ± | o | o | o |
| **Chloramphen** | ± | ± | ± | ± | + | + | + | + | + | + | + | + | + | + | + | + | + | + | + | ? | o | o | o | o |
| **Aminoglyco — Plazomicin** | o | o | o | o | + | + | + | ? | ? | ? | ? | ? | ? | o | o | o | o | o | o | o | o | o | o | ++ |
| **Amikacin** | o | o | o | o | ? | ? | ? | ? | ? | ? | ? | ? | ? | o | o | o | o | o | o | ? | ? | ? | o | ++ |
| **Tobramycin** | o | o | o | o | ? | ? | ? | ? | ? | ? | ? | ? | ? | o | o | o | o | o | ? | ? | ? | ? | o | o |
| **Gentamicin** | ± | ± | ± | ± | ± | ± | ± | ± | ± | ± | ± | o | ± | o | ± | ± | ± | o | ± | ? | ? | ? | ± | o |
| **Oral Cephalosporins — Cefditoren** | o | o | o | o | + | o | + | + | + | + | + | + | + | + | + | + | + | + | + | ? | ? | ? | o | o |
| **Cefdinir** | o | o | o | o | + | o | + | + | + | + | + | + | + | + | + | + | + | + | + | ? | ? | ? | o | o |
| **Cefpodoxime** | o | o | o | o | + | o | o | o | o | ? | ? | + | + | + | + | + | + | + | + | ? | ? | ? | o | o |
| **Ceftibuten** | o | o | o | o | o | o | o | o | o | ? | ? | o | ? | + | + | + | + | o | ? | ? | ? | ? | o | o |
| **Cefixime** | o | o | o | o | o | o | o | o | o | ? | ? | o | ? | + | + | + | + | + | o | ? | ? | ? | o | o |
| **Cefurox-Axe** | o | o | o | o | + | o | + | + | o | + | o | + | + | + | + | + | + | + | + | + | ? | ? | o | o |
| **Cefprozil** | o | o | o | o | + | o | + | + | ± | + | o | + | + | + | + | + | + | + | + | + | ? | ? | o | o |
| **Cefaclor** | o | o | o | o | + | o | ± | + | ± | + | o | + | + | + | + | + | + | ± | + | + | ? | ? | o | o |
| **Cephalexin** | o | o | o | o | + | o | ± | + | ± | + | o | + | + | + | + | + | + | ± | + | + | ? | ? | o | o |
| **Cefadroxil** | o | o | o | o | + | o | ± | + | ± | + | o | + | + | + | + | + | + | ± | + | + | ? | ? | o | o |

*Row groups (left labels): Other, Poly, Ox-lid, Glyco/Lipo, Tetracyclines, Macrolides, Aminoglyco, Oral Cephalosporins. Column groups (bottom labels): Aerobic gram-pos cocci, Aerobic gram-pos bacilli.*

**TABLE 4A (6)**

| Group | Drug | Aeromonas sp. | C. jejuni | C. freundii | C. koseri | E. aerogenes | E. cloacae | E. coli (S) | E. coli, Klebs ESBL | E. coli, Klebs KPC | E. coli, Klebs MBL | Enterics CRE, NOS | K. oxytoca | K. pneumoniae (S) | Morganella sp. | P. mirabilis | P. vulgaris | Providencia sp. | Salmonella sp. | Serratia sp. | Shigella sp. | Y. enterocolitica | Bartonella sp. | B. pertussis | B. burgdorferi | Brucella sp. | Capnocytophaga |
|---|---|---|---|---|---|---|---|---|---|---|---|---|---|---|---|---|---|---|---|---|---|---|---|---|---|---|---|
| Other | Quinu-Dalfo | O | O | O | O | O | O | O | O | O | O | O | O | O | O | O | O | O | O | O | O | O | O | O | O | O | O |
| | Metronidazole | O | O | O | O | O | O | O | O | O | O | O | O | O | O | O | O | O | O | O | O | O | O | O | O | O | O |
| | Fosfomycin (po) | O | + | + | + | +| | + | + | +| | +| | +| | +| | + | +| | O | +| | + | O | +| | O | +| | O | O | O | O | O | O |
| | Fosfomycin (IV) | ? | O | + | + | +| | + | + | +| | +| | +| | +| | +| | O | + | +| | O | O | +| | O | O | O | O | O | O | O | O |
| | Nitrofurantoin | O | O | +| | +| | O | +| | +| | O | +| | O | +| | + | O | O | O | O | O | O | O | O | O | O | O | O | O | O |
| | TMP-SMX | + | O | +| | +| | + | + | +| | +| | +| | O | +| | +| | +| | +| | +| | +| | +| | +| | +| | +| | +| | O | + | O | + | +| |
| | Rif (comb) | O | O | O | O | O | O | O | O | O | O | O | O | O | O | O | O | O | O | O | O | O | +| | O | O | +| | O |
| | Fusidic Acid | O | O | O | O | O | O | O | O | O | O | O | O | O | O | O | O | O | O | O | O | O | O | O | O | O | O |
| Poly | Colistin | + | O | + | + | + | + | + | + | + | + | + | + | + | O | O | O | O | + | O | + | + | O | O | O | O | O |
| | Polymyxin B | + | O | + | + | + | + | + | + | + | + | + | + | + | O | O | O | O | + | O | + | + | O | O | O | O | O |
| Ox-lid | Tedizolid | O | O | O | O | O | O | O | O | O | O | O | O | O | O | O | O | O | O | O | O | O | O | O | O | O | O |
| | Linezolid | O | O | O | O | O | O | O | O | O | O | O | O | O | O | O | O | O | O | O | O | O | O | O | O | O | O |
| Glyco/Lipo | Dalbavancin | O | O | O | O | O | O | O | O | O | O | O | O | O | O | O | O | O | O | O | O | O | O | O | O | O | O |
| | Oritavancin | O | O | O | O | O | O | O | O | O | O | O | O | O | O | O | O | O | O | O | O | O | O | O | O | O | O |
| | Telavancin | O | O | O | O | O | O | O | O | O | O | O | O | O | O | O | O | O | O | O | O | O | O | O | O | O | O |
| | Teicoplanin | O | O | O | O | O | O | O | O | O | O | O | O | O | O | O | O | O | O | O | O | O | O | O | O | O | O |
| | Vancomycin | O | O | O | O | O | O | O | O | O | O | O | O | O | O | O | O | O | O | O | O | O | O | O | O | O | O |
| | Daptomycin | O | O | O | O | O | O | O | O | O | O | O | O | O | O | O | O | O | O | O | O | O | O | O | O | O | O |
| Tetracyclines | Tigecycline | + | ? | + | + | + | + | + | + | + | + | + | + | + | O | O | O | O | + | + | + | ? | ? | O | ? | ? | ? |
| | Tetracycline | O | +| | O | O | O | O | +| | O | O | O | O | O | O | O | O | O | O | O | O | + | + | + | ? | + | + | + |
| | Omadacycline | + | ? | + | + | + | + | + | + | + | + | + | + | + | O | O | O | O | + | + | + | ? | ? | O | ? | ? | ? |
| | Minocycline | + | +| | O | O | O | O | +| | O | O | O | +| | +| | O | O | O | O | O | +| | O | +| | ? | + | ? | + | + | + |
| | Eravacycline | + | ? | + | + | + | + | + | + | + | + | + | + | + | O | O | O | O | + | + | + | ? | ? | O | ? | ? | ? |
| | Doxycycline | + | +| | O | O | O | O | O | O | O | O | O | O | O | O | O | O | O | +| | O | +| | ? | ++ | ? | ++ | +| | ? |
| Macrolides | Telithromycin | O | O | O | O | O | O | O | O | O | O | O | O | O | O | O | O | O | O | O | O | O | +| | ? | ? | O | ? |
| | Clarithromycin | O | + | O | O | O | O | O | O | O | O | O | O | O | O | O | O | O | O | O | O | O | +| | ++ | + | O | ? |
| | Azithromycin | O | ++ | O | O | O | +| | O | O | O | O | O | O | O | O | O | O | O | + | O | + | O | +| | ++ | + | O | ? |
| | Erythromycin | O | ++ | O | O | O | O | O | O | O | O | O | O | O | O | O | O | O | O | O | O | O | + | + | + | ? | ? |
| | Clindamycin | O | ? | O | O | O | O | O | O | O | O | O | O | O | O | O | O | O | O | O | O | O | O | O | O | O | ++ |
| | Chloramphen | ? | ? | ? | ? | O | O | + | + | O | O | O | + | + | ? | ? | ? | ? | + | O | + | + | ? | ? | ? | ? | + |
| Aminoglyco | Plazomicin | ? | ? | + | + | + | + | + | ++ | ++ | ++ | ++ | + | + | + | + | + | ? | + | + | ? | ? | O | O | O | ? | O |
| | Amikacin | + | + | + | + | + | + | + | +| | +| | +| | +| | + | + | + | + | + | + | + | + | + | + | O | O | O | ? | +| |
| | Tobramycin | + | + | + | + | + | + | + | +| | +| | +| | + | + | + | + | + | + | + | +| | + | + | + | O | O | O | O | +| |
| | Gentamicin | + | + | + | + | + | + | + | +| | +| | +| | + | + | + | + | + | + | + | + | + | + | + | ‡ | O | O | + | +| |
| Oral Cephalosporins | Cefditoren | ? | O | O | + | ? | O | + | O | O | O | O | ? | + | ? | ? | ? | ? | O | ? | + | ? | O | O | O | O | O |
| | Cefdinir | ? | O | + | + | O | O | + | O | O | O | O | + | + | O | + | + | O | O | ? | + | ? | O | O | O | O | O |
| | Cefpodoxime | ? | O | O | + | O | O | + | O | O | O | O | + | + | + | + | + | O | O | O | + | ? | O | O | O | O | O |
| | Ceftibuten | ? | O | + | + | O | O | + | O | O | O | O | + | + | + | + | + | + | O | O | + | + | O | O | O | O | O |
| | Cefixime | ? | O | + | + | O | O | + | O | O | O | O | + | + | + | + | + | O | O | O | + | + | O | O | O | O | O |
| | Cefurox-Axe | ? | O | O | + | O | O | + | O | O | O | O | + | + | O | + | O | O | O | O | + | ? | O | O | O | ‡ | O |
| | Cefprozil | ? | O | O | O | O | O | + | O | O | O | O | + | + | O | + | O | O | O | O | + | ? | O | O | O | O | O |
| | Cefaclor | ? | O | O | O | O | O | + | O | O | O | O | +| | + | O | + | O | O | O | O | + | O | O | O | O | O | O |
| | Cephalexin | O | O | O | O | O | O | +| | O | O | O | O | + | + | O | + | O | O | O | O | +| | O | O | O | O | O | O |
| | Cefadroxil | O | O | O | O | O | O | +| | O | O | O | O | + | +| | O | + | O | O | O | O | +| | O | O | O | O | O | O |
| | | Aerobic GNB - Enteric | | | | | | | | | | | | | | | | | | | | | Aerobic GNB - Non-enteric | | | | |

**TABLE 4A (7)**

| Organism | Quinu-Dalfo | Metronidazole | Fosfomycin (po) | Fosfomycin (IV) | Nitrofurantoin | TMP-SMX | Rif (comb) | Fusidic Acid | Colistin | Polymyxin B | Tedizolid | Linezolid | Dalbavancin | Oritavancin | Telavancin | Teicoplanin | Vancomycin | Daptomycin | Tigecycline | Tetracycline | Omadacycline | Minocycline | Eravacycline | Doxycycline | Telithromycin | Clarithromycin | Azithromycin | Erythromycin | Clindamycin | Chloramphen | Plazomicin | Amikacin | Tobramycin | Gentamicin | Cefditoren | Cefdinir | Cefpodoxime | Ceftibuten | Cefixime | Cefurox-Axe | Cefprozil | Cefaclor | Cephalexin | Cefadroxil |
|---|---|---|---|---|---|---|---|---|---|---|---|---|---|---|---|---|---|---|---|---|---|---|---|---|---|---|---|---|---|---|---|---|---|---|---|---|---|---|---|---|---|---|---|---|
| **Aerobic GNB - Non-enteric** *(continued)* | | | | | | | | | | | | | | | | | | | | | | | | | | | | | | | | | | | | | | | | | | | | |
| C. burnetii | o | o | o | o | o | + | +! | o | o | o | o | o | o | o | o | o | o | o | ? | + | ? | + | ? | ‡ | ? | + | + | + | o | + | o | o | o | o | o | o | o | o | o | o | o | o | o | o |
| Ehrlichia, Anaplas | o | o | o | o | o | o | +! | o | o | o | o | o | o | o | o | o | o | o | ? | + | ? | + | ? | ‡ | o | o | o | o | o | +! | o | o | o | o | o | o | o | o | o | o | o | o | o | o |
| Eikenella sp | o | o | o | o | o | o | o | o | o | o | o | o | o | o | o | o | o | o | ? | + | ? | + | ? | + | o | o | o | o | o | + | o | o | o | +! | ? | ? | + | + | + | + | + | +! | o | o |
| F. tularensis | o | o | o | o | o | o | o | o | o | o | o | o | o | o | o | o | o | o | ? | + | ? | + | ? | + | ? | ? | ? | ? | o | + | o | ? | + | ‡ | o | o | o | o | o | o | ? | ? | o | o |
| H. ducreyi | o | o | o | o | o | + | o | o | o | o | o | o | o | o | o | o | o | o | o | o | o | o | o | o | ? | +! | +! | +! | ? | + | o | o | o | o | o | o | o | o | o | o | o | o | o | o |
| H. influenzae | o | o | o | o | o | + | o | o | o | o | o | o | o | o | o | o | o | o | + | o | + | o | + | o | o | o | + | o | o | + | o | ? | o | o | + | + | + | + | + | + | o | + | o | o |
| Kingella sp. | o | o | o | o | o | ‡ | o | o | o | o | o | o | o | o | o | o | o | o | + | + | + | + | + | + | o | ? | ? | ? | o | + | o | o | o | + | + | + | + | + | + | + | + | + | o | o |
| K. granulomatis | o | o | o | o | o | + | o | o | o | o | o | o | o | o | o | o | o | o | ? | + | ? | + | ? | ‡ | ? | ‡ | ‡ | ? | o | o | o | o | o | o | o | o | o | o | o | o | o | o | o | o |
| Legionella sp. | o | o | o | o | o | ? | +! | o | o | o | o | o | o | o | o | o | o | o | ? | + | ? | + | ? | ‡ | ? | ‡ | ‡ | + | o | o | o | o | o | o | o | o | o | o | o | o | o | o | o | o |
| Leptospira sp. | o | o | o | o | o | o | o | o | o | o | o | o | o | o | o | o | o | o | ? | + | ? | + | ? | ‡ | + | + | + | + | o | o | o | o | o | o | o | o | o | o | o | o | o | o | o | o |
| M. catarrhalis | o | o | o | + | o | + | o | o | o | o | o | o | o | o | o | o | o | o | + | o | + | + | + | ‡ | + | + | + | + | + | + | o | o | o | +! | + | + | + | + | + | + | + | + | o | o |
| N. gonorrhoeae | o | o | o | o | o | o | o | o | o | o | o | o | o | o | o | o | o | o | ? | ? | ? | + | ? | ? | o | o | o | o | o | + | o | o | o | o | + | + | + | ? | + | ? | o | o | o | o |
| N. meningitidis | o | o | o | o | o | o | +! | o | o | o | o | o | o | o | o | o | o | o | ? | + | ? | + | ? | ‡ | o | o | + | o | o | + | o | o | o | o | + | + | + | o | + | + | o | o | o | o |
| P. multocida | o | o | o | o | o | + | o | o | o | o | o | o | o | o | o | o | o | o | + | + | + | + | + | + | o | + | + | + | o | + | o | o | o | + | + | + | + | + | + | + | ? | + | o | o |
| R. rickettsii | o | o | o | o | o | o | o | o | o | o | o | o | o | o | o | o | o | o | ? | + | ? | + | ? | ‡ | ? | o | o | o | o | ? | o | o | o | o | o | o | o | o | o | o | o | o | o | o |
| T. pallidum | o | o | o | o | o | o | o | o | o | o | o | o | o | o | o | o | o | o | ? | + | ? | + | ? | + | o | + | + | o | o | ? | o | o | o | o | o | o | o | o | o | o | o | o | o | o |
| V. cholera | o | o | o | o | o | ? | o | o | o | o | o | o | o | o | o | o | o | o | ? | + | ? | + | ? | + | o | o | + | ? | o | + | o | o | o | + | o | o | o | o | o | o | o | o | o | o |
| V. parahaemolyticus | o | o | o | o | o | ? | o | o | o | o | o | o | o | o | o | o | o | o | ? | + | ? | + | ? | + | o | o | + | o | o | + | o | ? | ? | ? | o | o | o | o | o | o | o | o | o | o |
| V. vulnificus | o | o | o | o | o | o | o | o | o | o | o | o | o | o | o | o | o | o | ? | + | ? | + | ? | + | o | o | o | o | o | + | o | ? | ? | ? | o | o | o | o | o | o | o | o | o | o |
| Y. pestis | o | o | o | o | o | + | o | o | o | o | o | o | o | o | o | o | o | o | ? | + | ? | + | ? | ‡ | o | o | ? | o | o | + | o | + | + | + | o | o | o | o | o | o | o | o | o | o |
| **Aerobic GNB non-fermenter** | | | | | | | | | | | | | | | | | | | | | | | | | | | | | | | | | | | | | | | | | | | | |
| A. baumannii | o | o | o | o | o | +! | o | o | + | o | o | o | o | o | o | o | o | o | + | +! | + | +! | + | o | o | o | o | o | o | o | +! | +! | o | + | o | o | o | o | o | o | o | o | o | o |
| B. cepacia | o | o | + | +! | o | +! | o | o | o | o | o | o | o | o | o | o | o | o | o | +! | o | +! | o | o | o | o | o | o | o | +! | +! | o | + | o | o | +! | o | o | o | o | o | o | o | o |
| P. aeruginosa | o | o | +! | +! | o | o | o | o | + | + | o | o | o | o | o | o | o | o | o | o | o | o | o | o | o | o | o | o | o | o | +! | + | + | + | o | o | o | o | o | o | o | o | o | o |
| S. maltophilia | o | o | o | o | o | ‡ | o | o | + | + | o | o | o | o | o | o | o | o | + | o | + | +! | + | + | o | o | o | o | o | o | o | o | o | o | o | o | o | o | o | o | o | o | o | o |

TABLE 4A (8)

Legend: o = inactive/not indicated · + = active · ++ = very active · ± = variable · ? = uncertain

| | Aerobic – cell wall-deficient | | | | | Anaerobic GNB | | | Anaerobic gram-positive | | | | |
|---|---|---|---|---|---|---|---|---|---|---|---|---|---|
| | C. trachomatis | Chlamydophila sp. | M. genitalium | M. pneumoniae | U. urealyticum | B. fragilis | F. necrophorum | P. melaninogenica | Actinomyces sp. | C. difficile | Clostridium sp. | P. acnes | Peptostreptococci |
| **Other** | | | | | | | | | | | | | |
| Quinu-Dalfo | o | o | o | o | o | o | o | o | + | o | + | + | ? |
| Metronidazole | o | o | o | o | o | ++ | ++ | ++ | o | + | + | o | ± |
| Fosfomycin (po) | o | o | o | o | o | o | o | o | o | o | o | o | o |
| Fosfomycin (IV) | o | o | o | o | o | o | o | o | o | o | o | o | + |
| Nitrofurantoin | o | o | o | o | o | o | o | o | o | o | o | o | o |
| TMP-SMX | o | o | o | o | o | o | o | o | o | o | o | ± | o |
| Rif (comb) | o | ± | o | o | o | o | o | o | o | o | o | o | o |
| Fusidic Acid | o | o | o | o | o | o | o | o | o | o | o | o | o |
| **Poly** | | | | | | | | | | | | | |
| Colistin | o | o | o | o | o | o | o | o | o | o | o | o | o |
| Polymyxin B | o | o | o | o | o | o | o | o | o | o | o | o | o |
| **Ox-id** | | | | | | | | | | | | | |
| Tedizolid | o | o | o | o | o | o | o | o | ? | o | o | o | ? |
| Linezolid | o | o | o | o | o | o | o | o | + | o | + | o | + |
| **Glyco/Lipo** | | | | | | | | | | | | | |
| Dalbavancin | o | o | o | o | o | o | o | o | o | o | + | + | + |
| Oritavancin | o | o | o | o | o | o | o | o | o | o | + | + | + |
| Telavancin | o | o | o | o | o | o | o | o | ? | o | + | + | + |
| Teicoplanin | o | o | o | o | o | o | o | o | o | o | + | + | + |
| Vancomycin | o | o | o | o | o | o | o | o | ? | o | ++ | + | + |
| Daptomycin | o | o | o | o | o | o | o | o | o | o | ± | + | + |
| **Tetracyclines** | | | | | | | | | | | | | |
| Tigecycline | o | + | + | ? | o | + | + | + | ? | o | + | + | + |
| Tetracycline | + | + | + | ± | ++ | ± | o | ± | + | o | + | + | + |
| Omadacycline | o | + | ? | + | ? | + | + | + | ? | o | + | + | + |
| Minocycline | + | + | ± | ++ | + | ± | o | + | + | o | + | + | + |
| Eravacycline | o | + | + | ? | + | + | + | + | ? | o | + | + | + |
| Doxycycline | ++ | ++ | ± | ++ | ++ | ± | o | + | + | o | + | + | + |
| **Macrolides** | | | | | | | | | | | | | |
| Telithromycin | ? | + | ? | ± | ? | o | o | o | ? | o | ? | ? | ? |
| Clarithromycin | + | + | ? | + | + | o | o | ± | ? | o | + | + | + |
| Azithromycin | ++ | + | ++ | ++ | ++ | o | o | ± | ? | o | ± | ± | ± |
| Erythromycin | + | + | ? | ± | ++ | o | o | ± | ++ | o | ± | ± | ± |
| Clindamycin | o | o | o | o | o | ± | o | + | ++ | o | ± | + | + |
| Chloramphen | o | o | + | o | o | + | + | + | + | o | + | + | + |
| **Aminoglyco** | | | | | | | | | | | | | |
| Plazomicin | o | o | o | o | o | o | o | o | o | o | o | o | o |
| Amikacin | o | o | o | o | o | o | o | o | o | o | o | ? | o |
| Tobramycin | o | o | o | o | o | o | o | o | o | o | o | ? | o |
| Gentamicin | o | o | o | o | o | o | o | o | o | o | ? | ? | o |
| **Oral Cephalosporins** | | | | | | | | | | | | | |
| Cefditoren | o | o | o | o | o | o | ? | ? | ? | ? | ? | ? | ? |
| Cefdinir | o | o | o | o | o | o | ? | ? | ? | ? | ? | ? | ? |
| Cefpodoxime | o | o | o | o | o | o | ? | ? | ? | ? | ? | ? | ? |
| Ceftibuten | o | o | o | o | o | o | ? | ? | ? | ? | ? | ? | ? |
| Cefixime | o | o | o | o | o | o | ? | ? | ? | ? | + | ? | ? |
| Cefurox-Axe | o | o | o | o | o | o | ? | ? | ? | o | + | + | + |
| Cefprozil | o | o | o | o | o | o | ? | ? | ? | o | + | + | + |
| Cefaclor | o | o | o | o | o | o | ? | ? | ? | o | + | + | + |
| Cephalexin | o | o | o | o | o | o | ? | ? | ? | ? | + | ? | ? |
| Cefadroxil | o | o | o | o | o | ? | ? | ? | ? | ? | + | + | + |

**TABLE 4B – ANTIFUNGAL ACTIVITY SPECTRA**

| | Fluconazole | Itraconazole | Voriconazole | Posaconazole | Isavuconazonium sulfate | Anidulafungin | Caspofungin | Micafungin | Amphotericin B |
|---|---|---|---|---|---|---|---|---|---|
| **Antifungal Drugs** | | | | | | | | | |
| **Fungi** | | | | | | | | | |
| Aspergillus fumigatus | 0 | ± | ++ | + | ++ | ± | ± | ± | + |
| Aspergillus terreus | 0 | ± | ++ | + | ++ | ± | ± | ± | 0 |
| Aspergillus flavus | 0 | ± | ++ | + | ++ | ± | ± | ± | + |
| Candida albicans | ++ | + | + | + | + | ++ | ++ | ++ | + |
| Candida dubliniensis | ++ | + | + | + | + | ++ | ++ | ++ | ++ |
| Candida glabrata | ± | ± | ± | ± | ± | ++ | ++ | ++ | ++ |
| Candida guilliermondii | ++ | ++ | ++ | ++ | + | ++ | ++ | ++ | ++ |
| Candida krusei | 0 | 0 | + | + | + | ++ | ++ | ++ | ++ |
| Candida lusitaniae | ++ | + | + | + | + | ++ | ++ | ++ | 0 |
| Candida parapsilosis | ++ | + | + | + | + | + | + | + | ++ |
| Candida tropicalis | ++ | + | + | + | + | ++ | ++ | ++ | ++ |
| Cryptococcus sp. | ++ | + | + | + | + | 0 | 0 | 0 | ++ |
| Dematiaceous molds | 0 | ++ | ++ | + | + | ± | ± | ± | + |
| Fusarium sp. | 0 | ± | ± | ± | ± | 0 | 0 | 0 | ± |
| Mucormycosis | 0 | 0 | 0 | + | + | 0 | 0 | 0 | ++ |
| Scedo apiospermum | 0 | 0 | + | ± | ± | 0 | 0 | 0 | 0 |
| Scedo (Lomentospora) prolificans | 0 | 0 | 0 | 0 | 0 | 0 | 0 | 0 | 0 |
| Trichosporon spp. | ± | + | + | + | + | 0 | 0 | 0 | + |
| **Dimorphic Fungi** | | | | | | | | | |
| Blastomyces | ± | ++ | + | + | ? | 0 | 0 | 0 | ++ |
| Coccidioides | ++ | ++ | + | + | ? | 0 | 0 | 0 | ++ |
| Histoplasma | ± | ++ | + | + | ? | 0 | 0 | 0 | ++ |
| Sporothrix | ± | ++ | + | + | ? | 0 | 0 | 0 | ++ |

**TABLE 4C – ANTIVIRAL ACTIVITY SPECTRA**

| | Adenovirus | BK Virus | Cytomegalovirus | Hepatitis B | Hepatitis C | Herpes simplex | HPV | Influenza A | Influenza B | JC Virus / PML | RSV | Smallpox | Monkeypox | Varicella-zoster |
|---|---|---|---|---|---|---|---|---|---|---|---|---|---|---|
| **Hepatitis B** | | | | | | | | | | | | | | |
| Adefovir | NA | NA | NA | ++ | NA | NA | NA | NA | NA | NA | NA | NA | NA | NA |
| Emtricitabine | NA | NA | NA | ± | NA | NA | NA | NA | NA | NA | NA | NA | NA | NA |
| Entecavir | NA | NA | NA | ++ | NA | NA | NA | NA | NA | NA | NA | NA | NA | NA |
| Lamivudine | NA | NA | NA | ± | NA | NA | NA | NA | NA | NA | NA | NA | NA | NA |
| Telbivudine | NA | NA | NA | ± | NA | NA | NA | NA | NA | NA | NA | NA | NA | NA |
| Tenofovir (TDF and TAF) | NA | NA | NA | ++ | NA | ± | NA | NA | NA | NA | NA | NA | NA | NA |
| **Hepatitis C** | | | | | | | | | | | | | | |
| Daclatasvir | NA | NA | NA | NA | ++ | NA | NA | NA | NA | NA | NA | NA | NA | NA |
| Dasabuvir | NA | NA | NA | NA | ++ | NA | NA | NA | NA | NA | NA | NA | NA | NA |
| Elbasvir | NA | NA | NA | NA | ++ | NA | NA | NA | NA | NA | NA | NA | NA | NA |
| Glecaprevir | NA | NA | NA | NA | ++ | NA | NA | NA | NA | NA | NA | NA | NA | NA |
| Grazoprevir | NA | NA | NA | NA | ++ | NA | NA | NA | NA | NA | NA | NA | NA | NA |
| Interferon alfa, peg | NA | NA | NA | ++ | + | NA | NA | NA | NA | NA | NA | NA | NA | NA |
| Ledipasvir | NA | NA | NA | NA | ++ | NA | NA | NA | NA | NA | NA | NA | NA | NA |
| Ombitasvir | NA | NA | NA | NA | ++ | NA | NA | NA | NA | NA | NA | NA | NA | NA |
| Paritaprevir | NA | NA | NA | NA | ++ | NA | NA | NA | NA | NA | NA | NA | NA | NA |
| Pibrentasvir | NA | NA | NA | NA | ++ | NA | NA | NA | NA | NA | NA | NA | NA | NA |
| Ribavirin | ± | NA | NA | 0 | + | NA | NA | N A | NA | NA | ± | NA | NA | NA |
| Simeprevir | NA | NA | NA | NA | + | NA | NA | NA | NA | NA | NA | NA | NA | NA |
| Sofosbuvir | NA | NA | NA | NA | ++ | NA | NA | NA | NA | NA | NA | NA | NA | NA |
| Velpatasvir | NA | NA | NA | NA | ++ | NA | NA | NA | NA | NA | NA | NA | NA | NA |
| Voxilaprevir | NA | NA | NA | NA | ++ | NA | NA | NA | NA | NA | NA | NA | NA | NA |
| **Influenza** | | | | | | | | | | | | | | |
| Amantadine | NA | NA | NA | NA | NA | NA | NA | 0 | 0 | NA | NA | NA | NA | NA |
| Baloxavir | NA | NA | NA | NA | NA | NA | NA | + | + | NA | NA | NA | NA | NA |
| Oseltamivir | NA | NA | NA | NA | NA | NA | NA | ++ | ++ | NA | NA | NA | NA | NA |
| Peramivir | NA | NA | NA | NA | NA | NA | NA | + | + | NA | NA | NA | NA | NA |
| Rimantadine | NA | NA | NA | NA | NA | NA | NA | 0 | 0 | NA | NA | NA | NA | NA |
| Zanamivir | NA | NA | NA | NA | NA | NA | NA | ++ | ++ | NA | NA | NA | NA | NA |
| **Herpes, CMV, VZV, misc.** | | | | | | | | | | | | | | |
| Acyclovir | NA | NA | 0 | NA | NA | ++ | NA | NA | NA | NA | NA | NA | NA | + |
| Cidofovir | + | + | ++ | NA | NA | NA | NA | NA | NA | + | NA | + | + | + |
| Famciclovir | NA | NA | 0 | NA | NA | ++ | NA | NA | NA | NA | NA | NA | NA | + |
| Foscarnet | NA | NA | ++ | NA | NA | + | NA | NA | NA | NA | NA | NA | NA | + |
| Ganciclovir | ± | NA | ++ | NA | NA | + | NA | NA | NA | NA | NA | NA | NA | + |
| Letermovir | NA | NA | ++ | NA | NA | NA | NA | NA | NA | NA | NA | NA | NA | NA |
| Valacyclovir | NA | NA | 0 | NA | NA | ++ | NA | NA | NA | NA | NA | NA | NA | ++ |
| Valganciclovir | ± | NA | ++ | NA | NA | NA | NA | NA | NA | NA | NA | NA | NA | + |
| **Pox Viruses** | | | | | | | | | | | | | | |
| Tecovirimat | NA | NA | NA | NA | NA | NA | NA | NA | NA | NA | NA | + | + | NA |
| **Topical Agents** | | | | | | | | | | | | | | |
| Imiquimod | NA | NA | NA | NA | NA | NA | ++ | NA | NA | NA | NA | NA | NA | NA |
| Penciclovir | NA | NA | 0 | NA | NA | + | NA | NA | NA | NA | NA | NA | NA | 0 |
| Podofilox | NA | NA | NA | NA | NA | NA | ++ | NA | NA | NA | NA | NA | NA | NA |
| Sinecatechins | NA | NA | NA | NA | NA | NA | + | NA | NA | NA | NA | NA | NA | NA |
| Trifluridine | NA | NA | NA | NA | NA | + | NA | NA | NA | NA | NA | NA | NA | NA |

TABLE 5A - TREATMENT OPTIONS FOR SYSTEMIC INFECTION DUE TO MULTI-DRUG RESISTANT GRAM-POSITIVE BACTERIA

| ORGANISM | RESISTANT TO | PRIMARY TREATMENT OPTIONS | ALTERNATIVE TREATMENT OPTIONS | COMMENTS |
|---|---|---|---|---|
| **Enterococcus faecium; Enterococcus faecalis** (Consultation suggested) For review of VRE treatment: *Infect Dis Clin North Am 30:415, 2016.* | Vancomycin (VRE), Ampicillin, Penicillin G, Gentamicin (high level resistance) | **E. faecium**, systemic infection, bacteremia: **Dapto** 10-12 mg/kg IV q24h + (**AMP** 2 gm IV q4h OR **Ceftaroline** 600 mg IV q8h). Less desirable alternatives: [**Linezolid** 600 mg po/IV q12h OR **Quinupristin-Dalfopristin** 7.5 mg/kg IV (central line)] + **AMP** 2 gm IV q4h | **E. faecalis** Resistance to AMP or Pen rare. If no resistance: **AMP** 2 gm IV q4h + **Ceftriaxone** 2 gm IV q12h. If Pen-resistant due to beta-lactamase: **Dapto** 8-12 mg/kg IV q12h + **AM-SB** 3 gm IV q6h. | **Addition of a beta lactam to Dapto reverses Dapto resistance & impedes development of resistance.** *E. faecalis* rarely resistance to penicillins. Linezolid 600 mg IV/po bid an alternative to Dapto for the treatment of VRE bacteremia, systemic infection, but data are conflicting as to which is better *(CID 61:871, 2015 and CID 61:879, 2015).* Dapto dose > 9 mg/kg is associated with lower mortality in treatment of VRE bacteremia *(CID 64:1026, 2017).* Linezolid should be used for treatment of VRE infections if Dapto MIC > 4 µg/mL. |
| **Staphylococcus aureus** (See *Table 6* for more details) | Vancomycin (VISA or VRSA) and all beta lactams (except Ceftaroline) | **Dapto** 6-12 mg/kg IV q24h or (**Dapto** 6-12 mg/kg IV q24h + **Ceftaroline** 600 mg IV q8h) *(AAC 56:5296, 2012).* | **Telavancin** 10 mg/kg IV q24h or **Linezolid** 600 mg IV/po q12h | **Confirm dapto susceptibility** as VISA strains may be non-susceptible. If prior vanco therapy (or persistent infection on vanco) there is significant chance of developing resistance to dapto *(JAC 66:1656, 2011).* Addition of an anti-staphylococcal beta-lactam (nafcillin or oxacillin) may restore susceptibility against Dapto-resistant MRSA *(AAC 54:3161, 2010).* Combination of Dapto + Oxacillin has been successful in clearing refractory MRSA bacteremia *(CID 53:158, 2011).* Dapto + Ceftaroline may also be effective. |
| **Streptococcus pneumoniae** | Penicillin G (MIC ≥4 µg/mL) | If no meningitis: **Ceftriaxone** 2 gm IV once daily OR **Ceftaroline** 600 mg IV q12h OR **Linezolid** 600 mg IV/po q12h | Meningitis: **Vanco** 15 mg/kg IV q8h OR **MER** 2 gm IV q8h | Ceftriaxone 2 gm IV q12h would also work for meningitis. |

**TABLE 5B: TREATMENT OPTIONS FOR SYSTEMIC INFECTION DUE TO CULTURE-IDENTIFIED MULTI-DRUG RESISTANT GRAM-NEGATIVE BACILLI**

Many of the treatment options for extensively drug-resistant GNB are not FDA-approved indications (NAI). Suggested options are based on a combination of in vitro data, animal models, observational studies or clinical trials for selected pathogens. For dosing, see specific topics in *Table 1* or drug listings in *Table 10A*.

| ORGANISM | RESISTANT TO | PRIMARY TREATMENT OPTIONS | ALTERNATIVE TREATMENT OPTIONS | COMMENTS |
|---|---|---|---|---|
| **Acinetobacter calcoaceticus-baumannii complex** | All beta-lactams (except Sulbactam), AG, FQ, TMP-SMX | *If susceptible:* **Cefepime**, **Ceftazidime**, **AM-SB**<br>*If MDR & suscept:* **MER** or **IMP** | *If critically ill:* **MER** + **AM-SB** + **Polymyxin B**/**Colistin** (*if UTI*) For dosing see *Table 1*. | For pneumonia, add nebulized Colistin 50-75 mg bid. Colistin + RIF and Colistin + MER failed in clinical trials (*CID 57:349, 2013; LnID 18:391, 2018*). Multiple mechanisms of resistance. |
| **Extended spectrum beta lactamase (ESBL)** produced by E. coli, K. pneumoniae, Enterobacteriaceae, P. aeruginosa | All cephalosporins, FQ, AG, TMP-SMX | **MER** or **IMP** | **Ceftolo-tazo**[a], **Ceftaz-avi**[a], **MER-vabor**[a] | Pip-tazo discordance: even if sensitive in vitro, may fail clinically. Pip-Tazo failed in a clinical trial vs. MER in ceftriaxone-resistant E. coli/K. pneumo (*JAMA 2018;320:979 & 984*). For UTI: Nitrofurantoin, Fosfomycin. |
| **OXA-48** producing Enterobacteriaceae | All penicillins, FQ, AG, TMP-SMX | *If sensitive:* **Cefepime**, **Ceftazidime** | *If critically ill:* **Ceftaz-avi** + **Aztreonam** | More common in areas bordering the Mediterranean Sea (*Clin Micro Rev 2014;27:241*). |
| **KPC** (serine carbapenemase) producing Enterobacteriaceae | All penicillins, cephalosporins, Aztreonam, carbapenems, FQ, AG, TMP-SMX | **Ceftaz-avi**[a], **MER-vabor** | None proven effective: ID consultation | MER + polymyxin failed in controlled clinical trial (*LnID 2018;18:391*). Check Plazomicin susceptibility. |
| **Metallo-carbapenemase** producing GNB | All beta lactams (except Aztreonam), FQ, AG, TMP-SMX | **Ceftaz-avi**[a] + **Aztreonam** | None proven effective: ID consultation | |
| **Stenotrophomonas maltophilia** | All beta lactams, FQ, AG | **TMP-SMX** | *If susceptible in vitro:* **FQ** | Ticar-clav no longer available.<br>Ref: *Sem Resp CCM 36:99, 2015* |

[a] Not FDA-approved indication

**TABLE 6 – SUGGESTED MANAGEMENT OF SUSPECTED OR CULTURE-POSITIVE**
**COMMUNITY-ASSOCIATED METHICILLIN-RESISTANT S. AUREUS INFECTIONS**

IDSA Guidelines: *CID 52 (Feb 1):1, 2011*. With the magnitude of the clinical problem and a number of new drugs, it is likely new data will require frequent revisions of the regimens suggested. See Sanford Guide digital content for most current recommendations. *(See page 2 for abbreviations.)*

NOTE: Distinction between community and hospital strains of MRSA blurring.

| CLINICAL ILLNESS | ABSCESS, NO IMMUNOSUPPRESSION, OUT-PATIENT CARE | PNEUMONIA | BACTEREMIA OR POSSIBLE ENDOCARDITIS OR BACTEREMIC SHOCK | TREATMENT FAILURE *(See footnote²)* |
|---|---|---|---|---|
| **Management**<br><br>*Drug doses in footnote¹.* | **TMP/SMX** 1 DS (2 DS if BMI >40) po bid OR **Clinda** 300 mg (450 mg for BMI >40) po tid *(NEJM 372:1093, 2015)*.<br><br>For larger abscesses, multiple lesions or systemic inflammatory response:<br><br>**I&D** + **Oritavancin** 1500 mg x 1 or **Dalbavancin** 1000 mg x 1 than 500 mg x 1 a wk later) an option for outpatient management of sicker patients with more extensive infection who might otherwise be admitted (see *NEJM 370:2180, 2014; NEJM 370:2169, 2014*). | **Vanco** IV or **Linezolid** IV | **Vanco** 15-20 mg/kg IV q8-12h. Confirm adequate vanco troughs of 15-20 μg/mL. Switch to alternative regimen if **Vanco** MIC >2 μg/mL.<br>If patient has slow response to vanco, consider alternative therapy.<br>**Dapto** 8-12 mg/kg q24h. | **Dapto** 8-12 mg/kg IV q24h; confirm in vitro susceptibility as prior vanco therapy may select for daptomycin non-susceptibility (MIC >1 μg/mL) & some VISA strains are daptomycin non-susceptible.<br>**Use combination therapy for bacteremia or endocarditis:** dapto + beta-lactam combination therapy (**Dapto** 8-12 mg/kg IV q24h + (**Nafcillin/Oxacillin** 2 gm IV q4h OR **Ceftaroline** 600 mg IV q8h) appears effective against MRSA strains as salvage therapy even if non-susceptible to dapto *(Int. J Antimicrob Agents, 42-450, 2013; AAC 54:3161, 2010; AAC 56:6192, 2013)*.<br>**Ceftaroline** 600 mg IV q8h *(AAC 61:e00215, 2017; Am J Health Syst Pharm. 74:201, 2017)*.<br>**Linezolid** 600 mg IV/po q12h. (Linezolid is bacteriostatic and should not be used as a single agent in suspected endovascular infection).<br>**Televancin** 10 mg/kg q24h IV *(CID 52:31, 2011; AAC 58:2030, 2014)*. |
| **Comments** | **Fusidic acid** 500 mg tid (not available in the US) + **RIF** also an option; do not use rifampin alone as resistance rapidly emerges. | Prospective study of **Linezolid** vs **Vanco** showed slightly higher cure rate with Linezolid, no difference in mortality *(CID 54:621, 2012)*. | TMP-SMX **NOT** recommended in bacteremia; inferior to Vanco *(BMJ 350:2215, 2015)*.<br>Adjunctive rifampin did not improve outcomes in patients with *S. aureus* bacteremia *(Lancet 391:668, 2018)*.<br>Patients not responding after 2-3 days should be evaluated for complicated infection and switched to **Vancomycin.** | |

¹ **Clindamycin:** 300 mg po tid. **Daptomycin:** 6 mg/kg IV q24h is the standard. FDA-approved dose for bacteremia and endocarditis but 8-12 mg/kg q24h is recommended by some and for treatment failures. **Doxycycline or Minocycline:** 100 mg po bid. **Linezolid:** 600 mg po/IV bid. **Quinupristin-Dalfopristin (Q-D):** 7.5 mg per /kg IV q8h via central line. **Rifampin:** Long serum half-life justifies dosing 600 mg q24h; however, frequency of nausea less with 300 mg po bid. **TMP-SMX-DS:** Standard dose 8-10 mg per kg per day. For 70 kg person = 700 mg TMP component per day. **TMP-SMX** contains 160 mg TMP and 800 mg SMX. The dose for treatment of CA-MRSA skin and soft tissue infections (SSTI) is 1 DS tablet twice daily. **Vancomycin:** 1 gm IV q12h; up to 45-60 mg/kg/day in divided doses may be required to achieve target trough concentrations of 15-20 mcg/mL recommended for serious infections.

² The median duration of bacteremia in endocarditis is 7-9 days in patients treated with vancomycin *(AnIM 115:674, 1991)*. Longer duration of bacteremia, greater likelihood of endocarditis *(JID 190:1140, 2004)*. Definition of failure unclear. Clinical response should be factored in. **Unsatisfactory clinical response especially if blood cultures remain positive >4 days.**

# TABLE 7 – ANTIBIOTIC HYPERSENSITIVITY REACTIONS & DRUG DESENSITIZATION METHODS

**Penicillin. Oral route (Pen VK) preferred.** 1/3 pts develop transient reaction, usually mild. **Perform in ICU setting. Discontinue β-blockers. Have IV line, epinephrine, ECG, spirometer available.** Desensitization works as long as pt receiving drug; allergy returns after discontinuance. History of Steven-Johnson, exfoliative dermatitis, erythroderma are contraindications. Skin testing for evaluation of Pen allergy: Testing with major determinant (benzyl Pen polylysine) and minor determinants has negative predictive value (97-99%). Risk of systemic reaction to skin testing <1% (*Ann Allergy Asth Immunol 106:1, 2011*). General refs: *CID 58:1140, 2014.*

- **Method:** Prepare dilutions using **Pen-VK** oral soln, 250 mg/5mL. Administer each dose @ 15 min intervals in 30 mL water/flavored bev. After Step 14 observe pt for 30 min, then give full therapeutic dose by route of choice. Ref: *Allergy, Prin & Prac, Mosby, 1993, pg. 1726.*

| Step | Dilution (mg/mL) | mL Administered | Dose/Step mg | Dose/Step units | Cumulative Dose Given mg | Cumulative Dose Given units |
|---|---|---|---|---|---|---|
| 1 | 0.5 | 0.1 | 0.05 | 80 | 0.05 | 80 |
| 2 | 0.5 | 0.2 | 0.1 | 160 | 0.15 | 240 |
| 3 | 0.5 | 0.4 | 0.2 | 320 | 0.35 | 560 |
| 4 | 0.5 | 0.8 | 0.4 | 640 | 0.75 | 1,200 |
| 5 | 0.5 | 1.6 | 0.8 | 1,280 | 1.55 | 2,480 |
| 6 | 0.5 | 3.2 | 1.6 | 2,560 | 3.15 | 5,040 |
| 7 | 0.5 | 6.4 | 3.2 | 5,120 | 6.35 | 10,160 |
| 8 | 5 | 1.2 | 6 | 9,600 | 12.35 | 19,760 |
| 9 | 5 | 2.4 | 12 | 19,200 | 24.35 | 38,960 |
| 10 | 5 | 4.8 | 24 | 38,400 | 48.35 | 77,360 |
| 11 | 50 | 1 | 50 | 80,000 | 98.35 | 157,360 |
| 12 | 50 | 2 | 100 | 160,000 | 198.35 | 317,360 |
| 13 | 50 | 4 | 200 | 320,000 | 398.35 | 637,360 |
| 14 | 50 | 8 | 400 | 640,000 | 798.35 | 1,277,360 |

**TMP-SMX.** Perform in hospital/clinic. Refs: *CID 20:849, 1995; AIDS 5:311, 1991.*

- **Method:** Use **TMP-SMX** oral susp. (40 mg TMP/200 mg SMX)/5 mL. Take with 6 oz water after each dose. Corticosteroids, antihistaminics NOT used.

| Hour | Dose (TMP/SMX) (mg) |
|---|---|
| 0 | 0.004/0.02 |
| 1 | 0.04/0.2 |
| 2 | 0.4/2 |
| 3 | 4/20 |
| 4 | 40/200 |
| 5 | 160/800 |

**Penicillin. Parenteral (Pen G) route.** Follow procedures/notes under Oral (Pen-VK) route. Ref: *Allergy, Prin & Prac, Mosby, 1993, pg. 1726.*

- **Method:** Administer **Pen G** IM, IV or sc as follows:

| Step | Dilution (units/mL) | mL Administered | Dose/Step (units) | Cumulative Dose Given (units) |
|---|---|---|---|---|
| 1 | 100 | 0.2 | 20 | 20 |
| 2 | 100 | 0.4 | 40 | 60 |
| 3 | 100 | 0.8 | 80 | 140 |
| 4 | 1,000 | 0.2 | 200 | 340 |
| 5 | 1,000 | 0.4 | 400 | 740 |
| 6 | 1,000 | 0.8 | 800 | 1,540 |
| 7 | 10,000 | 0.2 | 2,000 | 3,540 |
| 8 | 10,000 | 0.4 | 4,000 | 7,540 |
| 9 | 10,000 | 0.8 | 8,000 | 15,540 |
| 10 | 100,000 | 0.2 | 20,000 | 35,540 |
| 11 | 100,000 | 0.4 | 40,000 | 75,540 |
| 12 | 100,000 | 0.8 | 80,000 | 155,540 |
| 13 | 1,000,000 | 0.2 | 200,000 | 355,540 |
| 14 | 1,000,000 | 0.4 | 400,000 | 755,540 |
| 15 | 1,000,000 | 0.8 | 800,000 | 1,555,540 |

**Ceftriaxone.** Ref: *Allergol Immunopathol (Madr) 37:105, 2009.*

- **Method:** Infuse **Ceftriaxone** IV @ 20 min intervals as follows:

| Day | Dose (mg) |
|---|---|
| 1 | 0.001, then 0.01, then 0.1, then 1 |
| 2 | 1, then 5, then 10, then 50 |
| 3 | 100, then 250, then 500 |
| 4 | 1000 |

**Desensitization Methods for Other Drugs (References)**

- **Ceftazidime.** *Curr Opin All Clin Immunol 6(6): 476, 2006.*
- **Clindamycin.** *J Allergy Clin Immunol Pract 2018 Apr 12 [Epub ahead of print].*
- **Daptomycin.** *Ann All Asthma Immun 100:87, 2008.*
- **Doxycycline.** *(ID Cases 11:70, 2018; Ann Allergy Asthma Immunol 111:73, 2013.*
- **Flucloxacillin.** *AAC 2018 Sept 17 [Epub ahead of print].*
- **Imipenem-Cilastatin.** *Ann Pharmacother 37:513, 2003.*
- **Liposomal Amphotericin B.** *J Allergy Clin Immunol Pract 5:181, 2017.*
- **Meropenem.** *Ann Pharmacother 37:1424, 2003.*
- **Metronidazole.** *Allergy Rhinol 5:1, 2014.*
- **Vancomycin.** *Intern Med 45:317, 2006.*
- General review, including desensitization protocols for **Amp, Cefepime, CIP, Clarithro, Clinda, Dapto, Linezolid, Tobra** (*CID 58:1140, 2014*).

**TABLE 7 (2)**

**Ceftaroline.** 12-step IV desensitization protocol. Ref: *Open Forum Infect Dis 2:1, 2015.*
- Method: Cumulative drug infused: 600 mg. Total time required for all 12 steps: 318 minutes.

| Step | Conc (mg/mL) | Vol infused (mL) | Infusion duration (min) | Drug infused this step (mg) | Cumulative drug infused (mg) |
|---|---|---|---|---|---|
| 1 | 0.0002 | 5 | 15 | 0.001 | 0.001 |
| 2 | 0.0002 | 15 | 15 | 0.003 | 0.004 |
| 3 | 0.002 | 5 | 15 | 0.01 | 0.014 |
| 4 | 0.002 | 15 | 15 | 0.03 | 0.04 |
| 5 | 0.02 | 5 | 15 | 0.1 | 0.14 |
| 6 | 0.02 | 15 | 15 | 0.3 | 0.4 |
| 7 | 0.2 | 5 | 15 | 1 | 1.4 |
| 8 | 0.2 | 15 | 15 | 3 | 4.4 |
| 9 | 2 | 5 | 15 | 10 | 14.4 |
| 10 | 2 | 15 | 15 | 30 | 44.4 |
| 11 | 2 | 25 | 15 | 50 | 94.4 |
| 12 | 2 | 255 | 153 | 510 | 604.4 |

**Valganciclovir.** 12-step oral desensitization protocol. Ref: *Transplantation 98:e50, 2014.*
- Method: Administer doses at 15-minute intervals; entire protocol takes 165 minutes.
  Cumulative dose administered: 453.6 mg

| Step | Drug administered this step (mg) | Cumulative drug administered (mg) |
|---|---|---|
| 1 | 0.1 | 0.1 |
| 2 | 0.2 | 0.3 |
| 3 | 0.4 | 0.7 |
| 4 | 0.8 | 1.5 |
| 5 | 1.6 | 3.1 |
| 6 | 3.5 | 6.6 |
| 7 | 7 | 13.6 |
| 8 | 14 | 27.6 |
| 9 | 28 | 55.6 |
| 10 | 58 | 113.6 |
| 11 | 115 | 228.6 |
| 12 | 225 | 453.6 |

**TABLE 8 – PREGNANCY RISK AND SAFETY IN LACTATION**

| Drug | Risk Category (Old) | Use during Lactation |
|---|---|---|
| **Antibacterials** | | |
| Amikacin | D | Probably safe, monitor infant for GI toxicity |
| Azithromycin | B | Safe, monitor infant for GI toxicity |
| Aztreonam | B | Safe, monitor infant for GI toxicity |
| Cephalosporins | B | Safe, monitor infant for GI toxicity |
| Chloramphenicol | C | Avoid use |
| Ciprofloxacin | C | Avoid breastfeeding for 3-4 hrs after a dose, monitor infant for GI toxicity |
| Clarithromycin | C | Safe, monitor for GI toxicity |
| Clindamycin | B | Avoid use if possible, otherwise monitor infant for GI toxicity |
| Colistin (polymyxin E) | C | Probably safe with monitoring, but data limited |
| Dalbavancin | C | Probably safe with monitoring, but no data available |
| Daptomycin | B | Probably safe with monitoring, but data limited |
| Delafloxacin | No human data | No data |
| Doripenem | B | Probably safe with monitoring, but no data available |
| Doxycycline | D | Short-term use safe, monitor infant for GI toxicity |
| Eravacycline | Avoid during 2nd and 3rd trimesters | Avoid breastfeeding during treatment and for 4 days after last dose |
| Ertapenem | B | Safe |
| Erythromycin | B | Safe |
| Fidaxomicin | B | Probably safe |
| Fosfomycin | B | Probably safe with monitoring |
| Fusidic acid | - | Safety not established |
| Gatifloxacin | C | Short-term use safe |
| Gemifloxacin | C | Short-term use safe |
| Gentamicin | D | Probably safe |
| Imipenem | C | Safe, monitor infant for GI toxicity |
| Isepamicin | D | Safety not established, avoid use |
| Levofloxacin | C | Avoid breastfeeding for 4-6 hrs after a dose, monitor infant for GI toxicity |
| Linezolid | C | Probably safe with monitoring. Systemic exposure is low: in one pt, breast milk linezolid conc were 3.5-12.2 µg/mL and the infant's serum conc was <0.2 µg/mL (*JAC 72:2677, 2017*). |
| Meropenem | B | Probably safe with monitoring, but no data available |
| Meropenem-Vaborbactam | Humans ND, toxic in animals | Probably safe with monitoring, but no data available |
| Metronidazole | B | Data and opinions conflict; best to avoid |
| Minocycline | D | Short-term use safe, monitor infant for GI toxicity |
| Moxifloxacin | C | Short-term use safe, monitor infant for GI toxicity; avoid if possible |
| Netilmicin | D | Safety not established |
| Nitrofurantoin | B | Avoid if infant <8 days of age |
| Ofloxacin | C | Avoid breastfeeding for 4-6 hrs after a dose, monitor infant for GI toxicity |
| Omadacycline | Avoid during 2nd and 3rd trimesters | Avoid breastfeeding during treatment and for 4 days after last dose |
| Oritavancin | C | Probably safe with monitoring, but no data available; avoid if possible |
| Penicillins | B | Safe, monitor infant for GI toxicity |
| Plazomicin | No data | No data |
| Polymyxin B | C | Topical administration safe (no data with systemic use) |
| Quinupristin/ Dalfopristin | B | Probably safe with monitoring, but no data available; avoid if possible |
| Rifaximin | C | Probably safe with monitoring, but no data available; avoid if possible |
| Sarecycline | Do not use (risk of fetal harm, tooth discoloration, inhibition of bone growth) | No data; avoid use |
| Streptomycin | D | Probably safe, monitor infant for GI toxicity |
| Tedizolid | C | Probably safe with monitoring, but no data available; avoid if possible |
| Telavancin | C | Probably safe with monitoring, but no data available; avoid if possible |
| Telithromycin | C | Probably safe with monitoring, but no data available; avoid if possible |
| Tetracycline | D | Short-term use safe, monitor infant for GI toxicity |
| Tigecycline | D | Safety not established, avoid use |
| TMP-SMX | C | Risk of kernicterus in premature infants; avoid if infant G6PD-deficient |
| Tobramycin | D | Probably safe, monitor infant for GI toxicity |
| Vancomycin | C | Safe with monitoring |
| **Antifungals** | | |
| Amphotericin B (all products) | B | Probably safe, but no data available |
| Anidulafungin | B | Safety not established, avoid use |
| Caspofungin | C | Probably safe with monitoring, but no data available; avoid if possible |

TABLE 8 (2)

| Drug | Risk Category (Old) | Use during Lactation |
|---|---|---|
| **Antifungals** *(continued)* | | |
| Fluconazole (other regimens) | D | Safe with monitoring |
| Fluconazole (single dose) | C | Safe with monitoring |
| Flucytosine | C | Safety not established, avoid use |
| Griseofulvin | C | Safety not established, avoid use |
| Isavuconazonium sulfate | C | Avoid use |
| Itraconazole | C | Little data available, avoid if possible |
| Ketoconazole | C | Little data available, avoid if possible |
| Micafungin | C | Safety not established, avoid use |
| Posaconazole | C | Safety not established, avoid use |
| Terbinafine | B | Little data available, avoid if possible |
| Voriconazole | D | Safety not established, avoid use |
| **Antimycobacterials** | | |
| Amikacin | D | Probably safe, monitor infant for GI toxicity |
| Bedaquiline | B | Safety not established, avoid use |
| Capreomycin | C | Probably safe, monitor infant for GI toxicity |
| Clofazimine | C | May color breast milk pink; probably safe but avoid if possible |
| Cycloserine | C | Probably safe |
| Dapsone | C | Safe |
| Delamanid | Humans ND, toxic in animals | Safety not established, avoid use |
| Ethambutol | Safe | Probably safe |
| Ethionamide | C | Probably safe with monitoring |
| Isoniazid | C | Safe |
| Para-aminosalicylic acid | C | Probably safe |
| Pyrazinamide | C | Probably safe |
| Rifabutin | B | Probably safe |
| Rifampin | C | Probably safe |
| Rifapentine | C | Probably safe |
| Streptomycin | D | Probably safe |
| Thalidomide | X | Safety not established |
| **Antiparasitics** | | |
| Albendazole | C | Data limited; one-time dose considered safe by WHO |
| Artemether/ Lumefantrine | C | Data limited; probably safe, particularly if infant weighs at least 5 kg |
| Atovaquone | C | Data limited; probably safe, particularly if infant weighs at least 5 kg |
| Atovaquone/Proguanil | C | Data limited; probably safe, particularly if infant weighs at least 5 kg |
| Benznidazole | Avoid | Safe with monitoring |
| Chloroquine | C | Probably safe with monitoring, but data limited; avoid if possible |
| Dapsone | C | Safe, but avoid if infant G6PD-deficient |
| Eflornithine | C | Probably safe, monitor infant for toxicity |
| Ivermectin | C | Probably safe, monitor infant for toxicity |
| Mebendazole | C | Probably safe, monitor infant for toxicity |
| Mefloquine | B | Probably safe, monitor infant for toxicity |
| Miltefosine | D | Safety not established, avoid use |
| Moxidectin | Humans: insufficient data Animals: no embryo/ fetal toxicity | Safety not established; avoid use if possible |
| Nitazoxanide | B | Probably safe with monitoring, but data limited; avoid if possible |
| Pentamidine | C | Safety not established, avoid use |
| Praziquantel | B | Probably safe, monitor infant for toxicity |
| Primaquine | Avoid in pregnancy (risk of hemolysis if fetus G6PD-deficient) | Probably safe, monitor infant for toxicity |
| Pyrimethamine | C | Safe with monitoring |
| Quinidine | C | Probably safe, monitor infant for toxicity |
| Quinine | X | Probably safe, but avoid if infant G6PD-deficient |
| Secnidazole | No human data, safe in animals | Safety not established, avoid breastfeeding for 96 hours after dose |
| Sulfadoxine/ Pyrimethamine | C | Little data available, avoid use if possible |
| Tafenoquine | Not recommended (risk of hemolytic anemia if fetus G6PD-deficient) | Avoid breastfeeding x3 months after dose if infant G6PD-deficient or status unknown |
| Tinidazole | C | Safety not established, avoid use |

TABLE 8 (3) 95

| Drug | Risk Category (Old) | Use during Lactation |
|---|---|---|
| **Antivirals** | | |
| Acyclovir | B | Safe with monitoring |
| Adefovir | C | Safety not established, avoid use if possible |
| Amantadine | C | Avoid use |
| Cidofovir | C | Avoid use |
| Daclatasvir | No human data | Safety not established, avoid use if possible |
| Entecavir | C | Safety not established, avoid use if possible |
| Famciclovir | B | Safety not established, avoid use |
| Foscarnet | C | Safety not established, avoid use |
| Ganciclovir | C | Safety not established, avoid use |
| Interferons | C | Probably safe, monitor infant for toxicity |
| Letermovir | Humans ND, toxic in animals | Safety not established, avoid use if possible |
| Oseltamivir | C | Probably safe, monitor infant for toxicity |
| Peramivir | C | Safety not established, avoid use if possible |
| Ribavirin | X | No data, but probably safe with monitoring |
| Rimantadine | C | Avoid use |
| Simeprevir | C (X w/ribavirin) | Safety not established, avoid use if possible |
| Sofosbuvir | B (X w/ribavirin) | Safety not established, avoid use if possible |
| Tecovirimat | Humans ND, safe in animals | Safety not established, avoid use if possible |
| Telbivudine | B | Safety not established, avoid use if possible |
| Tenofovir AF (Vemlidy) | Humans ND, safe in animals | Safety not established, avoid use if possible |
| Valacyclovir | B | Safe with monitoring |
| Valganciclovir | C | Safety not established, avoid use |
| Zanamivir | C | Probably safe, but no data |
| **Antivirals (hep C combinations)** | | |
| Epclusa | Humans ND, safe in animals | Safety not established, avoid if possible |
| Harvoni | B | Safety not established |
| Mavyret | Humans ND, safe in animals | Safety not established, avoid use if possible |
| Technivie | B | Safety not established |
| Viekira Pak | B | Safety not established |
| Vosevi | Humans ND, safe in animals | Safety not established, avoid use if possible |
| Zepatier | Humans ND, safe in animals | Safety not established, avoid if possible |
| **Antiretrovirals (HIV-infected mothers are generally discouraged from breastfeeding their infants. When required, country-specific recommendations should be followed)** | | |
| Abacavir | C | |
| Atazanavir | B | |
| Darunavir | C | |
| Darunavir/ritonavir | Avoid in pregnancy (↓ exposure of DRV, RTV) | |
| Delavirdine | C | |
| Didanosine | B | |
| Dolutegravir | B | |
| Doravirine | Humans ND, safe in animals | |
| Efavirenz | D | |
| Elvitegravir | B | |
| Emtricitabine | B | |
| Enfuvirtide | B | |
| Etravirine | B | |
| Fosamprenavir | C | |
| Ibalizumab-uiyk | Human, animals: no data | |
| Indinavir | C | |
| Lamivudine | C | |
| Lopinavir/r | C | |
| Maraviroc | B | |
| Nelfinavir | B | |
| Nevirapine | B | |
| Raltegravir | C | |
| Rilpivirine | B | |
| Ritonavir | B | |

TABLE 8 (4)

| Drug | Risk Category (Old) | Use during Lactation |
|------|--------------------|--------------------|
| **Antiretrovirals** *(continued)* | | |
| Saquinavir | B | |
| Stavudine | C | |
| Tenofovir alafenamide (TAF) | No human data, safe in animals | Safety not established, avoid if possible |
| Tenofovir disoproxil (TDF) | B | |
| Tipranavir | C | |
| Zalcitabine | C | |
| Zidovudine | C | |
| **Antiretroviral Combinations** | | |
| Atripla (EFV-FTC-TAF) | D | |
| Biktarvy (BIC-FTC-TAF) | Humans ND, safe in animals | |
| Cimduo (3TC-TDF) | Humans: inadequate data, Animals: toxic in rabbits | |
| Combivir (3TC-ZDV) | C | |
| Complera (RPV-FTC-TDF) | B | |
| Descovy (FTC-TAF) | Humans ND, nontoxic in animals | |
| Epzicom (3TC-ABC) | Humans nontoxic, toxic in animals | |
| Evotaz (ATV-cobi) | B | |
| Genvoya (EVG-cobi-FTC-TAF) | Humans: inadequate data Animals: nontoxic | |
| Juluca (DTG-RPV) | Humans: inadequate data Animals: nontoxic | |
| Odefsey (RPV-FTC-TAF) | Humans: inadequate data Animals: nontoxic | |
| Prezcobix (DRV-cobi) | Avoid in pregnancy due to lower exposures of DRV and cobicistat | |
| Stribild (EVG-cobi-FTC-TDF) | B | |
| Symfi, Symfi Lo (EFV-3TC-TDF) | Risk of fetal harm from EFV; avoid in first trimester | |
| Symtuza (DRV-cobi-FTC-TAF) | Avoid in pregnancy due to lower exposures of DRV and RTV | |
| Temixys (3TC-TDF) | Humans: 3TC safe, TDF no data Animals: 3TC embryotoxic, TDF safe | |
| Triumeq (DTG-3TC-ABC) | C | |
| Trizivir (ABC-3TC-ZDV) | C | |
| Truvada (FTC-TDF) | B | |

## TABLE 9A – SELECTED PHARMACOLOGIC FEATURES OF ANTIMICROBIAL AGENTS

*For pharmacodynamics, see Table 9B; for Cytochrome P450 interactions, see Table 9C. Table terminology key at bottom of each page. Additional footnotes at end of Table 9A, page 108.*

| DRUG | REFERENCE DOSE (SINGLE OR MULTIPLE) | FOOD REC (PO DRUGS)[1] | ORAL ABS (%) | PEAK SERUM CONC[2] (µg/mL) | PROTEIN BINDING (%) | VOLUME OF DISTRIBUTION (Vd)[3] | AVG SERUM T½ (hr)[4] | BILE PEN (%)[5] | CSF/BLOOD[6] (%) | CSF PENETRATION[7] | AUC[8] (µg·hr/mL) | Tmax (hr) |
|---|---|---|---|---|---|---|---|---|---|---|---|---|
| **ANTIBACTERIALS** | | | | | | | | | | | | |
| **Aminoglycosides** | | | | | | | | | | | | |
| Amik, Gent, Kana, Tobra | See Table 10D | | | See Table 10D | 0-10 | 0.26 L/kg | 2-3 | 10-60 | 0-30 | No | | |
| Neomycin | | po | <3 | 0 | ND | ND | ND | ND | ND | ND | ND | ND |
| Plazomicin | 15 mg/kg IV q24h | Tab/soln ± food | - | 51-74 (15 mg/kg SD) | 20 | 18-31 L | 3.5 | ND | ND | ND | 226-257 (SD, 0-∞) | - |
| **Carbapenems** | | | | | | | | | | | | |
| Doripenem | 500 mg IV | | | 23 (SD) | 8.1 | 16.8 L Vss | 1 | 117 (0-611) | ND | ND | 36.3 | |
| Ertapenem | 1 gm IV | | | 154 (SD) | 95 | 0.12 L/kg Vss | 4 | 10 | ND | ND | 572.1 | |
| Imipenem | 500 mg IV | | | 40 (SD) | 15-25 | 0.27 L/kg | 1 | minimal | 8.5 | Possibly[9] | 42.2 | |
| Meropenem | 500 mg IV | | | 49 (SD) | 2 | 0.29 L/kg | 1 | 3-300 | ≈ 2 | Possibly[9] | 72.5 | |
| Meropenem/ Vaborbactam | Mer 2 gm/ Vab 2 gm IV q8h | | | Mer 43.4, Vab 55.6 (SS) | Mer 2, Vab 33 | Mer 20.2L, Vab 18.6 L (Vss) | Mer 1.2, Vab 1.7 | ND | ND | ND | Mer 138, Vab 196 (8 hr, SS) | |
| **Cephalosporins (IV)** | | | | | | | | | | | | |
| Cefazolin | 1 gm IV | | | 188 (SD) | 73-87 | 0.19 L/kg | 1.9 | 29-300 | 1-4 | No | 236 | |
| Cefepime | 2 gm IV | | | 164 (SD) | 20 | 18 L Vss | 2 | 10-20 | 10 | Yes | 284.8 | |
| Cefotaxime | 1 gm IV | | | 100 (SD) | 30-51 | 0.28 L/kg | 1.5 | 15-75 | 10 | Yes | 70 | |
| Cefotetan | 1 gm IV | | | 158 (SD) | 78-91 | 10.3 L | 4.2 | 2-21 | ND | ND | 504 | |
| Cefoxitin | 1 gm IV | | | 110 (SD) | 65-79 | 16.1 L Vss | 0.8 | 280 | 3 | No | | |
| Ceftaroline | 600 mg IV q12h | | | 21.3 (SS) | 20 | 20.3 L Vss | 2.7 | ND | ND | ND | 56.3 (12 hr) | |
| Ceftazidime/ Avibactam | 2.5 gm IV q8h | | | Ceftaz 90.4, Avi 14.6 (SS) | Ceftaz <10, Avi 5.7-8.2 | Ceftaz 17 L, Avi 22.2 L (Vss) | Ceftaz 2.8, Avi 2.7 | ND | ND | ND | Ceftaz 291, Avi 38.2 (8 hr) | |
| Ceftazidime | 1 gm IV | | | 69 (SD) | <10 | 0.24 L/kg Vss | 1.9 | 13-54 | 20-40 | Yes | 127 | |
| Ceftizoxime | 1 gm IV | | | 60 (SD) | 30 | 0.34 L/kg | 1.7 | 34-82 | ND | ND | 85 | |
| Ceftobiprole[NUS] | 500 mg IV | | | 33-34.2 (SD) | 16 | 18 L Vss | 2.9-3.3 | ND | ND | Yes | 116 | |
| Ceftolozane/ Tazobactam | 1.5 gm IV q8h | | | Ceftolo 74.4, Tazo 18 (SS) | Ceftolo 16-21, Tazo 30 | Ceftolo 13.5 L, Tazo 18.2 L (Vss) | Ceftolo 3.1, Tazo 1.0 | ND | ND | ND | Ceftolo 182, Tazo 25 (8 hr) | |
| Ceftriaxone | 1 gm IV | | | 150 (SD) | 85-95 | 5.8-13.5 L | 8 | 200-500 | 8-16 | Yes | 1006 | |
| Cefuroxime | 1.5 gm IV | | | 100 (SD) | 33-50 | 0.19 L/kg Vss | 1.5 | 35-80 | 17-88 | Marginal | 150 | |

**Food Effect (po dosing): + food** = take with food, **no food** = take without food, **± food** = take with or without food; **Oral % AB** = % absorbed; **Peak Serum Level: SD** = after single dose, **SS** = steady state after multiple doses; **Volume of Distribution (Vd): V/F** = Vd/oral bioavailability; **Vss** = Vd at steady state, **Vss/F** = Vd at steady state/oral bioavailability; **CSF Penetration:** therapeutic efficacy comment based on dose, usual susceptibility or target organism & penetration into CSF. **AUC** = area under drug concentration curve; **24hr** = AUC 0-24; **Tmax** = time to max plasma concentration.

**TABLE 9A (2)** *(Footnotes at the end of table)*

| DRUG | REFERENCE DOSE (SINGLE OR MULTIPLE) | FOOD REC (PO DRUGS)[1] | ORAL ABS (%)[1] | PEAK SERUM CONC[c] (µg/mL) | PROTEIN BINDING (%) | VOLUME OF DISTRIBUTION (Vd)[3] | AVG SERUM T½ (hr)[e] | BILE PEN (%)[g] | CSF/ BLOOD[e] (%) | CSF PENETRATION[b] | AUC[a] (µg·hr/mL) | Tmax (hr) |
|---|---|---|---|---|---|---|---|---|---|---|---|---|
| **ANTIBACTERIALS** *(continued)* | | | | | | | | | | | | |
| *Cephalosporins (po)* | | | | | | | | | | | | |
| Cefaclor | 500 mg po | Cap/susp ± food | 93 | 13 (SD) | 22-25 | 0.33 L/kg V/F | 0.8 | ≥60 | | | 20.5 | 0.5-1.0 |
| Cefaclor ER | 500 mg po | Tab + food | | 8.4 (SD) | 22-25 | | 0.8 | ≥60 | | | 18.1 | 2.5 |
| Cefadroxil | 500 mg po | Cap/tab/susp ± food | 90 | 16 (SD) | 20 | 0.31 L/kg V/F | 1.5 | 22 | | | 47.4 | ND |
| Cefdinir | 300 mg po | Cap/susp ± food | 25 | 1.6 (SD) | 60-70 | 0.35 L/kg V/F | 1.7 | | | | 7.1 | 2.9 |
| Cefditoren pivoxil | 400 mg po | Tab + food | 16 | 4 (SD) | 88 | 9.3 L Vss/F | 1.6 | | | | 20 | 1.5-3.0 |
| Cefixime | 400 mg po | Tab/susp ± food | 50 | 3-5 (SD) | 65 | 0.93 L/kg V/F | 3.1 | 800 | | | 25.8 | 4 |
| Cefpodoxime proxetil | 200 mg po | Tab + food, Susp ± food | 46 | 2.3 (SD) | 40 | 0.7 L/kg V/F | 2.3 | 115 | | | 14.5 | 2-3 |
| Cefprozil | 500 mg po | Tab/susp ± food | 95 | 10.5 (SD) | 36 | 0.23 L/kg Vss/F | 1.5 | | | | 25.7 | 1.5 |
| Ceftibuten | 400 mg po | Cap/susp no food | 80 | 15 (SD) | 65 | 0.21 L/kg V/F | 2.4 | | | | 73.7 | 2.6 |
| Cefuroxime axetil | 250 mg tab po | Susp + food, tab ± food | 52 | 4.1 (SD) | 50 | 0.66 L/kg V/F | 1.5 | | | | 12.9 | 2.5 |
| Cephalexin | 500 mg po | Cap/tab/susp ± food | 90 | 18 (SD) | 5-15 | 0.38 L/kg V/F | 1 | 216 | | | 29 | 1 |
| **Monobactams** | | | | | | | | | | | | |
| Aztreonam | 1 gm IV | | | 90 (SD) | 56 | 12.6 L Vss | 2 | 115-405 | 3-52 | ND | 271 | |
| **Penicillins** | | | | | | | | | | | | |
| Amox/Clav ER | 2 tabs [total 2000/125 mg] po | Tab + food | ND | 17/2.1 (SD) | 18/25 | 0.36/0.21 (both L/kg) | 1.4/1.0 | amox 100-3000 | ND | ND | 71.6/5.3 (0-∞) | 1.5/1.03 |
| Amox/Clav | 875/125 mg po | Cap/tab/susp ± food | 80/ 30-98 | 11.6/2.2 (SD) | 18/25 | 0.36/0.21 (both L/kg) | 1.4/1.0 | amox 100-3000 | ND | ND | 26.8/5.1 (0-∞) | ND |
| Amoxicillin ER | 775 mg po | Tab + food | | 6.6 (SD) | 20 | 0.36 L/kg | 1.2-1.5 | 100-3000 | | | 29.8 | 3.1 |
| Amoxicillin | 500 mg po | Cap/tab/susp ± food | 80 | 5.5-7.5 (SD) | 17 | 0.36 L/kg | 1.2 | 100-3000 | 13-14 | Yes (IV only) | 22 | 1-2 |
| Amp/Sulb | 3 gm IV | | | 109-150/ 48-88 (SD) | 28/38 | 0.29/0.3 (both L/kg) | 1.4/1.7 | amp 100-3000 | 13-14 | ND | 120/71 (0-∞) | |
| Ampicillin | 2 gm IV | | | 100 (SD) | 18-22 | 0.29 L/kg | 1.2 | 100-3000 | 13-14 | Yes | | |
| Benzathine Penicillin G | 1.2 million units IM | | | 0.15 (SD) | | | | | | | | |
| Cloxacillin[NUS] | 500 mg po | Cap no food | 50 | 7.5-14 (SD) | 95 | 0.1 L/kg | 0.5 | 5-8 | ND | ND | | 1-1.5 |
| Dicloxacillin | 500 mg po | Cap no food | 37 | 10-17 (SD) | 98 | 0.1 L/kg | 0.7 | >100 | 9-20 | Yes w/ high doses | ND | 1-1.5 |
| Nafcillin | 500 mg IV | | | 30 (SD) | 90-94 | 27.1 L Vss | 0.5-1 | 25 | 10-15 | Yes | 18.1 (0-∞) | |
| Oxacillin | 500 mg IV | Cap no food | 50 | 43 (SD) | 90-94 | 0.4 L/kg | 0.5-0.7 | 25 | 10-15 | Yes | | |
| Penicillin G | 2 million units IV | Cap no food | 50 | 20 (SD) | 65 | 0.35 L/kg | 0.5 | 500 | 5-10 | Yes: Pen-sens § pneumo | | |

**Food Effect (po dosing):** **+ food** = take with food, **no food** = take without food, **± food** = take with or without food; **Peak Serum Level:** **SD** = after single dose, **SS** = steady state after multiple doses; **Volume of Distribution (Vd):** **V/F** = Vd/oral bioavailability, **Vss** = Vd at steady state, **Vss/F** = Vd at steady state/oral bioavailability; **CSF Penetration:** therapeutic efficacy comment based on dose, usual susceptibility or target organism & penetration into CSF; **AUC** = area under drug concentration curve; **24hr** = AUC 0-24; **Tmax** = time to max plasma concentration.

**TABLE 9A (3)** (Footnotes at the end of table)

| DRUG | REFERENCE DOSE (SINGLE OR MULTIPLE) | FOOD REC (PO DRUGS)[1] | ORAL ABS (%) | PEAK SERUM CONC[2] (µg/mL) | PROTEIN BINDING (%) | VOLUME OF DISTRIBUTION (Vd)[3] | AVG SERUM T½ (hr)[4] | BILE PEN (%)[5] | CSF/ BLOOD[6] (%) | CSF PENETRATION[7] | AUC[8] (µg•hr/mL) | Tmax (hr) |
|---|---|---|---|---|---|---|---|---|---|---|---|---|
| **ANTIBACTERIALS** (continued) | | | | | | | | | | | | |
| **Penicillins** (continued) | | | | | | | | | | | | |
| Penicillin V | 500 mg po | Tab/soln no food | 60-73 | 5-6 (SD) | 65 | | 0.5 | | ND | ND | | ND |
| Pip/Tazo | 3.375 gm IV | | | 242/24 (SD) | 16/48 | 0.24/0.4 (both L/kg) | 1/1 | >100 | ND | ND | 242/25 | |
| Pivmecillinam | 400 mg po q12h | Tab ± food | 60-70 | 3 (400 mg) (SD) | 5-10 | 0.2-0.4 L/kg | 1 | ND | ND | ND | ND | |
| Temocillin | 2 gm IV | - | - | 150-200 (SD) | 70-85 | 0.2 L/kg | 4 | 800-1000 | 8-15 | | 785 (0-∞) | - |
| **Fluoroquinolones[10]** | | | | | | | | | | | | |
| Ciprofloxacin | 400 mg IV q12h | | | 4.6 (SS) | 20-40 | 2.4 L/kg | 4 | 2800-4500 | 26 | Inadequate for Strep | 25.4 (24 hr) | |
| Ciprofloxacin | 500 mg ER po q24h | Tab ± food | | 1.6 (SS) | 20-40 | 2.4 L/kg | 6.6 | | | | 8 (24 hr) | 1-4 |
| Ciprofloxacin | 750 mg po q12h | Tab/susp ± food | 70 | 3.6 (SS) | 20-40 | 2.4 L/kg | 4 | 2800-4500 | | | 31.6 (24 hr) | 1-2 |
| Delafloxacin | 300 mg IV or 450 mg po q12h | Tab ± food | 59 | po 7.45, IV 9.3 (SS) | 84 | 30-48 L Vss | 4.2-8.5 | ND | ND | ND | po 30.8, IV 23.4 (12 hr) | 1 |
| Gemifloxacin | 320 mg po q24h | Tab ± food | 71 | 1.6 (SS) | 55-73 | 2-12 L/kg Vss/F | 7 | | | | 9.9 (24 hr) | 0.5-2.0 |
| Levofloxacin | 750 mg po/IV q24h | Tab ± food, soln no food | 99 | po 8.6, IV 12.1 (SS) | 24-38 | 244 L Vss | 7 | | >50 | Yes (CID 49:1080, 2009) | po 90.7, IV 108 (24 hr) | po 1.6 |
| Moxifloxacin | 400 mg po/IV q24h | Tab ± food | 89 | 4.2-4.6 (SS) | 30-50 | 2.2 L/kg | 10-14 | | | No | po 48, IV 38 (24 hr) | po 1-3 |
| Norfloxacin | 400 mg po q24h | Tab no food | 30-40 | 1.5 (400 mg SD) | 10-15 | 1.7 L/kg | 3-4 | 700 | ND | | 6.4 (400 mg) | 1 |
| Ofloxacin | 400 mg po q12h | Tab ± food | 98 | 4.6-6.2 (SS) | 32 | 1-2.5 L/kg | 7 | | | No | 82.4 (24 hr) | 1-2 |
| Prulifloxacin[MUS] | 600 mg po | Tab ± food | ND | 1.6 (SD) | 45 | 1231 L | 10.6-12.1 | ND | ND | ND | 7.3 | 1 |
| **GLYCOPEPTIDES, LIPOGLYCOPEPTIDES, LIPOPEPTIDES** | | | | | | | | | | | | |
| Dalbavancin | 1 gm IV | | | 280-300 (SD) | 93-98 | 0.11 L/kg | 147-258 | ND | ND | ND | 23.443 | |
| Daptomycin | 4-6 mg/kg IV q24h | | | 58-99 (SS) | 92 | 0.1 L/kg Vss | 8.9 | ND | 0-8 | ND | 494-632 (24 hr) | |
| Oritavancin | 1200 mg IV | | | 138 (SD) | 85 | 87.6 L | 245 (terminal) | ND | ND | ND | 2800 (0-∞) | |
| Teicoplanin | 6 mg/kg IV | - | - | 40-50 (SD) | 90-95 | 0.9-1.6 L/kg Vss | 70-100 | ND | negligible | No | 500-600 (0-∞) | - |
| Telavancin | 10 mg/kg IV q24h | | | 108 (SS) | 90 | 0.13 L/kg | 8.1 | Low | 7-14 | Need high doses | 780 (24 hr) | |
| Vancomycin | 1 gm IV q12h | Tab ± food | | 20-50 (SS) | <10-55 | 0.7 L/kg | 4-6 | ND | negligible | | 500-600 if trough 20 (24 hr) | |

**Food Effect (po dosing): + food** = take with food, **± food** = take with or without food, **no food** = take without food; **Oral % AB** = % absorbed; **Peak Serum Level: SD** = after single dose, **SS** = steady state after multiple doses; **Volume of Distribution (Vd): V/F** = oral bioavailability, **Vss** = Vd at steady state, **Vss/F** = Vd at steady state/oral bioavailability, **CSF Penetration:** therapeutic efficacy comment based on dose, usual susceptibility of target organism & penetration into CSF; **24hr** = AUC 0-24; **AUC** = area under drug concentration curve; **Tmax** = time to max plasma concentration.

**TABLE 9A (4)** *(Footnotes at the end of table)*

| DRUG | REFERENCE DOSE (SINGLE OR MULTIPLE) | FOOD REC (PO DRUGS)¹ | ORAL ABS (%)² | PEAK SERUM CONC (µg/mL) | PROTEIN BINDING (%) | VOLUME OF DISTRIBUTION (Vd)³ | AVG SERUM T½ (hr)⁴ | BILE PEN (%)⁵ | CSF/ BLOOD (%)⁶ | CSF PENETRATION⁷ | AUC (µg•hr/mL) | Tmax (hr) |
|---|---|---|---|---|---|---|---|---|---|---|---|---|
| **MACROLIDES, AZALIDES, LINCOSAMIDES, KETOLIDES** | | | | | | | | | | | | |
| Azithromycin IV | 500 mg IV | | | 3.6 (SD) | 7-51 | 33.3 L/kg | 68 | High | | | 9.6 (24 hr, pre SS) | |
| Azithromycin | 500 mg po | Tab/susp ± food | 37 | 0.4 (SD) | 7-51 | 31.1 L/kg | 68 | High | | | 4.3 | 2.5 |
| Azithromycin ER | 2 gm po | Susp no food | ≈ 30 | 0.8 (SD) | 7-51 | 31.1 L/kg | 59 | High | | | 20 | 5 |
| Clarithromycin | 500 mg po q12h | Tab/susp ± food | 50 | 3-4 (SS) | 65-70 | 4 L/kg | 5-7 | 7000 | | | 20 (24 hr) | 2.0-2.5 |
| Clarithromycin ER | 1 gm ER po q24h | Tab ± food | ≈ 50 | 2-3 (SS) | 65-70 | | 5-7 | | | | | 5-8 |
| Clindamycin | 150 mg po | Cap ± food | 90 | 2.5 (SD) | 85-94 | 1.1 L/kg | 2.4 | 250-300 | | | ND | 0.75 |
| Clindamycin | 900 mg IV q8h | | | 14.1 (SS) | 85-94 | 1.1 L/kg | 2.4 | 250-300 | | | ND | |
| Erythromycin base, esters | 500 mg po | Tab/susp no food, DR caps ± food | 18-45 | 0.1-2 (SD) | 70-74 | 0.6 L/kg | 2-4 | | 2-13 | No | | delay rel: 3 |
| Erythromycin lactobionate | 500 mg IV | | | 3-4 (SD) | 70-74 | 0.6 L/kg | 2-4 | | | No | | |
| Telithromycin | 800 mg po q24h | Tab ± food | 57 | 2.3 (SS) | 60-70 | 2.9 L/kg | 10 | 7 | | | 12.5 (24 hr) | 1 |
| **MISCELLANEOUS ANTIBACTERIALS** | | | | | | | | | | | | |
| Chloramphenicol | 1 gm po q6h | Cap ± food | High | 18 (SS) | 25-50 | 0.8 L/kg | 4.1 | High | 45-89 | Yes | ND | |
| Fosfomycin (po) | 3 gm po | Sachet ± food | | 26 (SD) | <10 | 136.1 L Vss/F | 5.7 | ND | 20-50 | ND | 150 | 2 |
| Fosfomycin (IV) | 6 gm IV q6h | - | - | 276-370 (3 gm SD) | <10 | 9-30 L (Vss) | 1.9-3.9 | ND | ND | ND | 405-448 (3 gm SD) | - |
| Fusidic acid^MS | 500 mg po | Tab ± food | 91 | 30 (SD) | 95-99 | 0.3 L/kg | 15 | 100-200 | 45-89 | ND | 442 (0-∞) | 2-4 |
| Metronidazole | 500 mg IV/po q6h | ER tab no food, tab/cap ± food | 100 | 20-25 (SS) | 20 | 0.6-0.85 L/kg | 6-14 | 100 | 45-89 | ND | 560 (24 hr) | ER 6.8, regular 1.6 |
| Pristinamycin | 2 gm po | Tab ± food | ND | PIA 0.76, PIIA 0.58 (SD) | ND | ND | PIA 4.03, PIIA 2.83 | ND | ND | ND | PIA 2.2, PIIA 1.21 (2 gm SD, 0-∞) | PIA 3.25, PIIA 3.08 |
| Quinupristin-dalfopristin | 7.5 mg/kg IV q8h | | | Q 3.2/D 8 (SS) | ND | Q 0.45/D 0.24 (L/kg) Vss | Q 0.85/D 0.7 | ND | ND | ND | Q 7.2/D 10.6 (24 hr) | |
| Rifampin | 600 mg po | Cap no food | 70-90 | 7 (SD) | 80 | 0.65 L/kg Vss | 1.5-5 | 10,000 | 7-56 | Yes | 40-60 (24 hr) | 1.5-2 |
| Rifaximin | 200 mg po tid | Tab ± food | <0.4 | 0.0007-0.002 (SS) | 67.5 | | 2-5 | ND | ND | No | 0.008 | 1 |
| Secnidazole | 2 gm po | Granules ± food | ND | 45.4 (SS) | <5 | 42 L | 17 | ND | ND | ND | 1332 (2 gm SD) | 4 |
| TMP/SMX | 160/800 mg po q12h | Tab/susp ± food | 85 | 1-2/40-60 (SS) | 44/70 | 100-120 L/ 12-18 L | 11/9 | 100-200 | 50/40 | ND | ND | 1-4 |
| TMP/SMX | 160/800 mg IV q8h | | | 9/105 (SS) | 44/70 | 100-120 L/ 12-18 L | 11/9 | 40-70 | | | ND | 1-4 |
| Trimethoprim | 100 mg po | Tab ± food | 80 | 1 (SD) | 44 | 100-120 L/F | 8-15 | ND | | | ND | 1-4 |

**Food Effect (po dosing): + food** = take with food, **no food** = take without food, **± food** = take with or without food; **Oral % AB** = % absorbed; **Peak Serum Level: SD** = after single dose, **SS** = steady state after multiple doses; **Volume of Distribution (Vd): V/F** = Vd/oral bioavailability, **Vss** = Vd at steady state, **Vss/F** = Vd at steady state/oral bioavailability; **CSF Penetration:** therapeutic efficacy comment based on dose, usual susceptibility or target organism & penetration into CSF; **24hr** = AUC 0-24; **Tmax** = time to max plasma concentration.

**TABLE 9A (5)** (Footnotes at the end of table)

| DRUG | REFERENCE DOSE (SINGLE OR MULTIPLE) | FOOD REC (PO DRUGS)¹ | ORAL ABS (%) | PEAK SERUM CONC² (µg/mL) | PROTEIN BINDING (%) | VOLUME OF DISTRIBUTION (Vd)³ | AVG SERUM T½ (hr)⁴ | BILE PEN (%)⁵ | CSF/ BLOOD⁶ (%) | CSF PENETRATION⁷ | AUC⁸ (µg·hr/mL) | Tmax (hr) |
|---|---|---|---|---|---|---|---|---|---|---|---|---|
| **OXAZOLIDINONES** | | | | | | | | | | | | |
| Linezolid | 600 mg po/IV q12h | Tab/susp ± food | 100 | 15-20 (SS) | 31 | 40-50 L Vss | 5 | | 60-70 | Yes (AAC 50-3971, 2006) | po 276, IV 179 (24 hr) | po 1.3 |
| Tedizolid | 200 mg po/IV q24h | Tab ± food | 91 | po 2.2, IV 3.0 (SS) | 70-90 | 67-80 L Vss | 12 | ND | ND | ND | po 25.6, IV 29.2 (24 hr) | po 3, IV 1.1 |
| **POLYMYXINS** | | | | | | | | | | | | |
| Colistin (Polymyxin E) | 150 mg IV | | | 5-7.5 (SD) | ≈ 50 | 0.34 L/kg | colistimethate 1.5-2, Colistin >4 | 0 | | No | | |
| Polymyxin B | 1.5 mg/kg IV q12h | | | 2.8 (avg conc at SS) | 60 | ND | 4.5-6 (old data) | ND | ND | No | 66.9 (24 hr) | |
| **TETRACYCLINES, GLYCYLCYCLINES** | | | | | | | | | | | | |
| Doxycycline | 100 mg po | Tab/cap/susp + food | | 1.5-2.1 (SD) | 93 | 53-134 L Vss | 18 | 200-3200 | 26 | No | 31.7 (0-∞) | 2 |
| Eravacycline | 1 mg/kg IV q12h | - | - | 1.825 (SS) | 79-90 | 321 L (Vss) | 20 | ND | ND | ND | 6.31 (12 hr) | - |
| Minocycline | 200 mg po | Cap/tab ± food | ND | 2.0-3.5 (SS) | 76 | 80-114 L Vss | 16 | 200-3200 | ND | ND | 48.3 (0-∞) | 2,1 |
| Omadacycline | 100 mg IV (or 300 mg po) q24h | Tab no food | 35 | IV 2.12, po 0.95 (SS) | 20 | 190 L (Vss) | 15.5-16.8 | ND | ND | ND | IV 12.14, po 11.16 (24 hr) | po 2.5 |
| Sarecycline | 60-150 mg po q24h | Tab ± food | ND | ND | 62.5-74.7 | 91.4-97.0 (Vss) | 21-22 | ND | ND | ND | ND | 1.5-2.0 |
| Tetracycline | 250 mg po | Cap no food | ND | 1.5-2.2 (SD) | 20-65 | 1.3 L/kg | 6-12 | 200-3200 | Poor | No | 30 (0-∞) | 2-4 |
| Tigecycline | 50 mg IV q12h | | ND | 0.63 (SS) | 71-89 | 7-9 L/kg | 42 | 138 | 5.9-10.6 | No | 4.7 (24 hr) | |
| **ANTIFUNGALS** | | | | | | | | | | | | |
| **Benzofuran** | | | | | | | | | | | | |
| Griseofulvin (ultramicrosize) | 250 mg po | Tab + food (high fat) | 27-72 | 0.6-0.67 (SD) | ND | ND | 9-24 | ND | ND | ND | 8.6-9.0 (0-∞) | 4 |
| **Polyenes** | | | | | | | | | | | | |
| Ampho B deoxycholate | 0.4-0.7 mg/kg IV q24h | | | 0.5-3.5 (SS) | | 4 L/kg | 24 | | 0 | | 17 (24 hr) | |
| Ampho B lipid complex (ABLC) | 5 mg/kg IV q24h | | | 1-2.5 (SS) | | 131 L/kg | 173 | | | | 14 (24 hr) | |
| Ampho B liposomal | 5 mg/kg IV q24h | | | 83 (SS) | | 0.1-0.4 L/kg Vss | 6.8 | | | | 555 (24 hr) | |
| **Antimetabolites** | | | | | | | | | | | | |
| Flucytosine | 2.5 gm po | Cap ± food | 78-90 | 30-40 (SD) | ND | 0.6 L/kg | 3-5 | | 60-100 | Yes | ND | |
| **Azoles** | | | | | | | | | | | | |
| Fluconazole | 400-800 mg po/IV | Tab/susp ± food | 90 | 6.7-14 (SD) | 10 | 50 L V/F | 20-50 | | 50-94 | Yes | 140 (8 hr) after 3 mg/kg SD | po: 1-2 |

**Food Effect (po dosing): + food** = take with food, **no food** = take without food, **± food** = take with or without food; **Oral % AB** = % absorbed; **Peak Serum Level: SD** = after single dose, **SS** = steady state after multiple doses; **Volume of Distribution (Vd): V/F** = Vd/oral bioavailability, **Vss** = Vd at steady state, **Vss/F** = Vd at steady state/oral bioavailability; **CSF Penetration:** therapeutic efficacy comment based on dose, usual susceptibility or target organism & penetration into CSF; **24hr** = AUC 0-24; **Tmax** = time to max plasma concentration.

**TABLE 9A (6)** *(Footnotes at the end of table)*

| DRUG | REFERENCE DOSE (SINGLE OR MULTIPLE) | FOOD REC (PO DRUGS)[1] | ORAL ABS (%) | PEAK SERUM CONC[2] (μg/mL) | PROTEIN BINDING (%) | VOLUME OF DISTRIBUTION (Vd)[3] | AVG SERUM T½ (hr)[4] | BILE PEN (%)[5] | CSF/BLOOD[6] (%) | CSF PENETRATION[7] | AUC[a] (μg•hr/mL) | Tmax (hr) |
|---|---|---|---|---|---|---|---|---|---|---|---|---|
| **ANTIFUNGALS** *(continued)* | | | | | | | | | | | | |
| **Azoles** *(continued)* | | | | | | | | | | | | |
| Isavuconazonium sulfate (Isavuconazole) | 372 mg po/IV q24h (maint) | Cap ± food | 98 | 7.5 (SS) | 99 | 450 L Vss | 130 | ND | ND | ND | 121.4 (24 hr) | 2-3 |
| Itraconazole | 200 mg oral soln po q24h | Cap/tab + food, soln no food | 55+ | Itra 2.0, OH-Itra 2.0 (SS) | 99.8 | 796 L | 35 | ND | 0 | | Itra 29.3, OH-Itra 45.2 (24 hr) | Itra 2.5, OH-Itra 5.3 |
| Ketoconazole | 200 mg po | Tab ± food | variable | 3.5 (SD) | 99 | 1.2 L/kg | 8 | ND | <10 | No | 12 | 1-2 |
| Posaconazole oral susp | 400 mg po bid | Susp + food | ND | 0.2-1.0 (200 mg SD) | 98-99 | 226-295 L | 20-66 | ND | ND | Yes (JAC 56:745, 2005) | 9.1 (12 hr) | 3-5 |
| Posaconazole injection | 300 mg IV q24h | - | - | 3.3 (SS) | 98-99 | 226-295 L | 20-66 | ND | ND | Yes (JAC 56:745, 2005) | 36.1 (24 hr) | 1,5 |
| Posaconazole tab | 300 mg tab po q24h | Tab + food | 54 | 2.1-2.9 (SS) | 98-99 | 226-295 L | 20-66 | ND | ND | Yes (JAC 56:745, 2005) | 37.9 (24 hr) | 3-5 |
| Voriconazole | 200 mg IV q12h | Tab/susp no food | 96 | 3 (SS) | 58 | 4.6 L/kg Vss | variable | ND | 22-100 | Yes (CID 37:728, 2003) | 39.8 (24 hr) | 1-2 |
| **Echinocandins** | | | | | | | | | | | | |
| Anidulafungin | 100 mg IV q24h | | | 7.2 (SS) | >99 | 30-50 L | 26.5 | ND | | No | 112 (24 hr) | |
| Caspofungin | 50 mg IV q24h | | | 8.7 (SS) | 97 | 9.7 L Vss | 13 | ND | | No | 87.3 (24 hr) | |
| Micafungin | 100 mg IV q24h | | | 10.1 (SS) | >99 | 0.39 L/kg | 15-17 | | | No | 97 (24 hr) | |
| **ANTIMYCOBACTERIALS** | | | | | | | | | | | | |
| **First line, tuberculosis** | | | | | | | | | | | | |
| Ethambutol | 25 mg/kg po | Tab + food | 80 | 2-6 (SD) | 10-30 | 6 L/kg Vss/F | 4 | ND | 10-50 | No | 29.6 | 2-4 |
| Isoniazid (INH) | 300 mg po | Tab/syrup no food | 100 | 3-5 (SD) | <10 | 0.6-1.2 L/kg | 0.7-4 | ND | up to 90 | Yes | 20,1 | 1-2 |
| Pyrazinamide | 20-25 mg/kg po | Tab ± food | 95 | 30-50 (SD) | 5-10 | 9.7 L Vss | 10-16 | ND | 100 | Yes | 500 | 2 |
| Rifabutin | 300 mg po | Cap + food | 20 | 0.2-0.6 (SD) | 85 | 9.3 L/kg Vss | 32-67 | 300-500 | 30-70 | ND | 4.0 (24 hr) | 2.5-4.0 |
| Rifampin | 600 mg po | Cap no food | 70-90 | 7 (SD) | 80 | 0.65 L/kg Vss | 1.5-5 | 10,000 | 7-56 | ND | 40-60 (24 hr) | 1.5-2 |
| Rifapentine | 600 mg po q72h | Tab + food | ND | 15 (SS) | 98 | 70 L | 13-14 | ND | ND | ND | 320 (72 hr) | 4,8 |
| Streptomycin | 15 mg/kg IM | | | 25-50 (SD) | 0-10 | 0.26 L/kg | 2.5 | 10-60 | 0-30 | No | | |
| **Second line, tuberculosis** | | | | | | | | | | | | |
| Amikacin | 15 mg/kg IM | | | 25-50 (SD) | 0-10 | 0.26 L/kg | 2.5 | 10-60 | 0-30 | No | | |
| Bedaquiline | 400 mg po qd | Tab + food | ND | 3.3 (week 2) | >99 | ≈ 60 x total body water Vss | 24-30 (terminal 4-5 mo) | ND | ≈ 0 | No | 22 (24 hr) after 8 wks | 5 |
| Capreomycin | 1 gm IM | | | 30 (SD) | ND | 0.4 L/kg | 2-5 | ND | <10 | No | ND | 1-2 |
| Cycloserine | 250 mg po | Cap no food | 70-90 | 4-8 (SD) | <20 | 0.47 L/kg | 10 | ND | 54-79 | Yes | 110 | 1-2 |

**Food Effect (po dosing): ± food** = take with food, **no food** = take without food; **+ food** = take with or without food; **‡ food** = take with or without food at multiple doses; **Oral % AB** = % absorbed; **Peak Serum Level: SD** = after single dose, **SS** = steady state after multiple doses; **Volume of Distribution (Vd): V/F** = Vd/oral bioavailability; **Vss** = Vd at steady state; **Vss/F** = Vd at steady state/oral bioavailability; **CSF Penetration:** therapeutic efficacy comment based on dose, usual susceptibility of target organism & penetration into CSF; **AUC** = area under drug concentration curve; **24hr** = AUC 0-24; **Tmax** = time to max plasma concentration.

**TABLE 9A (7)** (Footnotes at the end of table)

| DRUG | REFERENCE DOSE (SINGLE OR MULTIPLE) | FOOD REC (PO DRUGS)[1] | ORAL ABS (%) | PEAK SERUM CONC[2] (µg/mL) | PROTEIN BINDING (%) | VOLUME OF DISTRIBUTION (Vd)[3] | AVG SERUM T½ (hr)[4] | BILE PEN (%)[5] | CSF/ BLOOD[6] (%) | CSF PENETRATION[7] | AUC[8] (µg*hr/mL) | Tmax (hr) |
|---|---|---|---|---|---|---|---|---|---|---|---|---|
| **ANTIMYCOBACTERIALS** *(continued)* | | | | | | | | | | | | |
| *Second line, tuberculosis (continued)* | | | | | | | | | | | | |
| Delamanid | 100 mg po q12h | Tab + food | 25-47 | ND | ≥99.5 | 2100 L V/F | 30-38 | ND | ND | ND | ND | ND |
| Ethionamide | 250 mg po | Tab ± food | near 100 | 2.2 (SD) | 30 | 93.5 L | 1.9 | ND | ≈100 | Yes | 7.7 (250 mg SD) | 1,5 |
| Kanamycin | 15 mg/kg IM | | | 25-50 (SD) | 0-10 | 0.26 L/kg | 2.5 | 10-60 | 0-30 | No | ND | |
| Para-aminosalicylic acid (PAS) | 4 g (granules)po | Granules + food | ND | 9-35 (SD) | 50-60 | 0.9-1.4 L/kg V/F | 0.75-1.0 | 10-60 | 10-50 | Marginal | 108 (4 gm SD, 0-∞) | 8 |
| **ANTIPARASITICS** | | | | | | | | | | | | |
| *Antimalarials* | | | | | | | | | | | | |
| Artemether/ lumefantrine | 4 tabs (80 mg/480 mg) | Tab + food | ND | Art 0.06-0.08, DHA 0.09-0.1, Lum 7.4-9.8 (SD) | Art 95.4, DHA 47-76, Lum 99.7 | ND | Art 1.6-2.2, DHA 1.6-2.2, Lum 101-119 | | | | Art 0.15-0.26, DHA 0.29, Lum 158-243 | Art 1.5-2, Lum 6-8 |
| Artesunate (AS) | 120 mg IV | - | - | DHA 2.4 (SD) | AS 62-75, DHA 66-82 | AS 0.1-0.3, DHA 0.5-1 L/kg | AS 2-4 min, DHA 0.5-1 hr | ND | <1 | No | DHA 2.1 (SD, 0-∞) | 25 min (to DHA) |
| Atovaquone | 750 mg bid | Susp + food | 47 | 24 (SS) | 99.9 | 0.6 L/kg Vss | 67 | ND | ND | ND | 801 (750 mg x1) | ND |
| Chloroquine phosphate | 300 mg base | Tab + food | 90 | 0.06-0.09 (SD) | 55 | 100-1000 L/kg | 45-55 days (terminal) | ND | ND | ND | ND | 1-6 |
| Dihydroartemisinin-piperaquine | Varies by body wt | Tab no food | ND | SD: DHA 0.75, PPQ 0.18 (dose?) | DHA 44-93, PPQ >99 | DHA 0.8 L/kg, PPQ 730 L/kg | DHA 1, PPQ 22 days | ND | ND | ND | SD: DHA 2 (0-∞), PPQ 1.7 (0-24) (dose?) | DHA 1-2, PPQ 5 |
| Mefloquine | 1.25 gm po | Tab + food | ND | 0.5-1.2 (SD) | 98 | 20 L/kg | 13-24 days | ND | ND | ND | 1.2-1.6 | 17 |
| Primaquine | 30 mg (base) po q24h x14 days | Tab + food | ND | 0.18-0.2 | ND | 3 L/kg | 3.7-9.6 | ND | ND | ND | ND | 2-3 |
| Proguanil[11] | 100 mg po | Tab + food | ND | ND | 75 | 1600-2600 L V/F | 12-21 | ND | ND | ND | ND | ND |
| Quinine sulfate | 648 mg po | Cap + food | 76-88 | 3.2 (SD) | 69-92 | 2.5-7.1 L/kg | 9.7-12.5 | ND | 2-7 | No | 28 (12 hr) | 2.8 |
| Tafenoquine | 200 mg po | Tab + food | ND | 0.15 (SD) | >99.5 | 1600-2500 L | 15 days (terminal) | ND | ND | ND | ND | 12-15 |
| **ANTIPARASITICS, Other** | | | | | | | | | | | | |
| Albendazole | 400 mg po | Tab + food | Poor | 0.5-1.6 (sulfoxide) | 70 | approx 260 L (Vss) | 8-12 | ND | ND | ND | ND | 2-5 (sulfoxide) |
| Antimony, pentavalent | 10-20 mg/kg IM/IV | - | - | 7.23-10.5 (10 mg/kg q24h, SS) | ND | ND | elim 2 hr, term 13 days | ND | ND | ND | 65.4 (10 mg/kg q24h) | IM 0.5-2 |
| Benznidazole (Arg) | 100 mg po | Tab + food | 92 | 2.2 | 44 | 39.2 L V/F | 13.3 | ND | ND | ND | 51.3 (0-Inf) | 2.9 |

**Food Effect (po dosing): + food** = take with food, **no food** = take without food; **± food** = take with or without food; **Oral % AB** = % absorbed; **Peak Serum Level: SD** = after single dose, **SS** = steady state after multiple doses; **Volume of Distribution (Vd): V/F** = Vd/oral bioavailability, **Vss** = Vd at steady state, **Vss/F** = Vd at steady state/oral bioavailability; **CSF Penetration:** therapeutic efficacy comment based on dose, usual susceptibility or target organism & penetration into CSF; **AUC** = area under drug concentration curve; **24hr** = AUC 0-24; **Tmax** = time to max plasma concentration.

TABLE 9A (8) *(Footnotes at the end of the table)*

| DRUG | REFERENCE DOSE (SINGLE OR MULTIPLE) | FOOD REC (PO DRUGS)[1] | ORAL ABS (%) | PEAK SERUM CONC[2] (μg/mL) | PROTEIN BINDING (%) | VOLUME OF DISTRIBUTION (Vd)[3] | AVG SERUM T½ (hr)[4] | BILE PEN (%)[5] | CSF/ BLOOD[6] (%) | CSF PENETRATION[7] | AUC[8] (μg·hr/mL) | Tmax (hr) |
|---|---|---|---|---|---|---|---|---|---|---|---|---|
| **ANTIPARASTICS, Other** *(continued)* | | | | | | | | | | | | |
| **Benznidazole (Bra)** | | | | | | | | | | | | |
| Dapsone | 100 mg po q24h | Tab ± food | 70-100 | 1.1 (SS) | 70 | 1.5 L/kg | 10-50 | ND | ND | ND | 52.6 (24 hr) | 2-6 |
| Diethylcarbamazine | 6 mg/kg po | Tab ± food | 80-85 | 1.93 (SD) | ND | 182 L V/F | 9 | ND | ND | ND | 23.8 (0-∞) | 1-2 |
| Ivermectin | 12 mg po | Tab no food | 60 | 0.05-0.08 (SD) | 93 | 3-3.5 L/kg | 20 | ND | ND | No | ND | 4 |
| Mebendazole | 100 mg po | Tab ± food | <10 | Negligible | 90-95 | 1-2 L/kg | 3-6 | ND | ND | ND | ND | 2-4 |
| Miltefosine | 50 mg po tid | Cap + food | ND | 76 (after 23 days) | 95 | 2421 L | 7-31 days | ND | ND | ND | 486 (8hr) | 2-8 |
| Moxidectin | 8 mg po x1 | Tab ± food | ND | 0.06 (SD) | ND | ND | 23 days | ND | ND | ND | 2.7-3.4 (0-∞) | 4 |
| Nitazoxanide | 500 mg po | Tab/susp + food | Susp 70% of tab | Nitazox 9-11, gluc 7.3-10.5 (SD) | Nitazox 99 | ND | Nitazox 1.3-1.8 | ND | | ND | Nitazox 40, gluc 46.5-63.0 | Nitazox, gluc: 1-4 |
| Praziquantel | 20 mg/kg po | Tab + food | 80 | 0.2-2.0 (SD) | 69 | 8000 L V/F | 0.8-1.5 | ND | ND | ND | 1.51 | 1-3 |
| Pentamidine | 4 mg/kg IV/IM q24h | - | - | 0.6 (SD) | | 200-400 L/kg (Vss) | terminal 11-12 days | ND | ND | ND | ND | IM: 1 |
| Pyrimethamine | 25 mg po | Tab ± food | High | 0.1-0.3 (SD) | 87 | 3 L/kg | 96 | ND | ND | ND | 0.75 (3 mg/kg IV SD) | 2-6 |
| Tinidazole | 2 gm po | Tab + food | 48 | 48 (SD) | 12 | 50 L | 13 | ND | ND | ND | 902 | 1.6 |
| **ANTIVIRALS (non-HIV)** | | | | | | | | | | | | |
| **Hepatitis B** | | | | | | | | | | | | |
| Adefovir | 10 mg po | Tab + food | 59 | 0.02 (SD) | ≤4 | 0.37 L/kg Vss | 7.5 | ND | ND | ND | 0.22 | 1.75 |
| Entecavir | 0.5 mg po q24h | Tab/soln no food | 100 | 4.2 ng/mL (SS) | 13 | >0.6 L/kg V/F | 128-149 (terminal) | ND | ND | ND | 0.014 (24 hr) | 0.5-1.5 |
| Telbivudine | 600 mg po q24h | Tab/soln ± food | ND | 3.7 (SS) | 3.3 | >0.6 L/kg V/F | 40-49 | ND | ND | ND | 26.1 (24 hr) | 2 |
| Tenofovir AF (Vemlidy) | 25 mg po q24h | Tab + food | ND | 0.27 (SS) | 80 | ND | 0.51 | ND | ND | ND | 0.27 (24 hr) | 0.48 |
| **Hepatitis C** | | | | | | | | | | | | |
| Daclatasvir | 60 mg po q24h | Tab ± food | 67 | 0.18 (Cmin, SS) | 99 | 47 Vss | 12-15 | ND | ND | ND | 11 (24 hr) | 2 |
| Dasabuvir | 250 mg po q12h | Tab + food | ND | 0.03-3.1 (10-1200 mg SD) | ND | ND | 5-8 | ND | ND | ND | ND | 3 |
| Elbasvir/ Grazoprevir | (Elba 50 + Grazo 100 mg) po q24h | Tab ± food | ND | Elba 0.121, Grazo 0.165 (SS) | Elba >99.9, Grazo >98.8 | ND | Elba 24, Grazo 31 | ND | ND | ND | Elba 1.92, Grazo 1.42 (24 hr) | Elba 3, Grazo 2 |
| Glecaprevir/ Pibrentasvir (Mavyret) | Gle 300 mg + Pib 120 mg q24h | Tab + food | ND | Gle 0.6, Pib 0.11 (SS) | Gle 97.5, Pib >99.9 | ND | Gle 6, Pib 13 | ND | ND | ND | Gle 4.8, Pib 1.43 (24 hr) | Gle 5, Pib 5 |
| Ledipasvir/ Sofosbuvir | 90 mg + Sofos 400 g po q24h | Tab ± food | ND | Ledip: 0.3 (SS) | Ledip: >99.8 | ND | Ledip: 47 | ND | ND | ND | Ledip: 7.3 (24hr) | Ledip: 4-4.5 |

**Food Effect (po dosing): + food** = take with food, **no food** = take without food, **± food** = take with or without food; **Oral % AB** = % absorbed; **Peak Serum Level: SD** = after single dose, **SS** = steady state after multiple doses. **Volume of Distribution (VD): V/F** = Vd/oral bioavailability; **Vss** = Vd at steady state, **Vss/F** = Vd at steady state/oral bioavailability; **CSF Penetration:** therapeutic efficacy comment based on dose, usual susceptibility or target organism & penetration into CSF; **AUC** = area under drug concentration curve; **24hr** = AUC 0-24; **Tmax** = time to max plasma concentration.

TABLE 9A (9) *(Footnotes at the end of table)*

| DRUG | REFERENCE DOSE (SINGLE OR MULTIPLE) | FOOD REC (PO DRUGS) | ORAL ABS (%) | PEAK SERUM CONC² (μg/mL) | VOLUME OF DISTRIBUTION (Vd)³ | PROTEIN BINDING (%) | AVG SERUM T½ (hr)⁴ | BILE PEN (%)⁵ | CSF/BLOOD⁶ (%) | CSF PENETRATION⁷ | AUC⁸ (μg•hr/mL) | Tmax (hr) |
|---|---|---|---|---|---|---|---|---|---|---|---|---|
| **ANTIVIRALS (non-HIV)** *(continued)* | | | | | | | | | | | | |
| **Hepatitis C** *(continued)* | | | | | | | | | | | | |
| Ombitasvir (with Paritaprevir/RTV) | 25 mg po q24h | Tab + food | ND | 0.56 (SS) | ND | ND | 28-34 | ND | ND | ND | 0.53 (24 hr) | 4-5 |
| Paritaprevir/RTV (with Ombitasvir) | 150 mg (+ RTV 100 mg) po q24h | Tab + food | ND | ND | ND | ND | 5.8 | ND | ND | ND | ND | 4,3 |
| Ribavirin | 600 mg po | Tab/cap/soln + food | 64 | 3.7 (SS) | 2825 L V/F | minimal | 44 (terminal 298) | ND | ND | ND | 228 (12 hr) | 2 |
| Simeprevir | 150 mg po | Cap + food | ND | ND | ND | >99.9 | 41 | ND | ND | ND | 57.5 (24 hr) | 4-6 |
| Sofosbuvir | 400 mg po q24h | Tab ± food | ND | Sofos: 0.6 (SS) | ND | Sofos: 61-65 | Sofos: 0.5-0.75 | ND | ND | ND | Sofos: 0.9 (24 hr) | 0.5-2 |
| Velpatasvir/Sofosbuvir | 100 mg (+ Sofos 400 mg) po q24h | Tab ± food | ND | Velpat: 0.26 (SS) | ND | Velpat: >99.5 | Velpat: 15 | ND | ND | ND | Velpat: 2.98 (24 hr) | Velpat: 3 |
| Voxilaprevir/Velpatasvir/Sofosbuvir (Vosevi) | Vox 100 + Vel 100 + Sof 400 mg q24h | Tab + food | ND | Vox 0.19, Vel 0.31, Sof 0.68 (SS) | ND | Vox >99, Vel >99, Sof 61-65 | Vox 33, Vel 17, Sof 0.5 | ND | ND | ND | Vox 2.6, Vel 4.0, Sof 1.7 (24 hr) | Vox 4, Vel 4, Sof 2 |
| **Herpesvirus** | | | | | | | | | | | | |
| Acyclovir | 400 mg po bid | Tab/cap/susp ± food | 10-20 | 1.21 (SS) | 0.7 L/kg | 9-33 | 2.5-3.5 | ND | ND | ND | 7.4 (24 hr) | 1.5-2 |
| Cidofovir (w/probenecid) | 5 mg/kg IV | Probenecid: ± food | | 19.6 (SD) | 0.441 L/kg Vss | <6 | 2.6 (diphosphate: 17-65) | ND | 0 | ND | 40.8 | 1,1 |
| Famciclovir | 500 mg po | Tab ± food | 77 | 3-4 (SD) | 1.1 L/kg (Penciclovir) | <20 | 2-3 (Penciclovir) | ND | ND | ND | 8.9 (Penciclovir) | 0.9 (Penciclovir) |
| Foscarnet | 60 mg/kg IV | | | 155 (SD) | 0.46 L/kg | 4 | 3 (terminal 18-88) | No | | | 2195 μM²•hr | |
| Ganciclovir | 5 mg/kg IV | | | 8.3 (SD) | 0.7 L/kg Vss | 1-2 | 3.5 | ND | ND | ND | 24.5 | 0.75-2.25 |
| Letermovir | 480 mg po/IV q24h | Tab ± food | 35-94 | 13 (po, SS) | 45.5 L Vss | 99 | 12 | ND | ND | ND | 71.5 (po, 24 hr) | |
| Valacyclovir | 1 gm po | Tab ± food | 55 | 5.6 (SD) | 0.7 L/kg | 13-18 | 3 | ND | ND | ND | 19.5 (Acyclovir) | |
| Valganciclovir | 900 mg po q24h | Tab/soln + food | 59 | 5.6 (SS) | 0.7 L/kg | 1-2 | 4 | ND | ND | ND | 29.1 (Ganciclo) | 1-3 (Ganciclo) |
| **Influenza** | | | | | | | | | | | | |
| Baloxavir marboxil (prodrug) | 40 mg po x1 | ND | ND | ND | ND | ND | 96 (baloxavir acid) | ND | ND | ND | ND | 4 (baloxavir acid) |
| Laninamivir (octanoate-prodrug) | 40 mg (prodrug) inhaled x1 | - | - | Lan: 0.024 (SD) | ND | Lan: <0.01 | Lan 64.7; Lan octanoate 1.8 | ND | ND | ND | Lan: 0.745 (0-∞) | Lan: 4 |

**Food Effect (po dosing): + food** = take with food, **± food** = take with or without food, **no food** = take without food. **Oral % AB** = % absorbed; **Peak Serum Level: SD** = after single dose, **SS** = steady state after multiple doses; **Volume of Distribution (Vd): V/F** = Vd/oral bioavailability; **Vss/F** = Vd at steady state, **Vss** = Vd at steady state/oral bioavailability; **CSF Penetration**: therapeutic efficacy comment based on dose, usual susceptibility or target organism & penetration into CSF; **AUC** = area under drug concentration curve; **24hr** = AUC 0-24; **Tmax** = time to max plasma concentration.

**TABLE 9A (10)** *(Footnotes at the end of table)*

| DRUG | REFERENCE DOSE (SINGLE OR MULTIPLE) | FOOD REC (PO DRUGS)¹ | ORAL ABS (%) | PEAK SERUM CONC² (µg/mL) | PROTEIN BINDING (%) | VOLUME OF DISTRIBUTION (Vd)³ | AVG SERUM T½ (hr)⁴ | BILE PEN (%)⁵ | CSF/ BLOOD⁶ (%) | CSF PENETRATION⁷ (%) | AUC⁸ (µg*hr/mL) | Tmax (hr) |
|---|---|---|---|---|---|---|---|---|---|---|---|---|
| **ANTIVIRALS (non-HIV) (continued)** | | | | | | | | | | | | |
| *Influenza (continued)* | | | | | | | | | | | | |
| Oseltamivir | 75 mg po bid | Cap/susp ± food | 75 | carboxylate 0.35 (SS) | 3 | carboxylate 23-26 L | carboxylate 6-10 | | | | carboxylate 5.4 (24 hr) | |
| Peramivir | 600 mg IV | | | 46.8 (SD) | <30 | 12.56 L | 20 | ND | ND | ND | 102.7 (0-∞) | |
| Rimantadine | 100 mg po q12h | Tab ± food | 75-95 | 0.4-0.5 (SS) | 40 | 17-19 L/kg | 25 | ND | ND | ND | 3.5 | 6 |
| **Other non-HIV antivirals** | | | | | | | | | | | | |
| Tecovirimat | 600 mg po q12h | Cap + food | ND | 2.11 (SS) | 77-82 | 1030 L (Vz/F) | 20 | ND | ND | ND | 28.8 (24 hr, SS) | 4-6 |
| **ANTIRETROVIRALS** | | | | | | | | | | | | |
| **NRTIs** | | | | | | | | | | | | |
| Abacavir (ABC) | 600 mg po q24h | Tab/soln ± food | 83 | 4.3 (SS) | 50 | 0.86 L/kg | 1.5 | 20.6 | 3 | 36 | 12 (24 hr) | 1.3 |
| Didanosine enteric coated (ddI) | 400 mg EC po q24h (pt ≥60 kg) | Cap/soln no food | 30-40 | ND | <5 | 308-363 L | 1.6 | 25-40 | 2 | ND | 2,6(24 hr) | 2 |
| Emtricitabine (FTC) | 200 mg po q24h | Cap/soln ± food | cap 93, soln 75 | 1.8 (SS) | <4 | ND | 10 | 39 | 3 | ND | 10 (24 hr) | 1-2 |
| Lamivudine (3TC) | 300 mg po q24h | Tab/soln ± food | 86 | 2.6 (SS) | <36 | 1.3 L/kg | 5-7 | 18 | 2 | ND | 11 (300 mg x1) | ND |
| Stavudine (d4T) | 40 mg po bid (pt ≥60 kg) | Cap/soln ± food | 86 | 0.54 (SS) | <5 | 46 L | 1.2-1.6 | 3,5 | 2 | 20 | 2.6 (24 hr) | 1 |
| Tenofovir alafenamide (TAF) | 25 mg po q24h | Tab ± food | ND | 0.16 (SS) | 80 | ND | 0.51 | ND | ND | ND | 0.21 (24hr) | 1 |
| Tenofovir disoproxil (TDF) | 300 mg po q24h | Tab ± food | 39 w/food | 0.3 (300 mg x1) | <7 | 1.2-1.3 L/kg Vss | 17 | >60 | 1 | ND | 2.3 (300 mg x1) | 1 |
| Zidovudine (ZDV) | 300 mg po bid | Tab/cap/syrup ± food | 60 | 1-2 (300 mg x1) | <38 | 1.6 L/kg | 0.5-3 | 11 | 4 | 2 | 2.1 (300 mg x1) | 0.5-1.5 |
| **NNRTIs** | | | | | | | | | | | | |
| Delavirdine (DLV) | 400 mg po tid | Tab ± food | 85 | 19 (SS) | 98 | ND | 5.8 | ND | 3 | ND | 180 µM*hr (24 hr) | 1 |
| Doravirine (DOR) | 100 mg po qd | Tab ± food | 64 | 0.962 (SS) | 76 | 60.5 L (Vss) | 15 | ND | ND | ND | 16.1 (24 hr) | 2 |
| Efavirenz (EFV) | 600 mg po q24h | Cap/tab no food | 42 | 4.1 (SS) | 99 | 252 L V/F | 40-55 | ND | 3 | ND | 184 µM*hr (24 hr) | 3-5 |
| Etravirine (ETR) | 200 mg po bid | Tab + food | ND | 0.3 (SS) | 99.9 | ND | 41 | ND | 2 | ND | 9 (24 hr) | 2.5-4.0 |
| Nevirapine (NVP) | 200 mg po bid | Tab/susp ± food | >90 | 2 (200 mg x1) | 60 | 1.21 L/kg Vss | 25-30 | ND | 4 | 63 | 110 (24 hr) | 4 |
| Rilpivirine (RPV) | 25 mg po qd | Tab + food | ND | 0.1-0.2 (25 mg x1) | 99.7 | 152 L | 45-50 | ND | ND | ND | 2.4 (24 hr) | 4-5 |

**Food Effect (po dosing): + food** = take with food, **no food** = take without food, **± food** = take with or without food; **Oral % AB** = % absorbed; **Peak Serum Level: SD** = after single dose, **SS** = steady state after multiple doses; **Volume of Distribution (Vd): V/F** = Vd/oral bioavailability; **Vss** = Vd at steady state, **Vss/F** = Vd at steady state/oral bioavailability; **AUC** = area under drug concentration curve; **24hr** = AUC 0-24; **Tmax** = time to max plasma concentration. **Bile Penetration** and penetration into CSF: **V/F** = Vd/oral bioavailability; **CSF Penetration:** therapeutic efficacy comment based on dose, usual susceptibility or target organism & penetration into CSF; **CSF/ Blood** = Vd at steady state.

**TABLE 9A (11)** *(Footnotes at the end of table)*

| DRUG | REFERENCE DOSE (SINGLE OR MULTIPLE) | FOOD REC (PO DRUGS)¹ | ORAL ABS (%) | PEAK SERUM CONC² (µg/mL) | PROTEIN BINDING (%) | VOLUME OF DISTRIBUTION (Vd)³ | AVG SERUM T½ (hr)⁴ | BILE PEN (%)⁵ | CSF/ BLOOD⁶ (%) | CSF PENETRATION⁷ | AUC⁸ (µg*hr/mL) | Tmax (hr) |
|---|---|---|---|---|---|---|---|---|---|---|---|---|
| **ANTIRETROVIRALS** *(continued)* | | | | | | | | | | | | |
| **PIs** | | | | | | | | | | | | |
| Atazanavir (ATV) | 400 mg po q24h | Cap/powder + food | Good | 2.3 (SS) | 86 | 88.3 L V/F | 7 | ND | 2 | ND | 22.3 (24 hr) | 2,5 |
| Cobicistat | 150 mg po q24h | Take with food | ND | 0.99 (SS) | 97-98 | ND | 4-Mar | ND | ND | ND | 7.6 (24 hr) | 3.5 |
| Darunavir (DRV) | 600 mg (+ RTV 100 mg) po bid | Tab/susp + food | 82 | 3.5 (SS) | 95 | 2 L/kg | 15 | ND | 3 | ND | 116.8 (24 hr) | 2.5-4.0 |
| Fosamprenavir (FPV) | 700 mg (+RTV 100 mg) po bid | Tab ± food; susp: adult no, peds + | ND | 6 (SS) | 90 | ND | 7,7 | ND | 3 | ND | 79.2 (24 hr) | 2,5 |
| Indinavir (IDV) | 800 mg (+ RTV 100 mg) po bid | Boosted cap + food | 65 | 20.2 µM (SS) | 60 | ND | 1.2-2.0 | ND | 4 | 11 | 249 µM*hr (24 hr) | 0,8 (fasting) |
| Lopinavir/RTV (LPV/r) | 400 mg/100 mg po bid | Tab ± food, soln + food | ND | 9.6 (SS) | 98-99 | ND | LPV 5-6 | ND | 3 | ND | LPV 186 (24 hr) | LPV 4 |
| Nelfinavir (NFV) | 1250 mg po bid | Tab/powder + food | 20-80 | 3-4 (SS) | 98 | 2-7 L/kg V/F | 3.5-5 | ND | 1 | 0 | 53 (24 hr) | ND |
| Ritonavir (RTV) | Boosting dose varies | Cap/powder + food | 65 | 11.2 (600 mg bid SS) | 98-99 | 0.41 L/kg V/F | 3-5 | ND | 1 | ND | 121.7 (600 mg soln SD) | soln 2-4 |
| Saquinavir (SQV) | 1 gm (+RTV 100 mg) po bid | Tab/cap + food | 4 (SQV alone) | 0.37 (SS) | 97 | 700 L Vss | 1-2 | ND | 1 | ND | 29.2 (24 hr) | ND |
| Tipranavir (TPV) | 500 mg (+RTV 200 mg) po bid | Cap/soln + food | Low | 47-57 (SS) | 99,9 | 7.7-10 L | 5.5-6 | ND | 1 | ND | 1600 µM*hr (24 hr) | 3 |
| **INSTIs** | | | | | | | | | | | | |
| Bictegravir (BIC) | 50 mg po q24h (as Biktarvy) | Tab ± food | ND | 6.15 (SS) | >99 | ND | 17,3 | ND | ND | ND | 102 (24 hr) | 2-4 |
| Dolutegravir (DTG) | 50 mg po q24h | Tab ± food | ND | 3.67 (SS) | >99 | 17.4 L V/F | 14 | ND | 4 | ND | 53.6 (24 hr) | 2-3 |
| Elvitegravir (EVG) | 85-150 mg po q24h | Tab + food | ND | 1.2-1.5 (SS) | 98-99 | ND | 8.7 (w/RTV) | ND | ND | ND | 18 (24 hr) | 4 |
| Raltegravir (RAL) | 400 mg po bid | Tab/susp ± food | ND | 11.2 µM (SS) | 83 | 287 L Vss/F | 9 | ND | 3 | 1-53.5 | 28.7 µM*hr (12 hr) | 3 |
| **Fusion, Entry Inhibitors** | | | | | | | | | | | | |
| Enfuvirtide (ENF, T20) | 90 mg sc bid | | 84 (sc %ab) | 5 (SS) | 92 | 5.5 L Vss | 3,8 | ND | 1 | ND | 97.4 (24 hr) | 4-8 |
| Maraviroc (MVC) | 300 mg po bid | Tab ± food | 33 | 0.3-0.9 (SS) | 76 | 194 L | 14-18 | ND | 3 | ND | 3 (24 hr) | 0.5-4.0 |
| **Monoclonal Antibodies** | | | | | | | | | | | | |
| Ibalizumab-uiyk | 2 gm IV load, then 800 mg IV q2 weeks | ND | ND | ND | ND | 4.8 L | Dose-dependent depending on dose (2.7-64 depending on dose) | ND | ND | ND | ND | ND |

**Food Effect (po dosing): + food** = take with food, **no food** = take without food, **± food** = take with or without food. **Oral % AB** = % absorbed; **Peak Serum Level: SD** = after single dose, **SS** = steady state after multiple doses; **Volume of Distribution (Vd): V/F** = Vd/oral bioavailability, **Vss/F** = Vd at steady state/oral bioavailability, **Vss** = Vd at steady state, **Vss/F** = Vd steady state/oral bioavailability; **CSF Penetration**: therapeutic efficacy comment based on dose, usual susceptibility or target organism & penetration into CSF; **24hr** = AUC 0-24; **AUC** = area under drug concentration curve; **Tmax** = time to max plasma concentration.

## TABLE 9A (12) (Footnotes at the end of table)

1 Refers to adult oral preparations unless otherwise noted; + food = take with food, no food = take without food, ± food = take with or without food
2 SD = after a single dose, SS = at steady state
3 V/F = Vd/oral bioavailability, Vss = Vd at steady state; Vss/F = Vd at steady state/oral bioavailability
4 Assumes CrCl >80 mL/min
5 (Peak concentration in serum) x 100. If blank, no data
6 CSF concentrations with inflammation
7 Judgment based on drug dose and organism susceptibility, CSF concentration ideally ≥10x MIC.
8 AUC = area under serum concentration vs. time curve; 12 hr = AUC 0-12, 24 hr = AUC 0-24
9 Concern over seizure potential (see Table 10B)
10 Take all FQs 2-4 hours before sucralfate or any multivalent cation (calcium, iron, zinc)
11 Given with Atovaquone as Malarone for malaria prophylaxis

## TABLE 9B – PHARMACODYNAMICS OF ANTIBACTERIALS*

| BACTERIAL KILLING/PERSISTENT EFFECT | DRUGS | THERAPY GOAL | PK/PD MEASUREMENT |
|---|---|---|---|
| Concentration-dependent/Prolonged persistent effect | Aminoglycosides; daptomycin; ketolides; quinolones; metro | High peak serum concentration | 24-hr AUC/MIC |
| Time-dependent/No persistent effect | Penicillins; cephalosporins; carbapenems; monobactams | Long duration of exposure | Time above MIC |
| Time-dependent/Moderate to long persistent effect | Clindamycin; erythro/azithro/clarithro; linezolid; tetracyclines; vancomycin | Enhanced amount of drug | 24-hr AUC/MIC |

* Adapted from Craig, WA: IDC No. Amer 17:479, 2003 & Drusano, G.L.: CID 44:79, 2007

## TABLE 9C – ENZYME -AND TRANSPORTER- MEDIATED INTERACTIONS OF ANTIMICROBIALS

>50% of all drugs are metabolized by one or more members of the CYP450 enzyme system. The metabolism of a drug that is a substrate of a particular CYP enzyme may be induced (accelerated) by another drug, resulting in under dosing and therapeutic failure. Conversely the metabolism of a drug may be inhibited (slowed) by another drug, resulting in overdosing and toxicity. A drug may act as substrate for more than one enzyme, or it may inhibit or induce multiple enzymes. Inhibition tends to be a relatively quick process related to the dose of the inhibitor, whereas induction occurs more slowly. Risk is amplified when two or more drugs that are enzyme inhibitors or inducers are administered. CYP450 enzymes commonly involved in drug interactions include CYP3A4, CYP2C9/19, CYP1A2, and CYP2D6.

Drug transporter systems may also be involved in drug interactions. Transporters are found in many tissues, such as the kidney and GI tract, and they work to pump drugs into cells (influx) or out of cells (efflux). Examples of important drug transporters systems include P-glycoprotein (PGP), organic anion transporter (OAT), and organic cation transporter (OCT).

Knowledge of these enzymes is useful in understanding clinically relevant drug interactions and can also assist in predicting previously unrecognized interactions. With respect to specific antimicrobials, always check for drug-drug interactions when ordering these inhibitors that may cause elevated serum concentrations: macrolides; ciprofloxacin, metronidazole, TMP-SMX, isoniazid, azole antifungals, antiretrovirals, and anti-HCV drugs. Nafcillin, rifampins, rifapentine, and certain antiretrovirals are known to induce metabolism and lead to treatment failure. If a drug interaction is recognized and no suitable alternative regimen exists, check serum concentration of the affected drug (if available), adjust dose, and monitor for toxicity. See Table 22A for common drug-drug interactions.

| DRUG | ISOZYME/TRANSPORTER THAT DRUG IS A SUBSTRATE OF | INHIBITED BY DRUG | INDUCED BY DRUG | IMPACT ON SERUM DRUG CONCENTRATIONS* |
|---|---|---|---|---|
| **Antibacterials** | | | | |
| Azithromycin | PGP | PGP (weak) | | mild ↑ |
| Cephalexin | MATE1 | | | No effect expected |
| Chloramphenicol | | 2C19, 3A4 | | ↑ |
| Ciprofloxacin | | 1A2; 3A4 (minor) | | ↑ |
| Clarithromycin | 3A4 | 3A4, PGP, OAT | | ↑ |
| Clindamycin | 3A4 | 3A4 | | No effect expected |

**TABLE 9C (2)**

| DRUG | Substrate | Inhibits | Induces | Impact |
|---|---|---|---|---|
| **Antibacterials** *(continued)* | | | | |
| Eravacycline | 3A4 | 3A4, PGP, OAT | | No effect expected |
| Erythromycin | 3A4, PGP | | 3A4? | ↑ |
| Flucloxacillin | | | | ↓ |
| Fusidic acid | 3A4 | 3A4, BCRP, OATP1B1 | | ↑ |
| Levofloxacin | | OCT | | ↑ |
| Meropenem | OAT1, OAT3 | | | No effect expected |
| Metronidazole | | 2C9 | | ↑ |
| Nafcillin | | | 2C9 (?), 3A4 | ↓ |
| Norfloxacin | | 1A2 (weak) | | mild ↑ |
| Omadacycline | PGP | | | No effect expected |
| Oritavancin | | 2C9 (weak), 2C19 (weak) | 2D6 (weak), 3A4 (weak) | mild ↑ or ↓ |
| Plazomicin | | MATE1, MATE2-K | | ↑ |
| Pristinamycin | | 3A4 | | ↑ |
| Quinupristin-Dalfopristin | | 3A4 | | ↓ |
| Rifampin | PGP, OATP1B1 | OAT, OATP1B1 | 1A2, 2B6, 2C8, 2C9, 2C19, 2D6 (weak), 3A4, PGP | ↓ |
| Rifaximin | 3A4, PGP, OAT1A2, OATP1B1/3 | PGP | | No effect expected |
| Sarecycline | | PGP | | |
| Telithromycin | | 3A4, PGP (?) | | ↑ |
| Tigecycline | PGP | | | No effect expected |
| TMP/SMX | SMX: 2C9 (major), 3A4 | TMP: 2C8; SMX: 2C9 | | ↑ |
| Trimethoprim | | 2C8 | | ↑ |
| **Antifungals** | | | | |
| Fluconazole | | 2C9, 2C19, 3A4 | | ↑ |
| Isavuconazole | 3A4 | 3A4, PGP, OCT2 | | ↑ |
| Itraconazole | 3A4 | 3A4, PGP | | ↑ |
| Ketoconazole | 3A4 | 3A4, PGP | | ↑ |
| Posaconazole | PGP | 3A4, PGP | | ↑ |
| Terbinafine | | 2D6 | | ↑ |
| Voriconazole | 2C9, 2C19, 3A4 | 2C9, 2C19, 3A4 | | ↑ |
| **Antimycobacterials (Rifampin listed above)** | | | | |
| Bedaquiline | 3A4 | | | No effect expected |
| Delamanid | 3A4 | | | No effect expected |
| Isoniazid (INH) | 2E1 | 2C19, 3A4 | | ↑ |
| Rifabutin | 3A4 | | 3A4 | ↓ |
| Rifapentine | | | 2C9, 3A4 | ↓ |
| Thalidomide | 2C19 | | | No effect expected |

TABLE 9C (3)

| DRUG | Substrate | Inhibits | Induces | Impact |
|---|---|---|---|---|
| **Antiparasitics** | | | | |
| Artemether/Lumefantrine | 3A4 (Art, Lum) | 2D6 (Lum) | 3A4 (Art) | ↑ or ↓ |
| Chloroquine | 2C8, 2D6 | 2D6 | | ↑ |
| Dapsone | 3A4 | | | No effect expected |
| Halofantrine | 3A4 | 2D6 | | ↑ |
| Mefloquine | 3A4, PGP | PGP | | ↑ |
| Praziquantel | 3A4 | | | No effect expected |
| Primaquine | 2D6, others? | | | No effect expected |
| Proguanil | 2C19 (→cycloguanil) | | | No effect expected |
| Quinine sulfate | main 3A4, also 1A2, 2C9, 2D6 | 2D6 | | ↑ |
| Tafenoquine | | OCT, MATE1, MATE2K | | No effect expected |
| Tinidazole | 3A4 | | | |
| **Antivirals (Hepatitis C)** | | | | |
| Daclatasvir | 3A4, PGP | 2C8, UGT1A1, OATP1B1, OATP1B3 | | ↑ |
| Dasabuvir | 3A4, PGP, OATP1B1 | BCRP | | ↑ |
| Elbasvir | CYP3A4, PGP | 3A4 (weak), PGP, BCRP, OATP1A1 (weak) | | ↑ |
| Glecaprevir | PGP, BCRP, OATP1/3 | 1A2 (weak), 3A4 (weak), PGP, BCRP, OATP1B1/3, UGT1A1 (weak) | | ↑ |
| Grazoprevir | CYP3A4, PGP, OATP1B1/3 | CYP3A4 (weak), BCRP | | |
| Ledipasvir | PGP, BCRP | PGP, BCRP | | ↑ |
| Ombitasvir | 3A4, PGP | 2C8, UGT1A1 | | ↑ |
| Paritaprevir | 2C8, 2D6, 3A4, PGP | UGT1A1, OATP1B1 | | ↑ |
| Pibrentasvir | PGP, BCRP | 1A2 (weak), 3A4 (weak), PGP, BCRP, OATP1B1/3, UGT1A1 (weak) | | ↑ |
| Simeprevir | 3A4, PGP, OAT | 1A2 (weak), 3A4, PGP, OAT | | ↑ |
| Sofosbuvir | PGP, BCRP | | | No effect expected |
| Velpatasvir | 2B6, 2C8, 3A4, PGP, BCRP, OATP1B1/3 | PGP, BCRP, OATP1B1/3, OATP2B1 | | ↑ |
| **Antivirals (Herpesvirus)** | | | | |
| Cidofovir | OAT1, OAT3 | | | No effect expected |
| Letermovir | 2D6, 3A4, OATP1B1/3 | 2C8, 3A4, OATP1B1/3 | 2C9, 2C19, 3A4 | ↑ or ↓ |
| **Antivirals (miscellaneous)** | | | | |
| Tecovirimat | UGT1A1, 1A4 | 2C8 (weak), 2C19 (weak), BCRP (weak) | 3A4 (weak) | ↑ or ↓ |
| **Antiretrovirals** | | | | |
| Atazanavir | 3A4, PGP | 1A2, 2C8, 3A4, UGT1A1 | | ↑ |
| Bictegravir (BIC) | 3A4, UGT1A1 | OCT2, MATE1 | | ↑ |
| Cobicistat (part of Stribild) | 2D6, 3A4 | 2D6, 3A4, PGP, BCRP, OATP1B1, OATP1B3 | | ↑ |
| Darunavir | 3A4 | 3A4 | | ↑ |

**TABLE 9C (4)**

| DRUG | Substrate | Inhibits | Induces | Impact |
|---|---|---|---|---|
| **Antiretrovirals** (continued) | | | | |
| Delavirdine | 2D6, 3A4 | 2C9, 2C19, 3A4 | | ↑ |
| Dolutegravir | 3A4, UGT1A1 | | | ↑ |
| Doravirine | 3A4 | | | No effect expected |
| Efavirenz | 2B6, 3A4 | 2B6, 2C9, 2C19 | 2C19, 3A4 | ↑ or ↓ |
| Elvitegravir (part of Stribild) | CYP3A4, UGT1A1/3 | PGP (weak) | 2C9 (weak) | mild ↑ or ↓ |
| Etravirine | 2C9, 2C19, 3A4 | 2C9, 2C19 (weak) | 3A4 | ↑ or ↓ |
| Fosamprenavir | 3A4 | 3A4 | | ↑ |
| Indinavir | 3A4, PGP | 3A4, PGP | | ↑ |
| Lamivudine | PGP, BCRP, MATE1, MATE2-K, OCT2 | | | No effect expected |
| Lopinavir | 3A4 | 3A4 | | ↑ |
| Maraviroc | 3A4, PGP | 2D6 | | ↑ |
| Nelfinavir | 2C19, 3A4, PGP | 3A4, PGP | 3A4 (?) | ↑ or ↓ |
| Nevirapine | 2B6, 3A4 | | 3A4 | ↓ |
| Raltegravir | UGT | | | No effect expected |
| Rilpivirine | 3A4 | | | No effect expected |
| Ritonavir | 3A4, PGP | 2D6, 3A4, PGP | 1A2, 2B6, 2C9, 3A4 (long term), PGP (long term), UGT | ↑ or ↓ |
| Saquinavir | 3A4, PGP | 3A4, PGP | | ↑ |
| Tenofovir alafenamide | PGP, BCRP, OATP1B/3 | | | No effect expected |
| Tenofovir disoproxil fum | PGP, BCRP | | | No effect expected |
| Tipranavir | 3A4, PGP | OAT | PGP (weak) | ↑ or ↓ |

*Refers to serum concentrations of companion drugs that may be affected by the listed antimicrobial. ↑=increase, ↓=decrease, blank=no drugs should be affected

**TERMINOLOGY:**
BCRP = breast cancer resistance protein
CYP450 nomenclature, e.g. 3A4: 3 = family, A = subfamily, 4 = gene
OAT = organic anion transporter
OATP = organic anion transporter polypeptide

OCT = organic cation transporter
PGP = P-glycoprotein
UGT = uridine diphosphate glucuronosyltransferase

**REFERENCES:**
Hansten PD, Horn JR. The Top 100 Drug Interactions: A Guide to Patient Management. Freeland (WA): H&H Publications, 2014; primary literature; package inserts.

## TABLE 10A – ANTIBIOTIC DOSAGE* AND SIDE-EFFECTS

| CLASS, AGENT, GENERIC NAME (TRADE NAME) | USUAL ADULT DOSAGE* | ADVERSE REACTIONS, COMMENTS (See Table 10B for Summary) |
|---|---|---|
| **NATURAL PENICILLINS** | | **Allergic reactions a major issue.** 10% of all hospital admissions give history of pen allergy; but only 10% have allergic reaction if given penicillin. Why? Possible reasons: inaccurate history, waning of immunity with age, aberrant response during viral illness. If given, **Bicillin L-A (Pen)** then observe for 20-30 min for allergic reaction to procaine. **Most serious reaction is immediate IgE-mediated anaphylaxis;** incidence only 0.05% but 5-10% fatal. Other IgE-mediated reactions: urticaria, angioedema, laryngeal edema, bronchospasm, abdominal pain with emesis, or hypotension. All appear within 4 hrs. Can form IgE antibody against either the beta-lactam ring or the R-group side chain. **Morbilliform rash after 72 hrs is not IgE-mediated and not serious.** |
| Benzathine penicillin G (Bicillin L-A) | 600,000–1.2 million units IM q2-4 wks | |
| Penicillin G | Low: 600,000–1.2 million units IM per day<br><br>High: ≥20 million units IV q24h(=12 gm) div q4h. | **Serious late allergic reactions:** Coombs-positive hemolytic anemia, neutropenia, thrombocytopenia, serum sickness, interstitial nephritis, hepatitis, eosinophilia, drug fever. |
| Penicillin V (250 & 500 mg caps) | 0.25–0.5 gm po bid, tid, qid before meals & at bedtime. Pen V preferred over Pen G for oral therapy due to greater acid stability. | **Cross-allergy to cephalosporins and carbapenems** varies from 0-11%. One factor is similarity, or lack of similarity, of side chains.<br>**For pen desensitization,** see Table 7. For skin testing, suggest referral to allergist.<br>High **CSF** concentrations cause seizures. Reduce dosage with renal impairment, see Table 17A.<br>Allergy refs: CID 55:1113, 2014; JAC 69:20-43, 2014; CID 58:1140, 2014. |
| **PENICILLINASE-RESISTANT PENICILLINS** | | |
| Dicloxacillin (Dynapen) (250 & 500 mg caps) | 0.125–0.5 gm po q6h before meals | Blood levels ~2 times greater than cloxacillin so preferred for po therapy. Hemorrhagic cystitis reported. |
| Flucloxacillin[NUS] (Floxapen, Lutropin, Staphcil) | 0.25–0.5 gm po q6h<br>1-2 gm IV q4h | Acute abdominal pain with GI bleeding without antibiotic-associated colitis also reported. Can impede warfarin. Cholestatic hepatitis occurs in 1/15,000 exposures. In age >55 yrs, females and therapy >2 wks duration. Can appear wks after end of therapy and take wks to resolve (JAC 66:1431, 2011). **Recommendation: use only in severe infection.** |
| Nafcillin (Unipen, Nafcil) | 1-2 gm IV/IM q4h. Due to >90% protein binding, need 12 gm/day for bacteremia. | Extravasation can result in tissue necrosis. With 200–300 mg per kg per day hypokalemia may occur. **Reversible neutropenia (over 10% with ≥21-day rx), occasionally WBC <1000 per day.** Can impede warfarin effect. |
| Oxacillin (Prostaphlin) | 1-2 gm IV/IM q4h. Due to >90% protein binding, need 12 gm/day for bacteremia. | **Hepatic dysfunction with ≥12 gm total day.** LFTs usually ↑ 24 days after start rx, reversible. In children, more rash and liver toxicity with oxacillin as compared to nafcillin (CID 34:50, 2002). |
| **AMINOPENICILLINS** | | |
| Amoxicillin (Amoxil, Polymox) | 250 mg-1 gm po tid | IV available in UK & Europe. IV amoxicillin rapidly converted to ampicillin. Rash with infectious mono—see Ampicillin. |
| Amoxicillin extended release (Moxatag) | One 775 mg tab po once daily | Increased risk of cross-allergenicity with oral cephalosporins with identical side-chains: cefadroxil, cefprozil. Allergic reactions, C. difficile associated diarrhea, false positive test for urine glucose with clinitest. |
| Amoxicillin-clavulanate (Augmentin)<br>AM-CL extra-strength peds suspension (ES-600)<br>AM-CL-ER—extended release adult tabs | See Comment for adult products<br>Peds Extra-Strength susp: 600/42.9 per 5 mL<br>Dose: 90/6.4 mg/kg div bid.<br>For adult formulations, see Comments<br>IV amox-clav available in Europe | With bid regimen, less clavulanate & less diarrhea. In pts with immediate allergic reaction to AM-CL, ⅓ due to Clav component (J Allergy Clin Immunol 125:502, 2010). **Hepatotoxicity linked to clavulanic acid; AM-CL causes 13-23% of drug-induced liver injury.** Onset delayed (avg 4 wks) (JAC 66:1431, 2011).<br>**Comparison adult Augmentin dosage regimens:**<br>  Augmentin      500/125      1 tab po tid<br>  Augmentin      875/125      1 tab po bid<br>  Augmentin      1000/125    1 tab po bid<br>  Augmentin-XR  1000/62.5   2 tabs po bid |
| Ampicillin (Principen) (250 & 500 mg caps) | 0.25–0.5 gm po q6h.<br>50-200 mg/kg IV/day. | A maculopapular rash occurs (not urticarial), **not true penicillin allergy,** in 65-100% pts with infectious mono, 90% with chronic lymphocytic leukemia, and 15-20% in pts taking allopurinol. Increased risk of true cross-allergenicity with oral cephalosporins with identical side chains: cefaclor, cephalexin, loracarbef. |

*NOTE: all dosage recommendations are for adults (unless otherwise indicated) & assume normal renal function.
(See page 2 for abbreviations)

**TABLE 10A (2)**

| CLASS, AGENT, GENERIC NAME (TRADE NAME) | USUAL ADULT DOSAGE* | ADVERSE REACTIONS, COMMENTS (See Table 10B for Summary) |
|---|---|---|
| **AMINOPENICILLINS** (continued) | | |
| Ampicillin-sulbactam (Unasyn) | 1.5-3 gm IV q6h. **For resistant Acinetobacter, 8 gm Amp/4 gm sulb IV over 4 hr q8h in combination with Meropenem and Polymyxin B.** | Supplied in vials: amp 2 gm, sulbactam 1 gm. Adjust dose for renal insufficiency, see Table 17A. For combination regimen dosing (Amp-sulb + MER + Polymyxin B), see Table 17, page 43. |
| **ANTIPSEUDOMONAL PENICILLINS** | | |
| Piperacillin-tazobactam (PIP-TZ) (Zosyn) *Prolonged infusion dosing, see Comment and Table 10E. Obesity dosing, see Table 17C.* | **Favor prolonged infusion:** load with 4.5 gm IV over 30 min, then 4 hrs later start 3.375 gm IV over 4 hrs & repeat q8h. Ties up IV line for 12 of 24 hrs. Old dose (except P. aeruginosa): 3.375 gm IV q6h or 4.5 gm q8h. Old P. aeruginosa dose: 3.375 gm q4h or 4.5 gm q6h. | Prolonged infusion references (CID 44:357, 2007; AAC 54:460, 2010). • Cystic fibrosis + P. aeruginosa infection: 350-450 mg/kg/day div q4-6h. For obesity dosing adjustment see Table 17C, page 250. Documented drug-induced thrombocytopenia (J Thromb Haemostasis 10:1069, 2012). Retrospective cohort review associated significantly greater risk of nephrotoxicity from PIP/TZ + Vancomycin compared with Cefepime + Vancomycin (AAC e1-e02099-16, 2017; CID 64: 116, 2017). |
| Temocillin^NUS | 2 gm IV q12h. | Semi-synthetic penicillin stable in presence of classical & ESBLs plus AmpC beta-lactamases. Source: www.eumedica.be |
| **CARBAPENEMS.** Review: AAC 55:4943, 2011. **NOTE: Cross allergenicity: In studies of pts with history of Pen-allergy but no confirmatory skin testing, 0-11% had allergic reactions with cephalosporin therapy** (JAC 54:1155, 2004). **In better studies, pts with positive skin tests for Pen allergy were given Carbapenem: no reaction in 9%** (J Allergy Clin Immunol 124:167, 2009). Of 12 pts with IgE-mediated reaction to ceph, 2 suffered rash & 1 an IgE reaction when given a carbapenem (CID 59:1113, 2014). Incidence of carbapenem-resistant GNB highest in Georgia, Maryland & New York (JAMA 314:1455 & 1479, 2015). | | |
| Doripenem (Doribax) Ref: CID 49:291, 2009. For prolonged infusion dosing, see Table 10E. | Intra-abdominal & complicated UTI: **500 mg IV q8h (1-hr infusion).** For prolonged infusion, see Table 10E, page 129. Do not use for pneumonia | Most common adverse reactions (≥5%): Headache, nausea, diarrhea, rash & phlebitis. Seizure reported in post-marketing surveillance. Can lower serum valproic acid levels. Adjust dose if renal impairment. Somewhat more stable in solution than **IMP** or **MER** (JAC 65:1023, 2010; CID 49:291, 2009). FDA safety announcement (01/05/12): Trial of DORI for the treatment of VAP stopped early due to safety concerns. Compared to IMP, patients receiving DORI were observed to have excess mortality and poorer cure rate. **NOTE: DORI is not approved to treat any type of pneumonia; DORI is not approved for doses greater than 500 mg q8h.** |
| Ertapenem (Invanz) | 1 gm IV/IM q24h. | Lidocaine diluent for IM use; ask about lidocaine allergy. Standard dosage may be inadequate in obesity (BMI ≥40). Reports of DRESS (drug rash eosinophilia systemic symptoms) Syndrome. Visual hallucinations reported (NZ Med J 122:76, 2009). No predictable activity vs. P. aeruginosa. |
| Imipenem + cilastatin (Primaxin) Ref: JAC 58:916, 2006 | 0.5 gm IV q6h: for P. aeruginosa: 1 gm q6-8h (See Comment). | For P. aeruginosa, increase dosage to 3 or 4 gm per day div, q8h or q6h. Continuous infusion of carbapenems more efficacious & safer (AAC 49:1881, 2005). **Seizures:** risk of seizures due to but greatest with carbapenems. No diff between IMP and MER (AAC 69:2043, 2014). Cilastatin blocks enzymatic degradation of imipenem in lumen of renal proximal tubule. Compared to other toxicities, seizure greatest with IMP, more in vitro resistance to IMP vs. Proteus sps, Providencia sps, Morganella sps, Acinetobacter sps. Compared to MER (Clin Micro Infect 10:147, 2004). |
| Meropenem (Merrem) | **0.5-1 gm IV q8h. Up to 2 gm IV q8h for meningitis. Prolonged infusion** in critically ill: If CrCl ≥50: 2 gm (over 3 hr) q8h If CrCl 30-49: 1 gm (over 3 hr) q8h If CrCl 10-29: 1 gm (over 3 hr) q12h (Inten Care Med 37:632, 2011) | **Seizures:** In meta-analysis, risk of seizures lowest with carbapenems among beta-lactams. No diff between IMP and MER (AAC 69:2043, 2014). Comments: Does not require a dehydropeptidase inhibitor (cilastatin). Activity vs aerobic gm-neg. slightly ↑ over IMP, activity vs staph & strep slightly ↓, anaerobes: B. ovatus, B. distasonis more resistant to meropenem. |
| Meropenem-vaborbactam (Vabomere) | 4 gm (2 gm meropenem + 2 gm vaborbactam) IV q8h infused over 3 hrs (with estimated eGFR >50 mL/min). | Combination of Meropenem with vaborbactam. Vaborbactam inhibits common serine beta-lactamases, ESBLs, KPCs, and AmpC but not metallo-beta-lactamases or oxacillinases with carbapenemase activity. Approved for the the treatment of complicated urinary tract infections in patients age ≥18 years caused by E. coli, K. pneumoniae, E. cloacae, and other susceptible aerobic gram-negative bacilli. **Contraindicated:** if known hypersensitivity to meropenem or beta lactams. **AEs:** hypersensitivity reactions, seizure potential, C. diff-associated diarrhea, thrombocytopenia, neuromotor impairment, phlebitis (infusion site), diarrhea, headache. **Major interactions:** valproic acid (concomitant use not recommended), probenecid. |

*NOTE: all dosage recommendations are for adults (unless otherwise indicated) & assume normal renal function.

(See page 2 for abbreviations)

TABLE 10A (3)

| CLASS, AGENT, GENERIC NAME (TRADE NAME) | USUAL ADULT DOSAGE[a] | ADVERSE REACTIONS, COMMENTS (See Table 10B for Summary) |
|---|---|---|
| **MONOBACTAMS** | | |
| Aztreonam (Azactam) | 1 gm q8h–2 gm IV q6h. | Can be used in pts with allergy to penicillins/cephalosporins with exception of Ceftazidime as **side-chains of Aztreonam and Ceftazidime are identical.** PK/PD (JAC 2016;71:2704). |
| Aztreonam for Inhalation (Cayston) | **75 mg inhaled tid x 28 days.** Use bronchodilator before each inhalation. | Improves respiratory symptoms in CF pts colonized with P. aeruginosa. Alternative to inhaled Tobra. AEs: bronchospasm, cough, wheezing. So far, no emergence of other resistant pathogens. Ref: Chest 135:1223, 2009. |
| **CEPHALOSPORINS (1st parenteral, then oral drugs). NOTE:** Prospective data demonstrate correlation between use of cephalosporins (esp. 3ʳᵈ generation) and ↑ risk of C. difficile toxin-induced diarrhea. May also ↑ risk of colonization with vancomycin-resistant enterococci. See Oral Cephalosporins, page 116, for important note on cross-allergenicity. | | |
| **1ˢᵗ Generation, Parenteral** | | |
| Cefazolin (Ancef, Kefzol) | **1–1.5 gm IV/IM q8h, occasionally 2 gm IV q8h for serious infections, e.g., MSSA bacteremia (max. 12 gm/day)** | **Do not give into lateral ventricles—seizures!** No activity vs. MRSA. Very low risk of cross-allergenicity with other cephalosporins or beta-lactams. |
| **2ⁿᵈ Generation, Parenteral (Cephamycins): May be active in vitro vs. ESBL-producing aerobic gram-negative bacilli. Do not use as there are no clinical data for efficacy.** | | |
| Cefotetan (Cefotan) | **1–3 gm IV/IM q12h. (max. dose not >6 gm q24h).** | Increasing resistance of B. fragilis, Prevotella bivia, Prevotella disiens (most common in pelvic infections); do not use for intra-abdominal infections. Methylthiotetrazole (MTT) side chain can inhibit vitamin K activation. Avoid alcohol—disulfiram reaction. |
| Cefoxitin (Mefoxin) | **1 gm q8h–2 gm IV/IM q6-8h.** | Increasing resistance of B. fragilis isolates. |
| Cefuroxime (Kefurox, Ceftin, Zinacef) | **0.75–1.5 gm IV/IM q8h.** | Improved activity against H. influenzae compared with 1st generation cephalosporins. See Cefuroxime axetil for oral preparation. |
| **3ʳᵈ Generation, Parenteral – Use correlates with incidence of C. difficile toxin diarrhea;** most are inactivated by ESBLs and amp C cephalosporinase from aerobic gram-negative bacilli. | | |
| Cefoperazone-Sulbactam[NUS] (Sulperazon) | **Usual dose (Cefoperazone comp) 1-2 gm IV q12h;** if larger doses, do not exceed 4 gm/day of sulbactam. | In SE Asia & elsewhere, used to treat intra-abdominal, biliary, & gyn. infections. Other uses due to broad spectrum of activity. Possible clotting problem due to side-chain. |
| Cefotaxime (Claforan) | **1 gm q8-12h to 2 gm IV q4h.** | Maximum daily dose: 12 gm; give as 4 gm IV q8h. Similar to ceftriaxone but, unlike ceftriaxone, but requires multiple daily doses. |
| Ceftizoxime (Cefizox) | From **1-2 gm q8-12h up to 2 gm IV q4h.** | Maximum daily dose: 12 gm; can give as 4 gm IV q8h. |
| Ceftobiprole[NUS] Similar activity to ceftaroline, incl MRSA | **0.5 gm IV over 2 hrs q8h** | Associated with caramel-like taste disturbance. Ref: Clin Microbiol Infections 13(Suppl 2):17 & 25, 2007. Hydrolyzed by ESBL & AmpC cephalosporinase. |
| Ceftriaxone (Rocephin) | Commonly used IV dosage in adults: **1-2 gm once daily** Purulent meningitis: **2 gm q12h.** Can give **IM** in 1% lidocaine. | **"Pseudocholelithiasis"** 2° to sludge in gallbladder by ultrasound (50%), symptomatic (9%) (NEJM 322:1821, 1990). More likely with ≥2 gm per day with pt on total parenteral nutrition and not eating (AnIM 115:712, 1991). Has led to cholecystectomy (JID 17:356, 1995) and gallstone pancreatitis (Ln 17:662, 1998). Can cause drug-induced thrombocytopenia (J Thrombo & Haemo 2012;17:169). Combination of Ceftriaxone & Lansoprazole led to 1.4 x increased risk of increased QTc to >500 msec (J Am Coll Cardio 2016;68:1756). For Ceftriaxone Desensitization, see Table 7, page 91. |

[a]NOTE: all dosage recommendations are for adults (unless otherwise indicated) & assume normal renal function.

**TABLE 10A (4)**

| CLASS, AGENT, GENERIC NAME (TRADE NAME) | USUAL ADULT DOSAGE* | ADVERSE REACTIONS, COMMENTS *(See Table 10B for Summary)* |
|---|---|---|
| **CEPHALOSPORINS** *(continued)* | | |
| **Antipseudomonal** | | |
| **Cefepime** (Maxipime) For obesity dosing, see *Table 17C* | **Usual dose: 1-2 gm IV q8-12h.** **Prolonged infusion dosing:** Initial dose: 15 mg/kg over 30 min, then immediately begin; If CrCl >60: 6 gm (over 24 hr) daily If CrCl 30-60: 4 gm (over 24 hr) daily If CrCl 11-29: 2 gm (over 24 hr) daily | Active vs. P. aeruginosa and many strains of Enterobacter, Serratia, C. freundii resistant to Ceftazidime, Cefotaxime, Aztreonam. More active vs MSSA than 3⁰ generation cephalosporins. Not "porin-dependent". Neutropenia after 14 days rx *(Scand J Infect Dis 42:156, 2010).* Failures vs. E. cloacae bacteremia with MIC of 4-8 mcg/mL *(AAC 2015;59:7558).* **FDA Safety warning (June 2012):** risk of non-convulsive status epilepticus, especially in pts with renal insufficiency when doses not adjusted. Seizure activity resolved after drug discontinuation and/or hemodialysis in the majority of pts. Postulated mechanism: binding to GABA receptors *(Scand J Infect Dis 46:272, 2014; Crit Care 17:R264, 2013.* |
| **Cefpirome**^NUS (HR 810) | **1-2 gm IV q12h** | Active against Enterobacteriaceae and aerobic Gram-positive cocci (not enterococci or MRSA). Has activity against some P. aeruginosa. No useful activity against anaerobic bacilli. |
| **Ceftazidime** (Fortaz, Tazicef) | **Usual dose: 1-2 gm IV/IM q8-12h.** **Prolonged infusion dosing:** Initial dose: 15 mg/kg over 30 min, then immediately begin: If CrCl >50.6 gm (over 24 hr) daily If CrCl 31-50: 4 gm (over 24 hr) daily If CrCl 10-30: 2 gm (over 24 hr) daily *(AAC 49:3550, 2005; Infect 37:418, 2009).* | Often used in healthcare-associated infections, where P. aeruginosa is a consideration. Use may result in ↑ incidence of C. difficile-assoc. diarrhea and/or selection of vancomycin-resistant E. faecium. Risk of cross-allergenicity with aztreonam (same side chain). |
| **Anti-staphylococcal (MRSA)** | | |
| **Ceftaroline fosamil** (Teflaro) | **600 mg IV q12h (5-60 min infusion)** Pneumonia/bacteremia 600 mg IV q8h^NAI. See Comment | **Avid binding to PBP 2a; active vs. MRSA.** Inactivated by Amp C & ESBL enzymes. Approved for MRSA skin and skin structure infections and used for MRSA pneumonia and bacteremia, but not approved indications *(J Infect Chemother 19:42, 2013).* Active in vitro vs. VISA, VRSA. Refs: *CID 52:1156, 2011.* Used successfully for bacteremia and bone/joint infections, but NAI *(AAC 59:2541, 2014).* Risk of neutropenia *(JAC 71:2010, 2016; AAC 60: 264, 2016).* |
| **ESBL resistant** | | |
| **Ceftolozane-tazobactam** (Zerbaxa) Ref: *CID 2016;63:234* | 1.5 gm (1/0.5 gm) IV q8h for gm-neg complicated UTI & complicated intra-abdominal (add Metro 500 mg IV q8h) infection. | Infuse over 1 hr. Active vs. P. aeruginosa *(AAC 2017;61:e0046517)* and many gm-neg bacteria producing beta-lactamases. Cross-reaction in Beta-lactam allergic pts. Decreased efficacy w/ CrCl 30-50 mL/min. |
| **ESBL and Serine-carbapenemase resistant** | | |
| **Ceftazidime-avibactam** (Avycaz) Ref: *CID 2016;63:234; JAC 2016;71:2713* | 2.5 gm (2 gm Ceftazidime/0.5 gm avibactam) IV over 2 hrs q8h for gram-negative complicated UTI & add metronidazole 500 mg q8h for complicated intra-abdominal infection. Also approved for suspect GNB causing nosocomial pneumonia *(UnID 2017;18:229 & 285).* | Active against ESBL- & KPC-producing metallo-carbapenemases. No activity vs. GNB-producing metallo-carbapenemases. Decreased efficacy in pts with w/ CrCl 30-50 mL/min (in clinical trials). |

*(See page 2 for abbreviations)*

*NOTE: all dosage recommendations are for adults (unless otherwise indicated) & assume normal renal function.

**TABLE 10A (5)**

| CLASS, AGENT, GENERIC NAME (TRADE NAME) | USUAL ADULT DOSAGE* | ADVERSE REACTIONS, COMMENTS (See Table 10B for Summary) |
|---|---|---|
| **CEPHALOSPORINS** (continued) | | |
| **Oral Cephalosporins** | | **Cross-Allergenicity: Patients with a history of IgE-mediated allergic reactions to penicillin (e.g., bronchospasm** |
| **1st Generation, Oral** | | **anaphylaxis), angioneurotic edema, immediate urticaria) should not receive a cephalosporin.** If the history is a |
| Cefadroxil (Duricef) (500 mg caps, 1 gm tabs) | 0.5–1 gm po q12h. | "measles-like" rash to penicillin, available data suggest a 5–10% risk of rash in such patients; there is no enhanced risk of anaphylaxis. |
| Cephalexin (Keflex) (250 & 500 mg tabs) | 0.25–1 gm po q6h (max 4 gm/day). | • In pts with history of Pen "reaction" and no skin testing, 0.2–8.4% react to a cephalosporin (Aller Asthma Proc 26:135, 2006). If positive Pen G skin test, only 2% given a cephalosporin will react. Can predict with cephalosporin skin testing, but not easily available (An Im IM 141:16, 2004; AJM 125:572, 2008). |
| **2nd Generation, Oral** | | • IgE antibodies against either ring structure or side chains; 80% pts lose IgE over 10 yrs post-reaction (J Aller Clin |
| Cefaclor (Ceclor, Raniclor) (250 & 500 mg caps) | 0.25–0.5 gm po q8h. | Immunol 103:918, 1999). Amox, Cefadroxil, Cefprozil have similar side chains; Amp, Cefaclor, Cephalexin, Cefradine have similar side chains. |
| Cefprozil (Cefzil) (250 & 500 mg tabs) | 0.25–0.5 gm po q12h. | • If Pen/Ceph skin testing not available or clinically no time, proceed with cephalosporin if history does not suggest IgE-mediated reaction, prior reaction more than 10 yrs ago or cephalosporin side chain differs from implicated Pen. |
| Cefuroxime axetil po (Ceftin) (125 & 250 mg tabs) | 0.125–0.5 gm po q12h. | Any of the cephalosporins can result in **C. difficile toxin-**mediated diarrhea/enterocolitis. The reported frequency of nausea/vomiting and non-C. difficile toxin diarrhea is summarized in Table 10B. |
| **3rd Generation, Oral** | | There are **few drug-specific adverse effects, e.g.:** |
| Cefdinir (Omnicef) (300 mg tab) | 300 mg po q12h or 600 mg po q24h. | **Cefaclor:** Serum sickness-like reaction 0.1–0.5%—arthralgia, rash, erythema multiforme but no adenopathy, proteinuria or demonstrable immune complexes. |
| Cefditoren pivoxil (Spectracef) (200 mg tab) | 400 mg po bid. | **Cefdinir:** Drug-iron complex causes red stools in roughly 1% of pts. |
| Cefixime (Suprax) (400 mg tab) | 0.4 gm po q12–24h. | **Cefditoren pivoxil:** Hydrolysis yields pivalate. Pivalate absorbed (70%) & becomes pivaloylcarnitine which is renally excreted; 39–63% in **serum carnitine concentrations.** Carnitine involved in fatty acid (FA) metabolism & FA transport |
| Cefpodoxime proxetil (Vantin) (100 & 200 mg tabs) | 0.1–0.2 gm po q12h. | into mitochondria. Hence, caution in patients with carnitine deficiency & do not use in patients with carnitine deficiency. Also contains caseinate |
| Ceftibuten (Cedax) (400 mg tab) | 0.4 gm po q24h. | (milk protein); **avoid if milk allergy** (not same as lactose intolerance). Avoid gastric acid for optimal absorption. **Cefpodoxime:** There are rare reports of acute liver injury, bloody diarrhea, pulmonary infiltrates with eosinophilia. |
| | | **Cephalexin:** Can cause false-neg. urine dipstick test for leukocytes. |

| **AMINOGLYCOSIDES AND RELATED ANTIBIOTICS** – See Table 10D, page 128, and Table 17A, page 235 | | |
|---|---|---|
| **GLYCOPEPTIDES, LIPOGLYCOPEPTIDES, LIPOPEPTIDES** | | |
| Dalbavancin (Dalvance) | 1000 mg IV over 30 mins; one week later, 500 mg IV over 30 min or 1500 mg IV over 30 min x 1 dose. Avoid use with saline, drug may precipitate out of solution. | **If CrCl<30:** 750 mg IV initial dose, then one week later 375 mg IV. **Hemodialysis:** Dose as for normal renal function. Red man syndrome can occur with rapid infusion. Potential cross-reaction in those with hypersensitivity to other glycopeptides. No activity vs. VRE. No drug-drug interactions. |
| Daptomycin (Cubicin) (Ref on resistance: JAC 2018;73-1). Case series success in treating right- & left-sided endocarditis with higher dose of 8–10 mg/kg/day (JAC 58:936 & 2921, 2013). In retrospective study, better survival in VRE bacteremia if dosed at ≥ 10 mg/kg/day (CID 2017;64:605). | **Skin/soft tissue:** 4 mg per kg IV over 2 or 30 minutes q24h **Bacteremia/right-sided endocarditis:** 6 mg per kg IV over 2 or 30 minutes q24h; up to 12 mg/kg IV q24h under study **Morbid obesity:** base dose on total body weight (AAC 51:2741, 2007); for other dosing see comment. See Table 17C, page 250. Dapto x ceftaroline may work as salvage therapy in pts with refractory MRSA bacteremia (AAC 57:66, 2013; AAC 56:5296, 2012). | **Pneumonia:** Dapto should not be used to treat pneumonia unless septic pneumonia in origin and is FDA approved for right-sided endocarditis with or without septic pneumonia/hematogenous pneumonia due to S. aureus. **Dapto Resistance:** Can occur de novo, after or during Vanco therapy, or after or during Dapto therapy (CID 50(Suppl 1):S10, 2010). Dapto MIC increases, MRSA more susceptible to TMP-SMX, nafcillin, oxacillin (AAC 54:5187, 2010; CID 53:158, 2011). **Potential muscle toxicity:** Suggest weekly CPK; DC dapto if CPK exceeds 10x normal level or if symptoms of myopathy and CPK >1,000. Package insert: stop statins during dapto rx. Dapto interferes with protime reagents & artificially prolongs the PT. (Blood Coag & Fibrinolysis 19:32, 2008). **Immune thrombocytopenia** reported (AAC 56:6480, 2012). Reversible neutropenia with low-dose daptomycin reported (CID 50:737, 2010; CID 50:e63, 2010). **Eosinophilic pneumonia:**/chronic steroid-dep pneumonia reported. |

(See page 2 for abbreviations) *NOTE: all dosage recommendations are for adults (unless otherwise indicated) & assume normal renal function.

| CLASS, AGENT, GENERIC NAME (TRADE NAME) | USUAL ADULT DOSAGE* | ADVERSE REACTIONS, COMMENTS (See Table 10B for Summary) |
|---|---|---|
| **GLYCOPEPTIDES, LIPOGLYCOPEPTIDES** *(continued)* | | |
| Oritavancin (Orbactiv) Review: CID 61:S27, 2015 | 1200 mg IV over 3 hr x 1 dose. Dilute in D5W; do not use saline | Artificially increases PT, INR & aPTT x 48 hr. **Drug-drug interactions with warfarin:** ↑ warfarin serum levels. Acute urticarial has occurred. No dose adjustment for renal or hepatic insuff. Not removed by hemodialysis. In vitro activity vs. VRE (AAC 56:1639, 2012). Hypersensitivity: fever (at 3 mg/kg 2.2%, at 24 mg per kg 8.2%), skin reactions 2.4%. Marked ↓ platelets (high dose ≥15 mg per kg per day). Red neck syndrome less common than with vancomycin. |
| Teicoplanin[NUS] (Targocid) | **For septic arthritis—maintenance dose 12 mg/kg per day; S. aureus endocarditis— trough serum levels 20 mcg/mL required 12 mg/kg q12h times 3 loading dose, then 12 mg/kg (q24h)** | |
| Telavancin (Vibativ) Lipoglycopeptide Ref: CID 60:787, 2015; CID 61(Suppl 2), 2015 | 10 mg/kg IV q24h if CrCl >50 mL/min. Reduce each dose over 1 hr. | **Avoid during pregnancy: teratogenic in animals.** Do pregnancy test before therapy. Adverse events: **dysgeusia (taste)** 33%; nausea 27%; vomiting 14%; headache 14%; ↑ creatinine (3.1%); foamy urine (13%); tinnitus if infused rapidly. In clin. trials, **evidence of renal injury in 3%** telavancin vs. 1% vanco. In practice, renal injury reported in 1/3 of 21 complicated pts (JAC 67:723, 2012). Interferes with PT, aPTT & INR for 18 hrs post-infusion. |
| Vancomycin (Vancocin) AAC 60:2601, 2016. See Comments for po dose. Continuous infusion dosing, see Table 10E | **Initial doses based on actual wt, including for obese pts.** Subsequent doses adjusted based on measured serum levels. **For critically ill pts, give loading dose of 25-30 mg/kg IV then 15-20 mg/kg IV q8-12h.** Target trough level is 15-20 mg/mL. For individual doses over 1 gm, infuse over 1.5-2 hrs. **Dosing for morbid obesity (BMI ≥40 kg/m2): If CrCl ≥50 mL/min & pt not critically ill:** 30 mg/kg/day divided q8-12h—no dose over 2 gm. Infuse doses of 1 gm or more over 1.5 hrs. Check trough levels. **Morbid obese & critically ill:** Loading dose 25-30 mg/kg (based on actual wt), then 15-20 mg/kg (actual wt) IV q8-12h. Infuse over 1.5-2 hrs. **Limit maximal single dose to 2 gm.** Oral tabs for C. difficile: 125 mg po q6h Generic drug now available | Vanco treatment failure of MRSA bacteremia with Vanco trough concentration <15 μg/mL & MIC >1 μg/mL (CID 52:975, 2011). IDSA Guideline supports target trough of 15-20 μg/mL (CID 52:e18, 2011). Pertinent issues:<br>• Max Vanco effect vs. MRSA when ratio of AUC/MIC >400 (CID 52:975, 2011).<br>• MIC values vary with method used, so hard to be sure/compare (CM 49:269, 2011)<br>• With MRSA Vanco MIC = 1 & Vanco dose >3 gm/day IV, AUC/MIC >400 in 80% with est. risk of nephrotoxicity of 25%. With MIC = 2 & 4 gm/day IV, AUC/MIC >400 in only 57% (nephrotoxicity risk 35%) (CID 52:969, 2011).<br>• Risk of AKI associated with concomitant PIP-TZ (AAC 2018;62:e00264).<br>• If pt clinically failing Vanco (regardless of MIC or AUC/MIC), choose active vs. MRSA: Ceftaroline, Daptomycin, Linezolid, Televancin. (See Table 5A.)<br>**Oral tabs for C. difficile colitis: 125 mg po q6h.** Commercial po formulation very expensive. Can compound po vanco from IV formulation (not recommended): 5 g, IV vanco powder + 47.5 mL sterile H2O, 0.2 gm saccharin, 0.05 gm stevia powder, 40 mL glycerin and then enough cherry syrup to yield 100 mL. = 50 mg/mL. Oral dose = 2.5 mL q6h po.<br>**Intrathecal dose:** 5-10 mg/day (infants); 10-20 mg/day (children & adults) to target CSF concentration of 10-20 mg/mL.<br>**Nephrotoxicity:** Risk increases with dose and duration; reversible (AAC 57:734, 2013).<br>**Red Neck Syndrome:** consequence of rapid infusion with non-specific histamine release. **Other adverse effects:** rash, immune thrombocytopenia (J Thrombo Haemostasis 11:169, 2012), fever, neutropenia. **IgA bullous dermatitis** (CID 38:442, 2004). **Obesity dosing:** Frequent under dosing (AJM 121:515, 2008). For obesity dosing adjustments, see Table 10C, page 250. For CrCl calculation for morbidly obese patient see Table 10D or Am J Health Sys Pharm 66:642, 2009. |
| **CHLORAMPHENICOL, CLINDAMYCIN(S), ERYTHROMYCIN GROUP, KETOLIDES, OXAZOLIDINONES, STREPTOGRAMINS, QUINUPRISTIN-DALFOPRISTIN** | | (max 4 gm/day) |
| Chloramphenicol (Chloromycetin) | 50-100 mg/kg/day po/IV div q6h (max 4 gm/day) | No oral drug distrib in US. Hematologic: (↓ RBC—1/3 pts, aplastic anemia 1:21,600 courses). Gray baby syndrome in premature infants, anaphylactoid reactions, optic neuritis or neuropathy (very rare), digital paresthesias, minor disulfiram-like reactions. Recent review suggests Chloro is probably less effective than current alternatives for serious infection: respiratory tract, enteric, meningitis (JAC 70:979, 2015). |
| Clindamycin (Cleocin) | 0.15-0.45 gm po q6h; 600-900 mg IV/IM q8h in obese child, calc dose based on total body wt (AAC 2017;61:e02014 16) | Based on number of exposed pts, these drugs are the most frequent cause of **C. difficile toxin-mediated diarrhea.** In most severe form can cause pseudomembranous colitis/toxic megacolon. Available as caps, IV soln, topical (for acne) & intravaginal suppositories & cream. **Used to inhibit synthesis of toxic shock syndrome toxins.** |
| Lincomycin (Lincocin) | 0.6 to 1 gm IV q8-12h | Rarely used. Risk of C difficile. Requires appropriate dilution and infusion time based on dose (see Package insert). |

**TABLE 10A (7)**

| CLASS, AGENT, GENERIC NAME (TRADE NAME) | USUAL ADULT DOSAGE* | ADVERSE REACTIONS, COMMENTS *(See Table 10B for Summary)* |
|---|---|---|
| **CHLORAMPHENICOL, CLINDAMYCIN(S), ERYTHROMYCIN GROUP, KETOLIDES, OXAZOLIDINONES, QUINUPRISTIN-DALFOPRISTIN** *(continued)* | | |
| **Erythromycin Group (Review drug interactions before use)** | | |
| **Azithromycin** (Zithromax) | po preps: Tabs 250 & 600 mg. Peds suspension: 100 & 200 mg per 5 mL. Adult ER suspension; **Zmax**: (Zmax): See note on specific indication, see Table 1. Acute otitis media *(page 12)*, acute exac. chronic bronchitis *(page 40)*, Comm-acq. pneumonia *(pages 42–43)*, & sinusitis *(page 53)*. | **Gastroparesis:** Erythro is alt drug for rx of gastroparesis. Initiates peristalsis by binding to motilin receptors & improves stomach emptying for approx 4 weeks; then effect; lost due to tachyphylaxis. Erythro dose: 1.5-3 mg/kg IV over 45 min q6h or 250 mg po liquid susp bid. Ref: *Gastro Clin NA 2015;44:97* |
| **Azithromycin ER** (Zmax) | | **Frequent drug-drug interactions:** see *Table 22A page 266.* Major concern is prolonged QT_c interval on EKG. **Prolonged QTc:** Erythro, clarithro & azithro all increase risk of ventricular tachycardia via increase in QTc interval. Can be congenital or acquired *(NEJM 358:169, 2008).* Caution if positive family history of sudden cardiac death, electrolyte abnormalities or concomitant drugs that prolong QTc. |
| | | **↑ risk QTc ≥500 msec: Risk amplified by other drugs** [macrolides, antiarrhythmics, & drug-drug interactions *(see FDs page 120 for list)*]. *www.qtdrugs.org & www.torsades.org.* Ref: *Am J Med 128:1362, 2015.* |
| **Erythromycin Base and esters** (Erythrocin)<br>IV name: E, lactobionate | **0.25 gm q6h–0.5 gm po/IV q6h:** | Cholestatic hepatitis in approx 1/1000 adults (in children) (over estolate). **Frequent drug-drug interactions:** (see *Table 22, page 266*). Azithro least likely to cause high levels, rhabdomyolysis *(Ann Int Med 158:869, 2013)*; concomitant clarithro & colchicine (gout) can cause fatal colchicine toxicity (pancytopenia, renal failure) *(CID 41:291, 2005).* Concomitant clarithro & Ca++ channel blockers increase risk of hypotension, kidney injury *(JAMA Int Med 174:1605, 2014).* |
| **Clarithromycin** (Biaxin)<br>or clarithro extended release (Biaxin XL) | **15–20 mg/kg up to 4 gm q24h. Infuse over 30- min.**<br>**0.5 gm q12h.**<br>**Extended release: Two 0.5 gm tabs po per day.** | Hypoglycemia with concomitant sulfonylureas *(JAMA Int Med 174:1605, 2014).* Transient reversible tinnitus or deafness with ≥4 gm per day of erythro IV in pts with renal or hepatic impairment. Reversible sensorineural hearing loss with Azithro *(J Otolaryngol 36:257, 2007).* Dosages of oral erythro preparations expressed as base equivalents. Variable amounts of erythro esters required to achieve same free erythro serum level. **Azithromycin** reported to exacerbate symptoms of myasthenia gravis. **FDA alerts:** clarithromycin use associated with increased cardio- and cerebro-vascular events, azithromycin use to prevent bronchiolitis obliterans after donor stem cell transplant associated with increased cancer relapse and death. Approved for C. difficile toxin-mediated diarrhea, including hypervirulent NAP1/B1/027 strains. Minimal GI absorption; |
| **Fidaxomicin** (Dificid)<br>(200 mg tab) | **One 200 mg tab po bid x 10 days with or without food** | high fecal concentrations. Limited activity vs. normal bowel flora. In trial vs. po Vanco, lower relapse rate vs. non-NAP-1 strains than Vanco *(NEJM 364:422, 2011)*, despite absence of IV arm. *(NEJM 355:2260, 2006).* No longer marketed in US. |
| **Ketolide:**<br>**Telithromycin** (Ketek)<br>*(Med Lett 46:66, 2004;*<br>*Drug Safety 31:561, 2008)* | **Two 400 mg tabs po q24h.**<br>300 mg tabs available. | Drug warnings: acute liver failure & serious liver injury post treatment. *(AnM 144:415. 447, 2006).* **Uncommon: blurred vision, 2° slow accommodation;** may cause exacerbation of **myasthenia gravis (Black Box Warning: Contraindicated in this disorder).** Liver, eye and myasthenia complications may be due to inhibition of nicotinic acetylcholine receptor at neuromuscular junction *(AAC 54:5399, 2010)*. Potential QT_c prolongation. Several **drug-drug interactions** *(Table 22A, page 256)* *(NEJM 355:2260, 2006).* |
| **Tedizolid phosphate** (Sivextro)<br>Ref: *CID 61:1315, 2015.* | **200 mg IV/po once daily. Infuse IV over 1 hr.** | IV dose reconstituted in 250 mL of normal saline; incompatible with lactated ringers as non-soluble in presence of divalent cations. SST clinical trial result *(JAMA 309:559 & 609, 2013).* Excreted by liver. No adjustment for hemodialysis or peritoneal dialysis *(Int J Antimicrob Ag 36:179, 2010; JAC doi:10.1093/jac/dkv184)* Increased risk on hemodialysis and peritoneal dialysis *(Int J Antimicrob Ag 36:179, 2010; JAC doi:10.1093/jac/dkv184)* |
| **Linezolid** (Zyvox)<br>(600 mg tab)<br>Review: *JAC 66(Suppl 4):3, 2011* | **po or IV dose: 600 mg q12h.**<br>Available as 600 mg tabs, oral suspension (100 mg per 5 mL), & IV solution. Special populations Refs: Renal insufficiency *(J Infect Chemother 17:70, 2011);* Liver transplant *(CID 42:434, 2006);* Cystic fibrosis *(AAC 48:281, 2004);* Burns *(J Burn Care Res 31:207, 2010);* Obesity: clinical failure with standard dose in 265 kg patient *(Ann Pharmacother 47:e25, 2013).* | **Reversible myelosuppression:** thrombocytopenia, anemia, & neutropenia reported. Most often after >2 wks of therapy. **Lactic acidosis: peripheral neuropathy, optic neuropathy:** After 4 or more wks of therapy. Data consistent with time and dose-dependent inhibition of intramitochondrial protein synthesis *(Pharmacotherapy 27:771, 2007).* Neuropathy, not reversible. Mitochondrial toxicity *(Lancet 388:465, 2002; AAC 50:2042, 2006).* **Inhibition of monoamine oxidase:** risk of severe hypertension if taken with foods rich in tyramine. Avoid concomitant pseudoephedrine, phenylpropanolamine, and caution with SSRIs! **Serotonin syndrome** (fever, agitation, mental status changes, tremors). Risk with concomitant SSRIs: *(CID 42:1578 and 43:180, 2006).* Incidence low *(AAC 57:5901, 2013).* **Other:** black tongue, acute interstitial nephritis *(IDCP 17:61, 2009);* teeth staining *(CID 2016;62:617).* **Rhabdomyolysis:** case probably related to linezolid in a patient receiving linezolid and rifampin for mult-drug therapy for XDR tuberculosis *(CID 54:1624, 2012).* **Resistance:** Linezolid resistant S. epidermidis and MRSA due to mutation of the 23S rRNA binding site *(JAC 68-4, 2013).* |

¹ **SSRI** = selective serotonin reuptake inhibitors, e.g., fluoxetine (Prozac).
*NOTE: all dosage recommendations are for adults (unless otherwise indicated) & assume normal renal function.*
*(See page 2 for abbreviations)*

**TABLE 10A (8)**

| CLASS, AGENT, GENERIC NAME (TRADE NAME) | USUAL ADULT DOSAGE* | ADVERSE REACTIONS, COMMENTS (See Table 10B for Summary) |
|---|---|---|
| **CHLORAMPHENICOL, CLINDAMYCIN(S), ERYTHROMYCIN GROUP, KETOLIDES, OXAZOLIDINONES, QUINUPRISTIN-DALFOPRISTIN** (continued) | | |
| Quinupristin + Dalfopristin (Synercid) (CID 36-473, 2003) | 7.5 mg per kg IV q12h for skin/skin structure infections, infused over 1 hour. [For previous indication of VRE infection, dose used was 7.5 mg per kg IV q8h). Give by central line. | Venous irritation (5%); none with central venous line. Asymptomatic ↑ in unconjugated bilirubin. **Arthralgia** 2%–50% (CID 36-476, 2003). **Note:** E. faecium susceptible; E. faecalis resistant. **Drug-drug interactions:** Cyclosporine, nifedipine, midazolam, many more—see Table 22A. |
| **TETRACYCLINES** | | |
| Doxycycline (Vibramycin, Doryx, Monodox, Adoxa, Periostat) (20, 50, 75, 100 mg tab) | **Adult:** 100 mg po/IV q12h; **Child (regardless of age): 4.4 mg/kg/day po/IV divided bid x max of 21 days** (considered safe, AAP Redbook 2018; J Ped 2015/166/1246). | Similar to other tetracyclines. ↑ nausea on empty stomach. Erosive esophagitis, esp. if taken at bedtime; **take with lots of water.** Phototoxicity & photo-onycholysis occur but less than with tetracycline. Deposition in teeth less than with tetracycline (JAC 2017;72:2887). Can be used in patients with renal failure. Pseudotumor cerebri (intracranial hypertension) can occur. Comments: Effective in treatment and prophylaxis for malaria, leptospirosis, typhus fevers. |
| Eravacycline (Xerava) Activity similar to omadacycline & tigecycline, see Table 4A) | 1 mg/kg IV infused over 60 min q12h x 4–14 days (increase to 1.5 mg/kg if co-administered with strong CYP3A4 inducer, e.g., RIF). Severe liver disease: (pg) Loading 1 mg/kg IV q12h x 1 day, then 1 mg/kg IV q24h. | Approved for complicated intra-abdominal infections in adults. **Warnings:** life-threatening hypersensitivity reactions if known tetracycline allergy; Pregnancy (2nd/3rd trimester) risk of tooth discoloration and bone growth inhibition. **Common AEs:** infusion site reactions, nausea, vomiting. |
| Minocycline (Minocin, Dynacin) (50, 75, 100 mg cap; 45, 90, 135 mg ext rel tab; IV prep) Contains Mg+, Monitor serum Mg+ levels if renal impairment. | **200 mg po/IV loading dose, then 100 mg po/IV q12h** IV minocycline available. | **Vestibular symptoms** (30–90% in some groups, none in others): vertigo 33%, ataxia 43%, nausea 50%, vomiting 3%, women less frequently than men. Phototoxicity pneumonitis. Hypersensitivity, ~34 cases reported (BMJ 310/1520, 1995). Can cause slate-grey **pigmentation** of the skin and other tissues with long-term use. **Intracranial hypertension** can occur. Comments: More effective than other tetracyclines vs staph and in prophylaxis of meningococcal disease. P. acnes: many resistant to other tetracyclines, not to mino. Induced autoimmunity reported in children treated for acne (J Ped 153:314, 2008). Active vs Nocardia asteroides, Mycobacterium marinum and many acinetobacter isolates. |
| Omadacycline (Nuzyra) Activity similar to eravacycline & tigecycline, see Table 4A) | **CABP/ABSSSI:** Loading: (IV/po): 200 mg IV infused over 60 min or 100 mg IV infused over 30 min twice on day 1; Maintenance: 100 mg IV infused over 30 min od or 300 mg po od. **ABSSSI:** (po): Loading: 450 mg po od days 1 & 2; Maintenance: 300 mg po od | Duration: 7–14 days. Breastfeeding not recommended during treatment and for 4 days after last dose. Fast for 4 hrs before dosing. No food for 2 hrs after dosing; no dairy products, antacids, multivitamins for 4 hrs after dosing. **Contraindication:** known tetracycline hypersensitivity. **Warnings:** Higher mortality risk in CAP vs. Moxi. Tooth discoloration/enamel dysplasia in 2nd half of pregnancy. Inhibition of bone growth in 2nd/3rd trimesters. **AEs:** increased AST, ALT, GGT; hypertension, headache; diarrhea, nausea, vomiting, constipation; infusion site reactions; insomnia. |
| Tetracycline, Oxytetracycline (Sumycin) (250, 500 mg cap) (CID 36-462, 2003) | **0.25–0.5 gm po q6h, 0.5–1 gm IV q12h** | GI (oral 10%, tetra 4%), anaphylactoid reaction (rare), deposition in teeth, negative N-balance, hepatotoxicity, vaginal agenesis, pseudotumor cerebri/encephalopathy. Outdated drug: Fanconi syndrome. See drug interactions, Table 22A. **Contraindicated in pregnancy, hepatotoxicity in mother, transplacental to fetus.** **Pregnancy:** IV dosage over 2 gm per day may be associated with fatal hepatotoxicity. (Ref: JAC 66:1431, 2011). |
| Tigecycline (Tygacil) Meta-analysis & editorial: Ln ID 11:804 & 834, 2011. Also CID 54:1699 & 1710, 2012. | **100 mg IV initially, then 50 mg IV q12h** with po food, if possible to decrease risk of nausea. If severe liver dis. (Child Pugh C) 100 mg IV initially, then 25 mg IV q12h | Derivative of tetracycline. High incidence of nausea (25%) & vomiting (20%) but only 1% of pts discontinued therapy. Pregnancy Category D. Do not use in children under age 18. Like other tetracyclines, may cause photosensitivity, pseudotumor cerebri, pancreatitis, a catabolic state (elevated BUN) and maybe hyperpigmentation (CID 45:136, 2007). Decreases serum fibrinogen (AAC 59:1650, 2015). Tetracycline, minocycline & tigecycline associated with acute pancreatitis (Int J Antimicrob Agents, 34:486, 2009). **Black Box Warning:** In meta-analysis of clinical trials, all cause mortality higher in pts treated with tigecycline (2.5%) vs. 1.8% in comparators. Cause of mortality risk difference of 0.6% (95% CI 0.1, 1.2) not established. Tigecycline should be reserved for use in situations when alternative treatments are not suitable (FDA MedWatch Sep 27, 2013). Poor result due to low serum levels (AAC 56:1065 & 1466, 2012); high doses superior to low doses for HAP (AAC 57:1756, 2013). |

*NOTE: all dosage recommendations are for adults (unless otherwise indicated) & assume normal renal function.

| CLASS, AGENT, GENERIC NAME (TRADE NAME) | USUAL ADULT DOSAGE* | ADVERSE REACTIONS, COMMENTS (See Table 10B for Summary) |
|---|---|---|
| **FLUOROQUINOLONES (FQs):** All can cause false-positive urine drug screen for opiates | | *(Pharmacother 26:435, 2006)*. Toxicity review: *Drugs Aging 27:193, 2010.* |
| Ciprofloxacin (CIP)<br>Ciprofloxacin-extended release<br>(CIP XR, Proquin XR)<br>(100, 250, 500, 750 mg tab;<br>500 mg ext rel tab) | Usual Parenteral Dose: **400 mg IV q12h**<br>For aerosolized exposure/cutaneous anthrax<br>Uncomplicated urinary tract infection/cystitis: (Oral) Dose:<br>**250 mg po bid** or CIP XR **500 mg po once daily**<br>Other indications (Oral): **500-750 mg po bid** | FQs are a common precipitant of **C. difficile toxin-mediated diarrhea**.<br>**CNS toxicity:** Overstimulation. Also based on animal cartilage injury in immature animals. Articular SEs in children est. at 2-3% (*UnID 3:537, 2003*). The exception is anthrax. Pathogenesis is believed to involve FQ chelation of Mg++ and damaging chondrites (*AAC 51:1022, 2007; Int J Antimicrob Agents 33:194, 2009*). No evidence of cartilage damage with Levo in children (*Pediatrics 134:e146, 2014*). |
| Delafloxacin (Baxdela)<br>450 mg tablets<br>IV for injection | **300 mg IV q12h** infused over 1 hr x 5-14 days<br>**450 mg po q12h x 5-14 days** | **CNS toxicity:** Poorly understood. Varies: lightheadedness, confusion, seizures. Trouble with attention/memory. Peripheral neuropathy occurs: rapid onset, potentially permanent injury. |
| Gatifloxacin (Tequin)[NUS]<br>See comments | Can switch from IV to po during course of rx. (See comment)<br>**200-400 mg IV/po q24h.** (See comment) | **Gem skin rash:** Macular rash after 8-10 days of rx. Incidence of rash with ≤5 days of therapy only 1.5%. Frequency highest females, < age 40, treated 14 days (22.6%). In men, < age 40, treated 14 days, frequency 77%. Mechanism unclear. Indication IV chelation to OC therapy. Ref: Diag Micro Infect Dis 68:140, 2010. |
| Gemifloxacin (Factive)<br>(320 mg tab) | **320 mg po q24h.** | **Hypoglycemia/hyperglycemia (dysglycemia):** Increased risk, esp. of hypoglycemia in diabetic pts from any of the marketed FQs (*CID 57:971, 2013*).<br>**Thrombocytopenia** in critically ill (*J Thrombo Haemostasis 11:169, 2012*).<br>**Opiate screen false-positives:** FQs can cause false-positive urine assay for opiates (*Ann Pharmacotherapy 38:1525, 2004*).<br>**Photosensitivity:** See Table 10C, page 127.<br>**QT, (corrected QT) interval prolongation:** ↑ QT, (>500 msec or >60 msec from baseline) is considered possible with any FQ (except Delaflox). ↑ QT, can lead to torsades de pointes and ventricular fibrillation. Overall risk is 4.7/10,000 person yrs (*CID 551:452, 2012*). Risk low with current marketed drugs. Risk ↑ in women, ↓ K+, ↓ mg++, bradycardia. (Refs.: *CID 43:1603, 2006*). Major problem is ↑ risk with concomitant drugs. |
| | | **Avoid concomitant drugs with potential to prolong QTc such as** (see www.qtdrugs.org; www.torsades.org): |
| Levofloxacin (Levaquin)<br>(250, 500, 750 mg tab) | **250-750 mg po/IV q24h.**<br>For most indications, 750 mg is preferred dose. po therapy: avoid concomitant dairy products, multivitamins, iron, antacids due to chelation by multivalent cations & interference with absorption. No dose adjustment for morbid obesity. | **Antiarrhythmics:** Amiodarone, Disopyramide, Dofetilide, Flecainide, Ibutilide, Procainamide, Quinidine, quinine, Sotalol<br>**Anti-Infectives:** Azoles (not Posa), Clarithro/erythro, FQs (not CIP), Halofantrine, NNRTIs, Protease Inhibitors, Pentamidine, Telavancin, Telithromycin<br>**Anti-Hypertensives:** Bepridil, Isradipine, Nicardipine, Moexipril<br>**CNS Drugs:** Fluoxetine, Haloperidol, Phenothiazines, Pimozide, Quetiapine, Risperidone, Sertraline, Tricyclics, Venlafaxine, Ziprasidone<br>**Misc:** Dolasetron, Droperidol, Fosphenytoin, Indapamide, Methadone, Naratriptan, Ondansetron, Salmeterol, Sumatriptan, Tamoxifen, Tizanidine |
| Moxifloxacin (Avelox) | **400 mg po/IV q24h.** Note: no need to increase dose for morbid obesity (*AAC 66:2330, 2011*).<br>Ophthalmic solution (Vigamox). | **Tendinopathy:** Over age 60, approx. 2-6% of all Achilles tendon ruptures attributable to use of FQ (*ArIM 163:1801, 2003*). ↑ risk with concomitant steroid, renal disease or post-transplant (heart, lung, kidney) (*CID 36:1404, 2003*).<br>**Chelation:** Risk of chelation of oral FQs by multivalent cations (**Ca++, Mg++, Fe++, Zn++**). Avoid dairy products, multivitamins *Clin Pharmacokinet 40 (Suppl 1) 33-2001*). |
| Ofloxacin (Floxin) | **200-400 mg po bid.**<br>Ophthalmic solution (Ocuflox) | **Allergic Reactions:** Rare (150,000), IgE-mediated; urticaria, anaphylaxis, 3 pts with Moxi had immediate reactions but tolerated CIP (*Ann Pharmacother 44:740, 2010*).<br>**Myasthenia gravis:** Any of the FQs may exacerbate muscle weakness in pts. with myasthenia gravis.<br>**Carpal tunnel syndrome:** Inconsistent data.<br>**Retinal detachment:** Pharmacoepidemiological study found increased risk of CTS with FQ use (*CID 65: 684, 2017*).<br>**Pseudotumor cerebri:** Significant risk ratio (4-5) reported (*Neurology 207:89-892*). |

*NOTE: all dosage recommendations are for adults (unless otherwise indicated) & assume normal renal function.

**TABLE 10A (10)**

| CLASS, AGENT, GENERIC NAME (TRADE NAME) | USUAL ADULT DOSAGE* | ADVERSE REACTIONS, COMMENTS (See Table 10B for Summary) |
|---|---|---|
| **FLUOROQUINOLONES (FQs)** (continued) | | |
| **Prulifloxacin**<br>Ref: Drugs 64:2221, 2004. | Tablets: 250 and 600 mg.<br>Usual dose: **600 mg po once daily** | **Contraindications:** persons with celiac disease, pregnancy, nursing mothers, persons with seizure disorder<br>**AEs:** similar to other FQs |
| **POLYMYXINS (POLYPEPTIDES) Note:** Proteus sp., Providencia sp., Serratia sp., B. cepacia are intrinsically resistant to polymyxins. Review: CID 59:88, 2014. | | |
| **Polymyxin B** (Poly-Rx)<br>1 mg = 10,000 international units<br>**Where available, Polymyxin B preferred over Colistin.** | Doses based on actual body weight.<br>**LOADING DOSE:** 2.5 mg/kg IV over 2 hrs.<br>**MAINTENANCE DOSE:** 12 hrs later 1.5 mg/kg over 1 hr, then repeat q12h.<br>No dose reduction for renal insufficiency.<br>**Intrathecal therapy for meningitis:** 5 mg/day into CSF x 3-4 days, then 5 mg every other day x 2 or more weeks. | **Adverse effects: Neurologic:** rare, but serious, is neuromuscular blockade; other, circumoral paresthesias, extremity numbness, blurred vision, drowsy, irritable, ataxia; can manifest as respiratory arrest (Chest 141:515, 2012).<br>**Renal:** reversible acute tubular necrosis. Renal injury in 42% (Polymyxin B) vs. 60% (Colistin) (CID 57:1300, 2013).<br>**Skin:** Hyperpigmentation in 8% of 249 pts (J Clin Pharm Ther 2017;42:573).<br><br>PK study showed no need to reduce dose for renal insufficiency (CID 57:524, 2013).<br>**Polymyxin B preferred over Colistin** (except for UTI) (see Comment under Colistin for rationale).<br>Combination therapy (polymyxin + carbapenem) failed in controlled clinical trial (LnID 2018;18:391). |

*NOTE: all dosage recommendations are for adults (unless otherwise indicated) & assume normal renal function.

TABLE 10A (11)

| CLASS, AGENT, GENERIC NAME (TRADE NAME) | USUAL ADULT DOSAGE* | ADVERSE REACTIONS, COMMENTS (See Table 10B for Summary) |
|---|---|---|
| **POLYMYXINS (POLYPEPTIDES)** | (continued) | |
| **Colistin, Polymyxin E** (Colymycin)<br><br>Polymyxin E (Colistin) and Polymyxin B are polymyxin class parenteral antibiotics active against multi-drug resistant (MDR) gram negative bacilli, e.g., *A. baumannii*, *P. aeruginosa*, *E. coli*, *K. pneumoniae*.<br><br>**Resistance issues:**<br>*Serratia* sp. *Proteus* sp. *Providencia* sp., *Morganella* sp., and *B. cepacia* are intrinsically resistant to polymyxins. Pan-resistant strains of Enterobacteriaceae with resistance to colistin mediated by plasmid-encoded gene mcr-1 (*AAC 60: 2443, 2016*) have been identified worldwide.<br><br>Colistin is the preferred polymyxin for:<br>Urinary tract infections (UTIs) & adjunctive inhalation therapy for pneumonia caused by MDR gram-negative bacilli.<br><br>For all other infections, Polymyxin B: equivalent efficacy, faster attainment of target serum conc, less inter-patient variability in PK, no dose adjustment for renal impair. and lower risk of renal toxicity (*AAC 60: 2443, 2016*; and *AAC 2017;61:e02339-16*). | **Formulation and conversion:** Colistin is formulated as a prodrug, colistimethate. Product vials may be labeled as international units (IU) or mg of prodrug or mg of **colistin base activity (CBA)** of active drug. **Always dose based on the CBA.** *To avoid dosing errors read product labels carefully!* **Conversions** (*CID 2014, 56:139*): 1 mg CBA = 30,000 IU colistimethate (prodrug).<br><br>Dosing recommendations continue to evolve. At present, there are 3 sets of dosing guidance: **PK Study Group:** creatinine clearance (CrCl)-based dosing (*CID 2017;64:565*); **European Medicines Agency (EMA):** CrCl-based dosing (*CID 2016, 62:552*); **U.S. FDA:** weight- and CrCl-based dosing, as found in the package insert (June 2016). Complicated calculation-based dosing has been replaced by simpler CrCl-based dosing using CrCl levels as benchmarks. The PK Study Group recommendations use finer divisions between CrCl levels; the EMA recommendations use broader divisions. See Comments.<br><br>For severe systemic infection and patients not on dialysis of any kind: (Note: for dosing in patients on intermittent hemodialysis or CRRT, see Table 17A):<br><br>1. **Loading Dose:** Administer a Colistin loading dose IV, then begin daily maintenance dosing 12 hours later. Loading dose formula: 4 x body weight in kg. Use lower of ideal or actual weight. May result in loading dose > 300 mg CBA. Start daily maintenance dose 12 hrs. later.<br><br>2. **Maintenance Dose:** Then, **Total Daily maintenance dose: Divide daily dose to bid or tid** (from Total Daily maintenance dose [Comments]: Editors prefer PK Study Group). Once daily dosing not recommended due to potential for toxicity and lack of efficacy data.<br><br>**Other adult dosing:**<br>Inhaled therapy: 50-75 mg CBA in 3-4 mL saline via vibrating mesh nebulizer 2-3 times/day: concentration in lung epithelial lining is 100-1000x greater with inhaled dosing vs. IV dosing alone<br><br>**Meningitis:** (intraventricular or intrathecal dose): 10 mg/day x several weeks; intrathecal dose often combined with IV dose<br><br>**Pediatric dosing:**<br>Systemic infection: 2.5-5 mg/kg/day in 2-4 divided doses (based on ideal body weight).<br>Cystic Fibrosis: 3-8 mg/kg/day in 3 divided doses (based on ideal body weight).<br><br>**Note: Resistance and allergy issues.** The plasmid-encoded colistin resistance gene, mcr-1, has been found in *E. coli* and *Klebsiella* spp. Resistance is due to modification of the lipid A target of the polymyxins. Strains may also produce metallo-carbapenemases, resulting in pan-resistance (*CID 2016, 16:287; Lancet 2016, 16:1293; mBio 2017, 8:e00543-17*). For treatment of MDR gram-neg. pathogens, no clear alternatives for a companion drug with colistin. Combination therapy with Rifampin did not improve clinical response or 30-day mortality in patients with Acinetobacter infections (*CID 2013, 57:349; Epidemiol Infect 2013, 141:1214*). In vitro and in vivo exposure to polymyxins prevented emergence of resistance and augmented sub-populations. In vitro, minocycline prevented resistance to polymyxins. Tigecycline may function similarly, but no data. Colistin activity but no clinical trial data. | **Nephrotoxicity** (*Pharmacotherapy 35:28, 2015*): Reversible acute tubular necrosis due to localization of drug in proximal tubular cells: *AAC 2015; 61:e02339-16*. Depending on criteria, incidence of toxicity varies, average around 25%. Risk factors: length of therapy, daily dose, and cumulative dose; exposure to concomitant nephrotoxins; obesity, diabetes mellitus, age and hypertension. In animal models, high dose ascorbic acid and melatonin prevented toxicity. In critically ill, the benefit of patient salvage may exceed the risk of nephrotoxicity.<br><br>**Neurotoxicity:** Frequent vertigo, facial paresthesias, abnormal vision, confusion, ataxia. Rarely, neuromuscular blockade results in respiratory failure; may unmask or exacerbate myasthenia gravis. In cystic fibrosis patients, 29% experienced paresthesias, ataxia or both.<br><br>**Other:** Maybe hyper-pigmentation (*CID 45:136, 2007*).<br><br>**Discussion and critiques of current dosing recommendations.** The PK Study Group favors the EMA recommendations over the current (June 2016) U.S. FDA approved dosing (*CID 2016, 62:552*). The weight- and CrCl-based approach in the FDA approved dosing is more complicated than either the PK Study Group or EMA recommendations. The PK Study Group recommendations are based on PK study of 214 critically ill patients (*CID 2017; 64:565*). In patients with CrCl >80 mL/min, EMA recommended doses failed to achieve target serum concentration in 66% of patients versus less than 10% in patients with CrCl < 80 mL/min (*CID 2016, 62:552*) due to rapid renal clearance of colistimethate prodrug with less time for conversion to active colistin.<br><br>**Total Daily maintenance dose:**<br><br>(see table below) |

**Total Daily maintenance dose:**

| CrCl (mL/min) | PK Study Group (doses div bid or tid)* | EMA (doses div bid or tid)* | U.S. FDA (Wt - IBW)* |
|---|---|---|---|
| ≥90 | 360 mg/day | 300 mg/day | 2.5-5 mg/kg/day div 2-4 doses |
| 80 to <90 | 340 mg/day | | |
| 70 to <80 | 300 mg/day | | 2.5-3.8 mg/kg/day div 2 doses |
| 60 to <70 | 275 mg/day | | |
| 50 to <60 | 245 mg/day | | |
| 40 to <50 | 220 mg/day | 183-250 mg/day | 2.5 mg/kg once daily or div |
| 30 to <40 | 195 mg/day | | |
| 20 to <30 | 175 mg/day | 150-183 mg/day | 1.5 mg/kg q36h |
| 10 to <20 | 160 mg/day | | |
| 5 to <10 | 145 mg/day | 117 mg/day | N/R |
| <5 | 130 mg/day | | |

\* All doses are stated as colistin base activity (CBA) in mg.<br>IBW = ideal body weight

(See page 2 for abbreviations)

*NOTE: all dosage recommendations are for adults (unless otherwise indicated) & assume normal renal function.

**TABLE 10A (12)**

| CLASS, AGENT, GENERIC NAME (TRADE NAME) | USUAL ADULT DOSAGE* | ADVERSE REACTIONS, COMMENTS (See Table 10B for Summary) |
|---|---|---|
| **MISCELLANEOUS AGENTS** | | |
| Fosfomycin (Monurol) (3 gm packet) | 3 gm with water po times 1 dose. For emergency use: single patient, IND for IV use. From FDA: 1-888-463-6332. | Diarrhea in 9% compared to 6% of pts given nitrofurantoin and 2.3% given TMP-SMX. Available outside U.S., IV & po, for treatment of multi-drug resistant bacteria. For MDR-GNB: 6-12 gm/day IV divided q6-8h. Ref: *Int J Antimicrob Ag 37:415, 2011.* |
| Fusidic acid[NUS] (Fucidin, Taksta) | 500 mg po/IV tid (Denmark & Canada) US: loading dose of 1500 mg po bid x 1 day, then 600 mg po bid | Activity vs. MRSA of importance. Approved outside the U.S.; currently in U.S. clinical trials. Ref for proposed US regimen: *CID 52 (Suppl 7):S520, 2011.* |
| Methenamine hippurate (Hiprex, Urex) | 1 gm po qid | Nausea and vomiting, skin rash or dysuria. Overall ~3%. Methenamine requires (pH ≤5.5) urine to liberate formaldehyde. Use of agents to acidify urine no longer recommended; do not use to treat pyelonephritis. **Comment:** Do not force fluids; may dilute formaldehyde. Of no value in pts with chronic Foley. If urine pH >5.5, co-administer ascorbic acid (1–2 gm q4h) to acidify the urine; cranberry juice (1200–4000 mL per day) has been used; results 120-mile. |
| Methenamine mandelate (Mandelamine) | 1 gm po qid | Do not use concomitantly with sulfonamides (precipitate), or in presence of renal or severe hepatic dysfunction. |
| Metronidazole (Flagyl) (250, 375, 500 mg tab/cap) Prevotella sp: some resistance (*JAC 2018;73:265*). | Anaerobic infections: usually IV, 7.5 mg per kg (~500 mg) q6h (not to exceed 4 gm q24h). With long T½, can use IV at 15 mg per kg q12h. If life-threatening, use loading dose of IV 15 mg per kg. Oral dose: 500 mg qid; extended release tabs available 750 mg | **Common AEs:** nausea (12%), metallic taste, "furry" tongue. **Avoid alcohol during 48 hrs after last dose to avoid disulfiram reaction (N/V, flushing, tachycardia, dyspnea).** Neurologic AEs with high dose/long Rx: peripheral, autonomic and optic neuropathy. **Aseptic meningitis, encephalopathy, seizures & reversible cerebellar lesion** reported (*NEJM 374:1465, 2016*); *CID 2017;64:525*. Risk of hypoglycemia with concomitant sulfonylureas. Can use IV soln as enema for C. diff colitis. **Resistant anaerobic organisms:** Actinomyces, Peptostreptococci. **Once-daily IV dosing of** 1,500 mg: based on long serum T1/2; standard in Europe (*JAC 19:410, 2007*). **Safe to use in pregnancy** (*Curr Drug Safety 2015;10:170*). |
| Nitazoxanide | See Table 13B, page 173 | |
| Nitrofurantoin Systematic rev: *JAC 70:2456, 2015* | Active UTI: Furadantin/Macrobid 50-100 mg po qid x 5-7 days OR Macrobid 100 mg po bid x 5-7 days Decreased UTI suppression: 50-100 mg at bedtime | Absorption ↑ with meals. Increased activity in acid urine, much reduced at pH 8 or over. Nausea and vomiting, peripheral neuropathy, pancreatitis. **Pulmonary reactions** (with chronic rx): acute ARDS type, **chronic desquamative interstitial pneumonia with fibrosis.** Intrahepatic cholestasis & **hepatitis** (DRESS) hypersensitivity syndrome reported (*Weth J Med 67:147, 2009*). Drug rash, eosinophilia, similar to chronic active. Hemolytic anemia in G6PD deficiency. Birth defects: increased risk reported (*Arch Ped Adolesc Med 163:978, 2009*). Should not be used in infants <1 month of age. |
| Rifampin (Rimactane, Rifadin) (150, 300 mg cap) | 300 mg po/IV bid or 600 mg po/IV qd. Rapid selection of resistant bacteria if used as monotherapy | Causes orange-brown discoloration of sweat, urine, tears, contact lens. **Many important drug-drug interactions;** see *Table 22A.* Immune complex flu-like syndrome: fever, headache, myalgias, arthralgia—especially with intermittent rx. Drug induced immune hemolytic/thrombocytopenia (*J Thrombosis & Haemostasis 2012;11:169*). Can cause interstitial nephritis. Risk-benefit of adding RIF to standard therapies for S. aureus endocarditis (*AAC 52:2463, 2008*). See also, *Antimycobacterial Agents, Table 12B, page 157.* |
| Rifaximin (Xifaxan) (200, 550 mg tab) | Traveler's diarrhea: 200 mg tab po tid times 3 days. Hepatic encephalopathy: 550 mg tab po bid. C. diff diarrhea as "chaser": 400 mg po bid | For traveler's diarrhea and hepatic encephalopathy (*AAC 54:3618, 2010; NEJM 362:1071, 2010*). In general, adverse events equal to or less than placebo. Monitor INR in those taking warfarin. Systemic exposure may increase with severe hepatic disease or P-glycoprotein inhibitors. |
| Secnidazole (Solosec) | 2 gm packet (granules): sprinkle on applesauce, yogurt or pudding and consume mixture within 30 min without chewing granules. Follow with glass of water to aid swallowing. | Nitroimidazole for treatment of bacterial vaginosis in adults. Vulvo-vaginal candidiasis may develop requiring antifungal therapy. Potential carcinogenicity seen in rodent studies. Avoid chronic use. **AEs:** Vulvo-vaginal candidiasis (≥2%), headache, nausea, dysgeusia, vomiting, diarrhea, abdominal pain, vulvo-vaginal pruritus. |
| Sulfonamides (e.g., sulfisoxazole (Gantrisin), sulfamethoxazole (Gantanol), (Truxazole), sulfadiazine) | Dose varies with indications. See Nocardia & Toxoplasmosis | **CNS:** fever, headache, dizziness; **Derm:** mild rash to life threatening Stevens-Johnson syndrome, toxic epidermal necrolysis (*Br J Derm 2016;174:1194*), photosensitivity. **Hem:** agranulocytosis, aplastic anemia, **Cross-allergenicity:** other sulfa drugs, diuretics, crystalluria—older sulfonamides (can occur with sulfadiazine-need ≥1500 mL po fluid/day); **Other:** serum sickness, hemolysis if G6PD def, polyarteritis, SLE reported. |

*NOTE: all dosage recommendations are for adults (unless otherwise indicated) & assume normal renal function.

*See page 2 for abbreviations.)

**TABLE 10A (13)**

| CLASS, AGENT, GENERIC NAME (TRADE NAME) | USUAL ADULT DOSAGE* | ADVERSE REACTIONS, COMMENTS *(See Table 10B for Summary)* |
|---|---|---|
| **MISCELLANEOUS AGENTS** *(continued)* | | |
| **Tinidazole** (Tindamax) | **Tabs 250, 500 mg.** Dose for giardiasis: 2 gm po times 1 with food. | **Adverse reactions:** metallic taste 3.7%, nausea 3.2%, anorexia/vomiting 1.5%. All higher with multi-day dosing. Avoid alcohol during 3 to 7 days. after last dose: cause disulfiram reaction, flushing, N/V, tachycardia. |
| **Trimethoprim** (Trimpex, Proloprim, and others). (100, 200 mg tab) | 100 mg po q12h or 200 mg q24h. | **CNS:** drug fever, aseptic meningitis; **Derm:** rash (3-7% at 200 mg/day), photoxicity, Stevens-Johnson syndrome (rare), toxic epidermal necrolysis (rare); **Renal:** ↑K+ (↑Na+, ↑Cr). Hem: neutropenia, thrombocytopenia, methemoglobinemia. ACE inhibitors & aldactone increase serum K+. Higher incidence & severity when combined. Increased risk of death. *BMJ 2014; 349:g6196.* Mechanism: *JAMA 2015; 314:2406.* |
| **Trimethoprim (TMP)–Sulfamethoxazole (SMX)** (Bactrim, Septra, Sulfatrim, Cotrimoxazole) Single-strength (SS) is 80 TMP/400 SMX, double-strength (DS) 160 TMP/800 SMX | **Standard po rx: 1 DS tab bid. P. jirovecii IV rx (base on TMP component):** standard 8–10 mg per kg IV per day divided q6h, q8h, or q12h. For shigellosis: 2.5 mg per kg IV q6h. | Adverse reactions in 10%: GI nausea, vomiting, anorexia. Skin: Rash, urticaria, photosensitivity. More serious (1–10%): death (*BMJ 2014; 349:g6196, 2014*). TMP, ACE inhibitors & aldactone increase serum K+. Higher incidence of severity when combined. Increased risk of death (*BMJ 2014; 349:g6196, 2014*). Stevens-Johnson syndrome & toxic epidermal necrolysis. Skin reactions may represent toxic metabolites of SMX rather than allergy (*Ann Pharmacotherapy 32:381, 1998*). Daily ascorbic acid 0.5–1.0 gm may promote detoxification (*JAIDS 36:1041, 2004*). Risk of **hypoglycemia** with concomitant sulfonylureas. **Sweet's Syndrome** can occur.<br>Hyperkalemia: Both TMP & ACE inhibitors can block renal tubular secretions of K+ & lead to dangerous hyperkalemia (*BMJ 349:g6196, 2014*).<br>TMP one etiology of **aseptic meningitis**. Report of psychosis during treatment of PCP (*JAC 65:1117, 2011*).<br>TMP-SMX contains sulfites and may trigger asthma in sulfite-sensitive pts. Frequent drug. cause of thrombocytopenia. No cross allergenicity with other sulfonamide non-antibiotic drugs (*NEJM 349:1628, 2003*). **For TMP-SMX desensitization**, see *Table 7, page 91.* |
| **Topical Antimicrobial Agents Active vs. S. aureus & Strep. pyogenes** *(CID 49:1541, 2009)* | | **Review of topical antiseptics, antibiotics** *(CID 49:1541, 2009)* |
| **Bacitracin** (Baciguent) | 20% bacitracin zinc ointment, apply 1-5 x/day. | Active vs. staph, strep & clostridium. Contact dermatitis occurs. Available without prescription. |
| **Fusidic acid**‡ ointment | 2% ointment, apply tid | Available in Canada and Europe (*Leo Laboratories*). Active vs. S. aureus & S. pyogenes. |
| **Mupirocin** (Bactroban) | **Skin cream or ointment 2%: Apply tid times 10 days. Nasal ointment 2%: apply bid times 5 days.** | Skin cream: itch, burning, stinging 1-1.5%; Nasal: headache 9%, rhinitis 6%, respiratory congestion 5%. Not active vs. enterococci or gm-neg bacteria. Summary of resistance: *JAC 70:2681, 2015.* If large amounts used in azotemic pts, can accumulate polyethylene glycol (*CID 49:1541, 2009*). |
| **Polymyxin B–Bacitracin** (Polysporin) | 5000 units/gm; 400 units/gm. Apply 1-4x/day | Polymyxin active vs. some gm-neg bacteria but not Proteus sp., Serratia sp. or gm-pos bacteria. See Bacitracin & polymyxin B comments above. Available without prescription. |
| **Polymyxin B–Bacitracin—Neomycin** (Neosporin, triple antibiotic ointment (TAO)) | 5000 units/gm; 400 units/gm; 3.5 mg/gm. Apply 1-3x/day. | See Bacitracin & polymyxin B comments above. Neomycin active vs. gm-neg bacteria and staphylococci: not active vs. streptococci. Contact dermatitis incidence 1%; risk of nephro- & oto-toxicity if absorbed. TAO spectrum broader than mupirocin and active mupirocin-resistant strains (*JAMID 54:63, 2006*). Available without prescription. |
| **Retapamulin** (Altabax) | 1% ointment; apply 5, 10 & 15 gm tubes. | Microbiologic success in 90% S. aureus infections and 97% of S. pyogenes infections (*J Am Acad Derm 55:1003, 2006*). Package insert says for **MSSA only** (not enough MRSA pts in clinical trials). Active vs. some mupirocin-resistant S. aureus strains. Resistance can occur (see *Clin Micro Infect Dis 36: 322, 2017*). |
| **Silver sulfadiazine** | 1% cream, apply once or twice daily. | A sulfonamide but the active ingredient is released silver ions. Activity vs. gram-pos & gram-neg bacteria (including P. aeruginosa). Often used to prevent infection in 2nd/3rd degree burns. Rarely, may stain into the skin. |

*NOTE: all dosage recommendations are for adults (unless otherwise indicated) & assume normal renal function.

*Footnote:* *NOTE: all dosage recommendations are for adults (unless otherwise indicated) & assume normal renal function.

(See page 2 for abbreviations)

## TABLE 10B – SELECTED ANTIBACTERIAL AGENTS—ADVERSE REACTIONS—OVERVIEW

Adverse reactions in individual patients represent all-or-none occurrences, even if rare. After selection of an agent, the physician should read the manufacturer's package insert [statements in the product labeling (package insert)] must be approved by the FDA]. For unique reactions, see the individual drug (*Table 10A*). For drug-drug interactions, see *Table 22A*.

**Numbers = frequency of occurrence (%); + = occurs, ++ = significant adverse reaction; 0 = not reported; R = rare, defined as <1%.**

**NOTE: Important reactions in bold print. A blank means no data found. Any antibacterial can precipitate C. difficile colitis.**

| ADVERSE REACTIONS (AR) For unique ARs, see individual drug, *Table 10A* | PENICILLINASE-RESISTANT ANTI-STAPH. PENICILLINS | | | | AMINOPENICILLINS | | | | AP PENS | CARBAPENEMS | | | | MONOBACTAMS | AMINOGLYCO-SIDES | MISC. | |
|---|---|---|---|---|---|---|---|---|---|---|---|---|---|---|---|---|---|
| | Penicillin G, V | Dicloxacillin | Nafcillin | Oxacillin | Amoxicillin | Amox-Clav | Ampicillin | Amp-Sulb | Pip-Taz | Doripenem | Ertapenem | Imipenem | Meropenem | Aztreonam | Amikacin Gentamicin Kanamycin Netilmicin[AUS] Tobramycin | Linezolid | Tedizolid |
| Rx stopped due to AR | | | | | 2-4.4 | | | | 3.2 | 3.4 | | | 1.2 | <1 | | | 0.5 |
| Rash | 3 | 4 | 4 | 4 | 5 | 3 | 5 | 2 | 4 | 1-5 | + | 1 | + | 2 | | 2 | |
| + Coombs | 3 | O | R | R | + | O | + | O | + | R | 1 | 2 | + | R | | | |
| Neutropenia | + | R | + | R | R | + | R | + | + | R | 1 | 2 | + | + | | 1.1 | 0.5 |
| Eosinophilia[1] | + | + | 22 | 22 | 2 | 22 | 22 | 22 | + | R | + | + | + | 8 | | | |
| Thrombocytopenia | R | O | O | R | R | R | R | R | + | + | 3 | 2 | 2 | R | | 3 | 2.3 |
| Nausea/vomiting | | + | O | O | 2 | 3 | 2 | + | 7 | 4-12 | 3 | 2 | 4 | R | | 6/4 | 8/3 |
| Diarrhea | R | + | O | O | **5** | **9** | **10** | **2** | 11 | 6-11 | 6 | 2 | 5 | 2 | | 8.3 | 10 |
| ↑ LFTs | R | + | + | + | R | + | R | + | + | + | 6 | 4 | 5 | 4 | | 5-10 | 6 |
| ↑ BUN, Cr | R | O | O | + | R | R | R | R | + | + | 6 | 2 | 4 | 2 | 5-25 | | |
| Seizures | R | O | O | O | O | R | R | R | O | *See footnote[2]* | | + | | + | | R | |
| Ototoxicity | O | O | O | O | O | O | O | O | O | R | | | | O | – 3-14 | | |
| Vestibular | O | O | O | O | O | O | O | O | O | O | | | | O | 4-6 | | |

[1] Eosinophilia in 25% of pts; of those 30% have clinical event (rash 30%, renal injury 15%, liver injury 6%, DRESS in 0.8% (J Allergy Clin Immunol doi 10.1076/j.jaci.2015.04.005).

[2] All β-lactams in high concentration can cause seizures. IMP 10x more neurotoxic than benz. penicillin (JAC 22:687, 1988). In clinical trial of IMP for pediatric meningitis, trial stopped due to seizures in 7/25 IMP recipients; hard to interpret as purulent meningitis causes seizures (PIDJ 10:122, 1991). Risk with IMP ↓ with careful attention to dosage (Epilepsia 42:1590, 2001).

**Postulated mechanism:** Drug binding to GABA$_A$ receptor. IMP binds with greater affinity than MER.

**Package insert, percent seizures:** ERTA 0.5, IMP 0.4, MER 0.7. However, in 3 clinical trials of MER for bacterial meningitis, no drug-related seizures (Scand J Inf Dis 31:3, 1999; Drug Safety 22:191, 2000). In meta-analysis, seizure risk low but greatest with carbapenems vs. other beta-lactams. No difference in incidence between IMP & MER (JAC 69:2043, 2014).

## TABLE 10B (2)

### CEPHALOSPORINS/CEPHAMYCINS

| ADVERSE REACTIONS (AR) For unique ARs, see individual drug, Table 10A | Cefazolin | Cefotetan | Cefoxitin | Cefuroxime | Cefotaxime | Ceftazidime | Ceftaz-avi | Ceftizoxime | Ceftriaxone | Cefepime | Ceftaroline | Ceftobiprole^NUS | Ceftolo-tazo | Cefaclor/Cef.ER/Loracarbef^NUS | Cefadroxil | Cefdinir | Cefixime | Cefpodoxime | Cefprozil | Ceftibuten | Cefditoren pivoxil | Cefuroxime axetil | Cephalexin |
|---|---|---|---|---|---|---|---|---|---|---|---|---|---|---|---|---|---|---|---|---|---|---|---|
| Rx stopped due to AR | + | 3 | | | 2 | 2 | <5 | 2 | 2 | 1.5 | 2.7 | 4 | 2 | 1 | | 3 | 1 | 2.7 | 1 | 2 | 2 | 2.2 | 2.2 |
| Rash | 3 | + | 2 | R | 2 | 2 | R | 2 | 2 | 2 | 3 | 2.7 | R | R | + | R | R | R | 1 | R | R | R | 1 |
| + Coombs | 3 | + | 2 | R | 6 | 4 | 2 | | | 14 | 9.8 | | <1 | R | + | R | R | R | R | 5 | R | R | 3 |
| Neutropenia | + | | 2 | R | + | | | + | | | | + | | | | | R | R | 2 | | R | R | |
| Eosinophilia | + | 3 | 3 | 7 | 1 | 8 | <5 | + | 6 | 1 | | + | | 2 | | | | 3 | | | | 1 | 9 |
| Thrombocytopenia | + | ++ | | | | | <5 | + | + | + | | + | | | | | R | R | | R | | | |
| ↑ PT/PTT | | ++ | | | | R | | R | R | + | 4/2 | + | 3/1 | | | | 7 | 4 | | | | | |
| Nausea/vomiting | 4 | 4 | 2 | R | R | 1 | 2 | | | 1 | 5 | 9.1/4.8 | 2 | 1-4 | | 15 | 16 | 7 | 4 | 3 | 6/1 | 1 | |
| Diarrhea | 4 | 1 | 3 | R | 1 | | 4 | 3 | 3 | | 2 | <2 | 1.7 | 3 | + | 1 | R | 4 | 2 | 3 | 1.4 | 3 | |
| ↑ LFTs | + | | | 4 | | 6 | | 4 | 3 | | | R | | + | | 15 | | | 2 | | | | + |
| Hepatic failure | 0 | 0 | 0 | 0 | 0 | | | 0 | 0 | 0 | | R | 1.5 | + | | | | 4 | | | R | R | + |
| ↑ BUN, Cr | 0 | | 0 | 0 | 0 | R | 1.5 | 0 | 1 | + | | 4.5 | 1.5 | 3 | | 2 | | 4 | | | R | R | + |
| Headache | 0 | 3 | 0 | 4 | 0 | 1 | 10 | 3 | R | 2 | 2 | 6 | 6 | 3 | | 2 | R | 1 | R | R | 2 | R | + |

### MACROLIDES / FLUOROQUINOLONES / OTHER AGENTS

| ADVERSE REACTIONS (AR) For unique ARs, see individual drug, Table 10A | Azithromycin, Reg. & ER | Clarithromycin, Reg. & ER | Erythromycin | Ciprofloxacin/ CIP XR | Gatifloxacin^NUS | Gemifloxacin | Levofloxacin | Moxifloxacin | Ofloxacin | Chloramphenicol | Clindamycin | Polymyxin B & E (Colistin) | Daptomycin | Dalbavancin | Oritavancin | Metronidazole | Quinupristin-Dalfopristin | Rifampin | Telavancin | Tetracycline/ Doxy/Mino | Tigecycline | TMP-SMX | Vancomycin |
|---|---|---|---|---|---|---|---|---|---|---|---|---|---|---|---|---|---|---|---|---|---|---|---|
| Rx stopped due to AR | 1 | R | 1 | 3.5 | 3 | 2.2 | 2.9 | 4 | 4 | | | | 2.8 | 3 | 3.8 | | R | | 5 | | 5 | | |
| Rash | R | 3 | + | 3 | R | 1-2[3] | 2 | R | 2 | + | + | + | 4 | 2.7 | <1.5 | + | R | R | 4 | + | 2.4 | + | 3 |
| Nausea/vomiting | 5 | 3 | 25 | 5 | 8/<3 | 2.7 | 7/2 | 7/2 | 7 | + | 7 | | 6.3 | 6/3 | 9.9/4.6 | 12 | | + | 27/14 | + | 30/20 | + | + |
| Diarrhea | 5 | 3-6 | 8 | 2 | 3.6 | 5 | 5 | 5 | 4 | + | 7 | | 3.7 | 4.4 | 3.7 | | 2 | + | 7 | + | 13 | + | + |
| ↑ LFTs | R | R | + | 2 | R | 1.5 | 0.1-1 | 2 | 2 | + | + | | 2.8 | 0.8 | 2.8 | + | 2 | + | 3 | + | 4 | + | |
| ↑ BUN, Cr | + | 4 | + | 1 | R | | | R | R | | 0 | ++ | R | | | | | + | 3 | + | 2 | + | 5 |
| Dizziness, light headedness | R | 2 | | R | 3 | 0.8 | 3 | 2 | 3 | | | | 2.7 | | 2.7 | + | | | | + | 3.5 | + | |
| Headache | R | 2 | | 1 | 4 | 1.2 | 6 | 2 | | | + | | 4.7 | | 7.1 | | | + | | + | | + | + |

[3] Highest frequency: females <40 years of age after 14 days of rx; with 5 days or less of Gemi; incidence of rash <1.5%.

## TABLE 10C – ANTIMICROBIAL AGENTS ASSOCIATED WITH PHOTOSENSITIVITY

The following drugs (listed alphabetically) are known to cause photosensitivity in some individuals. Note that photosensitivity lasts for several days after the last dose of the drug, at least for tetracyclines. There is no intent to indicate relative frequency or severity of reactions. *Ref: Drug Saf 34:821, 2011.*

| DRUG OR CLASS | COMMENT |
|---|---|
| Antiparasitic drugs | Pyrimethamine (one report), Quinine (may cross-react with quinidine) |
| Azole antifungals | Voriconazole, Itraconazole, Ketoconazole, but not Fluconazole |
| Cefotaxime | Manifested as photodistributed telangiectasia |
| Ceftazidime | Increased susceptibility to sunburn observed |
| Dapsone | Confirmed by rechallenge |
| Efavirenz | Three reports |
| Flucytosine | Two reports |
| Fluoroquinolones | Worst offenders have halogen atom at position 8; lowest risk: Delaflox |
| Griseofulvin | Not thought to be a potent photosensitizer |
| Isoniazid | Confirmed by rechallenge |
| Pyrazinamide | Confirmed by rechallenge |
| Saquinavir | One report |
| Tetracyclines | Least common with Minocycline; common with Doxycycline |
| Trimethoprim | Alone and in combination with Sulfamethoxazole |

## TABLE 10D – AMINOGLYCOSIDE ONCE-DAILY AND MULTIPLE DAILY DOSING REGIMENS
### (If estimated CrCl <90 mL/min or if on dialysis, see Table 17A, page 235)

- General Note: dosages are given as **once daily dose (OD)** and **multiple daily doses (MDD)**.

- For **calculation of dosing weight in non-obese patients** use **Ideal Body Weight (IBW):**

  Female: 45.5 kg + 2.3 kg per inch over 60 inch height = dosing weight in kg;

  Male: 50 kg + 2.3 kg per inch over 60 inch height = dosing weight in kg.

- **Adjustment for calculation of dosing weight in obese patients** (actual body weight (ABW) is ≥30% above IBW): IBW + 0.4 (ABW minus IBW)= adjusted weight (*Pharmacotherapy 27:1081, 2007; CID 25:112, 1997*).

- If estimated CrCl >90 mL/min or if on dialysis, **use doses in this table. If CrCl <90 mL/min, use doses in Table 17A, page 235.**

- For **non-obese patients, calculate estimated creatinine clearance (CrCl) as follows:**

$$\frac{(140 \text{ minus age/IBW in kg})}{72 \times \text{serum creatinine}} = \frac{\text{CrCl in mL/min for men.}}{\text{Multiply answer by 0.85 for women (estimated)}}$$

- For **morbidly obese patients, calculate estimated creatinine clearance (CrCl) as follows** (*AJM 84:1053, 1988*):

$$\frac{(137 \text{ minus age}) \times [(0.285 \times \text{wt in kg}) + (12.1 \times \text{ht in meters}^2)]}{51 \times \text{serum creatinine}} = \text{CrCl (obese male)}$$

$$\frac{(146 \text{ minus age}) \times [(0.287 \times \text{wt in kg}) + (9.74 \times \text{ht in meters}^2)]}{60 \times \text{serum creatinine}} = \text{CrCl (obese female)}$$

| DRUG | MDD AND OD IV REGIMENS/ TARGETED PEAK (P) AND TROUGH (T) SERUM LEVELS | COMMENTS For more data on once-daily dosing, see AAC 55:2528, 2011 and Table 17A, page 235 |
|---|---|---|
| Gentamicin (Garamycin), Tobramycin (Nebcin) | MDD: 2 mg per kg load, then 1.7 mg per kg q8h<br>   P 4-10 mcg/mL, T 1-2 mcg per mL<br>OD: 5.1 (7 if critically ill) mg per kg q24h<br>   P 16-24 mcg per mL, T <1 mcg per mL | All aminoglycosides have potential to cause tubular necrosis and renal failure, deafness due to cochlear toxicity, vertigo due to damage to vestibular organs, and rarely neuromuscular blockade. Risk minimal with oral or topical application due to small % absorption unless tissues altered by disease. |
| Kanamycin (Kantrex), Amikacin (Amikin), Streptomycin | MDD: 7.5 mg per kg q12h<br>   P 15-30 mcg per mL, T 5-10 mcg per mL<br>OD: 15 mg per kg q24h<br>   P 56-64 mcg per mL, T <1 mcg per mL | Risk of nephrotoxicity ↑ with concomitant administration of cyclosporine, vancomycin, ampho B, radiocontrast.<br>Risk of nephrotoxicity ↓ by once-daily dosing method (especially if baseline renal function normal).<br>In general, same factors influence risk of ototoxicity.<br>**NOTE: There is no known method to eliminate risk of aminoglycoside nephro/ototoxicity. Proper rx attempts to ↓ the % risk.** |
| Netilmicin[NUS] | MDD: 2 mg per kg q8h<br>   P 4-10 mcg per mL, T 1-2 mcg per mL<br>OD: 6.5 mg per kg q24h<br>   P 22-30 mcg per mL, T <1 mcg per mL | The clinical trial data of OD aminoglycosides have been reviewed extensively by meta-analysis (*CID 24:816, 1997*).<br>**Serum levels:** Collect peak serum level (PSL) exactly 1 hr after the start of the infusion of the 3rd dose in critically ill pts. PSL after the 1st dose in volume of distribution and renal function may change rapidly |
| Plazomicin (Zemdri) | OD: Severe infections 15 mg per kg q24h, less severe 8 mg per kg q24h<br>P: 74 mcg per mL, T: <1 mcg per mL | |
| Isepamicin[NUS] | Only OD: Severe infections 15 mg per kg q24h, less severe 8 mg per kg q24h | One in 500 patients (Europe) have mitochondrial mutation that predicts cochlear toxicity (*NEJM 360:640 & 642, 2009*). Aspirin supplement (3 gm/day) attenuated risk of cochlear injury from gentamicin (*NEJM 354:1856, 2006*). Vestibular injury usually bilateral & hence no vertigo but imbalance & oscillopsia (*Med J Aust 196:701, 2012*). |
| Spectinomycin (Trobicin)[NUS] | 2 gm IM times 1-gonococcal infections | |
| Neomycin-oral | Prophylaxis GI surgery: 1 gm po times 3 with erytho, see Table 15B, page 219<br>For hepatic coma: 4-12 gm per day po | |

**Tobramycin–inhaled** (Tobi): See *Cystic Fibrosis, Table 1, page 46 & Table 10F, page 130*. Adverse effects few: transient voice alteration (13%) and transient tinnitus (3%).

**Paromomycin–oral:** See *Entamoeba and Cryptosporidia, Table 13A, page 160*.

## TABLE 10E – PROLONGED OR CONTINUOUS INFUSION DOSING OF SELECTED ANTIBIOTICS

**Prolonged or continuous infusion of beta-lactams is at least as successful as intermittent dosing.** Hence, this approach can be part of stewardship programs as supported by recent publications.

**Antibiotic stability is a concern.** Factors influencing stability include drug concentration, IV infusion diluent (e.g. NS vs. D5W), type of infusion device, and storage temperature (Ref & Ref 36:723, 2011). Portable pumps worn close to the body expose antibiotics to temperatures closer to body temperature (37°C) than to room temperature (around 25°C). Carbapenems are particularly unstable and may require wrapping of infusion pumps in cold packs or frequent changes of infusion bags or cartridges.

A meta-analysis of observational studies found reduced mortality among patients treated with extended or continuous infusion of carbapenems or piperacillin-tazobactam (pooled data) as compared to standard intermittent regimens. The results were similar for extended and continuous regimens when considered separately. There was a mortality benefit with piperacillin-tazobactam but not carbapenems (CID 56:272, 2013). The lower mortality could, at least in part, be due to closer professional supervision engendered by a study environment. On the other hand, a small prospective randomized controlled study of continuous vs. intermittent Pip-Tazo, and meropenem found a higher clinical cure rate and a trend toward lower mortality in the continuous infusion patients (CID 56:236, 2013).

| DRUG/METHOD | MINIMUM STABILITY | RECOMMENDED DOSE | COMMENTS |
|---|---|---|---|
| **Ampicillin-sulbactam** (Prolonged) | @ 37°C: In NS at 24 hr amp 77%, sulb 93% (IJAA 6:S31, 1996)<br>@ 25°C: 8 hr (NS)ᵃ<br>@ 4°C: 48 hr (NS)ᵃ<br>ᵃ(amp/sulb conc ≤ 30 mg/15 mg per mL) | 12 gm (8 gm amp + 4 gm sulb) IV over 4 hours q8h | Recommended dose is for VAP due to Acinetobacter. High dose found safe and effective in observational studies (Scand J ID 39:38, 2007; J Infect 56:432, 2008). The need for a high-dose prolonged-infusion sulbactam regimen is supported by pharmacodynamic computer simulation studies using serum concentration measurements in healthy volunteers (AAC 57:3441, 2013). Recommended dose is for patients with normal renal function. |
| **Cefepime** (Continuous) | @ 37°C: 8 hours<br>@ 25°C: 24 hours<br>@ 4°C: 24 hours | Initial dose: 15 mg/kg over 30 min, then immediately begin:<br>• If CrCl >60: 6 gm (over 24 hr) daily<br>• If CrCl 30-60: 4 gm (over 24 hr) daily<br>• If CrCl 11-29: 2 gm (over 24 hr) daily | CrCl adjustments extrapolated from prescribing information, not clinical data.<br>Refs: JAC 57:1017, 2006; Am. J. Health Syst. Pharm. 68:319, 2011. |
| **Ceftazidime** (Continuous) | @ 37°C: 8 hours<br>@ 25°C: 24 hours<br>@ 4°C: 24 hours | Initial dose: 15 mg/kg over 30 min, then immediately begin:<br>• If CrCl >50: 6 gm (over 24 hr) daily<br>• If CrCl 31-50: 4 gm (over 24 hr) daily<br>• If CrCl 10-30: 2 gm (over 24 hr) daily | CrCl adjustments extrapolated from prescribing information, not clinical data.<br>Refs: Br J Clin Pharmacol 50:184, 2000; IJAA 17:497, 2001; AAC 49:3550, 2005; Infect 37: 418, 2009; JAC 68:900, 2013. |
| **Doripenem** (Prolonged) | @ 37°C: 8 hours (in NS)<br>@ 25°C: 24 hours (in NS)<br>@ 4°C: 24 hours (in NS) | • If CrCl ≥50: 500 mg (over 4 hr) q8h<br>• If CrCl 30-49: 250 mg (over 4 hr) q8h<br>• If CrCl 10-29: 250 mg (over 4 hr) q12h | Based on a single study (Crit Care Med 36:1089, 2008). |
| **Meropenem** (Prolonged) | @ 37°C: <4 hours<br>@ 25°C: 4 hours<br>@ 4°C: 24 hours | • If CrCl ≥50: 2 gm (over 3 hr) q8h<br>• If CrCl 30-49: 1 gm (over 3 hr) q8h<br>• If CrCl 10-29: 1 gm (over 3 hr) q12h | Initial 1 gm dose reasonable but not used by most investigators.<br>Ref: Intens Care Med 37:632, 2011. |
| **PIP-TZ** (Prolonged) | @ 37°C: 24 hours<br>@ 25°C: 24 hours<br>@ 4°C: no data | Initial dose: 4.5 gm over 30 min, then 4 hrs later start:<br>• If CrCl ≥20: 3.375 gm (over 4 hr) q8h<br>• If CrCl <20: 3.375 gm (over 4 hr) q12h | Reasonable to begin first infusion 4 hrs after initial dose.<br>Refs: CID 44:357, 2007; AAC 54:460, 2010.<br>See CID 56:236, 245 & 272, 2013. In obese patients (>120 kg), may need higher doses: 6.75 gm or even 9 gm (over 4 hrs) q8h to achieve adequate serum levels of tazobactam (Int J Antimicrob Agts 41:52, 2013). |
| **Temocillin** | @ 37°C: 24 hours<br>@ 25°C: 24 hours<br>These apply to Temocillin 4 gm/48 mL dilution (JAC 61:382, 2008) | Initial dose: 2 gm over 30 min, then immediately begin:<br>• If CrCl >50: 6 gm (over 24 hr) daily<br>• If CrCl 31-50: 3 gm (over 24 hr) daily<br>• If CrCl 10-30: 1.5 gm (over 24 hr) daily<br>• If CrCl <10: 750 mg (over 24 hr) daily<br>CVVH: 750 mg (over 24 hr) daily | CVVH: 750 mg (over 24 hr) daily offers higher probability of reaching desired PK/PD targets than conventional q8h dosing. This study not designed to assess clinical efficacy (JAC 70:891, 2015). |

## TABLE 1OE (2)

| DRUG/METHOD | MINIMUM STABILITY | RECOMMENDED DOSE | COMMENTS |
|---|---|---|---|
| Vancomycin (Continuous) | @ 37°C: 48 hours<br>@ 25°C: 48 hours<br>@ 4°C: 58 days<br>(at conc 10 µg/mL) | Loading dose of 15-20 mg/kg over 30-60 minutes, then 30 mg/kg by continuous infusion over 24 hrs. No data on pts with renal impairment. | Adjust dose to target plateau concentration of 20-25 µg/mL. Higher plateau concentrations (30-40 µg/mL) achieved with more aggressive dosing increase the risk of nephrotoxicity (*Clin Micro Inf 19:E98, 2013*). The AUC/MIC ratio is superior to T-MIC for predicting Vancomycin efficacy. Successful treatment of MRSA is associated with a steady-state AUC$_{24}$/MIC of ≥400. Vancomycin administration by continuous infusion is gaining acceptance as a treatment option although limited clinical data demonstrate no improvement in efficacy over intermittent infusion although target concentrations are more rapidly achieved with less variability (*JAC 68:743, 2013; Ann Pharmacother 47:279, 2013*). A recent meta-analysis suggests decreased nephrotoxicity compared to intermittent infusion but definitive conclusions are premature (*JAC 67:17, 2012*). With continuous infusion the AUC$_{24}$ can be calculated by multiplying a single concentration measured at state state by 24 (*JAC 62:e02042, 2018*). |

## TABLE 1OF – INHALATION ANTIBIOTICS

There are many reasons to consider inhaled antibiotics as an adjunct to parenteral therapy: • spectrum of activity that includes MDR GNB • documented high drug concentration in lung epithelial alveolar lining fluid • benefit in animal models of pneumonia • improved drug delivery (nebulizer) systems • Low risk of serious AEs. Refs: *Adv Drug Del Rev 2015;85-65* (review); *Chest 2017, 151:737* (clinical debate). The European Medicines Agency (EMA) has approved Colistin dry powder for inhalation.

| INHALED DRUG | DELIVERY SYSTEM | DOSE | COMMENT |
|---|---|---|---|
| Amikacin + Ceftazidime | Vibrating plate nebulizer | AMK: 25 mg/kg once daily x 3 days<br>Ceftaz: 15 mg/kg q3h x 8 days | Radiographic and clinical cure of *P. aeruginosa* ventilator-associated pneumonia (VAP) similar to IV AMK/Ceftaz, including strains with intermediate resistance (*AJRCCM 184:106, 2011*). |
| Aztreonam (Cayston) | Altera vibrating mesh nebulizer | 75 mg tid x 28 days (every other month) | Improves pulmonary function, reduces frequency of exacerbations, and improves symptoms in cystic fibrosis (CF) pts (*Exp Opin Pharmacother 14:2115, 2013*). Cost per treatment cycle about $6070. |
| Colistin (colistimethate) dry powder (EMA approved)<br><br>Note: Polymyxin B is not used for inhalation due to toxicity to lung epithelial cells (*AAC 2017;61:e02690-16*) | Vibrating mesh (*AAC 2014;58:7337*) | 50-75 mg CBA in 3-4 mL saline via vibrating mesh nebulizer 2-3 times/day; concentration in lung epithelial lining is 100-1000x greater with inhaled dosing vs. IV dosing alone.<br>See *AAC 2014; 58:7337.* | • Efficacious vs. *P. aeruginosa* pneumonia in mouse model (*AAC 2017;61:e02025-16*)<br>• Favorable PK in 6 cystic fibrosis (CF) pts (*AAC 2014;58:2570*) and 12 ICU pneumonia pts (*AAC 2014;58:7337*)<br>• Recommended by IDSA HAP/VAP Guidelines as adjunctive rx for GNB susceptible to only polymyxins and AG (*CID 2016;63:e61*) |
| Fosfomycin + Tobramycin (FTI) 4:1 wt/wt | eFlow vibrating mesh nebulizer | FTI 160/40 or 80/20 bid x 28 days | Both doses maintained improvements in FEV1 following a 28-day inhaled aztreonam run-in (vs. placebo) in CF patients with *P. aeruginosa*; FTI 80/20 better tolerated than 160/40 (*AJRCCM 185:171, 2012*). |
| Levofloxacin | eFlow vibrating mesh nebulizer | 240 mg bid x 28 days | Reduced sputum density of *P. aeruginosa*, need for other antibiotics, and improved pulmonary function compared to placebo in CF pts (*AJRCCM 183:1510, 2011*). |
| Liposomal Amikacin (Arikayce) | Lamira Nebulizer System | 590 mg q24h | For refractory MAC when limited or no alternative treatment options. |
| Tobramycin (TOBI, Bethkis) | PARI LC PLUS jet nebulizer | 300 mg bid x 28 days (every other month) | Cost: about $6700 for one treatment cycle (*Med Lett 56:51, 2014*). Major AEs: bronchospasm, voice alteration, transient tinnitus. |
| Tobramycin (TOBI Podhaler) | 28 mg dry powder caps | 4 caps (112 mg) bid x 28 days (every other month) | Improvement in FEV1 similar to Tobra inhaled solution in CF patients with chronic *P. aeruginosa* but more airway irritation with the powder. Cost of one month treatment cycle about $6700 (*Med Lett 56:51, 2014*). |

**TABLE 11A – TREATMENT OF FUNGAL INFECTIONS**
For Antifungal Activity Spectra, see *Table 4B, page 86*

| TYPE OF INFECTION/ORGANISM/ SITE OF INFECTION | ANTIMICROBIAL AGENTS OF CHOICE | | COMMENTS |
|---|---|---|---|
| | PRIMARY | ALTERNATIVE | |
| **Aspergillosis** (A. fumigatus most common, also A. flavus and others) *(See NEJM 360:1870, 2009; Chest 146:1358, 2014).* | | | |
| **Allergic bronchopulmonary aspergillosis (ABPA)** Clinical deterioration (wheezing, pulmonary infiltrates, bronchiectasis & fibrosis. Airway colonization w/fungus. ↑ serum IgE, ↑ blood eosinophils, ↑ serum IgE, ↑ specific serum antibodies. | Acute asthma attacks associated with ABPA. **Corticosteroids** | Rx of ABPA: **Itra** soln 200 mg po bid times 16 wks or longer | Itra decreases number of exacerbations requiring corticosteroids with improved immunological markers, improved lung function & exercise tolerance *(CID 63:433, 2016).* |
| **Allergic fungal sinusitis:** relapsing chronic sinusitis; nasal polyps without bony invasion; asthma, eczema or allergic rhinitis; ↑ IgE levels and isolation of Aspergillus sp. or other dematiaceous sp. (Alternaria, Cladosporium, etc.) | **Rx controversial:** systemic corticosteroids + surgical debridement (relapse common). | For failures try **Itra** 200 mg po bid times 12 mos or **Flu** nasal spray. | Controversial area. |
| **Aspergilloma (fungus ball)** | No therapy or surgical resection. Efficacy of antimicrobial agents not proven. | | Aspergillus may complicate pulmonary sequestration. |
| **Invasive, pulmonary (IPA) or extrapulmonary:** Post-transplantation and post-chemotherapy in neutropenic pts w/prolonged neutropenia. Common pneumonia in transplant recipients. Usually acute (<30 days); complication in allogeneic bone marrow & liver transplantation. High mortality *(CID 44:531, 2007).*

**Typical x-ray/CT lung lesions** (halo sign, cavitation, or macronodules) *(CID 44:373, 2007).*
**Galactomannan antigen immunoassay:** Detects aspergillus cell wall polysaccharide. Adjunct to diagnosis in neutropenic pts. Serum sens/spec. varies from 71-86% sens/80-92% spec. BAL fluid 60-100% sens/68-100% spec. False neg. if receiving antifungals. False pos. if colonized by aspergillus or infected by Fusarium, histo or blasto *(JAMA 298:2178-1175).*
**Better diagnostic strategy:** combination of serum galactomannan & aspergillus PCR (not routinely) *(LnID 13:519, 2013).*
**Beta D-Glucan** in fungal cell wall. Can detect with immunoassay. Many false positives + low sensitivity *(JCM 51:3478, 2013).* | **Primary therapy** *(See CID 63:433, 2016):*
**Vori** 6 mg/kg IV q12h on day 1; then either (4 mg/kg IV q12h) or (200 mg po q12h for body weight ≥40 kg, but 100 mg po q12h for body weight <40 kg) (use actual wt). Goal trough (day 4): 1.0-5.5 mg/L associated with improved response rates and reduced adverse effects *(Clin Infect Dis 55:1080, 2012).*

**Alternative therapies:**
**Isavuconazonium sulfate** loading dose of 372 mg (equivalent to isavuconazole 200 mg) IV/po q8 x 6 doses then 372 mg IV/po daily
OR
**Liposomal Ampho B (LAB)** (L-AmB) 3-5 mg/kg/day IV;
OR
**Ampho B lipid complex** (ABLC) 5 mg/kg/d IV;
OR
**Caspo** 70 mg/day IV load then 50 mg/day thereafter;
OR
**Mica**^AA 100 mg bid *(JAC 64:840, 2009– based on PK/PD study);*
OR
**Posa**^AA 200 mg qid, then 400 mg bid after stabilization of disease.

In documented azole-resistant invasive aspergillosis, most experts suggest change to either **Liposomal Ampho B** or combination of **Vori + echinocandin** *(IJID 2017;276(S3):S436)* | **Vori**, both a substrate and an inhibitor of CYP2C19, CYP2C9, and CYP3A4, has potential for deleterious drug interactions (e.g., with protease inhibitors). Review concomitant medications. Measure serum level with prolonged therapy or for patients with possible drug-drug interactions. In patients with CrCl <50 mL/min, po may be preferred due to concerns for nephrotoxicity of IV vehicle in renal dysfunction. *(Clin Infect Dis 54:913, 2012)*
**Isavuconazole** (prodrug isavuconazonium sulfate): A randomized control trial of isavuconazole vs. Voriconazole for invasive aspergillosis demonstrated that isavuconazole is non-inferior to voriconazole for the treatment of invasive aspergillosis *(Ln 2016;387:760).*
**Ampho B: not recommended except as a lipid formulation**, either L-AMB or ABLC. 10 mg/kg and 3 mg/kg doses of L-AMB are equally efficacious with greater toxicity of higher dose *(CID 2007; 44:1289–97).* One comparative trial found greater toxicity with ABLC than with L-AMB. 34.6% vs 9.4% adverse events and 21.2% vs 8% nephrotoxicity *(Cancer 112:1282, 2008).* Vori preferred as primary therapy
**Posaconazole:** 42% response rate in open-label trial of patients refractory/ intolerant to conventional therapy *(CID 44:2, 2007).* Concern for cross-resistance with azole-non-responders. Measurement of serum concentrations advisable.
**Caspofungin:** ~50% response rate in IPA. Licensed for salvage therapy.
**Micafungin:** Favorable responses to micafungin as a single agent in 6/12 patients in primary therapy group and 9/22 in the salvage therapy group *(J Infect 53: 337, 2006).*
**Combination therapy:** RCT of Voriconazole plus Anidulafungin vs. Voriconazole alone (Ann Intern Med 162:81, 2015). Subgroup of patients with invasive aspergillosis whose diagnosis was established by radiographic findings and GM positivity had lower mortality with combination therapy. Combination therapy should be strongly considered although further data is needed to determine which patients would benefit the most. Some experts would recommend addition of echinocandin to amphotericin-based regimen or other azoles as well. |

*See page 2 for abbreviations. All dosage recommendations are for adults (unless otherwise indicated) and assume normal renal function.*

**TABLE 11A (2)**

| TYPE OF INFECTION/ORGANISM/ SITE OF INFECTION | ANTIMICROBIAL AGENTS OF CHOICE | | COMMENTS |
|---|---|---|---|
| | **PRIMARY** | **ALTERNATIVE** | |
| **Blastomycosis** *(CID 46: 1801, 2008)* (Blastomyces dermatitidis.) Cutaneous, pulmonary or extrapulmonary. | **LAB,** 3-5 mg/kg per day; OR **Ampho B,** 0.7-1 mg/kg per day, for 1-2 weeks, **then Itra** oral sol'n 200 mg tid for 3 days followed by Itra 200 mg bid for 6-12 months | **Itra** oral sol'n 200 mg tid for 3 days then once or twice per day for 6-12 months for mild to moderate disease; OR **Flu** 400-800 mg per day for those intolerant to Itra | Serum levels of **Itra** should be determined after 2 weeks to ensure adequate drug exposure. Flu less effective than Itra; role of Vori or Posa unclear but active in vitro. Can look for Blastomyces in antigen in urine as aid to diagnosis. |
| **Blastomycosis:** CNS disease *(CID 50:797, 2010)* | **LAB** 5 mg/kg per day for 4-6 weeks, followed by **Flu** 800 mg per day | **Itra** oral sol'n 200 mg bid or tid; OR **Vori** 200-400 mg q12h | Flu and Vori have excellent CNS penetration, to counterbalance their slightly reduced activity compared to Itra. Treat for at least 12 months and until CSF has normalized. Monitor serum Itra levels to assure adequate drug concentrations. More favorable outcome with Voriconazole *(CID 50:797, 2010).* |
| **Candidiasis:** Candida is a common cause of nosocomial bloodstream infection. *C. albicans* & non-albicans species show ↓ susceptibility to antifungal agents (esp. fluconazole). In immunocompromised pts where antifungal prophylaxis (esp. fluconazole) is widely used. Oral, esophageal, or vaginal candidiasis is a major manifestation of advanced HIV & represents common AIDS-defining diagnosis. See CID 62:e1, 2016 for updated IDSA Guidelines. | | | |
| **Candidiasis: Bloodstream infection (*C. albicans & C. glabrata*)** | | | |
| **Bloodstream: non-neutropenic patient** Remove all intravascular catheters if possible; replace catheters at a new site (not over a wire). Higher mortality associated with delay in therapy *(CID 43:25, 2006).* | **Caspo** 70 mg IV loading dose, then 50 mg IV daily; OR **Mica** 100 mg IV daily; OR **Anidula** 200 mg IV loading dose then 100 mg IV daily. Note: Reduce **Caspo** dose for renal impairment | **Flu** 800 mg (12 mg/kg) loading dose, then 400 mg (6 mg/kg) daily IV OR **Lipid-based Ampho** B 3-5 mg/kg IV daily; OR **Vori** 400 mg (6 mg/kg) IV twice daily for 2 doses then 200 mg q12h. | **Echinocandin** is recommended for empiric therapy, particularly for patients with recent azole exposure or with moderately severe or severe illness, hemodynamic instability. **An echinocandin should be used for treatment of** *Candida glabrata* **unless susceptibility to fluconazole or voriconazole has been confirmed.** Echinocandin preferred empiric therapy in centers with high prevalence of non-albicans candida species. Echinocandins vs. polyenes or azole associated with better survival *(Clin Infect Dis 54:1110, 2012).* A double-blind randomized trial of anidulafungin (n=127) and fluconazole (n=118) showed an 88% microbiologic response rate (119/135 candida species) with anidulafungin vs a 76% (99/130 candida species) with fluconazole (p=0.02) *(NEJM 356: 2472, 2007).* |
| ***Candida auris:*** This is an emerging **multi-drug resistant** Candida species able to cause a wide-range of infections. It can misidentified as *Candida haemulonii* or *Saccharomyces cerevisiae.* Molecular methods are needed to confirm species. Often resistant to azoles and amphotericin, some are also echinocandin resistant *(CID 2018;66:306).* | **Funduscopic examination** within first week of therapy to exclude ophthalmic involvement. Ocular disease present in ~15% of patients with candidemia, but endophthalmitis is uncommon (~2%) *(CID 53:262, 2011).* Intraocular injections of Ampho B required for endophthalmitis as echinocandins have poor penetration into the eye. For **septic thrombophlebitis,** catheter removal and incision and drainage and resection of the vein, as needed, are recommended, duration of therapy at least 2 weeks after last positive blood culture. | | **Fluconazole** is not recommended for empiric therapy but could be considered recommended for patients with mild-to-moderate illness, hemodynamically stable, with no recent azole exposure. **Fluconazole not recommended for treatment of documented** *C. krusei:* use an echinocandin or voriconazole or posaconazole; (note: echinocandins have better in vitro activity than either Vori or Posa against *C. glabrata).* **Fluconazole recommended for treatment of** *Candida parapsilosis* because of reduced susceptibility of this species to echinocandins. Transition from echinocandin to fluconazole for stable patients with *Candida albicans* or other azole-susceptible species. **Voriconazole** with little advantage over fluconazole (more drug-drug interactions) except for oral step-down therapy of *Candida krusei* or voriconazole-susceptible *Candida glabrata.* Recommended **duration of therapy** is 14 days after last positive blood culture. Duration of systemic therapy should be extended to 4-6 weeks for eye involvement. |
| Multi-drug resistant Candida species *(JID 2017;216(S3):S445).* | | | |

*See page 2 for abbreviations. All dosage recommendations are for adults (unless otherwise indicated) and assume normal renal function.*

TABLE 11A (3)

| TYPE OF INFECTION/ORGANISM/ SITE OF INFECTION | ANTIMICROBIAL AGENTS OF CHOICE | | COMMENTS |
|---|---|---|---|
| | PRIMARY | ALTERNATIVE | |
| **Candidiasis: Bloodstream infection** (continued) | | | |
| **Bloodstream: neutropenic patient** Remove all intravascular catheters if possible; replace catheters at a new site (not over a wire). | **Caspo** 70 mg (1 mg/kg) loading dose, then 50 mg IV daily, 35 mg for moderate hepatic insufficiency; OR **Mica** 100 mg IV daily; OR **Anidula** 200 mg IV loading dose then 100 mg IV daily; OR **Lipid-based Ampho B** 3-5 mg/kg IV daily. | **Flu** 800 mg (12 mg/kg) loading dose, then 400 mg daily IV po; OR **Vori** 400 mg (6 mg/kg) IV twice daily for 2 doses then 200 mg (3 mg/kg) IV q12h. | **Duration of therapy** in absence of metastatic complications is for 2 weeks after last positive blood culture, resolution of signs, and resolution of neutropenia. Perform funduscopic examination after recovery of white count as signs of ophthalmic involvement may not be seen during neutropenia. *See comments above for recommendations concerning choice of specific agents.* |
| **Candidiasis: Bone and joint infections** | | | |
| **Osteomyelitis** | **Flu** 400 mg (6 mg/kg) daily IV or po; OR **Lipid-based Ampho B** 3-5 mg/kg daily x several weeks, then oral fluconazole. | **Caspo**, **Mica** or **Anidula** or **Ampho B** 0.5-1 mg/kg IV daily x several weeks then oral **Flu**. | Treat for a total of 6-12 months. **Surgical debridement** often necessary; **remove hardware** whenever possible. |
| **Septic arthritis** | **Flu** 400 mg (6 mg/kg) daily IV or po; OR **Lipid-based Ampho B** 3-5 mg/kg IV daily x several weeks, then oral fluconazole. | **Caspo**, **Mica** or **Anidula** or **Ampho B** 0.5-1 mg/kg IV daily for several weeks then **Flu**. | **Surgical debridement** in all cases; removal of prosthetic joints whenever possible. Treat for at least 6 weeks and indefinitely if retained hardware. |
| **Candidiasis: Cardiovascular infections** | | | |
| **Endocarditis, Myocarditis, Pericarditis** (See Eur J Clin Microbiol Infect Dis 27:519, 2008) | **Caspo** 50-150 mg/day IV; OR **Mica** 100-150 mg/day IV; OR **Anidula** 100-200 mg/day IV; OR **Lipid-based Ampho B** 3-5 mg/kg IV daily + **Flucytosine** 25 mg/kg po qid. | **Ampho B** 0.6-1 mg/kg IV daily + **Flucytosine** 25 mg/kg po qid | Consider use of higher doses of echinocandins for endocarditis or other endovascular infections. Can switch to **Fluconazole 400-800 mg orally in stable patients** with negative blood cultures and fluconazole susceptible organism. *See Med 90:237, 2011.* Valve replacement strongly recommended, particularly if prosthetic valve endocarditis. Duration of therapy not well defined, but treat for at least 6 weeks after valve replacement and longer in those with complications (e.g., perivalvular or myocardial abscess, extensive disease, delayed resolution of candidemia). Pericarditis: Pericardial window or pericardiectomy also is recommended. Long-term (life-long?) suppression with Fluconazole 400-800 mg daily for native valve endocarditis and no valve replacement; life-long suppression for prosthetic valve endocarditis if no valve replacement. |
| **Candidiasis: Mucosal, esophageal, and oropharyngeal** | | | |
| **Candida esophagitis** Primarily encountered in HIV-positive patients Dysphagia or odynophagia predictive of esophageal candidiasis. | **Flu** 200-400 (3-6 mg/kg) mg IV/po daily; OR (**Caspo** 50 mg IV daily; OR **Mica** 150 mg IV daily; OR **Anidula** 200 mg IV loading dose then 100 mg IV daily); OR **Ampho B** 0.5 mg/kg IV daily. | An azole (**Itra** solution 200 mg daily; OR **Posa** suspension 400 mg bid x 3 days then 400 mg daily or **Vori** IV/po 200 mg q12h. | **Duration of therapy** 14-21 days. IV Echinocandin or Ampho B for patients unable to tolerate oral therapy. For Fluconazole refractory disease, Itra (80% will respond). Posa, Vori, an Echinocandin, or Ampho B. Echinocandins associated with higher relapse rate than fluconazole. ART recommended. Suppressive therapy with fluconazole 200 mg 3x/wk until CD4 >200/mm³. |

*See page 2 for abbreviations. All dosage recommendations are for adults (unless otherwise indicated) and assume normal/renal function.*

TABLE 11A (4)

| TYPE OF INFECTION/ORGANISM/ SITE OF INFECTION | ANTIMICROBIAL AGENTS OF CHOICE | | COMMENTS |
|---|---|---|---|
| | PRIMARY | ALTERNATIVE | |
| **Candidiasis: Mucosal, esophageal, and oropharyngeal** (continued) | | | |
| Oropharyngeal candidiasis | | | |
| Non-AIDS patient | Clotrimazole troches 10 mg 5 x daily; OR Nystatin suspension or pastilles po qid; OR Flu 100-200 mg daily. | Itra solution 200 mg daily; OR Posa suspension 400 mg bid for 3 days then 400 mg daily; or Vori 200 mg q12h; OR Capso 70 mg loading dose then 50 mg IV daily; or Mica 100 mg IV daily; or Anidula 200 mg IV loading dose then 100 mg IV daily); OR Ampho B 0.3 mg/kg daily. | Duration of therapy 7-14 days. Clotrimazole or nystatin recommended for mild disease; Fluconazole preferred for moderate-to-severe disease. Alternative agents reserved for refractory disease. |
| AIDS patient | Flu 100-200 mg po daily x 7-14 days. | Same as for non-AIDS patient x 7-14 days. | ART in HIV-positive patients. Suppressive therapy until CD4 >200/mm³; but if required fluconazole 100 mg po thrice weekly. Oral Itra, Posa, or Vori for 28 days for Fluconazole-refractory disease. IV echinocandin also an option. Dysphagia or odynophagia predictive of esophageal candidiasis. |
| Vulvovaginitis | | | |
| Non-AIDS Patient | Topical azole therapy: Butoconazole 2% cream (5 gm) q24h at bedtime x 3 days or 2% cream SR 5 gm x 1; OR Clotrimazole 100 mg vaginal tabs (2 at bedtime x 3 days) or 1% cream (5 gm) at bedtime times 7 days (14 days may ↑ cure rate) or 100 mg vaginal tab x 7 days or 500 mg vaginal tab x 1; OR Miconazole 200 mg vaginal suppos (1 at bedtime x 3 days) or 100 mg vaginal suppos. q24h x 7 days or 2% cream (5 gm) at bedtime x 7 days; OR Terconazole 80 mg vaginal tab (1 at bedtime x 3 days) or 0.4% cream (5 gm) at bedtime x 7 days or 0.8% cream 5 gm intravaginal q24h x 3 days; OR Tioconazole 6.5% vag. ointment x 1 dose. Oral therapy: Flu 150 mg po x 1; OR If severe, Flu 150 mg q72h x 3 OR Itra 200 mg po bid x 1 day. | Recurrent vulvovaginal candidiasis: Fluconazole 150 mg weekly for 6 months. If severe can induce with Flu 150 mg q10-14 days, then weekly. |
| AIDS Patient | Topical azoles (clotrimazole, buto, mico, tico, or tercon) x3-7d; OR Topical Nystatin 100,000 units/day as vaginal tablet x14d; OR Flu 150 mg po x1/dw. | Flu 150 mg po x 1. | For recurrent disease 10-14 days of topical azole or oral Flu 150 mg, then Flu 150 mg po weekly for 6 mos. |
| **Candidiasis: Other infections** | | | |
| CNS Infection | Lipid-based Ampho B 3-5 mg/kg IV daily + 5-FC 25 mg/kg po qid. | Flu 400-800 mg (6-12 mg/kg) IV or po. | Removal of intraventricular devices recommended. Flu 400-800 mg as step-down therapy in the stable patient and in patient intolerant of Ampho B. Experience too limited to recommend echinocandins at this time. Treatment duration for several weeks until resolution of CSF, radiographic, and clinical abnormalities. |
| Cutaneous (including paronychia, Table 1, page 29) | Apply topical Ampho B, Clotrimazole, Econazole, Miconazole, or Nystatin 3-4 x daily for 7-14 days or ketoconazole 400 mg po once daily x 14 days. Ciclopirox olamine 1% cream/lotion; apply topically bid x 7-14 days. | | |

See page 2 for abbreviations. All dosage recommendations are for adults (unless otherwise indicated) and assume normal renal function.

## TABLE 11A (5)

| TYPE OF INFECTION/ORGANISM/ SITE OF INFECTION | ANTIMICROBIAL AGENTS OF CHOICE | | COMMENTS |
|---|---|---|---|
| | PRIMARY | ALTERNATIVE | |
| **Candidiasis: Other infections** (continued) | | | |
| **Endophthalmitis /Chorioretinitis**<br>• Occurs in 10% of candidemia, thus ophthalmologic consult for all pts<br>• Diagnosis: typical white exudates on retinal exam and/or positive vitrectomy culture<br>• Chorioretinitis accounts for 85% of ocular disease while endophthalmitis occurs in only 15% (Clin Infect Dis 53:262, 2011). | Chorioretinitis or Endophthalmitis: Lipid-based **Ampho B** 3-5 mg/kg daily **+ Fluctosine** 25 mg/kg qid OR **Vori** 6 mg/kg/IV q12 x 2 doses and then 4 mg/kg po/IV q12. Consider intravitreal **Ampho B** 5-10 mcg in 0.1 mL for sight threatening disease. | Chorioretinitis or Endophthalmitis: **Flu** 6-12 mg/kg IV daily (poor activity against C. glabrata or C. krusei) and consider intravitreal **Ampho B** 5-10 mcg in 0.1 mL for sight-threatening disease. Consider vitrectomy in advanced disease. Clin Infect Dis. 52:648, 2011. | **Duration of therapy:** 4-6 weeks or longer, based on resolution determined by repeated examinations.<br>Vitrectomy may be necessary for those with vitritis or endophthalmitis (Br J Ophthalmol 92:466, 2008; Pharmacotherapy 27:1711, 2007). |
| **Neonatal candidiasis** | **Ampho B** 1 mg/kg IV daily; OR **Flu** 12 mg/kg IV daily. | Lipid-based **Ampho B** 3-5 mg/kg IV daily. | **Lumbar puncture** to rule out CNS disease, **dilated retinal examination**, abdominal ultrasound and **intravascular catheter removal** strongly recommended. Lipid-based Ampho B used only if there is no renal involvement. Echinocandins considered 3cd line therapy. **Duration of therapy is at least 3 weeks.** |
| **Peritonitis** (Chronic Ambulatory Peritoneal Dialysis)<br>See Table 19, page 252. | **Flu** 400 mg po q24h x 2-3 wks; or **Caspo** 70 mg IV on day 1 followed by 50 mg IV q24h x 14 days; or **Mica** 100 mg IV q24h x 14 days. | **Ampho B**, continuous intraperitoneal dosing at 1.5 mg/L of dialysis fluid x 4-6 wks. | Remove cath immediately or if no clinical improvement in 4-7 days. |
| **Candidiasis: Urinary tract infections** | | | |
| **Cystitis**<br>**Asymptomatic**<br>See CID 52:S427, 2011; CID 52:S452, 2011. | If possible, remove catheter or stent. No therapy indicated except in patients undergoing a urologic procedure. | **Ampho B** 0.5 mg/kg IV at high risk for dissemination or undergoing a urologic procedure. | **High risk patients** (neonates and neutropenic patients), should be managed as outlined for treatment of bloodstream infection. For patients undergoing urologic procedures, Flu 200 mg (3 mg/kg) IV/po daily or Ampho B 0.5 mg/kg IV daily (for flu-resistant organisms) for several days pre- and post-procedure.<br>Concentration of echinocandins is low: case reports of efficacy versus azole resistant organisms (Can J Infect Dis Med Microbiol 18:149, 2007;<br>CID 44:e46, 2007).<br>Persistent candiduria in immunocompromised pt warrants ultrasound or CT of kidneys to rule out fungus ball. |
| **Symptomatic** | **Flu** 200 mg (3 mg/kg) IV/po daily x 14 days. | **Ampho B** 0.5 mg/kg IV daily (for fluconazole resistant organisms) x 7-10 days. | |
| **Pyelonephritis** | **Flu** 200-400 mg (3-6 mg/kg) po once daily. | **Ampho B** 0.5 mg/kg daily IV + 5-FC 25 mg/kg qid. | **Treat for 2 weeks.** For suspected disseminated disease treat as if bloodstream infection is present. |
| **Chromoblastomycosis**<br>(Clin Exp Dermatol, 34:849, 2009).<br>(Cladophialophora, Phialophora, or Fonsecaea).<br>Cutaneous (usually feet, legs): raised scaly lesions, most common in tropical areas | If lesions small & few, surgical **excision** or **cryosurgery with liquid nitrogen**. If lesions chronic, extensive, burrowing: **Itraconazole**. | **Itra** 200-400 mg oral soln q24h or 400 mg pulse therapy once daily for 1 week of each month x 6-12 months (or until response)[NM]. | **Terbinafine**[NM] 500-1000 mg once daily alone or in combination with **Itra** 200-400 oral soln mg; or **Posa** (800 mg) po may be effective. Anecdotal report of efficacy of topical imiquimod 5% 5x/wk (CID 58:1734, 2014). |

*See page 2 for abbreviations. All dosage recommendations are for adults (unless otherwise indicated) and assume normal renal/renal function.*

**TABLE 11A (6)**

| TYPE OF INFECTION/ORGANISM/ SITE OF INFECTION | ANTIMICROBIAL AGENTS OF CHOICE | | COMMENTS |
|---|---|---|---|
| | **PRIMARY** | **ALTERNATIVE** | |
| **Coccidioidomycosis** (Coccidioides immitis) IDSA Guidelines: CID 63: e112, 2016; see also Mayo Clin Proc 83:343, 2008) | | | |
| **Primary pulmonary** (San Joaquin or Valley Fever): **For pts at low risk of persistence/complication.** | **Antifungal rx not generally recommended.** Treat if fever, wt loss and/or fatigue that does not resolve within 4-8 wks. | | Uncomplicated pulmonary in normal host most common in endemic areas (Emerg Infect Dis 12:958, 2006). Influenza-like illness of 1-2 wks duration. |
| **Primary pulmonary in pts with ↑ risk for complications or dissemination. Rx indicated:** • Immunosuppressive disease, post-transplantation, hematological malignancies or therapies (steroids, TNF-α antagonists) • Pregnancy in 3rd trimester. • Diabetes • CF antibody >1:16 • Pulmonary infiltrates • Dissemination (identification of spherules or culture of organism from ulcer, joint effusion, pus from subcutaneous abscess or bone biopsy, etc.) | **Mild to moderate severity:** Itra solution 200 mg po or IV bid; OR **Flu** 400 mg po q24h x 3-12 mos **Locally severe or disseminated disease Ampho B** 0.6-1 mg/kg per day x 7 days then 0.8 mg/kg every other day or liposomal **Ampho B** 3-5 mg/kg/d IV or **ABLC** 5 mg/kg IV, until clinical improvement (usually several wks or longer) in disseminated disease followed by **Itra** or **Flu** for at least 1 year. Some use combination of Ampho B & Flu for progressive severe disease; **Consultation with specialist recommended:** surgery may be required. Suppression in HIV+ patients until CD4 >250 & infection controlled; controlled series lacking. **Flu** 200 mg po q24h or Itra oral soln 200 mg po bid (MvCosis 56:42, 2003). | | **Ampho B cure rate 50-70%. Responses to azoles are similar.** Itra may have slight advantage esp. in soft tissue infection. Relapse rates after rx 40%. Relapse rate if ↑↑↑ CF titer ≥1:256. Following CF titers are important; rising titers warrant retreatment. **Posaconazole** reported successful in 73% of pts with refractory non-meningeal cocci (Chest 132:952, 2007). Not frontline therapy. Treatment of pediatric cocci to include salvage therapy with Vori & Caspo (Ped Infect Dis J 26:1573, 1579 & 1567, 2013). Can detect delayed hypersensitivity with skin test antigen called Spherusol; helpful if history of Valley Fever. |
| **Meningitis:** occurs in 1/3 to 1/2 of pts with disseminated coccidioidomycosis | | | |
| Adult (IDSA Guideline: CID 42:103, 2006) | **Flu** 400-1,000 mg po q24h indefinitely. | **Ampho B** IV as for pulmonary (above) + 0.1-0.3 mg daily intra- | **80% relapse rate, continue flucon indefinitely. Voriconazole** successful in high doses (6 mg/kg IV q12h) followed by oral |
| Child (Cryptococcus neoformans, C. gattii) | **Flu** (Pediatric dose not established, 6 mg per kg po q24h used) | thecal (with gradual increase of intrathecal amino B, see CID 2017;64:e79). Small retrospective study suggests benefit from reservoir device. **OR** Itra oral soln 400-800 mg q24h **OR Vori** (See Comment) | suppression (200 mg po q24h). For practical aspects of intrathecal ampho B, see CID 2017;64:e79). Small retrospective study suggests benefit from adjunctive corticosteroids (CID 2017;65:338). |
| **Cryptococcosis** (IDSA Guideline: CID 50:291, 2010. | | | |
| **Non-meningeal (non-AIDS)** Risk 57% in organ transplant & those receiving other forms of immunosuppressive agents (EID 13:953, 2007) | **Flu** 400 mg/day IV or x 8 wks to 6 mos. **For more severe disease: Ampho B** 0.5-0.8 mg/kg per day IV till response then change to **Flu** 400 mg po q24h x 8-10 wks course | **Itra** 200-400 mg solution q24h x 6-12 mo OR (**Ampho B** 0.3 mg/kg per day x 6 wks) (use ideal body wt) | **Flu alone 90% effective for meningeal and non-meningeal forms.** Fluconazole as effective as Ampho B. Addition of **interferon**-g (IFN-γ-1b 50 mcg per M² subcut. 3x per wk x 9 wks) to liposomal Ampho B assoc. with response in pt failing antifungal rx (CID 38: 910, 2004). Posaconazole 400-800 mg po daily effective in a small series with response in (CID 45:562, 2007; Chest 132:952, 2007. |
| **Meningitis (non-AIDS)** IDSA Guidelines: CID 50:291, 2010. | **Induction phase: (Liposomal Ampho B** 3-4 mg/kg IV q24h or **Ampho B lipid complex** 5 mg/kg IV q24h) + **Flucytosine** 25 mg/kg po q6h • Duration: Minimum 2 weeks for transplant recipients and minimum 4 weeks in non-immunocompromised patients. o Treat until patient is afebrile and cultures are negative. o Need to monitor intracranial pressure; if over 25 cm, need to remove CSF. See comment. • Consolidation phase: **Flu** 400-800 mg po daily x 8 weeks • Maintenance phase: **Flu** 200 mg po daily x 6-12 months | | **C. gattii** meningitis reported in the Pacific Northwest (EID 13:42, 2007); severity of disease and prognosis appear to be worse than with C. neoformans; initial therapy with **Ampho B + Flucytosine** recommended. C. gattii less susceptible to flucon than C. neoformans Outcomes in both AIDS and non-AIDS cryptococcal meningitis improved with Ampho B + 5-FC induction therapy for 14 days in those with neurological abnormalities or high organism burden (PLoS ONE 3:e2870, 2008). **If CSF opening pressure >25 cm H₂O, repeat LP to drain fluid to control pressure.** |

See page 2 for abbreviations. All dosage recommendations are for adults (unless otherwise indicated) and assume normal renal function.

**TABLE 11A (7)**

| TYPE OF INFECTION/ORGANISM/ SITE OF INFECTION | ANTIMICROBIAL AGENTS OF CHOICE | | COMMENTS |
|---|---|---|---|
| | PRIMARY | ALTERNATIVE | |
| **Cryptococcosis** (continued) | | | |
| **HIV/AIDS: Cryptococcemia and/or Meningitis** | | | |
| **Treatment** See *Clin Infect Dis 50:291, 2010* (IDSA Guidelines). ↓ with ARV but still common presenting OI in newly diagnosed AIDS pts. Cryptococcal infection may be manifested by positive blood culture or positive serum cryptococcal antigen (CRAG: >95% sens). CRAG no help in monitoring response to therapy. With ARV, symptoms of acute meningitis may return: immune reconstitution inflammatory syndrome (IRIS). ↑ CSF pressure (**>250 mm H2O**) associated with high mortality: lower with CSF removal. If frequent LPs not possible, ventriculoperitoneal shunts an option (*Surg Neurol 63:529 & 531, 2005*). | **Ampho B** 0.7 mg/kg IV q24h + **Flucytosine** 25 mg/kg po q6h for at least two weeks or longer until CSF is sterilized. *See Comment.* **Consolidation therapy:** Flu 400-800 mg po q24h to complete a 10-wks course then suppression *(see below)*. Deferring ART for 5 wks after initiation cryptococcal meningitis therapy significantly improved survival as compared to starting ART during the first 2 wks (*NEJM 370:2487, 2014*). | **Ampho B** IV or **Liposomal Ampho B** IV+ **Flu** 400-800 mg po or IV daily, **OR Ampho B** 0.7 mg/kg IV q24h daily, **OR Ampho B** 4 mg/kg IV q24h alone; **OR Flu** ≥800 mg/day (1200 mg preferred) (po or IV) + **Flucytosine** 25 mg/kg po q6h for 4-6 weeks. *Then* | • Outcome of treatment: treatment failure associated with dissemination of infection & high serum antigen titer, indicative of high burden of organisms and lack of 5FC use during inductive Rx, abnormal neurological evaluation & underlying hematological malignancy. Mortality rates still high, particularly in those with concomitant pneumonia (*PLOS Medicine 4:e42, 2007*). Early Dx essential for improved outcome (*Postgrad Med 121:107, 2009*). <br>• Ampho B + 5FC treatment ↓ crypto CFUs more rapidly than ampho + Flu or Ampho + 5FC + Flu. Ampho B 1 mg/kg/d alone much more rapidly fungicidal in vivo than Flu 400 mg/kg/d (*CID 45:76681, 2007*). Use of lipid-based Ampho B associated with lower mortality compared to Ampho B deoxycholate in solid organ transplant recipients (*CID 48:1566, 2009*). <br>• Monitor 5-FC levels: peak 70-80 mg/L, trough 30-40 mg/L. Higher levels assoc. with bone marrow toxicity. No difference in outcome if given IV or po (*AAC 51:1038, 2007*). <br>• Failure of Flu may rarely be due to resistant organism, especially if burden of organism high at initiation of Rx. Although 200 mg qd = 400 mg qd of Flu: median survival 76 & 82 days respectively, authors prefer 400 mg po qd (*BMC Infect Dis 6:118, 2006*). <br>• Trend toward improved outcomes with fluconazole 400-800 mg combined with Ampho B versus Ampho B alone in AIDS patients (*CID 48:1775, 2009*). Role of other azoles uncertain: successful outcomes were observed in 14/29 (48%) subjects with cryptococcal meningitis treated with posaconazole (*JAC 56:745, 2005*). Voriconazole also may be effective. <br>• **When to initiate antiretroviral therapy (ART)?** Defer ART to allow for 5 weeks of anti-fungal treatment. When ART was started 1-2 weeks after diagnosis of cryptococcal meningitis mortality was increased when compared to initiation of ART >5 weeks after diagnosis (*NEJM 370:2487, 2014*). |
| **Suppression** (chronic maintenance therapy) Discontinuation of antifungal rx can be considered among pts who remain asymptomatic, with CD4 >100-200/mm³ on ART. Some authorities recommend ≥6 months. Some perform a lumbar puncture before discontinuation of maintenance rx. Reappearance of pos. serum CRAG may predict relapse | **Flu** 200 mg/day po [If CD4 count rises to >100/mm³ with effective antiretroviral rx, some authorities recommend dc suppressive rx. See www.hivatis.org. Authors would dc if CSF culture negative.] | **Itra** 200 mg po q12h (Flu intolerant or failure. No data on Vori for maintenance. | Itraconazole less effective than fluconazole & not recommended because of higher relapse rate (23% vs 4%). Recurrence rate of 0.4 to 3.9 per 100 patient-years with discontinuation of suppressive therapy in 100 patients on ARV with CD4 >100 cells/mm³. |

*See page 2 for abbreviations. All dosage recommendations are for adults (unless otherwise indicated) and assume normal renal function.*

**TABLE 11A (8)**

| TYPE OF INFECTION/ORGANISM/ SITE OF INFECTION | ANTIMICROBIAL AGENTS OF CHOICE | | COMMENTS |
|---|---|---|---|
| | PRIMARY | ALTERNATIVE | |
| **Dermatophytosis** | | | |
| **Onychomycosis** (Tinea unguium) (primarily cosmetic) Laser rx FDA approved: modestly effective, expensive (Med Lett 55:15, 2013). Review: JAMA 2018,319:397. | **Fingernail Rx Options: Terbinafine** 250 mg po q24h [children <20 kg: 62.5 mg/day, 20–40 kg: 125 mg/day, >40 kg: 250 mg/day] x 6 wks (79% effective) OR **Itra** 200 mg po q24h x 3 mos. OR **Itra** 200 mg po bid x 1 wk/mo x 2 mos **Flu** 150–300 mg po q wk x 3–6 mos. Note: Cure rates for all options are low. | | **Toenail Rx Options: Terbinafine** 250 mg po q24h [children <20 kg: 62.5 mg/day, 20–40 kg: 125 mg/day, >40 kg: 250 mg/day] x 12 wks (76% effective) OR **Itra** 200 mg po q24h x 3 mos (59% effective) OR **Efinaconazole** 10% solution applied to nail once daily for 48 wks OR **Itra** 200 mg bid x 1 wk/mo. x 3–4 mos (63% effective) OR **Flu** 150–300 mg po q wk. x 6–12 mos (48% effective) OR topical **Tavaborole** (Kerydin) or topical **Efinaconazole** (Jublia). |
| **Tinea capitis ("ringworm")** (Trichophyton tonsurans, Microsporum canis, N. America, other sp. elsewhere) (PIDJ 18:191, 1999) | **Terbinafine** 250 mg po q24h x 2–4 wks (adults) 250 mg (or less for children) 10–20 kg: 62.5 mg q24h x 2 wks 20–40 kg: 125 mg q24h x 2 weeks >40 kg: 250 mg q24h x 2 weeks | **Itra** 5 mg/kg per day x 4 wks OR **Flu** 6 mg/kg q wk x 8–12 wks. **Griseo:** adults 500 mg po q24h; children age >2 years: Micro susp: 20–25 mg/kg/day; Ultramicro tabs: 10–15 mg/kg/day Dur: at least 6 wks, continue until clear | Durations of therapy are approx. twice as long for M. canis. All agents with similar cure rates (60–100%) in clinical studies. Addition of topical ketoconazole or selenium sulfate shampoo reduces transmissibility (Int J Dermatol 39:261, 2000). |
| **Tinea corporis, cruris, or pedis** (Trichophyton rubrum, T. mentagrophytes, Epidermophyton floccosum) "Athlete's foot, jock itch", and ringworm | **Topical rx:** Generally applied 2x/day. Available as creams, ointments, sprays, by prescription & "over the counter." Apply 2x/day for 2–3 wks. Recommend: Lotrimin Ultra & Lamisil AT: contain butenafine & terbinafine—both are fungicidal | **Terbinafine** 250 mg po q24h x 2 wks OR **Keto** 200 mg po q24h x 4 wks OR **Flu** 150 mg po 1x/wk for 2–4 wks **Griseo:** adults 500 mg po q24h times 4–6 wks, children 10–20 mg/kg per day. Duration: 2–4 wks for corporis, 4–8 wks for pedis. | **Keto** po often effective in severe recalcitrant infection. Follow for hepatotoxicity; many drug-drug interactions. |
| **Tinea versicolor** (Malassezia furfur or Pityrosporum orbiculare) Rule out erythrasma—see Table 1, page 58 | **Keto** (400 mg po single dose) or **Itra** (200 mg q24h x 7 days) or (2% cream 1x q24h x 2 wks) | **Flu** 400 mg po single dose or **Itra** 400 mg q24h x 3–7 days | **Keto** (po) times 1 dose was 97% effective in 1 study. Another alternative: **Selenium sulfide** (Selsun), 2.5% lotion, apply as lather, leave on 10 min then wash off. 1/day x 7 day or 3–5/wk times 2–4 wks |
| **Fusariosis** Third most common cause of invasive mold infections, after Aspergillus and Mucorales and related molds, in patients with hematologic malignancies (Mycoses 52:197, 2009). Pneumonia, skin infections, bone and joint infections, and disseminated disease occur in severely immunocompromised patients. In contrast to other molds, blood cultures are frequently positive. Fusarium solani, F. oxysporum, F. verticillioides and F. moniliforme account for approx. 90% of isolates (Clin Micro Rev 20: 695, 2007). Frequently fatal, outcome depends on decreasing the level of immunosuppression. | **Lipid-based Ampho B** 5–10 mg/kg/d IV. OR **Ampho B** 1–1.5 mg/kg/d IV. | **Posa** 400 mg po bid with meals (if not meals, 200 mg qid); OR **Vori** IV: 6 mg per kg q12h times 1 day, then 4 mg per kg q12h; po: 400 mg q12h, then 200 mg q12h. See comments. | Surgical **debridement** for localized disease. Fusarium spp. resistance to most antifungal agents, including echinocandins. F. solani and F. verticillioides typically are resistant to azoles. F. oxysporum and F. moniliforme may be susceptible to voriconazole and posaconazole. Role of combination therapy not well defined but case reports of response (Mycoses 50: 227, 2007). Given variability in susceptibility, can consider combination therapy with Vori and Ampho B awaiting speciation. Outcome dependent on reduction or discontinuation of immuno-suppression. Duration of therapy depends on response; long-term suppressive therapy for patients remaining in immunosuppression. |

[1] **Serious but rare cases of hepatic failure** have been reported in pts receiving Terbinafine & should not be used in those with chronic or active liver disease (see Table 11B, page 145).

[2] Use of Itraconazole has been associated with myocardial dysfunction and with onset of congestive heart failure.

See page 2 for abbreviations. All dosage recommendations are for adults (unless otherwise indicated) and assume normal renal function.

TABLE 11A (9)

| TYPE OF INFECTION/ORGANISM/ SITE OF INFECTION | ANTIMICROBIAL AGENTS OF CHOICE | | COMMENTS |
|---|---|---|---|
| | PRIMARY | ALTERNATIVE | |
| **Histoplasmosis** (Histoplasma capsulatum). *See IDSA Guideline: CID 45:807, 2007.* Best diagnostic test is urinary, serum, or CSF histoplasma antigen: MiraVista Diagnostics (1-866-647-2847). | | | |
| Acute pulmonary histoplasmosis | **Mild to moderate disease, symptoms <4 wks:** No rx; If symptoms last over one month, **Itra** oral soln 200 mg po tid for 3 days then once or twice daily for 6-12 wks. <br><br> **Moderately severe or severe: Liposomal Ampho B**, 3-5 mg/kg/d IV or **ABLC** 5 mg/kg/d IV or Ampho B 0.7-1.0 mg/kg/d for 1-2 wks, then Itra 200 mg tid for 3 days, then bid for 12 wks. + **methylprednisolone** 0.5-1 mg/kg/d for 1-2 wks. | | Ampho B for patients at low risk of nephrotoxicity. Check for Itra drug-drug interactions. |
| Chronic cavitary pulmonary histoplasmosis | **Itra** oral soln 200 mg po tid for 3 days then once or twice daily for at least 12 mos (some prefer 18-24 mos). | | Document therapeutic Itraconazole blood levels at 2 wks. Relapses occur in 9-15% of patients. |
| Mediastinal lymphadenitis, mediastinal granuloma, pericarditis; and rheumatologic syndromes | **Mild cases:** Antifungal therapy not indicated. Nonsteroidal anti-inflammatory drug for pericarditis or rheumatologic syndromes. <br><br> If no response to non-steroidals, **Prednisone** 0.5-1 mg/kg/d tapered over 1-2 weeks for <br> 1) pericarditis with hemodynamic compromise, <br> 2) lymphadenitis with obstruction or compression syndromes, or <br> 3) severe rheumatologic syndromes. <br><br> **Itra** 200 oral soln mg po once or twice daily for 6-12 wks for moderately severe to severe cases, if of prednisone is administered. | | |
| Progressive disseminated histoplasmosis | **Mild to moderate disease: Itra** 200 mg po tid for 3 days then bid for at least 12 mos. <br><br> **Moderately severe to severe disease: Liposomal Ampho B**, 3 mg/kg/d or **ABLC** 5 mg/kg/d for 1-2 weeks then **Itra** 200 mg tid for 3 days, then bid for at least 12 mos. | | **Ampho B** 0.7-1.0 mg/kg/d may be used for patients at low risk of nephrotoxicity. Confirm therapeutic Itra blood levels. Azoles are teratogenic; Itra should be avoided in pregnancy; use a lipid Ampho formulation. Urinary antigen levels useful for monitoring response to therapy and relapse. |
| CNS histoplasmosis | **Liposomal Ampho B**, 5 mg/kg/d, for a total of 175 mg/kg over 4-6 wks, then **Itra** 200 mg 2-3x a day for at least 12 mos. Vori likely effective for CNS disease. (*Arch Neurology 65: 666, 2008; J Antimicro Chemo 57:1235, 2006*). | | Monitor CNS histo antigen, monitor Itra blood levels. PCR may be better for dx than histo antigen. Absorption of Itra (check levels) and CNS penetration may be an issue; case reports of success with Fluconazole (*Braz J Infect Dis 12:555, 2008*) and Posaconazole (*Drugs 65:1553, 2005*) following Ampho B therapy. |
| Prophylaxis (immunocompromised patients) | **Itra** 200 mg po daily. Check for Itra drug-drug interactions (*Table 22A*). | | Consider primary **prophylaxis** in **HIV-infected** patients with <150 CD4 cells/mm³ in high prevalence areas. <br> Secondary prophylaxis (i.e. suppressive therapy) indicated in HIV-infected patients with <150 CD4 cells/mm³ and other immunocompromised patients in who immunosuppression cannot be reversed |

*See page 2 for abbreviations. All dosage recommendations are for adults (unless otherwise indicated) and assume normal renal function.*

TABLE 11A (10)

| TYPE OF INFECTION/ORGANISM/ SITE OF INFECTION | ANTIMICROBIAL AGENTS OF CHOICE | | COMMENTS |
|---|---|---|---|
| | PRIMARY | ALTERNATIVE | |
| **Madura foot** (*See Nocardia & Scedosporium*) | | | |
| **Mucormycosis** & other related species—Rhizopus, Rhizomucor, Lichtheimia (*CID 54:1629, 2012*). Rhinocerebral, pulmonary due to angioinvasion with tissue necrosis.<br><br>Key to successful rx: early dx with symptoms suggestive of sinusitis (or painful pain or numbness): think mucor with palatal ulcers, &/or black eschars, onset unilateral blindness in immunocompromised or diabetic pt. Rapidly fatal without rx. Dx by culture of tissue or stain: wide ribbon-like, non-septated hyphae with variation in diameter & right angle branching.<br>Diabetics are predisposed to mucormycosis due to microangiopathy & ketoacidosis.<br>Iron overload also predisposes: iron stimulates fungal growth. | Liposomal Ampho B 5-10 mg/kg/day, OR Ampho B 1-1.5 mg/kg/day. | Posa 400 mg bid with meals (if not taking meals, 200 mg po qid)^NAI or Isavuconazole sulfate loading dose of 372 mg (equivalent to isavuconazole 200 mg) IV/po q8 x 6 doses then 372 mg IV/po daily | **Ampho B** (ABLC) monotherapy relatively ineffective with 20% success rate vs 69% for other polyenes (*CID 47:364, 2008*). Complete or partial response rates of 60-80% in **Posa** salvage protocols (*JAC 61, Suppl 1, i35, 2008*).<br>**Isavuconazole:** Approved for treatment of invasive mucor infection based on historical controls (*Ln 2016;387760*).<br>**Combination therapy:** Adjunctive echinocandin to liposomal Amphotericin B is promising given safety profile, synergy in murine models, and observational clinical data (*Clin Infect Dis 54(S1):S73, 2012*). Adjunctive Deferasirox therapy to liposomal Amphotericin B failed to demonstrate benefit (*J Antimicrob Chemother, 67:715, 2012*).<br>Resistant to **Vori:** prolonged use of voriconazole prophylaxis predisposes to mucormycosis infections.<br>Total duration of therapy based on: 1) resolution of clinical signs and symptoms of infection, 2) resolution or stabilization of radiographic abnormalities, and 3) resolution of underlying immunosuppression. Posaconazole for secondary prophylaxis for those on immunosuppressive therapy (*CID 48:1743, 2009*). |
| **Paracoccidioidomycosis** (South American blastomycosis) P. brasiliensis (*Dermatol Clin 26:257, 2008; Expert Rev Anti Infect Ther 6:251, 2008*). Important cause of death from fungal infection in HIV-infected patients in Brazil (*Mem Inst Oswaldo Cruz 104:513, 2009*). | Mild-moderate disease: **Itra** 200 mg po daily for 6-9 months for mild and x 12-18 months for moderate disease.<br>Severe disease: **Ampho B** 0.7-1 mg/kg IV daily to a cumulative total 30 mg/kg followed by **Itra** 200 mg po daily for at least 12 months | **Keto** 200-400 mg daily x 6-18 months; OR **Ampho B** total dose >30 mg/kg OR **TMP/SMX** 800/160 mg bid-tid x 30 days, then 400/80 mg/day indefinitely (up to 3-5 years) | Improvement in >90% pts on Itra or Keto.^NAI<br>**Ampho B** reserved for severe cases and for those intolerant to other agents. TMP-SMX suppression life-long in HIV+. Check for Itra or Keto drug interactions. |
| **Lobomycosis** (keloidal blastomycosis)/ P. loboi | Surgical excision, clofazimine or itra. | | |
| **Penicilliosis** (Talaromyces marneffei, formerly Penicillium marneffei):<br>Common disseminated fungal infection in AIDS pts in SE Asia (esp. Thailand & Vietnam). | **Ampho B** 0.5-1 mg/kg per day times 2 wks followed by **Itra** 400 mg/day x 10 wks followed by 200 mg/day indefinitely in AIDS pts. | For less sick patients **Itra** oral sol'n 200 mg tid x 3 days, then 200 mg bid x 12 wks, then 200 mg q24h.<br>(Oral sol'n better absorbed) | 3rd most common OI in AIDS pts following TBc and cryptococcal meningitis. Prolonged fever, lymphadenopathy, hepatomegaly. Skin nodules are umbilicated (mimic cryptococcal infection or molluscum contagiosum). Preliminary data suggests Vori effective: *CID 43:1060, 2006*. |
| **Phaeohyphomycosis, Black molds, Dematiaceous fungi** (*See Clin Microbiol Rev 27:527, 2014.*) Opportunistic infection in immunocompromised hosts (e.g., HIV/AIDS, Transplants). Most often presents with skin and soft tissue infection or mycetoma but can cause disease in bone and joint, brain abscess, endocarditis, and disseminated disease. Most clinically relevant species are within the genera of Exophiala, Cladophialophora, Coniosporium, Cyphellophora, Fonsecaea, Phialophora, and Rhinocladiella. | Surgery + Itra oral sol'n 400 mg/day po, duration not defined, probably 6 mo^NAI | Voriconazole 6 mg/kg bid x 1 day and then 4 mg/kg po bid, or Posaconazole (suspension) 400 mg bid | Both Vori and Posa have demonstrated efficacy (*Med Mycol 48:769, 2010; Med Mycol 43:91, 2005*) often in addition to surgical therapy. Consider obtaining anti-fungal susceptibility testing. |

*See page 2 for abbreviations. All dosage recommendations are for adults (unless otherwise indicated) and assume normal renal function.*

**TABLE 11A (11)**

| TYPE OF INFECTION/ORGANISM/ SITE OF INFECTION | ANTIMICROBIAL AGENTS OF CHOICE | | COMMENTS |
|---|---|---|---|
| | PRIMARY | ALTERNATIVE | |
| **Pneumocystis pneumonia (PJP)** caused by **Pneumocystis jirovecii.** Ref: *JAMA 301:2578, 2009.* | | | |
| **Not acutely ill,** able to take po meds. PaO₂ >70 mmHg Diagnosis: sputum PCR, Serum Beta-D Glucan may help; reasonable sensitivity & specificity, but also many false positives *(JCM 51:3476, 2013).* | **(TMP-SMX-DS,** 2 tabs po q8h x 21 days) OR **(Dapsone** 100 mg po q24h + **TMP** 5 mg/kg po tid x 21 days) | **[Clinda** 300-450 mg po q6h + **Primaquine** 15 mg base po q24h] x 21 days OR **Atovaquone** suspension 750 mg po bid with food x 21 days | Mutations in gene of the enzyme target (dihydropteroate synthetase) of sulfamethoxazole identified. Unclear whether mutations result in resist to TMP-SMX or dapsone + TMP *(EID 10:1721, 2004).* Dapsone ref: *CID 27:191, 1998.* **After 21 days, chronic suppression in AIDS pts (see below—*post-treatment suppression*).** |
| **Acutely ill,** po rx not possible. PaO₂ <70 mmHg. Still unclear whether antiretroviral therapy should be started during treatment of PCP *(CID 46: 634, 2008).* | **NOTE:** Concomitant use of corticosteroids usually reserved for sicker pts with PaO₂ <70 (see below) | | |
| | **[Prednisone** (15-30 min. before **TMP-SMX**): 40 mg po bid times 5 days, then 40 mg po q24h times 5 days, then 20 mg po q24h times 11 days] + **[TMP-SMX** (15 mg of TMP component per kg per day) IV div. q6-8h times 21 days]. Can substitute IV prednisolone (reduce dose 25%) for po prednisone | **Prednisone** as in primary rx + **[Clinda** 600 mg IV q8h) + (**Primaquine** 30 mg base po q24h)] times 21 days OR **Pentamidine** 4 mg per kg per day IV times 21 days. **Caspo** active in animal models: *CID 36:1445, 2003* | **After 21 days, chronic suppression in AIDS pts** *(see post-treatment suppression).* PJP can occur in absence of HIV infection & steroids *(CID 25:215 & 219, 1997).* Wait 4-8 days before declaring treatment failure& switching to clinda + primaquine or pentamidine *(JAIDS 48:63, 2008),* or adding caspofungin *(Transplant 84:685, 2007).* |
| **Primary prophylaxis and post-treatment suppression** | **(TMP-SMX-DS** or **-SS,** 1 tab po q24h or 1 DS 3x/wk) OR **(Dapsone** 100 mg po q24h). DC when CD4 >200 x/3 mos *(NEJM 344:159, 2001).* | **(Pentamidine** 300 mg in 6 mL sterile water by aerosol q4 wks) OR **(Dapsone** 200 mg po + **Pyrimethamine** 75 mg po + **folinic acid** 25 mg po —all once a week)** or **Atovaquone** 1500 mg po q24h with food. | TMP-SMX-DS regimen provides cross-protection vs Toxo and other bacterial infections. Dapsone + pyrimethamine protects vs Toxo. Atovaquone suspension 1500 mg once daily as effective as daily dapsone *(NEJM 339:1889, 1998)* or inhaled pentamidine *(JID 180:369, 1999).* |
| **Scedosporium species (Scedosporium apiospermum [Pseudallescheria boydii] and Scedosporium prolificans [now Lomentospora prolificans])** Infection occurs via inhalation or inoculation of skin. Normal hosts often have cutaneous disease. Immunocompromised hosts can have pulmonary colonization → invasive disease in lung or skin → disseminated disease. | *Scedosporium apiospermum:* **Vori** 6 mg/kg IV/po q12h on day 1, then 4 mg/kg IV/po q12h. *Scedosporium prolificans:* Surgical debridement and reduction of immunosuppression, consider addition of Vori as above although usually resistant. | **Posa** 400 mg po bid with meals (may be less active) | Surgical debridement should be considered in most cases. S. apiospermum is resistant Amphotericin B and Scedosporium prolificans is resistant to all antifungal agents. Synergy with Terbinafine and echinocandins has been reported in vitro although clinical data is limited *(AAC 56:2635, 2012).* S. prolificans osteomyelitis responded to miltefosine *(CID 48:1257, 2009)* in a case report. Consider susceptibility testing. Treatment guidelines/review: *Clin Microbiol Infect 3:27, 2014. Clin Microbiol Rev 21:157, 2008.* |

*See page 2 for abbreviations. All dosage recommendations are for adults (unless otherwise indicated) and assume normal renal function.*

**TABLE 11A (12)**

| TYPE OF INFECTION/ORGANISM/ SITE OF INFECTION | ANTIMICROBIAL AGENTS OF CHOICE | | COMMENTS |
|---|---|---|---|
| | PRIMARY | ALTERNATIVE | |
| **Sporotrichosis** (IDSA Guideline: CID 45:1255, 2007.) | | | |
| Cutaneous/Lymphocutaneous | **Itra** oral sol'n po 200 mg/day for 2-4 wks after all lesions resolved, usually 3-6 mos. | If no response, **Itra** 200 mg po bid or **Terbinafine** 500 mg po bid or **SSKI** 5 drops (eye drops) tid & increase to 40-50 drops tid | **Flu** 400-800 mg daily only if no response to primary or alternative suggestions. Pregnancy or nursing: local hyperthermia (see below). |
| Osteoarticular | **Itra** oral sol'n 200 mg po bid x 12 mos. | **Liposomal Ampho B** 3-5 mg/kg/d IV or **ABLC** 5 mg/kg/d IV or **Ampho B Deoxycholate** 0.7-1 mg/kg IV daily; if response, change to **Itra** oral sol'n 200 mg po bid x total 12 mos. | After 2 wks of therapy, document adequate serum levels of Itraconazole. |
| Pulmonary | If severe, **Lipid Ampho B** 3-5 mg/kg IV or **standard Ampho B** 0.7-1 mg/kg IV once daily until response, then **Itra** 200 mg po bid. Total of 12 mos. | Less severe: **Itra** 200 mg po bid x 12 mos. | After 2 weeks of therapy document adequate serum levels of Itra. Surgical resection plus Ampho B for localized pulmonary disease. |
| Meningeal or Disseminated | **Lipid Ampho B** 5 mg/kg IV once daily x 4-6 wks, then—if better—**Itra** 200 mg po bid for total of 12 mos. | AIDS/Other immunosuppressed pts: chronic therapy with **Itra** oral sol'n 200 mg po once daily. | After 2 weeks, document adequate serum levels of Itra. |
| Pregnancy and children | Pregnancy: Cutaneous—local hyperthermia. Severe: **Lipid Ampho B** 3-5 mg/kg IV once daily. **Avoid Itraconazole.** | **Children:** Cutaneous: **Itra** 6-10 mg/kg (max of 400 mg) daily. Alternative is **SSKI** 1 drop tid increasing to max of 1 drop/kg or 40-50 drops tid/day, whichever is lowest. | For children with disseminated sporotrichosis: Standard **Ampho B** 0.7 mg/kg IV once daily & after response, **Itra** 6-10 mg/kg (max 400 mg) once daily. |

See page 2 for abbreviations. All dosage recommendations are for adults (unless otherwise indicated) and assume normal renal function.

**TABLE 11B – ANTIFUNGAL DRUGS: DOSAGE, ADVERSE EFFECTS, COMMENTS**

| DRUG NAME, GENERIC (TRADE)/ USUAL DOSAGE | ADVERSE EFFECTS/COMMENTS |
|---|---|
| **Non-lipid Amphotericin B deoxycholate** (Fungizone): 0.5–0.7 mg/kg IV per day as single infusion.<br><br>Ampho B predictably not active vs. Scedosporium, Candida lusitaniae & Aspergillus terreus | **Admin:** Ampho B is a colloidal suspension that must be prepared in electrolyte-free D5W at 0.1 mg/mL to avoid precipitation. No need to protect suspensions from light. Infusions cause chills/fever, myalgia, anorexia, nausea, rarely hemodynamic collapse/hypotension. Postulated due to proinflammatory cytokines, doesn't appear to be histamine release (Pharmacol 23:966, 2003). **Infusion duration usu. 4+ hrs.** No difference for chills/fever occurred sooner with 1 hr infus. except chills/fever occurred sooner with 1 hr infus. **Severe rigors respond to meperidine (25–50 mg IV).** Febrile reactions ↓ with repeat doses. Rare pulmonary reactions (severe dyspnea & focal infiltrates suggest pulmonary edema) assoc with rapid infus., esp leukocyte transfusions. Premedication with acetaminophen, diphenhydramine, hydrocortisone (25–50 mg) and heparin (1000 units) had no influence on rigors/fever. If cytokine postulate correct, NSAIDs or high-dose steroids may prove effective although their use may risk worsening infection under rx or increased risk of **nephrotoxicity** (i.e., NSAIDs). Clinical side effects ↓ with ↑ age.<br>**Toxicity:** Major concern is **nephrotoxicity.** Manifest initially by kaliuresis and **hypokalemia**, then fall in serum bicarbonate (may proceed to renal tubular acidosis), ↓ in renal erythropoietin and anemia, and rising BUN/serum creatinine. To minimize the nephrotoxicity, avoid other nephrotoxins, eg, Can reduce risk of renal injury by **(a) pre- & post-infusion saline infusion with 500 mL saline (if clinical status allows salt load), (b)** avoidance of other nephrotoxins, eg, radiocontrast, aminoglycosides, cis-platinum, cyclosporine. |
| **Lipid-based Ampho B products:** **Amphotericin B lipid complex (ABLC)** (Abelcet): 5 mg/kg per day as single infusion | **Admin:** Consists of Ampho B complexed with 2 lipid bilayer ribbons. Compared to standard Ampho B, larger volume of distribution, rapid blood clearance and high tissue concentrations (liver, spleen, lung). Dosage: **5 mg/kg once daily;** infuse at 2.5 mg/kg per hr; adult and ped. dose the same. Saline pre- and post-dose lessens toxicity. Do NOT use with saline in an in-line filter.<br>**Toxicity:** Fever and chills 14–18%; nausea 9%, vomiting 8%; serum creatinine ↑ in 11%; renal failure 5%; anemia 4%; ↓ K 5%; rash 4%. A fatal fat embolism following ABLC infusion (Exp Mol Path 177:246, 2004). Majority of pts intolerant of conventional Ampho B can tolerate ABLC (CID 56:701, 2013). |
| **Liposomal Amphotericin B (LAB),** AmBisome): 3–5 mg/kg IV per day as single infusion. If intolerant, majority IV with lipid form (CID 56:701, 2013). | **Admin:** Consists of vesicular bilayer liposome with Ampho B intercalated within the membrane. Dosage: **3–5 mg/kg per day IV** as single dose infused over a period of approx. 120 min. If tolerated, infusion time reduced to 60 min. (See footnote.)<br>**Major toxicity:** Gen less than Ampho B. Nephrotoxicity 18.7% vs 33.7% for Ampho B, chills 47% vs 75%, nausea 39.7% vs 38.7%, vomiting 31.8% vs 43.9%, rash 24% for both, ↓ La 18.4% vs 20.9%, ↓ K 20.4% vs 25.6%, ↓ mg 20.4% vs 25.6%. Acute reactions common with liposomal Ampho B. 20–40%. 86% occur within 5 min of infusion, incl chest pain, dyspnea, hypoxia or severe abdom, flank or leg pain; 14% dev flushing & urticaria near end of 4 hr infusion. All responded to diphenhydramine (1 mg/kg) & interruption of infusion. Reactions may be due to complement activation by liposome (CID 36:1213, 2003). |
| **Caspofungin** (Cancidas): 70 mg IV x 1 day 1 followed by 50 mg IV q24h (up to 35 x 70 mg IV q24h for severe hepatic insufficiency) | An echinocandin which inhibits synthesis of β-(1,3)-D-glucan. Fungicidal against Candida (MIC <2 mcg/mL) including those resistant to other antifungals & active against aspergillus. Effective rx of esophageal candidiasis & invasive aspergillosis in pts refractory or intolerant of other antifungals. Serum levels on rx: dosages ↑ peak 12, trough 1.3 (24 hrs) mcg/mL. **Toxicity:** remarkably non-toxic. Most common adverse effect: pruritus at infusion site & headache, fever, chills, vomiting, & diarrhea assoc with infusion. ↑ serum creatinine in 3% on caspo vs 21% short-course Ampho B in 422 pts with candidemia (Lu, Oct. 12, 2005, online). Drug metab in liver & dosage ↓ to 35 mg in moderate to severe hepatic failure. Class C for preg (embryotoxic in rats & rabbits). See Table 22A, page 256 for drug-drug interactions, incl cyclosporine (hepatic toxicity) & tacrolimus (drug level monitoring recommended). Reversible thrombocytopenia reported (Pharmacother 24:1408, 2004). **No drug in CSF, urine or vitreous humor of the eye.** |
| **Micafungin** (Mycamine): 50 mg IV q24h for prophylaxis post-bone marrow stem cell trans; 100 mg IV q24h candidemia, 150 mg IV q24h candida esophagitis. | Approved for rx of esophageal candidiasis & C. krusei. Active against most strains of candida sp. & aspergillus sp. incl those refractory to fluconazole such as C. glabrata & C. krusei. No dosage adjust for severe renal failure or moderate hepatic impairment. Watch for drug-drug interactions with sirolimus or nifedipine. Micafungin well tolerated & common adverse events incl nausea 2.8%, vomiting 2.4%, & headache 2.4%. Transient ↑ LFTs, BUN, creatinine reported; rare cases of significant hepatitis & renal insufficiency. See CID 42:1171, 2006. **No drug in CSF or urine.** |

[1] Published data from patients intolerant of or refractory to conventional Ampho B deoxycholate. **None of the lipid Ampho B preps has shown superior efficacy compared to Ampho B in prospective trials (except liposomal Ampho B was more effective vs Ampho B in rx of disseminated histoplasmosis at 2 wks). Dosage equivalency has not been established** (CID 36:1500, 2003). Nephrotoxicity ↓ with all lipid Ampho B preps. Compared with Abelcet (70% vs 36%) but higher frequency of mild hepatic toxicity with AmBisome (59% vs 38%, p<0.05). Mild elevations in serum creatinine were observed in 1/3 of both (BJ Hemat 103:198, 1998; Focus on Fungal Inf 49, 1999; Bone Marrow Tx 20:39, 1997; CID 26:1383, 1998).

[2] Toxicity grade: the slower the infusion, the higher the tolerated Ampho B infusion-assoc. toxicity (rigors). At higher doses (70% vs 36%) but higher frequency of mild hepatic toxicity with AmBisome

[3] HSCT = hematopoietic stem cell transplant.

See page 2 for abbreviations. All dosage recommendations are for adults (unless otherwise indicated) and assume normal/renal function.

**TABLE 11B (2)**

| DRUG NAME, GENERIC (TRADE)/ USUAL DOSAGE | ADVERSE EFFECTS/COMMENTS |
|---|---|
| **Anidulafungin** (Eraxis)<br>For Candidemia: 200 mg IV on day 1 followed by 100 mg/day IV. Esophageal candida: 100 mg IV x 1, then 50 mg IV once/d | An echinocandin with antifungal activity (cidal) against candida sp. & aspergillus sp. including Ampho B- & triazole-resistant strains. FDA approved for treatment of esophageal candidiasis (EC), candidemia, and other complicated Candida infections. Effective in rx of invasive candidiasis/candidemia in 245 pts (75.6% vs 60.2%). Like other echinocandins, remarkably non-toxic; most common side-effects: nausea, vomiting, ↓ mg, ↓ K & headache in 11–13% of pts. No dose adjustments for renal or hepatic insufficiency. See *CID 43:215, 2006.* **No drug in CSF or urine.** |
| **Fluconazole** (Diflucan)<br>100 mg tabs<br>150 mg tabs<br>200 mg tabs<br>400 mg tabs<br>Oral suspension: 50 mg per 5 mL | IV/oral dose because of excellent bioavailability. **Pharmacology:** absorbed po, water solubility enables IV. For peak serum levels *(see Table 9A, page 101).* T½ 30hr (range 20–50 hr). 12% protein bound. **CSF levels 50–90% of serum in normals.** ↑ in meningitis. No effect on mammalian steroid metabolism. **Drug-drug interactions common,** *see Table 22A.* Side-effects overall 16% (more common in HIV+ pts (21%)). Nausea 3.7%, headache 1.9%, skin rash 1.8%, abdominal pain 1.7%, diarrhea 1.5%, ↑ SGOT 20%. Alopecia (scalp, pubic crest) in 12–20% pts at 2400 mg po q24h after median of 3 mos (reversible in approx. 6mo). Rare: severe hepatotoxicity (↑ SGOT, reversible); skin rash 7%, aplastic anemia (rare—2 or 3 cases). False ↑ in serum creatinine on EKTACHEM analyzer. **Note: Candida krusei and Candida glabrata resistant to Flu.** |
| **Flucytosine** (Ancobon, 5-FC)<br>500 mg cap<br>**Expensive:** $11,000 for 100 capsules (Sep 2015 US price) | AEs: Overall 30%. GI 6% (diarrhea, anorexia, nausea, vomiting); hematologic 22% (leukopenia, thrombocytopenia, when serum level >100 mcg/mL, (esp. in azotemic pts)); hepatotoxicity (asymptomatic ↑ SGOT, reversible). Interferes with warfarin drugs. Increases blood and urine porphyrins, should not be used in patients with porphyria. Minor disulfiram-like reactions. Exacerbation of systemic lupus erythematosus.<br>Bioavailability 100%. Good levels in CSF, eye & urine. |
| **Griseofulvin**<br>(Fulvicin, Grifulvin, Grisactin)<br>500 mg, susp 125 mg/mL | Photosensitivity, urticaria, GI upset, fatigue, headache, leukopenia (rare). Increases blood and urine porphyrins, should not be used in patients with porphyria. Minor disulfiram-like reactions.<br>Not a recommended in 1st trimester of pregnancy. Local reactions: 0.5–1.5%: dyspareunia, mild vaginal or vulvar erythema, burning, pruritus, urticaria, rash. Rarely similar symptoms in sexual partner. |
| **Imidazoles,** topical<br>For vaginal and/or skin use | |
| **Isavuconazonium sulfate**<br>(prodrug **Isavuconazole**) (Cresemba)<br>po: 186 mg caps<br>IV: 372 mg vials<br>No drug in CSF.<br>Ref: *Med Lett 2016,58-33* | Azole antifungal agent for treatment of invasive aspergillosis and invasive mucormycosis in adults. **Contraindications:** Coadministration with strong CYP3A4 inhibitors, e.g., Ketoconazole or high-dose Ritonavir; or strong CYP3A4 inducers, e.g., Rifampin, carbamazepine, St. John's wort, or long-acting barbiturates is contraindicated. The drug in CSF.<br>**Dosing: Isavuconazonium sulfate** loading dose of 372 mg (equivalent to Isavuconazole 200 mg) IV/po q8 x 6 doses then 372 mg IV/po daily.<br>**AEs:** Most common: nausea, vomiting, diarrhea, headache, elevated liver chemistry tests, hypokalemia, constipation, dyspnea, cough, peripheral edema, and back pain.<br>Hepatic: increased ALT, AST. **Teratogenic.** |
| **Itraconazole** (Sporanox)<br>100 mg cap<br>10 mg/mL oral solution.<br>IV usual dose 200 mg bid x 4 doses followed by 200 mg q24h for a max of 14 days | **Itraconazole tablet & solution forms not interchangeable; solution preferred.** Many authorities recommend measuring drug serum concentration after 2 wks to ensure satisfactory absorption. To obtain highest plasma concentration, tablet is given with food & acidic drinks (e.g., cola) while solution is taken in fasted state; under these conditions, the peak conc. of capsule is approx. 3 mcg/mL & of solution 5.4 mcg/mL. Peak levels reached faster (2.2 vs 5 hrs) with solution. **Peak plasma concentrations after IV injection (200 mg) compared to oral capsule (200 mg): 2.8 mcg/mL (on day 7 of rx) vs 2 mcg/mL (on day 36 of rx).** Protein-binding for both preparations is over 99%, which explains virtual absence of penetration into CSF **(do not use to treat meningitis).** Adverse effects: nausea 10%, diarrhea 8%, vomiting 6%, & abdominal discomfort 5.7%. Allergic rash 8.6%, ↑ bilirubin 6%, edema 3.5%, & hepatitis 2.7% reported. ↑ doses may produce hypokalemia 8% & ↑ blood pressure 3.2%. Delirium, peripheral neuropathy & rash reported (*J New Microbiol: Drug Saf 27:329, 2004*). **Reported to produce impairment of left ventricular function.** Severe liver failure rare transplant in pt's receiving pulse rx for onychomycosis in pts with possible ↑ risk. Reported 24 cases with 11 deaths out of 50 mill people who received the drug prior to 2001. Other concern, as with fluconazole and ketoconazole, is **drug-drug interactions,** *see Table 22A.* Some can be life-threatening. |
| **Ketoconazole** (Nizoral)<br>200 mg tab | **Gastric acid required for absorption**—cimetidine, omeprazole, antacids block absorption. In achlorhydria, dissolve tablet in 4 mL 0.2N HCl, drink with a straw. Coca-Cola ↑ absorption by 65%. CSF levels "none". **Drug-drug interactions important,** *see Table 22A.* **Some interactions can be life-threatening.**<br>**Dose-dependent nausea and vomiting.**<br>Liver toxicity of hepatocellular type reported in about 1:10,000 exposed pts—usually after several days to weeks of exposure.<br>At doses of ≥800 mg/day serum testosterone and plasma cortisol levels fall. With high doses, adrenal (Addisonian) crisis reported. |
| **Miconazole** (Monistat IV)<br>200 mg tab—*not available in U.S.* | IV miconazole indicated in patient critically ill with Scedosporium (Pseudallescheria boydii) infection. Very toxic due to vehicle needed to get drug into solution. |

*See page 2 for abbreviations. All dosage recommendations are for adults (unless otherwise indicated) and assume normal renal function.*

**TABLE 11B (3)**

| DRUG NAME, GENERIC (TRADE)/ USUAL DOSAGE | ADVERSE EFFECTS/COMMENTS |
|---|---|
| **Nystatin** (Mycostatin)<br>30 gm cream<br>500,000 units oral tab | Topical: virtually no adverse effects. Less effective than imidazoles and triazoles.<br>po: large doses may cause occasional GI distress and diarrhea. |
| **Posaconazole** (Noxafil)<br>**Suspension** (40 mg/mL): 400 mg po bid with meals (if not taking meals, 200 mg po qid). 200 mg po tid (with food) for prophylaxis.<br>**Delayed-release tabs** (100 mg): 300 mg bid x 1 day and then 300 mg daily for prophylaxis.<br>**Intravenous formulation**: 300 mg IV bid x 1 day, then 300 mg IV daily (for prophylaxis). Takes 7–10 days to achieve steady state. No IV formulation. | **Suspension is dosed differently than delayed-release tablets (not interchangeable) – check dose carefully.** An oral triazole with activity against a wide range of fungi refractory to other antifungal rx including: aspergillosis, mucormycosis (variability by species), fusariosis, Scedosporium (Pseudallescheria), phaeohyphomycosis, histoplasmosis, refractory candidiasis, refractory coccidioidomycosis, refractory cryptococcosis, & refractory chromoblastomycosis. **Should be taken with high fat meal for maximum absorption.** Approved for prophylaxis of invasive aspergillosis and candidiasis. Clinical response in 75% of 176 AIDS pts with azole-refractory oral/esophageal candidiasis. Posaconazole has similar side-effects than other triazoles: nausea 9%, vomiting 6%, abd. pain 5%, headache 5%, diarrhea, ↑ ALT, AST, & rash (3% each). In pts rx for >6 mos, serious side-effects have included adrenal insufficiency, nephrotoxicity, & QTc interval prolongation. Significant drug-drug interactions; inhibits CYP3A4 (see Table 22A). Consider monitoring serum concentrations (AAC 53:24, 2009). **100 mg delayed-release tablets:** loading dose of 300 mg (three 100 mg delayed-release tablets) starting on the second day of therapy. Approved for prophylaxis only and not treatment. Tablets allow patients to achieve better levels than the suspension. Treatment dose unknown but clinical trials of other doses achieve therapeutic levels. The intravenous formulation was recently approved for prophylaxis at 300 mg IV daily after a loading dose of 300 mg bid x 1 day. Consider therapeutic drug monitoring with a goal trough of >0.7 for prophylaxis and >1.0 for treatment. |
| **Terbinafine** (Lamisil)<br>250 mg tab<br><br>Discontinued in U.S. in May 2017. | In pts given **terbinafine** for onychomycosis, rare cases (8) of idiosyncratic & symptomatic hepatic injury & more rarely liver failure leading to death or liver transplant. The drug is **not recommended** for pts with **chronic or active liver disease;** hepatotoxicity may occur in pts with or without pre-existing disease. Pretreatment serum transaminases (ALT & AST) advised & alternate rx used for those with abnormal levels. Pts started on terbinafine should be warned about symptoms suggesting liver dysfunction (persistent nausea, anorexia, fatigue, vomiting, RUQ pain, jaundice, dark urine or pale stools). If symptoms develop, drug should be discontinued & liver function immediately evaluated. In controlled trials, changes in ocular lens and retina reported—clinical significance unknown. Major drug interaction is 100% ↑ in rate of clearance by rifampin. **AEs:** usually mild, transient and rarely cause discontinuation of rx, % with AE, terbinafine vs placebo: nausea/diarrhea 2.8–5.6 vs 2.9; rash 5.6 vs 2.2; taste disturbance 2.8 vs 0.7. Inhibits CYP2D6 enzymes (see Table 22A). An acute generalized exanthematous pustulosis and subacute cutaneous lupus erythematosus reported. |
| **Voriconazole** (Vfend)<br>**IV: Loading dose 6 mg per kg q12h times 1 day,** then **4 mg per kg q12h IV** for invasive aspergillus & serious mold infections; **3 mg per kg IV** q12h for serious candida infections.<br>**Oral:** **>40 kg body weight:** 400 mg po q12h, then 200 mg po q12h **≤40 kg body weight:** 200 mg po q12h, then 100 mg po q12h<br>**Take oral dose 1 hour before or 1 hour after eating.**<br>Oral suspension (40 mg per mL). Oral suspension dosing: Same as for oral tabs.<br>Reduce to ½ maintenance dose for moderate hepatic insufficiency. | A triazole with activity against Aspergillus sp., **including Ampho resistant strains of A. terreus.** Active vs Candida sp. (including krusei), Fusarium sp. & various molds. Steady state serum levels reach 2.5–4 mcg per mL. Up to 20% of patients with subtherapeutic levels with oral administration; check levels for suspected treatment failure, life threatening infections. 300 mg bid oral dose or 8 mg/kg/d IV dose may be required to achieve target steady-state drug concentrations of 1–6 mcg/mL. **Toxicity** similar to other azoles/triazoles including uncommon serious hepatic toxicity (hepatitis, cholestasis & fulminant hepatic failure. Liver function tests should be monitored during rx & drug dc'd if abnormalities develop. **Photosensitivity is common and can be severe.** Many reports of associated skin cancers. Strongly recommend sun protective measures. CID 58:997, 2014 & hallucinations & anaphylactoid infusion reactions with fever and hypertension. 1 case of QT prolongation with ventricular tachycardia in a 15 y/o pt with ALL reported. **Approx. 21% experience a transient visual disturbance** including IV or po ("altered/visual perception", blurred or colored visual change or photophobia) within 30–60 minutes. Visual changes may **not clear at night for outpatient rx).** Persistent visual changes occur rarely. Cause unknown. In patients with CrCl <50 mL per mL, the intravenous vehicle (SBECD-sulfobutylether-β-cyclodextrin) may accumulate but not obviously toxic (CID 54:913, 2012). Hallucinations, hypoglycemia, electrolyte disturbance & pneumonitis attributed to 1 drug concentrations. Potential for drug-drug interactions high—see Table 22A. **With prolonged use, fluoride in drug can cause a painful periostitis.** (CID 59:1237, 2014)<br>**NOTE: Not in urine in active form. No activity vs. mucormycosis.** |

## TABLE 12A – TREATMENT OF MYCOBACTERIAL INFECTIONS*
*(IDSA, ATS, CDC): CID 64:e1, 2017.*

**Diagnosis of M. tuberculosis, Updated Guidelines** *(IDSA, ATS, CDC): CID 64:e1, 2017.*

**Tuberculin skin test (TST). Same as PPD** *(Chest 138:1456, 2010)* Criteria for positive TST after 5 tuberculin units (intermediate PPD) read at 48-72 hours:
- ≥5 mm induration: + HIV; immunosuppressed, ≥15 mg prednisone per day, recent close contact
- ≥10 mm induration: foreign-born, countries with high prevalence; healed TBc on chest x-ray, recent IVD Users; low income; NH residents; chronic illness; silicosis
- ≥15 mm induration: otherwise healthy

Two-stage to detect sluggish positivity: if 1st PPD + but <10 mm induration, do 2nd PPD. Response to 2nd PPD can also happen in 1 wk.

**BCG vaccine as child:** If ≥10 mm induration and from country with TB, should be attributed to MTB. Prior BCG may result in booster effect in 2-stage TST. Routine anergy testing not recommended.

**Interferon Gamma Release Assays (IGRAs):** IGRAs detect sensitivities to MTB by measuring IFN-γ release in response to MTB antigens (for review see *JAMA 308:241, 2012 and MMWR 59 (RR-5):1, 2010*):
- Approved tests: T-SPOT.TB (Oxford Immunotec) and QuantiFERON-TB Gold and QuantiFERON-TB Gold Plus (Qiagen).
- May be used in place of TST in all situations in which TST is indicated.
- CDC recommends IGRA over TST in most circumstances the exception being children age < 5 years (although some experts recommend age < 3 years.

IGRAs are relatively specific for MTB and do not cross-react with BCG or most nontuberculous mycobacteria. CDC recommends IGRA over TST for persons unlikely to return for reading TST & for persons who have received BCG. IGRA or TST may be used without preference for recent contacts of TB with special utility for follow-up testing since IGRAs do not produce "booster effect".
- May also be used as preference over TBc for occupational exposures.
- As with TST, testing with IGRAs in low prevalence populations will result in false-positive results *(CID 52:234, 2011)*.
- Manufacturer's IFN-gamma cutoff ≥0.35 IU/mL for QFT-GIT may be too low for low prevalence settings, inflating positivity and conversion rates, and a higher cut-off may be more appropriate *(Am J Respir Crit Care Med 188:1005, 2013)*. For detailed discussion of IGRAs, see *MMWR 59 (RR-5), 2010 and JAMA 308:241, 2012.* False positive IGRA *(JCM 54:845, 2016)*.

**Rapid (24-hr or less) diagnostic tests** for MTB: (1) The Amplified Mycobacterium tuberculosis Direct Test amplifies and detects MTB ribosomal RNA; (2) the AMPLICOR Mycobacterium tuberculosis Test amplifies and detects MTB DNA. Both tests have sensitivities >95% in sputum samples that are AFB-positive. In negative smears, sensitivity remains >95% but sensitivity is 40-77% *(MMWR 58:7, 2009, CID 49:1, 2009, CID 60:1377, 2015)*; (3) BIOMIC MTB/RIF assay (Cepheid) fully automated real-time PCR test; real-time PCR test for detection of M. tuberculosis in respiratory specimens (not available in the U.S.), with performance characteristics similar to other rapid tests *(J Clin Microbiol 51:3225, 2013)*.

**Xpert MTB/RIF** is a rapid test (2 hrs) for MTB in sputum samples which also detects RIF resistance with specificity of 99.2% and sensitivity of 72.5% in smear negative patients *(NEJM 363:1005, 2010)*. Current antibody-based and ELISA-based rapid tests for TBc not recommended by WHO because they are less accurate than microscopy ± culture *(Lancet ID 11:36, 2011)*.

**Xpert MTB/RIF Ultra (Xpert Ultra)** (not yet available in the US) *(Lancet Infect Dis 018 Jan;18(1):76-84)*: Higher sensitivity than Xpert MTB/RIF for detection of M. tuberculosis in smear-negative specimens, pediatric patients, HIV-infected patients, and in extra-pulmonary disease; slightly lower specificity than Xpert MTB/RIF. Recommended by WHO as initial diagnostic test for suspected tuberculosis and meningitis *(Lancet Infect Dis 2018 Jan;18(1):58-75)*.

| CAUSATIVE AGENT/ DISEASE | MODIFYING CIRCUMSTANCES | INITIAL THERAPY | SUGGESTED REGIMENS |
| --- | --- | --- | --- |
| | | | CONTINUATION PHASE OF THERAPY |
| I. **Mycobacterium tuberculosis exposure** baseline TST/IGRA **negative** (household members & other close contacts of potentially infectious cases) | Neonate– Rx essential NOTE: If fever, abnormal CXR (pleural effusion, hilar adenopathy, infiltrate at baseline, treat for active TBc and not with INH alone. | INH (10 mg/kg day for 8-10 wks) RIF 10-20 mg/kg/d also an option *(NEJM 379:454, 2018)* | Repeat tuberculin skin test (TST) in 8-12 wks: if TST neg & CXR normal & infant age at exposure >6 mos., stop INH. If TST (≥5 mm) or age ≤ 6 mos., treat with INH for total of 9 mos. (4 mos if RIF used). If follow-up CXR abnormal, treat for active TB. |
| | As for neonate for + 8-10 wks | | If repeat TST at 8-10 wks is negative, stop. |
| | Children <5 years of age– Rx indicated | | If repeat TST ≥5 mm, continue INH for total of 9 mos. |
| | Older children & adults– Risk 2-4% 1st yr | | TST at 3 mos, if TST is positive, treat with INH for 9 mos. If INH not given initially, repeat TST at 8-10 wks. Pts at high risk of progression (e.g., HIV+, immunosuppressed or on immunosuppressive therapy) and no evidence of active infection should be treated for LTBI *(see Category I below)*. For others repeat TST/IGRA at 8-10 wks: no rx if repeat TST/IGRA neg. |

*See page 2 for abbreviations*   * Dosages are for adults (unless otherwise indicated) and assume normal renal function   † **DOT** = directly observed therapy; **SAT** = self-administered therapy

**TABLE 12A (2)**

| CAUSATIVE AGENT/ DISEASE | MODIFYING CIRCUMSTANCES | SUGGESTED REGIMENS | |
|---|---|---|---|
| | | INITIAL THERAPY | ALTERNATIVE |
| **II. Tuberculosis (LTBI, positive TST or IGRA as above, active TB ruled out)**<br><br>See FIGURE 1 for treatment algorithm for pt with abnormal baseline CXR (e.g., upper lobe fibronodular disease) suspected active TB.)<br><br>Review:<br>NEJM 372:2127, 2015<br><br>Estimating risk of active TB in pts with positive TST or IGRA (www.tst3d.com) | Age no longer an exclusion, all persons with LTBI should be offered therapy. If pre-anti-TNF therapy, recommend at least one month of treatment for LBTI prior to start of anti-TNF therapy (*Arth Care & Res 64:625, 2012*). Overall, regimens containing a rifamycin (RIF, RBF or RFP) are most effective at preventing active tuberculosis (*AnIM 161:419 & 449, 2014*).<br><br>For patients on **Isoniazid (INH)** educate and monitor clinically for signs and symptoms of hepatitis. Baseline lab testing of liver function at start of therapy not routinely indicated but is indicated for patients with HIV infection, pregnant women, and women within 3 mo of delivery, persons with a history of chronic liver disease, persons who use alcohol regularly, and persons at risk for chronic liver disease.<br><br>Lab monitoring of liver function during therapy is indicated if baseline liver function tests are abnormal, if risk factors for hepatic disease are present, or to evaluate for possible adverse effects. | **INH** po once daily (adult: 5 mg/kg/day, max 300 mg/day; child: 10-15 mg/kg/day not to exceed 300 mg/day) x 9 mos. For current recommendations for monitoring hepatotoxicity on INH see *MMWR 59:227, 2010*. Supplemental pyridoxine 50 mg/day for HIV+ patients.<br><br>**3HP**: a 12 dose once weekly 3-month regimen of INH + Rifapentine (RFP)(3HP): INH po 15 mg/kg (max dose 900 mg) and RFP (wt-based dose): 10-14 kg: 300 mg; 14.1-25 kg: 450 mg; 25.1-32 kg: 600 mg; 32.1-49.9 kg: 750 mg; 50 kg: 900 mg. Recommended for treatment of LTBI 1) in adults; 2) in persons with LTBI aged 2-17 years; 3) in persons who have HIV infection, including persons with AIDS, and are taking antiretroviral medications with acceptable drug-drug interactions with rifapentine; and 4) by DOT† or SAT† in persons aged ≥2 years (*MMWR 67:723, 2018*). Not recommended for children age <2 yrs.<br><br>HIV Note: Increase in flu-like sx when INH/RFP combined with dolutegravir (*CID 2018;67:193*). | **INH** 300 mg once daily for 6 mo (but slightly less effective than 9 mos.; not recommended in children, HIV+ persons, or those with fibrotic lesions on chest film).<br><br>**INH** 2x/wk (adult: 15 mg/kg, max 900 mg; child: 20-30 mg/kg, max dose 900 mg) x 9 mo.<br><br>**RIF** once daily po (adult: 10 mg/kg/day, max dose 600 mg/day; child: 10-20 mg/kg/day, max dose 600 mg/day) for 4 mos (*NEJM 379:440, 454, 2018*).<br><br>**INH + RIF** once daily x 3 mos (*AnIM 2017;167:248*).<br><br>Rates of flu-like symptoms, cutaneous reactions, and severe drug reactions (rare, 0.3%) higher with 3 mo INH-RFP than with 9 mo INH (*CID 61:527, 2015*), but hepatotoxicity higher with INH (1.8% vs. 0.4%) (*Int J Tuberc Lung Dis 19:1039, 2015*). |
| | Pregnancy | Regimens as above. Once active disease is excluded may delay initiation of therapy until after delivery unless patient is recent contact to an active case. HIV+. Supplemental pyridoxine 10-25 mg/d recommended | |
| **LTBI, suspected INH-resistant organism** | | **RIF** once daily po (adult: 10 mg/kg, max dose 600 mg/day; child: 10-20 mg/kg/day, max dose 600 mg/day) for 4 mos. | **RFB** 300 mg once daily po may be substituted for RIF (in HIV+ patient on anti-retrovirals, dose may need to be adjusted for drug interactions). |
| **LTBI, suspected INH and RIF resistant organism** | | **Moxi** 400 mg once daily + **EMB** 15 mg/kg once daily x 12 months | **Levo** 500 mg once daily + (**EMB** 15 mg/kg or **PZA** 25 mg/kg) once daily x 12 months.<br>**NOTE:** PZA combo regimen, although perhaps most efficacious, poorly tolerated and may be overall less effective than FQ + EMB (*CID 64:1670, 2017*) |

\* Dosages are for adults (unless otherwise indicated) and assume normal renal function    † **DOT** = directly observed therapy;   **SAT** = self-administered therapy

**TABLE 12A (3)**

SEE COMMENTS FOR DOSAGE AND DIRECTLY OBSERVED THERAPY (DOT) REGIMENS

| CAUSATIVE AGENT/ DISEASE | MODIFYING CIRCUM-STANCES | SUGGESTED REGIMENS | | | | | | | COMMENTS |
|---|---|---|---|---|---|---|---|---|---|
| | | INITIAL THERAPY | | CONTINUATION PHASE OF THERAPY (in vitro susceptibility known) | | | Range of Total Doses (min. duration) | | |
| | | Regimen: in order of preference | Drugs | Interval/Doses (min. duration) | Regimen | Drugs | Interval/Doses (min. duration) | | |

**III. Mycobacterium tuberculosis**

**A. Pulmonary TB**
General reference on rx in adults & children; *MMWR* 52 (RR-11):1, 2003. In pts with newly diagnosed HIV and TB, Rx for both should be started as soon as possible (*NEJM* 362:697, 2010).

**Isolation essential!** Hospitalized pts. with suspected or documented active TB should be isolated in single rooms using airborne precautions until deemed non-infectious. DC isolation if 3 negative AFB smears or 1-2 neg NAAT (Xpert MTB/RIF) (*CID* 59:1353 & 1361, 2014).

**USE DOT REGIMENS IF POSSIBLE**

Rate of INH resistance known to be <4% (drug-susceptible organisms)

| Regimen | Drugs | Interval/Doses (min. duration) | Regimen | Drugs | Interval/Doses (min. duration) | Range of Total Doses (min. duration) |
|---|---|---|---|---|---|---|
| 1 (See Figure 2 page 152) | INH RIF PZA EMB | 7 days per wk times 56 doses (8 wks.) or 5 days per wk (DOT) times 40 doses (8 wks.) | 1a | INH/ RIF[b] | 7 days per wk times 126 doses (18 wks.) or 5 days per wk (DOT) times 90 doses (18 wks.). If cavitary disease, treat for 9 mos. | 182-130 (26 wks) |
| | | | 1b | INH/ RIF | 2 times per wk times 36 doses (18 wks) | 92-76 (26 wks) (Not AIDS pts.) |
| | | | 1c | INH/ RPF | 1 time per wk times 18 doses (18 wks) (only if HIV-neg) | 74-58 (26 wks) |
| 2 (See Figure 2 page 152) | INH RIF PZA EMB | 7 days per wk times 14 doses (2 wks.), then 2 times per wk times 12 doses (6 wks.) or 5 days per wk (DOT) times 10 doses (2 wks.) then 2 times per wk times 12 doses (6 wks) | 2a | INH/ RIF | 2 times per wk times 36 doses (18 wks) | 62-58 (26 wks) (Not AIDS pts.) |
| | | | 2b[a] | INH/ RPF | 1 time per wk times 18 doses (18 wks) (only if HIV-neg) | 44-40 (26 wks) |
| 3 (See Figure 2 page 152) | INH RIF PZA EMB | 3 times per wk times 24 doses (8 wks) | 3a | INH/ RIF | 3 times per wk times 54 doses (18 wks) | 78 (26 wks) |
| 4 (See Figure 2 page 152) | INH RIF EMB | 7 days per wk times 56 doses (8 wks) or 5 days per wk (DOT) times 40 doses (8 wks) | 4a | INH/ RIF | 7 days per wk times 217 doses (31 wks) or 5 days per wk (DOT) times 155 doses (31 wks) | 273-195 (39 wks) |
| | | | 4b | INH/ RIF | 2 times per wk times 62 doses (31 wks) | 119-102 (39 wks) |

**COMMENTS**

Dose in mg per kg (max. q24h dose)

| Regimen* Q24h: | INH | RIF | PZA | EMB | SM | RFB |
|---|---|---|---|---|---|---|
| Child | 10-20 (300) | 10-20 (600) | 15-30 (2000) | 15-25 | 20-40 (1000) | 10-20 |
| Adult | 5 (300) | 10 (600) | 15-30 (2000) | 15-25 | 15 (1000) | 5 (300) |

**2 times per wk (DOT):**

| | INH | RIF | PZA | EMB | SM | RFB |
|---|---|---|---|---|---|---|
| Child | 20-40 (900) | 10-20 (600) | 50-70 (4000) | 50 | 25-30 (1500) | 10-20 (300) |
| Adult | 15 (900) | 10 (600) | 50-70 (3000) | 50 | 25-30 (1500) | 5 (300) |

**3 times per wk (DOT):**

| | INH | RIF | PZA | EMB | SM | RFB |
|---|---|---|---|---|---|---|
| Child | 20-40 (900) | 10-20 (600) | 50-70 (3000) | 25-30 | 25-30 (1500) | NA |
| Adult | 15 (900) | 10 (600) | 50-70 (3000) | 25-30 | 25-30 (1500) | NA |

**Second-line anti-TB agents can be dosed as follows to facilitate DOT:** Cycloserine 500-750 mg po q24h (5 times per wk)
Ethionamide 500-750 mg po q24h (5 times per wk)
Kanamycin or capreomycin 15 mg per kg IM/IV q24h (3-5 times per wk)
Ciprofloxacin 750 mg po q24h (5 times per wk)
Ofloxacin 600-800 mg po q24h (5 times per wk)
Levofloxacin 750 mg po q24h (5 times per wk) (*CID* 21:1245, 1995)

**Risk factors for drug-resistant (MDR) TB:** Recent immigration from Latin America or Asia or living in area of resistance (≥4%) or previous rx without Rx; exposure to known MDR TB. Incidence of MDR TB in US **steady** from 2000. Incidence of primary drug resistance is part. high (>25%) in parts of China, Thailand, Russia, Estonia & Latvia; ~80% of US MDR cases in foreign born.

**NOTE:** Thrice weekly therapy for both the initial and continuation phase and twice weekly therapy in the continuation phase have higher rates of relapse and microbiological failure, acquired drug resistance compared to daily therapy (*CID* 64:1211, 2017).

(continued on next page)

(continued on next page)

*Dosages are for adults (unless otherwise indicated) and assume normal renal function    † DOT = directly observed therapy; SAT = self-administered therapy

See page 2 for abbreviations    * Dosages are for adults (unless otherwise indicated) and assume normal renal function

**TABLE 12A (4)**

| CAUSATIVE AGENT/ DISEASE | MODIFYING CIRCUM-STANCES | SUGGESTED REGIMEN[b] | DURATION OF TREATMENT (mos.)[a] | SPECIFIC COMMENTS[c] | COMMENTS |
|---|---|---|---|---|---|
| **III. Mycobacterium tuberculosis** | | | | | *(continued from previous page)* |
| **A. Pulmonary TB** *(continued from previous page)* | INH (± SM) resistance | RIF, PZA, EMB (a FQ may strengthen the regimen for pts with extensive disease) | 6 | INH should be stopped in cases of INH resistance. Outcome similar for drug susceptible and INH-mono-resistant strains *(CID 48:179, 2009).* | **Alternatives for resistant strains: Moxi** and **levo are FQs of choice,** not CIP. FQ resistance may be seen in pts previously treated with FQ. WHO recommends using moxi (if MIC ≤ 2) if resistant to earlier generation FQs *(AAC 54:4765, 2010).* |
| | | | | | **Linezolid** 600 mg once daily has excellent in vitro activity, including MDR strains and effective in selected cases of MDR TB and XDR TB but watch for toxicity *(NEJM 367:1508, 2012).* |
| **Multidrug-Resistant Tuberculosis** (MDR TB): Defined as resistant to at least 2 drugs including INH & RIF. Pt clusters with high mortality *(NEJM 363:1050, 2010).* | Resistance to INH & RIF (± SM) | FQ, PZA, EMB, AMK or capreomycin (SM only if confirmed susceptible), see Comment | WHO (2016) recommends 7 drugs pending drug suscept. results: INH EMB, Moxi, SM, ETH, PZA, CLO x 9-11 mos. *(CID 2017:65:1206 & 1212)* | Extended rx is needed to ↓ the risk of relapse. In cases with extensive disease, the use of an additional agent (alternative agents) may be prudent to ↓ the risk of failure & additional acquired drug resistance. Resectional surgery may be appropriate. | **Clofazimine** 100 mg is one component of a multiple drug regimen may improve outcome *(CID 60:1361, 2015).* |
| | | | | | **Bedaquiline** recently FDA approved for treatment of MDR TB based on efficacy in Phase 2 trials *(NEJM 360:2397, 2009; AAC 56:3271, 2012; NEJM 371:689, 723, 2014).* Dose is 400 mg once daily for 2 weeks then 200 mg tiw for 22 weeks administered with food, and always in combination with other anti-TB meds. |
| **Extensively Drug-Resistant TB** (XDR-TB): Defined as resistant to INH & RIF plus any FQ and at least 1 of the 3 second-line drugs: capreomycin, kanamycin or amikacin *(MMWR 56:250, 2007; CID 51:1379, 2010).* | Resistance to INH, RIF (± SM), & EMB or PZA | FQ (EMB or PZA if active), AMK or capreomycin (SM only if confirmed susceptible) | 24 | Use the first-line agents to which there is susceptibility. Add 2 or more alternative agents in case of extensive disease. Surgery should be considered. Survival ↑ in pts receiving active FQ & surgical intervention *(AJRCCM 169:1103, 2004).* | The investigational agent, **delamanid** *(NEJM 366:2151, 2012; Eur Respir J 45:1498, 2015),* at a dose of 100 mg bid, granted conditional approval for treatment of MDR-TB as one component of an optimized background regimen by the European Medicines Agency. |
| | Resistance to RIF | INH, EMB, FQ supplemented with PZA for the first 2 mos. (an IA may be included for the first 2-3 mos. for pts with extensive disease) | 12-18 | Extended use of an IA may be feasible. An all-oral regimen times 12-18 mos. should be effective but is less well studied. Use of an injectable agent (IA) when effective may shorten duration (e.g., to 12 mos.). An IA may be added in the initial 2 mos. of rx. | **Consultation with experts in MDR-TB management** strongly advised for use of this agent. For MDR-TB and XDR-TB, do drug susceptibility testing for ethambutol, PZA & other 2nd line drugs if possible *(CID 59:1364, 2014)* |
| | XDR-TB | Expert consultation strongly advised See comments | 18-24 | Therapy requires administration of 4-6 drugs to which infecting organism is susceptible, including multiple second-line drugs *(AJRCCM 56:250, 2007).* Increased mortality seen primarily in HIV+ patients. Cure with outpatient therapy likely in non-HIV+ patients when regimens of 4 or 5 or more drugs to which organism is susceptible are employed *(NEJM 359:563, 2008; CID 47:496, 2008).* Successful sputum culture conversion correlates to initial susceptibility to FQs and kanamycin *(CID 46:42, 2008).* Bedaquiline *(CID 60:188, 2015)* and Linezolid are options. | |

*See page 2 for abbreviations*     [a] Dosages are for adults (unless otherwise indicated) and assume normal renal function     † **DOT** = directly observed therapy     **SAT** = self-administered therapy

**TABLE 12A (5)**

| CAUSATIVE AGENT/DISEASE; MODIFYING CIRCUMSTANCES | SUGGESTED REGIMENS | | COMMENTS |
|---|---|---|---|
| | INITIAL THERAPY | CONTINUATION PHASE OF THERAPY (in vitro susceptibility known) | |

**III. Mycobacterium tuberculosis** (continued)

| CAUSATIVE AGENT/DISEASE; MODIFYING CIRCUMSTANCES | INITIAL THERAPY | CONTINUATION PHASE OF THERAPY (in vitro susceptibility known) | COMMENTS |
|---|---|---|---|
| **B. Extrapulmonary TB** Steroids: see **Comment** | **INH + RIF (or RFB) + PZA + EMB** q24h x 2 months. Some add pyridoxine 25–50 mg q24h | **INH + RIF (or RFB)** | IDSA recommends 6 mos for lymph node, pleural, pericarditis, disseminated disease, genitourinary & peritoneal TB; 6–9 mos for bone & joint; 9–12 mos for CNS (including meningeal) TBc. **Corticosteroids** "strongly rec" only for meningeal TBc (*MMWR 52(RR-11):1, 2003*). TBc not recommended for pericarditis (*NEJM 371:1121 & 1155, 2014*). |
| **C. Tuberculous meningitis** Excellent review of clinical aspects and therapy (*IDSA guidelines; Clin Infect Dis, Aug 10) (pii: ciw376. [Epub ahead of print], 2016*) | **(INH + RIF + EMB + PZA) +** prednisone 60 mg/day x 4 wks, then 30 mg/day x 4 wks, then 15 mg/day x 4 wks, then 7.5 mg/day x 1 wk | May omit **EMB** when susceptibility to INH and RIF established. Can D/C PZA after 2 months. Treat for total of 12 months. *See Table 9, page 102,* for CSF drug penetration. Initial reg of **INH + RIF + SM + PZA** also effective, even in patients with INH resistant organisms. | **3 drugs often rec for initial rx; we prefer 4** (*J Infect 59:167, 2009*). Infection with MDR TB ↑ mortality & morbidity. Adjunctive corticosteroids improve survival (*Cochrane Database Syst Rev, Apr 28;4:CD002244, 2016*) and strongly recommended: Adult - dexamethasone 0.4 mg/kg/day week 1, 0.3 mg/kg/day week 2, 0.2 mg/kg/day week 3, 0.1 mg/kg/day week 4, then tapered to stop over 3-4 weeks. Child - dexamethasone 0.6 mg/kg/day or prednisolone 4 mg/kg/day for 4 weeks then tapered to stop over 4 weeks. |
| **D. Tuberculosis during pregnancy** | **INH + RIF + EMB** x 9 mos | | SM should not be substituted for EMB due to toxicity. AMK, capreomycin, kanamycin, FQs also contraindicated. PZA is recommended for routine use in pregnant women by the WHO but has not been used in U.S. due to lack of safety data, although PZA has been used in some US health jurisdictions without reported adverse events. If PZA is not included in the initial treatment regimen, the minimum duration of therapy is 9 months. Pyridoxine, 25 mg/day, should be administered. |
| **E. Treatment failure or relapse** Usually due to poor compliance or resistant organisms, or subtherapeutic drug levels (*CID 55:169, 2012*). | Directly observed therapy (DOT). Check susceptibilities. (*See section III. A, page 148 & above*) | | Pts whose sputum is culture-positive after 5–6 mos. = treatment failures. Failures may be due to non-compliance or resistant organisms. Non-compliance common, therefore institute DOT. If isolates show resistance, modify regimen to include at least 2 (preferably 3) new active agents, ones that the patient has not previously received if at all possible. Patients with MDR-TB usually convert sputum within 12 weeks of successful therapy. |
| **F. HIV infection or AIDS— pulmonary or extrapulmonary** All HIV infected patients with TB should be treated with ARVs. If CD4 <50, initiation of ARVs within 2 weeks of starting TB meds associated with improved survival (*Ann Intern Med 163:32, 2015*). If CD4 >50 no proven survival benefit with early ARVs: initiate ARVs at 2-4 weeks of TB meds for moderately severe or severe TB, 8-12 weeks for less severe TB. | **INH + RIF (or RFB) + PZA** q24h x 2 mos. Add pyridoxine 50 mg q24h | **INH + RIF (or RFB)** q24h x 4 months (total 6 mos.). Treat up to 9 mos in pts with delayed response, cavitary disease. 6 mos + **RIF (or RFB)** q24h to regimens that include INH | 1. Co-administration of RIF not recommended for these anti-retroviral drugs: nevirapine, etravirine, rilpivirine, maraviroc, elvitegravir (integrase inhibitor), Stribild), all HIV protease inhibitors. Use RFB instead. 2. RIF may be coadministered with efavirenz; nucleoside reverse transcriptase inhibitors. Coadministration with raltegravir or dolutegravir OK but if necessary increase raltegravir dose to 800 mg q12h; RIF + dolutegravir OK at 50 mg bid of latter. 3. Because of possibility of developing resistance to RIF or RFB in pts with low CD4 cell counts who receive wkly or biwkly (2x/wk) therapy, daily dosing (preferred), or at a min 3x/wk dosing (failure rate likely higher) rec for initial or continuation phase of rx. 4. Clinical & microbiologic response similar to that of HIV-neg patient. 5. Post-treatment suppression not necessary for drug-susceptible strains. 6. In RBPCT, prednisone reduced IRIS from 47% to 33% (*NEJM 2018;379:1915*). |
| **Concomitant protease inhibitor (PI) therapy** | **INH 300 mg q24h + RFB** (150 mg q24h or 300 mg two/wk) + **EMB 15 mg/kg q24h + PZA 25 mg/kg q24h** x 2 mos; then INH + RFB x 4 mos. (up to 7 mos.) | **INH + RFB** x 4 mos. (7 mos. in slow responders, cavitary disease) | Rifamycins induce cytochrome CYP450 enzymes (RIF > RFP > RFB) & reduce serum levels of concomitantly administered PIs. Conversely, PIs inhibit CYP450 & cause ↑ serum levels of RFP & RFB. If dose of RFB is not reduced, toxicity ↑. |

**TABLE 12A (6)**

**FIGURE 1: TREATMENT ALGORITHM FOR ACTIVE, CULTURE-NEGATIVE PULMONARY TUBERCULOSIS AND INACTIVE TUBERCULOSIS** *(modified from MMWR 52(RR-11):1, 2003).*

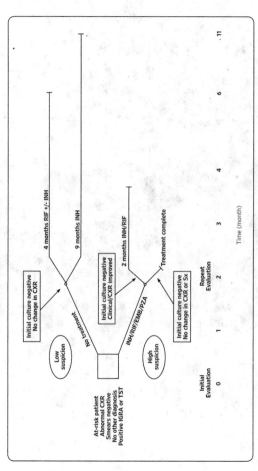

Patients at high clinical suspicion of active TB should be started on 4-drug therapy, pending results of cultures. If cultures are negative and there is no change in symptoms or CXR, the 4-drug regimen can be stopped and no further therapy is required. If cultures are negative and there is clinical or CXR improvement, continue INH/RIF for 2 additional months. For patients at low suspicion for active TB, treat for LTBI once cultures are negative.

*See page 2 for abbreviations*     * Dosages are for adults (unless otherwise indicated) and assume normal renal function     † **DOT** = directly observed therapy; **SAT** = self-administered therapy

152

TABLE 12A (7)
FIGURE 2: TREATMENT ALGORITHM FOR CULTURE-POSITIVE PULMONARY TUBERCULOSIS [Modified from MMWR 52(RR-11):1, 2003]

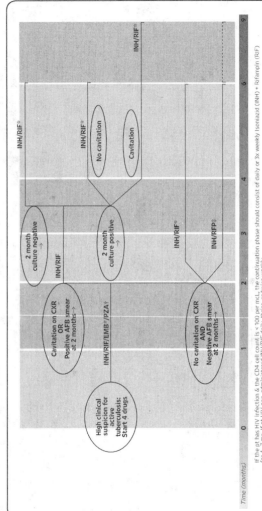

If the pt has HIV infection & the CD4 cell count is < 100 per mcL, the continuation phase should consist of daily or 3x weekly Isoniazid (INH) + Rifampin (RIF) for 4-7 mo. If pt HIV-neg, administered INH/RIF daily, thrice, or twice weekly.

※ EMB may be discontinued in <2 months if drug susceptibility testing indicates no drug resistance.
† PZA may be discontinued after 2 months (56 doses).
‡ Once weekly INH/RFP, do not use in HIV-infected patients with tuberculosis or in patients with extrapulmonary tuberculosis. Therapy should be extended to 9 months if 2 mo. culture is positive.

See page 2 for abbreviations    ※ Dosages are for adults (unless otherwise indicated) and assume normal renal function    † DOT = directly observed therapy; SAT = self-administered therapy

**TABLE 12A (8)**

| CAUSATIVE AGENT/DISEASE | MODIFYING CIRCUMSTANCES | SUGGESTED REGIMENS PRIMARY/ALTERNATIVE | | COMMENTS |
|---|---|---|---|---|
| **IV. Nontuberculous Mycobacteria (NTM)** *(See ATS Consensus: AJRCCM 175:367, 2007; EID 17:506, 2011)* | | | | |
| **A. Mycobacterium bovis** | | | | The M. tuberculosis complex includes M. bovis, and regimens effective for MTB (except PZA based) also likely to be effective for M. bovis. **All isolates resistant to PZA.** Isolation not required. Increased prevalence of extrapulmonary disease in U.S. born Hispanic populations and elsewhere *(CID 47:168, 2008; EID 14:909, 2008; EID 17:457, 2011)* |
| **B. Bacillus Calmette-Guerin (BCG)** (derived from M. bovis) | Only fever (>38.5°C) for 12–24 hrs | **INH + RIF + EMB** x 2 months then **INH + RIF** x 7 months | | Intravesical BCG effective in superficial bladder tumors and carcinoma in situ. With sepsis, consider initial adjunctive prednisolone. Also susceptible to RFB, CIP, oflox, levo, moxi, streptomycin, amikacin, capreomycin. **Resistant to PZA.** |
| | Systemic illness or sepsis | **INH 300 mg q24h** times 3 months Same as for M. bovis. | | BCG may cause regional adenitis or pulmonary disease in HIV-infected children. **Resistant to PZA.** |
| **C. Mycobacterium avium-intracellulare complex** (MAC, MAI, or Battey bacillus) *ATS/IDSA Consensus Statement: AJRCCM 175:367, 2007. See http://aidsinfo.nih.gov/guidelines/html/4/adult-and-adolescent-oi-prevention-and-treatment-guidelines/0 for updated CDC recommendations for AIDS patients.* | **Immunocompetent patients** | | | |
| | Nodular/Bronchiectatic disease | **Clarithro 1000 mg or Azithro 500 mg** tiw **+ EMB 25 mg/kg tiw +** **RIF 600 mg or RFB 300 mg]** tiw | | Intermittent (tiw) therapy not recommended for patients with cavitary disease, patients who have been previously treated or patients with moderate of severe disease. Intermittent therapy may be an option in mild bronchiectatic form of the disease *(Am J Respir Crit Care Med 191:96, 2015).* The primary microbiologic goal of therapy is 12 months of negative sputum cultures on therapy. |
| | Cavitary disease or severe nodular/bronchiectatic disease | **Clarithro 500–1000 mg/day (lower dose for wt <50 kg) or Azithro 250 mg/day) + EMB 15 mg/kg/day + [RIF 600 mg/day or RFB 150–300 mg/day] ± [Strep or AMK]** If sputum remains MAC+, can add FDA-approved inhalations of liposomal AMK per day | | **"Classic" pulmonary MAC:** Men 50–75, smokers, COPD. May be associated with hot tub use *(Chest Med 23:675, 2002).* **"New" pulmonary MAC:** Women 30–70, scoliosis, mitral valve prolapse, (bronchiectasis), pectus excavatum ("Lady Windermere syndrome") and fibronodular disease in elderly women *(AJM 113:756, 2002).* May also be associated with interferon gamma deficiency *(AJM 115:576, 2010).* For cervicofacial lymphadenitis (localized) in immunocompetent children, surgical excision is as effective as chemotherapy *(CID 44:1057, 2007).* Moxifloxacin and gatifloxacin, active in vitro & in vivo *(AAC 51:4071, 2007).* |
| | **HIV infection:** **Primary prophylaxis**—Pt's CD4 count <50–100 per mm³ Discontinue when CD4 count >100 per mm³ in response to ART | **Azithro 1200 mg po weekly** OR **Clarithro 500 mg po bid** | **RFB 300 mg po q24h** OR **Azithro 1200 mg po weekly + RIF 300 mg po q24h** | Many drug-drug interactions, see *Table 22A, page 256.* Drug-resistant MAI disease seen in 29–58% of pts in whom disease develops while taking clarithro prophylaxis & in 11% of those on azithro but has not been observed with RFB prophylaxis. Clarithro resistance more likely in pts with extremely low CD4 counts at initiation. Need to be sure no active MTB; RFB used for prophylaxis may promote selection of rifamycin-resistant MTB. |
| | **Treatment** Either presumptive dx or after + culture of blood, bone marrow, or usually, sterile body fluids, eg liver | **Clarithro 500 mg po bid + EMB 15 mg/kg/day +/- RFB 300 mg po q24h (adjust dose)** | **Azithro 500 mg po/day + EMB 15 mg/kg/day +/- RFB 300–450 mg po/day** | Addition of a third or fourth drug should be considered for patients with advanced immunosuppression (CD4 count <50 cells/µL, high mycobacterial loads (>2 log CFU/mL of blood), or in the absence of effective ART: AMK 10–15 mg/kg IV daily; Strep 1 gm IV or IM daily; CIP 500–750 mg PO bid; Levo 500 mg PO daily; Moxi 400 mg PO daily. Testing of susceptibility to clarithromycin and azithromycin is recommended. Short term (4–8 weeks) of systemic corticosteroid (equivalent to 20–40 mg of prednisone) can be used for IRIS. |

*See page 2 for abbreviations*          * Dosages are for adults (unless otherwise indicated) and assume normal renal function          † **DOT** = directly observed therapy;  **SAT** = self-administered therapy

**TABLE 12A (9)**

| CAUSATIVE AGENT/DISEASE | MODIFYING CIRCUMSTANCES | SUGGESTED REGIMENS PRIMARY/ALTERNATIVE | | COMMENTS |
|---|---|---|---|---|

**IV. Nontuberculous Mycobacteria (NTM)** (continued)

| CAUSATIVE AGENT/DISEASE | MODIFYING CIRCUMSTANCES | PRIMARY | ALTERNATIVE | COMMENTS |
|---|---|---|---|---|
| **C. Mycobacterium avium-intracellulare complex** (continued) | Chronic post-treatment suppression—secondary prophylaxis | **Always necessary.** (Clarithro or azithro) + EMB 15 mg/kg/day (dosage above) | Clarithro or Azithro + or RFB (dosage above) | Recurrences almost universal without chronic suppression. Can discontinue if no signs and symptoms of MAC disease and sustained (>6 months) CD4 count >100 cells/µL in response to ART. |
| **D. Mycobacterium celatum** | Treatment; optimal regimen not defined | May be susceptible to clarithro, FQ. Treat as if MAC. | | Isolated from pulmonary lesions and blood in AIDS patients. Easily confused with M. xenopi (and MAC). |
| **E. Mycobacterium abscessus** | Treatment; Surgical debridement may facilitate clarithro rx in subcutaneous abscess and is important adjunct to rx. For role of surgery in M. abscessus pulmonary disease, see CID 52:565, 2011. | **Cutaneous infection:** Surgical debridement + Azithro 500 mg once daily x 4-6 months OR Azithro 500 mg once daily + Moxi 400 mg once daily x 4-6 months<br><br>**Pulmonary or disseminated disease:**<br>**Intensive phase: (Imipenem** 1000 mg IV q12h or **Cefoxitin** 8-12 gm/day IV in 2-3 divided doses) + **Azithro** 250-500 mg once daily + **Amikacin** 15 mg/kg once daily IV (adjust dose to obtain a peak serum concentration of 20-30 µg/mL and a trough of < 5-10 µg/mL) + **Tigecycline** 100 mg loading dose then 50 mg q12h IV; treat for 2-3 months depending on severity of infection, clinical response, tolerability and toxicity, ideally with the goal of converting sputum cultures to negative.<br>**Continuation phase: Azithro** 250-500 mg + one or two other oral agents depending on tolerability and disease severity; optimal duration of therapy is unknown but target is 12 months after sputum cultures convert to negative. | | **M. abscessus** is a complex of 3 species: M. abscessus, M. massiliense, M. bolletii. Treatment outcomes poor with half or more of patients remaining culture-positive or relapsing with infection due to strains with inducible macrolide resistance, i.e., M. abscessus subspecies abscessus (CID 64:301, 309, 2017). Inducible resistance to macrolides seen in M. abscessus subspecies massiliense due to non-functional macrolide resistance gene; Outcomes better with infection from this species compared to other members of the complex (Int J Tuberc Lung Dis 18:1141, 2014). 2-4 week regimen of IV **amikacin** + IV **cefoxitin** (or **IMP**) + an oral macrolide (**clarithro** 1000 mg/d or **azithro** 250 mg/d) followed by oral macrolide administered for 12-15 months after culture conversion at end of treatment) in many patients remaining culture-positive pulmonary infection highly effective (98% culture conversion at end of treatment) in one study (Chest 150:1211, 2016). M. abscessus subspecies susceptibilities: Amikacin (70%), Clarithromycin (95%) (however, M. abscessus subspecies abscessus often has inducible resistance requiring prolonged incubation for detection), Cefoxitin (70%), Rifabutin, Ciprofloxacin, Doxycycline (EID 21:doi:10.3201/2109.141634, 2015) Linezolid, Clofazimine.<br>Pulmonary and disseminated disease notoriously refractory to therapy and outcomes are poor with half or more of patients remaining culture-positive or relapsing particularly with infection due to strains with inducible macrolide resistance such as M. abscessus subspecies abscessus; long-term suppressive therapy often needed to control symptoms or disease progression (Int J Tuberc Lung Dis 18:1141, 2014).<br>Significant toxicity (Int J Tuberc Lung Dis. 2017; 21:818) and uncertain efficacy of Amikacin (AAC 2016;60(10):6374-6 and AAC 2017;61(11). pii: e01206-17). Inhalation therapy with nebulised Amikacin may be an option for refractory cases or as an adjunct during the continuation phase, although lack of a commercially available product and lack of quality data on efficacy, tolerability, and duration of treatment are limitations. |
| **Mycobacterium chelonae** | Rapid grower assoc. with skin, wound, soft tissue infection; rarely disseminated/pulmonary | Skin: **Clarithro** 500 mg po bid x 6 mo. Complicated/disseminated: **Clarithro** + **Tobra** or **IMP** or **Linezolid**) x 2-8 wks, then **Clarithro** to complete 6-12 mo. | | **M. chelonae** susceptible to AMK (80%), clarithro, azithro, tobramycin (100%), IMP (60%), moxifloxacin, CIP, Mino, Doxy, linezolid (94%) (CID 42:1756, 2006). Resistant to cefoxitin, FQ. Tigecycline highly active in vitro and successfully used as salvage for M. chelonae infection in combination regimens (J Antimicrob Chemother 69:1945, 2014). |
| **F. Mycobacterium fortuitum** | Treatment; optimal regimen not defined. Surgical excision of infected areas. | AMK + Cefoxitin + Probenecid 2-6 wks, then po TMP-SMX, or doxy 2-6 mos. Usually responds to 6-12 mos of oral rx with 2 drugs to which it is susceptible. | | **Resistant to all standard anti-Tbc drugs.** Sensitive in vitro to doxycycline, minocycline, cefoxitin, IMP, AMK, TMP-SMX, CIP, oflox, azithro, clarithro, linezolid, tigecycline, but some strains resistant to clarithromycin, rifabutin. For rapid mycobacterial pulmonary disease, see some strains resistant to clarithro; active in vitro until sputum cultures negative for at least 12 months (Am J RCCM 175:367, 2007). Disseminated disease associated with auto-antibodies to interferon-γ (Intern Med 53:1361, 2014). |

See page 2 for abbreviations

* Dosages are for adults (unless otherwise indicated) and assume normal renal function    † **DOT** = directly observed therapy; **SAT** = self-administered therapy

**TABLE 12A (10)**

| CAUSATIVE AGENT/DISEASE | MODIFYING CIRCUMSTANCES | SUGGESTED REGIMENS PRIMARY/ALTERNATIVE | COMMENTS |
|---|---|---|---|
| **IV. Nontuberculous Mycobacteria (NTM)** *(continued)* | | | |
| **G. Mycobacterium haemophilum** | Regimen(s) not defined. In animal model, **Clarithro** + **Rifabutin** effective. Combination of **CIP** + **RFB** + **Clarithro** reported effective but clinical experience limited *(CID 52:488, 2011).* Surgical debridement may be necessary. | | Clinical: Ulcerating skin lesions, synovitis, osteomyelitis, cervicofacial lymphadenitis in children. Associated with permanent eyebrow makeup *(CID 52:488, 2011).* Lab: Requires supplemented media to isolate. Sensitive in vitro to: CIP, cycloserine, rifabutin, moxifloxacin. Over ½ resistant to: INH, RIF, EMB, PZA. For localized cervicofacial lymphadenitis in immunocompetent children, surgical excision as effective as chemotherapy *(CID 44:1057, 2007)* or "watchful waiting" *(CID 52:180, 2011).* |
| **H. Mycobacterium genavense** | 2 or more drugs: **Clarithro, EMB, RFB; CLO, Amikacin, Moxifloxacin** as alternatives. | | Seen in AIDS patients with CD4 <50 and in non-HIV severely immunocompromised hosts. *For review see Clin Microbiol Infect 19:432, 2013.* |
| **I. Mycobacterium gordonae** | Rarely a true pathogen. | | Frequent colonizer, not associated with disease. In vitro: sensitive to EMB, RIF, AMK, CIP, clarithro, linezolid. Resistant to INH. Surgical excision. |
| **J. Mycobacterium kansasii** | [**Clarithro** 500 mg or **Clarithro** 1000 mg) + **RIF** 600 mg + **EMB** 15 mg/kg] po q24h | **INH** 300 mg + **Pyridoxine** 50 mg + **RIF** 600 mg + **EMB** 15 mg/kg) po q24h.<br>**For Rifampin resistant organism:**<br>[**INH** 900 mg + **Pyridoxine** 50 mg + **EMB** 15 mg/kg + (**Moxi** 400 mg or **Azithro** 500 mg or **Clarithro** 1000 mg)] po q24h | **All isolates are resistant to PZA.** Treat until sputum cultures have been negative for 12 mo. For HIV+ patients on a protease inhibitor, substitute Rifabutin (150 mg/day) for Rifampin |
| **K. Mycobacterium marinum** | Two active agents for 1-2 months after surgical incision: **Clarithro** 500 mg bid + **EMB** 25 mg/kg q24h or **RIF** 600 mg q24h + **EMB** 25 mg/kg q24h Surgical excision. | | For deep tissue involvement use a three drug combination therapy with Rifampin 600 mg q24h + [Minocycline 100–200 mg q24h or Doxycycline 100–200 mg q24h] + Clarithromycin 500 mg bid. Monotherapy may be considered for minimal disease: Minocycline 100–200 mg q24h or Doxycycline 100–200 mg q24h; or TMP-SMX 160/800 mg bid. |
| **L. Mycobacterium scrofulaceum** | Surgical excision. Chemotherapy seldom indicated. Although regimens not defined, **Clarithro** + **CLO** with or without **EMB**, **INH**, **RIF**, **strep** + **cycloserine** have also been used. | | In vitro resistant to INH, RIF, EMB, PZA, AMK, CIP. Susceptible to clarithro, strep, erythromycin. |
| **M. Mycobacterium simiae** | Regimen(s) not defined. Start 4 drugs as for disseminated MAC | | Most isolates resistant to all 1st-line anti-TBc drugs. Isolates often not clinically significant. |
| **N. Mycobacterium ulcerans (Buruli ulcer)** | WHO recommends **RIF** + **SM** for 8 weeks. **RIF**+ **CIP** recommended as alternatives by WHO *(CMN 31:119, 2009).* | | Susceptible in vitro to RIF, strep, CLO, clarithro, CIP, ofloxacin, amikacin, moxi, linezolid. Australian guidelines *(MJA 200:267, 2014)* recommend oral combination of RiF + Clarithro or RiF + a FQ (moxifloxacin or CIP). Surgery not required for cure and reserved for those declining or intolerant of antibiotic, debridement of necrotic tissue, large defects. |
| **O. Mycobacterium xenopi** | Regimen(s) not defined. **Clarithro** 500 mg bid + **RIF** 600 mg or **Rifabutin** 300 mg + **EMB** 15 mg/kg once daily + **INH** 300 mg once daily. | | In vitro: susceptible to clarithro and many standard antimycobacterial drugs. MOXI active in vitro and may be an alternative. |

**TABLE 12A (11)**

| CAUSATIVE AGENT/DISEASE | MODIFYING CIRCUMSTANCES | SUGGESTED REGIMENS | | COMMENTS |
|---|---|---|---|---|
| | | PRIMARY/ALTERNATIVE | | |
| **IV. Nontuberculous Mycobacteria (NTM)** *(continued)* | | | | |
| **P. Mycobacterium leprae (leprosy)** Classification: *CID 44:1096, 2007.* Overview: *Lancet ID. 11:464, 2011.* | | There are 2 sets of therapeutic recommendations here: one from USA (National Hansen's Disease Program [NHDP], Baton Rouge, LA) and one from WHO. Both are based on expert recommendations and neither has been subjected to controlled clinical trial. | | |
| **Paucibacillary Forms:** **(Intermediate, Tuberculoid, Borderline tuberculoid)** | (Dapsone 100 mg/day + RIF 600 mg po/day) for 12 months | (Dapsone 100 mg/day (unsupervised) + RIF 600 mg 1x/mo (supervised)) for 6 mos | | Side effects overall 0.4% |
| **Single lesion paucibacillary** | Treat as paucibacillary leprosy for 12 months. | Single dose ROM therapy: (RIF 600 mg + Oflox 400 mg + Mino 100 mg). (*Ln 353:655, 1999.*) | | |
| **Multibacillary forms:** **Borderline** **Borderline-lepromatous** **Lepromatous** See *Comment for erythema nodosum leprosum (ENL)* Rev: *Lancet 363:1209, 2004* | (Dapsone 100 mg/day + CLO 50 mg/day + RIF 600 mg/day) for 24 mos **Alternative regimen:** (Dapsone 100 mg/day + RIF 600 mg/day + Minocycline 100 mg/day) for 24 mos if CLO is refused or unavailable. | (Dapsone 100 mg/day + CLO 50 mg/day (both unsupervised) + RIF 600 mg + CLO 300 mg once monthly (supervised)). Continue regimen for 12 months. | | Side-effects overall 5.1%. For **erythema nodosum leprosum:** prednisone 60–80 mg/day or thalidomide 100–400 mg/day. Thalidomide available in US at 1-800-4-CELGENE. Altho thalidomide effective, WHO no longer rec because of potential toxicity however the majority of leprosy experts feel thalidomide remains drug of choice for ENL under strict supervision. **CLO (Clofazimine)** available from NHDP under IND protocol; contact at 1-800-642-2477. **Ethionamide** (250 mg q24h) or prothionamide (375 mg q24h) may be subbed for CLO. Etanercept effective in one case refractory to above standard therapy (*CID 52:e133, 2011*). Regimens incorporating clarithro, minocycline, dapsone monotherapy have been reported due to emergence of resistance (*CID 52:e127, 2011*), but older patients previously treated with dapsone monotherapy may remain on lifelong maintenance therapy. Moxi highly active in vitro and produces rapid clinical response (*AAC 52:3113, 2008*). |

See page 2 for abbreviations          * Dosages are for adults (unless otherwise indicated) and assume normal renal function          † **DOT** = directly observed therapy          **SAT** = self-administered therapy

See Comment for erythema nodosum leprosum (ENL) and assume normal renal function

## TABLE 12B - DOSAGE AND ADVERSE EFFECTS OF ANTIMYCOBACTERIAL DRUGS

| AGENT (TRADE NAME)[1] | ROUTE/[1]° DRUG RESISTANCE (RES) US[2-6] | USUAL DOSAGE[3] | SIDE-EFFECTS, TOXICITY AND PRECAUTIONS | SURVEILLANCE |
|---|---|---|---|---|
| **FIRST LINE DRUGS** | | | | |
| Ethambutol (Myambutol) (100, 400 mg tab) | RES: 0.3% (0-0.7%) po 400 mg tab | 25 mg/kg/day for 2 mos then 15 mg/kg/day q24h as 1 dose (<50% protein binding) [Bacteriostatic to both extra-cellular & intracellular organisms] | **Optic neuritis** with decreased visual acuity, central scotomata, and loss of green and red perception; peripheral neuropathy and headache (~1%), rashes (rare), arthralgia (rare), hyperuricemia (rare). Anaphylactoid reaction (rare). *Comment*: Primarily used to inhibit resistance. Disrupts outer cell membrane in M. avium with ↑ activity to other drugs. | Monthly visual acuity & red/green with dose >15 mg/kg/day. ≥10% loss considered significant. Usually reversible if drug discontinued |
| Isoniazid (INH) (Nydrazid, Laniazid, Teebaconin) (50, 100, 300 mg tab) | RES: 4.1% (2.6-8.5%) po 300 mg tab IM 100 mg/mL in 10 mL (IV route not FDA-approved but has been used, esp. in AIDS) | Q24h dose: 5-10 mg/kg/day up to 300 mg/day as 1 dose. 2x/wk dose: 15 mg/kg (900 mg max dose) (<10% protein binding) [Bactericidal to both extracellular and intracellular organisms] Add pyridoxine in alcoholic, pregnant, or malnourished pts. | Overall ~1%. **Hep** (children 10% mild ↑ SGOT; normalizes with continued rx, age <20 yrs rare; 20-34 yrs 1.2%; ≥50 yrs 2.3%) (also ↑ with q24h alcohol & previous exposure to Hep C (usually asymptomatic–*CID 26:292, 2003*)). May be fatal. With prodromal sx, dark urine do LFTs; discontinue if SGOT >3-5x normal. **pyridoxine 10 mg q24h will decrease incidence**; peripheral neuropathy (17% on 6 mg/kg per day, less on 300 mg, incidence ↑ in slow acetylators); **Peripheral neuropathy**, optic neuritis, toxic encephalopathy, psychosis, muscle twitching, dizziness, coma (all rare); allergic skin rashes, fever, minor disulfiram-like reaction, flushing after Swiss cheese; blood dyscrasias (rare); + antinuclear (20%). **Drug-drug interactions** common, see *Table 22A*. | Pre-rx liver functions. Repeat if symptoms (fatigue, weakness, malaise, anorexia, nausea or vomiting) >3 days (*AJRCCM 152: 1705, 1995*). Some recommend SGOT at 2, 4, 6 mos esp. if age >50 yrs. Clinical evaluation every mo. |
| Pyrazinamide (500 mg tab) | po 500 mg tab | 25 mg per kg per day (maximum 2.5 gm per day) q24h as 1 dose [Bactericidal for intracellular organisms] | **Arthralgia; hyperuricemia** (with or without symptoms); hepatitis (not over 2% if recommended dose not exceeded); gastric irritation; photosensitivity (rare). | Pre-rx liver functions. Monthly SGOT, uric acid. Measure serum uric acid if symptomatic gouty attack occurs. |
| Rifamate[4]– combination tablet | 2 tablets single dose q24h | 2 tablets single dose q24h | 1 tablet contains 150 mg INH, 300 mg RIF | As with individual drugs |
| Rifampin (Rifadin, Rimactane, Rifocin) (100, 300, 450, 600 mg cap) | RES: 0.3% (0-0.3%) po 300 mg cap (IV available, Merrell-Dow) | 10.0 mg per kg per day up to 600 mg per day q24h as 1 dose (60-90% protein binding) [Bactericidal to all populations of organisms] | INH/RIF in ~3% for toxicity; gastrointestinal irritation, antibiotic-associated colitis, drug fever (1%), pruritus with or without skin rash (1%), anaphylactoid reactions in HIV+ pts, mental confusion, thrombocytopenia (1%), leukopenia (1%), hemolytic anemia, transient **abnormalities in liver function**. **"Flu syndrome"** (fever, chills, headache, bone pain, shortness of breath) seen if q24h dose irregularly or if q24h dose restarted after an interval of no rx. **Discolors urine, tears, sweat, contact lens an orange-brownish color**. May cause drug-induced lupus erythematosus (*Ln 349: 1521, 1977*). | Pre-rx liver functions. Repeat if symptoms, **Multiple significant drug-drug interactions**, see *Table 22A*. |
| Rifater[4]– combination tablet (See Side-Effects) | po (1 hr before meal) | Wt ≤55 kg, 6 tablets single dose q24h | 1 tablet contains 50 mg INH, 120 mg RIF, 300 mg PZA. Used in 1st 2 months of rx (PZA 25 mg per kg per day). Purpose is convenience in dosing, ↑ compliance (*AnIM 122: 951, 1995*) but cost 1.58 more, side-effects = individual drugs. | As with individual drugs, PZA 25 mg per kg |
| Streptomycin (IV/IM sol'n) | RES: 3.9% (2.7-7.6%) IM (or IV) | 15 mg per kg IM q24h, 0.75-1.0 gm per day initially for 60-90 days, then 1.0 gm 2-3 times per week (15 mg per kg per day) q24h as 1 dose | Overall 8%. **Ototoxicity**: vestibular dysfunction (vertigo); paresthesias; dizziness & nausea (all less in pts receiving 2-3 doses per week); tinnitus and high frequency loss (1%); nephrotoxicity (rare); peripheral neuropathy (rare); allergic skin rashes (4-5%); drug fever. Available from X-Gen Pharmaceuticals, *607-732-4411*. Ref: re: IV–*CID 19:1750, 1994*. Toxicity similar with IM vs IV dosing (*CID 38:1538, 2004*). | Monthly audiogram. In older pts, serum creatinine or BUN at start of rx and weekly if pt stable |

[1] Note: Malabsorption of antimycobacterial drugs may occur in patients with AIDS enteropathy. For review of adverse effects, see *AJRCCM 167:1472, 2003*.

[2] **RES** = % resistance of M. tuberculosis

[3] Dosages are for adults (unless otherwise indicated) and assume normal renal function     † **DOT** = directly observed therapy;  **SAT** = self-administered therapy

§ Mean (range) (higher in Hispanics, Asians, and patients <10 years old)

*See page 2 for abbreviations*

TABLE 12B (2)

| AGENT (TRADE NAME)[1] | USUAL DOSAGE* | ROUTE/10 DRUG RESISTANCE (RES) US§[1] | SIDE-EFFECTS, TOXICITY AND PRECAUTIONS | SURVEILLANCE |
|---|---|---|---|---|
| **SECOND LINE DRUGS** (more difficult to use and/or less effective than first line drugs) | | | | |
| **Amikacin** (Amikin) (IV sol'n) | 7.5–10.0 mg per kg q24h [Bactericidal for extracellular organisms] | RES: (est. 0.1%) IM/IV 500 mg vial | See Table 10B, page 125 & Table 10D, page 128 Toxicity similar with old vs td dosing (CID 38:1538, 2004). | Monthly audiogram. Serum creatinine or BUN weekly if pt stable |
| **Amikacin liposomal suspension** (for inhalation) | One daily oral inhalation | Via inhalation | Risk of respiratory AEs: hypersensitivity, pneumonitis, hemoptysis, bronchospasm. | |
| **Bedaquiline** (Sirturo) (100 mg tab) JAC 69:2310, 2014; NEJM 371:723, 2014; CID 60:188, 2015: | Directly observed therapy (DOT): 400 mg once daily for 2 weeks, then 200 mg 3 times weekly for 22 weeks, taken with food and always used in combination with other anti-TB medications. | Does not exhibit cross-resistance to other TB drugs; always use in combination with other TB drugs to prevent selection of resistant mutants | Most common: nausea, vomiting, arthralgia, headache, hyperuricemia. Elevated transaminases. Bedaquiline in clinical trials was administered as one component of a multiple drug regimen, so side-effects were common, yet difficult to assign to a particular drug. Resistance reported: CID 2015;66:1625. | Moderate QTc increases (average of 10-16 ms over the 24 weeks of therapy). Potential risks of pancreatitis, myopathy, myocardial injury, severe hepatotoxicity. |
| **Capreomycin sulfate** (Capastat sulfate) | 1 gm per day (15 mg per kg per day) q24h as 1 dose | RES: 0.1% (0–0.9%) IM/IV | Nephrotoxicity (36%), ototoxicity (auditory 11%), eosinophilia, leukopenia, skin rash, fever, hypokalemia, neuromuscular blockade. | Monthly audiogram, biweekly serum creatinine or BUN |
| **Ciprofloxacin** (Cipro) (250, 500, 750 mg tab) | 750 mg bid | 500 mg or 750 mg po IV 200-400 mg daily | TB not a FDA-approved indication for CIP. Desired CIP serum levels 4–6 mcg per mL. See Table 10A, page 120 & Table 10B, page 126 for adverse effects. | None |
| **Clofazimine** (Lamprene) (50, 100 mg cap) | 50 mg per day (unsupervised) + 300 mg 1 time per month supervised or 100 mg per day | 50 mg (with meals) | Skin: **pigmentation (pink-brownish black)** 75–100%; dryness 20%, pruritus 5%. GI: abdominal pain 50% (rarely severe leading to exploratory laparoscopy), splenic infarction (VR), bowel obstruction (VR), GI bleeding (VR). Eye: conjunctival irritation, retinal crystal deposits. | None |
| **Cycloserine** (Seromycin) (250 mg tab) | 750–1000 mg per day (15 mg per kg per day) 2–4 doses per day [Bacteriostatic for both extra-cellular & intracellular organisms] | RES: 0.1% (0–0.3%) 250 mg cap | Convulsions, **psychoses** (5–10% of those receiving 1.0 gm per day); headache; somnolence; hyperreflexia; increased CSF protein and pressure, **peripheral neuropathy.** 100 mg pyridoxine (or more) q24h should be given concomitantly. Contraindicated in epileptics. | None |
| **Dapsone** (25, 100 mg tab) | 100 mg per day | 100 mg per day | Blood: ↓ hemoglobin (1-2 gm) & ↑ retics (2-12%), in most pts. Hemolysis in G6PD deficiency; ↑ hemolysis due to concomitant atazanavir (AAC 56:1081, 2012). **Methemoglobinemia.** CNS: peripheral neuropathy (rare). GI: nausea, vomiting. Renal: albuminuria, nephrotic syndrome. Erythema nodosum leprosum in pts rx for leprosy (½ of 1st year pts). Hypersensitivity syndrome in 0.5-3.6% (See Surveillance). | Hypersensitivity syndrome: fever, rash, eosinophilia, lymphadenopathy, hepatitis, pneumonitis. Genetic marker identified (NEJM 369:1620, 2013). |
| **Ethionamide** (Trecator-SC) (120, 250 mg tab) | 500–1000 mg per day (15–20 mg per kg per day) divided 1-3 doses per day [Bacteriostatic for extracellular organisms only] | RES: 0.8% (0–1.5%) 250 mg tab | **Gastrointestinal irritation** (up to 50% on large dose); goiter; peripheral neuropathy (rare); convulsions (rare); changes in affect (rare); difficulty in diabetes control; rashes; hepatitis; purpura; stomatitis; gynecomastia; menstrual irregularity. Give drug with meals or antacids; 50–100 mg pyridoxine per day concomitantly; SGOT monthly. Possibly teratogenic. | None |

*See page 2 for abbreviations*    * Dosages are for adults (unless otherwise indicated) and assume normal renal function    † **DOT** = directly observed therapy;    **SAT** = self-administered therapy

§ Mean (range) (higher in Hispanics, Asians, and patients <10 years old)

**TABLE 12B (3)**

| AGENT (TRADE NAME)[1] | USUAL DOSAGE* | ROUTE/§ DRUG RESISTANCE (RES) US°§ | SIDE-EFFECTS, TOXICITY AND PRECAUTIONS | SURVEILLANCE |
|---|---|---|---|---|
| **SECOND LINE DRUGS** *(continued)* | | | | |
| **Linezolid** (Zyvox) (600 mg tab, oral suspension 100 mg/mL) | 600 mg once daily | PO or IV | Not FDA-approved indication. High rate of adverse events (>80% with 4 months or longer of therapy, myelosuppression, peripheral neuropathy, optic neuropathy). Avoid tyramine-containing foods, soy products, adrenergic agents (e.g., pseudoephedrine, phenylpropanolamine). MOA inhibitors, SSRIs. 600 mg >300 mg dose for toxicity; consider reducing dose to 300 mg for toxicity or after 4 mos of therapy or culture-conversion to reduce toxicity. | Baseline and monthly complete blood count, visual acuity checks, screen for symptoms of peripheral neuropathy, neurologic examination. |
| **Moxifloxacin** (Avelox) (400 mg tab) | 400 mg qd | 400 mg cap | Not FDA-approved indication. Concomitant administration of rifampin reduces serum levels of moxi (*CID 45:1001, 2007*). | None |
| **Ofloxacin** (Floxin) (200, 300, 400 mg tab) | 400 mg bid | 400 mg cap | Not FDA-approved indication. Overall adverse effects 11%, 4% discontinued due to side-effects. GI: nausea 3%, diarrhea 1%. **CNS:** insomnia 3%, headache 1%, dizziness 1%. | None |
| **Para-aminosalicylic acid** (PAS, Paser) (Na+ or K+ salt) (4 gm cap) | 4–6 gm bid (200 mg per kg per day) [Bacteriostatic for extracellular organisms only] | RES: 0.8% (0–1.5%) 450 mg tab (see Comment) | **Gastrointestinal irritation** (10–15%); goitrogenic action (rare); depressed prothrombin activity (rare); G6PD-mediated hemolytic anemia (rare), drug fever, rashes, hepatitis, myalgia, arthralgia. Retards hepatic enzyme induction, may ↓ INH hepatotoxicity. Available from CDC, (404) 639-3670, Jacobus Pharm. Co. (609) 921-7447. | None |
| **Rifabutin** (Mycobutin) (150 mg cap) | 300 mg per day (prophylaxis or treatment) | 150 mg tab | Polymyalgia, polyarthralgia, granulocytopenia. Uveitis rare with 300 mg/day but increases to 8-38% if higher dose or combined with clarithro, PI or azole antifungal. Reddish urine, orange skin (pseudojaundice). | None |
| **Rifapentine** (Priftin) (150 mg tab) | 600 mg twice weekly for 1st 2 mos., then 600 mg q week | 150 mg tab | Similar to other rifabutins. (See *RIF, RFB*). Hyperuricemia seen in 21%. Causes red-orange discoloration of body fluids. Flu-like illness in pts given weekly Rifapentine + INH for latent MTB (*CID 61:527, 2015*). | None |
| **Thalidomide** (Thalomid) (50, 100, 200 mg cap) | 100–300 mg po q24h (may use up to 400 mg po q24h for severe erythema nodosum leprosum) | 50 mg tab | **Contraindicated in pregnancy. Causes severe life-threatening birth defects. Both male and female patients must use barrier contraceptive methods (Pregnancy Category X).** Frequently causes drowsiness or somnolence. May cause peripheral neuropathy. (*AJM 108>487, 2000*) For review, see *Ln 363:1803, 2004.* | In US: contact Celgene (800-4-CELGENE) |

* Dosages are for adults (unless otherwise indicated) and assume normal renal function
§ Mean (range) (higher in Hispanics, Asians, and patients <10 years old)

**DOT** = directly observed therapy    **SAT** = self-administered therapy

*See page 2 for abbreviations*

# TABLE 13A – TREATMENT OF PARASITIC INFECTIONS

- **See Table 13D for sources for antiparasitic drugs not otherwise commercially available.**
- The following resources are available through the Centers for Disease Control and Prevention (CDC). General advice for parasitic diseases other than malaria: Website is www.cdc.gov. For Parasitic Diseases Public Inquiries: (+1) (404) 718-4745 (day), (+1) (770) 488-7100 after hours. For CDC Drug Service: 8:00a.m. – 4:30 p.m. EST: (+1) (404) 639-3717. See www.cdc.gov/laboratory/drugservice/index.html For malaria: Prophylaxis advice: (+1) (770) 488-7788; or after hours (+1) (770) 488-7100; toll-free (US) 1-855-856-4713; website: www.cdc.gov/malaria
- **NOTE: All dosage regimens are for adults with normal renal function unless otherwise stated.** Many of the suggested regimens are not FDA approved.
- For licensed drugs, suggest checking package inserts to verify dosage and side-effects. Occasionally, post-licensure data may alter dosage as compared to package inserts.

| INFECTING ORGANISM | SUGGESTED REGIMENS | | COMMENTS |
| --- | --- | --- | --- |
| | PRIMARY | ALTERNATIVE | |
| **PROTOZOA—INTESTINAL** (non-pathogenic: E. hartmanni, E. dispar, E. moshkovskii, E. coli, Iodamoeba bütschlii, Endolimax nana, Chilomastix mesnili) | | | |
| **Balantidium coli** | Tetracycline 500 mg qid x 10 days | Metronidazole 750 mg po tid x 5 days | Another alternative: Iodoquinol 650 mg po tid x 20 days. |
| **Blastocystis hominis**<br>Ref: Trends Parasitol 28:305, 2012;<br>Trends Parasitol. 2018; 34:369 | Metronidazole 1.5 gm po 1x/day x 10 days or 750 mg po tid x 10 days (need to treat is dubious). | Alternatives: **Iodoquinol** 650 mg po tid x 20 days or **TMP-SMX-DS**, one bid x 7 days or **Nitazoxanide** 500 mg po bid x 3 days | Role as pathogen unclear; may serve as marker of exposure to contaminated food/water. Some genotypes may be more virulent. |
| **Cryptosporidium parvum & hominis**<br>Ref: Curr Opin Infect Dis 23:494, 2010 | **Immunocompetent—No HIV:** Nitazoxanide 500 mg po bid x 3 days (expensive) | **HIV with immunodeficiency:** Effective antiretroviral therapy best therapy. **Nitazoxanide** no clinical or parasite response compared to placebo. | **Nitazoxanide:** Approved in liquid formulation for rx of children 4 500 mg tabs for adults who are immunocompetent. Ref: CID 40:1173, 2005. **C. hominis** assoc. with 1 in post-infection eye & joint pain, recurrent headache, & dizzy spells (CID 39:504, 2004). |
| **Cyclospora cayetanensis; cyclosporiasis**<br>(Clin Micro Rev 23:218, 2010) | **Immunocompetent pts:** TMP-SMX-DS tab 1 po bid x 7–10 days. Other options: see Comments. | **AIDS pts:** TMP-SMX-DS tab 1 po qid for up to 3-4 wks. immunocompromised pts: may require suppressive rx with **TMP-SMX** DS 1 tab 3x/wk | **Metronidazole** failed in prospective random placebo-control DS study (CID 58:1692, 2014). In vitro tinidazole, metronidazole most active. AAC 56:467, 2012 |
| **Dientamoeba fragilis**<br>Ref: A JTMH 82:614, 2010;<br>J Clin Microbiol pii: JCM.00400-16, 2016 | **Iodoquinol** 650 mg po tid x 20 days or **Paromomycin** 25-35 mg/kg/day po in 3 div doses x 7 days or **Metronidazole** 750 mg tid x 10 days. | For treatment failures: **Tetracycline** 500 mg po qid x 10 days + **Iodoquinol** 650 mg po bid x 10 days **OR** (**Iodoquinol** + **Paromomycin**) May try second course of Iodoquinol | If sulfa-allergic **CIP** 500 mg po bid x 7 days but results inconsistent. Biliary disease described in HIV pts. |
| **Entamoeba histolytica; amebiasis.** If available, use stool PCR for diagnosis. E. histolytica, E. dispar, E. moshkovskii, are microscopically identical; antigen testing needed to distinguish. | | | |
| Asymptomatic cyst passer | **Paromomycin** 25-35 mg/kg/day po in 3 divided doses x 7 days **OR Iodoquinol** 650 mg po tid x 20 days. | **Diloxanide furoate** (Furamide) 500 mg po tid x 10 days. | General review: Open Forum Infect Dise 2018, 5:ofy161. Colitis can mimic ulcerative colitis; ameboma can mimic adenocarcinoma of colon. **Nitazoxanide** 500 mg po bid x 3 days may be effective (JID 184:381, 2001 & Tran R Soc Trop Med & Hyg 101:1025, 2007). |
| Patient with diarrhea/dysentery, mild/moderate disease. Oral therapy possible | **Metronidazole** 500–750 mg po tid x 7-10 days or **Tinidazole** 2 gm daily x 3 days, followed by: Either (**Paromomycin** 25-35 mg/kg/day po divided in 3 doses x 7 days) or [**Iodoquinol** 650 mg po tid x 20 days] to clear intestinal cysts. See comment. | | |
| Severe or extraintestinal infection, e.g., hepatic abscess | (**Metronidazole** 750 mg **IV to po** tid x 10 days or **Tinidazole** 2 gm 1x/day x 5 days) followed by **Paromomycin** 25-35 mg/kg/day po divided in 3 doses x 7 days or **Iodoquinol** 650 mg po tid x 20 days. | | Serology positive (antibody present) with extraintestinal disease. |

For source of drug, see Table 13D, page 177.

* For source of drug, see Table 13D, page 177.

**TABLE 13A (2)**

| INFECTING ORGANISM | SUGGESTED REGIMENS | | COMMENTS |
|---|---|---|---|
| | **PRIMARY** | **ALTERNATIVE** | |
| **PROTOZOA—INTESTINAL** (continued) | | | |
| **Giardia duodenalis** also known as **Giardia lamblia, Giardia intestinalis.** | **Tinidazole** 2 gm po x 1 | **Metronidazole** 250 mg po tid x 5 days; **Nitazoxanide** 500 mg po bid x 3 days; Albendazole 400 mg po once daily with food x 5 days. Cochrane Database Syst Rev.2012 Dec 12: 12:CD007787. | **Refractory pts:** Quinacrine 100 mg po tid x 5 days or (**metro 750 mg po + quinacrine 100 mg po**) or (**Paromomycin** 10 mg/kg po) 3x/day x 3 wks (CID 33:22, 2001) giardia genetically heterogeneous (J Clin Invest 123:2346, 2013). **Pregnancy: Paromomycin** 25-35 mg/kg/day po in 3 divided doses x 5-10 days. |
| **Cystoisospora belli (formerly Isospora belli)** Diagnosis requires special order: AFB stain of stool | **Immunocompetent: TMP-SMX-DS** tab 1 po bid x 7-10 days; **Immunocompromised: TMP-SMX-DS** tid for up to 4 wks. If CD4<200 may not respond; need ART. | **CIP** 500 mg po bid x 7 days is second-line alternative (AnIM 132:885, 2000). OR **Pyrimethamine** 50-75 mg/day + Folinic acid 10-25 mg/day (po). | **Chronic suppression in AIDS pts:** either **TMP-SMX-DS** 1 tab po 3x/wk OR tab 1 po daily OR (**Pyrimethamine** 25 mg/day po + **Folinic acid** 10 mg/day po) OR as 2nd-line alternative: **CIP** 500 mg po 3x/wk. |
| **Microsporidiosis** | For HIV pts: antiretroviral therapy key. | | |
| **Ocular:** Encephalitozoon hellum or cuniculi, Vittaforma (Nosema) corneae, Nosema ocularum | **Albendazole** 400 mg po bid x 3 wks plus fumagillin eye drops (see Comment). | In HIV pts, reports of response of E. hellium to **Fumagillin** eyedrops (see Comment). For V. corneae, may need keratoplasty. | To obtain fumagillin: 800-292-6773 or www.leiterrx.com. Neutropenia & thrombocytopenia serious adverse events. |
| **Intestinal** (diarrhea): Enterocytozoon bieneusi (HIV), Encephalitozoon (Septata) intestinalis | **Albendazole** 400 mg po bid x 3 wks; peds dose: 15 mg/kg per day div. into 2 daily doses x 7 days for E. intestinalis. Fumagillin equally effective. | Oral **Fumagillin** 20 mg po tid reported effective for **E. bieneusi** (NEJM 346:1963, 2002) (see Comment). Albendazole not effective. | Dx: Most labs use modified trichrome stain. Need electron micrographs for species identification. FA and PCR methods in development. Peds dose ref.: PIDJ 23:915, 2004 |
| **Disseminated:** E. hellum, cuniculi or intestinalis; Pleistophora sp., others in Comment. Ref: JCM 52:3839, 2014. | **Albendazole** 400 mg po bid x 3 wks. Fumagillin 20 mg po tid (not available in US) | No established rx for Pleistophora sp. | For Trachipleistophora sp., try itraconazole + albendazole (NEJM 351:42, 2004). Other pathogens: Brachiola vesicularum & algerae (NEJM 351:42, 2004). |
| **PROTOZOA—EXTRAINTESTINAL** | | | |
| **Amebic meningoencephalitis** (Clin Infect Dis 51:e7, 2010 (Balamuthia). CDC no longer provides miltefosine. See www.lmpavido.com | | | |
| **Acanthamoeba sp.**— no proven rx Rev.: FEMS Immunol Med Micro 50:1, 2007 | Adult IV therapy: (**Pentamidine + Fluconazole**) + **Miltefosine** + **TMP-SMX**. Metronidazole, and Azithromycin | | For Acanthamoeba keratitis: miltefosine or voriconazole. Need brain tissue for dx. |
| **Balamuthia mandrillaris** | **Albendazole** + (**Fluconazole** or **Itraconazole**) + **Miltefosine** 50 mg po tid ± **pentamidine** (poorly tolerated). | | Need brain tissue for dx. |
| **Naegleria fowleri.** >95% mortality. Ref. MMWR 57:573, 2008. | **Amphotericin B** 1.5 mg/kg/day ± intrathecal + **Rifampin** 10 mg/kg/day + **Fluconazole** 10 mg/kg/day IV/po. **Miltefosine** 50 mg po tid + **Azithromycin** 500 mg IV/po. Duration of therapy is empiric as there are few survivors | | |
| **Babesia microti** (US), **Babesia duncani** (US West Coast), and **Babesia divergens** (EU) (NEJM 366:366-2397, 2012) | **For mild-to-moderate disease: Atovaquone** 750 mg po bid + **Azithro** 500 mg po on day 1, then 250-1000 mg po daily for total of 7-10 days. If relapse, treat x 6 wks & until blood smear neg x 2 wks. | **For severe babesiosis: (Clindamycin** 600 mg po tid) + **Quinine** 650 mg po tid x 7-10 days For adults, can give **Clinda** IV 1.2 gm bid. | Overwhelming infection in asplenic patients. treat for >6 more weeks (CID 46:370, 2008). Transfusion related cases occur. |

* For source of drug, see Table 130, page 177.

162

**TABLE 13A (3)**

| INFECTING ORGANISM | SUGGESTED REGIMENS | | COMMENTS |
|---|---|---|---|
| | PRIMARY | ALTERNATIVE | |

**PROTOZOA—EXTRAINTESTINAL** *(continued)*

**Leishmaniasis** (*Suggest consultation— CDC (+1) 404-718-4745*). Therapy needs individualization according to species and many options for each manifestation. **Note: Miltefosine available directly from Profounda, Inc. (+1 407-270-7790), www.impavido.com.** Definitive guidelines from IDSA/ASTMH *academic.oup.com/cid/article/63/12/e202/2645609* and include geographic distribution maps for each species. Diagnosis of cutaneous disease: Sample full depth punch biopsy from raised edge of ulcer. PCR mandatory to speciate; culture and histology also available. Rapid diagnosis often possible using needle aspirate, slit skin smear, brushings, or scraping of lesion edge with giemsa staining. Serology not useful.

| | | | |
|---|---|---|---|
| **Cutaneous:**<br>Mild Disease 4 or less lesions (1 cm or more), none > or = to 5 cm in diameter, no lesions in cosmetically sensitive areas, no lesions over joints or genitalia; may observe.<br><br>Otherwise, consider Complex Disease which includes: failure of previous treatment, or substantial local or lymphatic nodules, or large regional lymphadenopathy. | **Mild Disease** in travelers frequently responds to observation or local therapy and is considered an acceptable approach if patient agrees.<br>**Paromomycin⁵** 15% paromomycin and 12% MBCL ointment bid x 10 days rest for 10 days and then 10 more days; cryotherapy (freeze up to 3 x with liquid nitrogen); Intralesional Antimony up to 5 mL into lesions weekly x 8-10 wks with cryotherapy at end of each treatment. CDC antimony IND does not cover intralesional use, common outside US.<br>**Alternative: Miltefosine** (w/food) 50 mg po bid (wt 30-44 kg); 50 mg tid (wt ≥45 kg). Treat for 28 days. Response in about 70% of pts. | **Moderate Disease:**<br>**Sodium stibogluconate⁵** (Pentostam) or **Meglumine antimoniate** (Glucantime) 20 mg/kg/day Sb IV x 20 days. Dilute in 120 mL of D5W and infuse over 1-2 hrs OR Liposomal **Amphotericin B** (3 mg/kg IV once daily days 1-5 and 10.<br>Alternatives: **Fluconazole** 200 mg po daily x 6 weeks (for *L. mexicana, L. panamensis, L. major*) or **Ketoconazole** 600 mg po daily x 30 days (*L. mexicana*) or **Miltefosine** (dose as for mild disease). Some experts use **Ampho B** 0.5-1 mg/kg IV daily or qod to total dose of 15-30 mg/kg | Observation, oral therapy, topical paromomycin⁵ only when low potential for mucosal spread; never use for lesions of any severity which are or may be *L. brasiliensis, L. panamensis* or *L. guyanensis* which always require therapy as per mucosal leishmaniasis below.<br>Generic pentavalent antimony varies in quality and safety. Mild disease in travelers frequently responds to observation (*CID 57:370, 2013*) and is acceptable per IDSA/ASTMH guidelines. Monitor for gradual healing. Miltefosine is preg cat D (do not use in pregnancy). |
| **Leishmaniasis, Mucosal (Espundia)**<br>All cutaneous lesions due to *L. brasiliensis, L. guyanensis,* or *L. panamensis* is proven or possible. | • **Cutaneous *L. brasiliensis* of any severity:**<br>○ **[Sodium Stibogluconate** (Pentostam) or **Meglumine antimoniate** (Glucantime)] 20 mg/kg/ day IV/IM x 20 days<br>○ **Liposomal Ampho B** (3 mg/kg IV once daily days 1-5 and days 14, 21 of days) [1-5 and days 14, 21 of days]<br>• **Mucosal: Pentavalent antimony (Sb⁵)** 20 mg/day Sb IV x 28 days for mucosal disease, or **Liposomal Amphotericin B** (regimens vary) with total cumulative dose of 20-60 mg/kg or **Amphotericin B** 0.5-1 mg/kg IV daily or qod to total dose of 20-45 mg/kg. | **Miltefosine⁵** (w/food) 50 mg po bid (wt 30-44 kg); 50 mg tid (wt ≥45 kg). Treat for 28 days. Complete resolution in 62% of pts. | Antimony available from CDC drug service. *See Table 13D for contact information.*<br>Miltefosine has variable activity against mucosal disease according to geographic location. Expert consultation needed. |
| **Visceral leishmaniasis (Kala-Azar)**<br>New World & Old World<br>*L. donovani:* India, Africa<br>*L. infantum:* Mediterranean<br>*L. chagasi:* New World (identical to *L. infantum*) | *Immunocompetent:* **Liposomal Ampho B** 3 mg/kg once daily days 1-5 & days 14, 21 (increase to 40 mg/kg total dose for East African VL)<br>HIV/AIDS: **Liposomal Ampho B** 4 mg/kg od on days 1-5, 10, 17, 24, 31, 38 (*Curr Opin Infect Dis 26:1, 2013*). | **Standard Ampho B** 1 mg/kg IV daily x 15-20 days or qod x 8 wks to total of 15-20 mg/kg) OR **pentavalent antimony⁵** 20 mg/kg/day IV x 28 days OR **Miltefosine⁵** (w/food) 50 mg po bid (wt 30-44 kg; 50 mg tid (wt ≥45 kg). | In HIV patients, need suppression with Amphotericin B q 2-4 wks. While CD4 remains <200. VL from South Asia is resistant to antimony. Miltefosine may be less effective against *L. infantum-chagasi* and less efficacy data for *L. donovani* in Africa. |

---

⁵ For source of drug, see *Table 13D, page 177.*

TABLE 13A (4)

| INFECTING ORGANISM | SUGGESTED REGIMENS | | COMMENTS |
|---|---|---|---|
| | PRIMARY | ALTERNATIVE | |

**PROTOZOA—EXTRAINTESTINAL** (continued)

**Malaria (Plasmodia species)—NOTE:** CDC Malaria info— prophylaxis/treatment (770) 488-7788. After hours: 770-488-7100. US toll-free 1-855-856-4713. CDC offers species confirmation and drug resistance testing. Refs: JAMA 297:2251, 2264 & 2272, 2007. See: www.cdc.gov/malaria Review of rapid diagnostic tests: CID 54:1637, 2012.

**Prophylaxis**—Drugs plus personal protection: screens, nets, 35% DEET skin repellent (avoid >50% DEET) (JAMA 2016:316:766), permethrin spray on clothing and mosquito nets. Country risk from CDC (https://www.cdc.gov/malaria/travelers/country_table/b.html) or WHO (http://www.who.int/ith/ith-country-list.pdf?ua=1)

| | | | |
|---|---|---|---|
| **For areas free of chloroquine (CQ)-resistant P. falciparum:** Central America (west of Panama Canal), Caribbean, Korea, Middle East (most). | CQ phosphate 500 mg (300 mg base) po per wk starting 1-2 weeks before travel, during travel & 4 wks post-travel **or** Atovaquone-Proguanil (AP) 1 adult tab per day (1 day prior to, during, & 7 days post-travel) or Tafenoquine 200 mg once daily x3 days (starting 3 days before travel) then 200 mg once weekly (starting 7 days after last loading regimen dose) then a 200 mg one-time dose (7 days after last dose in malaria area) G6PD-normal travelers. Note: **CQ** may exacerbate psoriasis. | **CQ Peds dose:** 8.3 mg/kg (5 mg/kg of base) po 1x/wk up to 300 mg (base) max. dose **or AP** by weight (peds dose): 5-8 kg, ¼ adult tab; 9-10 kg, ⅜ tab; 11-20 kg, 1 tab; 21-30 kg, 2 tabs; 31-40 kg, 3 tabs; >40 kg, 1 adult tab per day. **Adults:** Doxy or MQ as below. | AP must be taken with food for adequate absorption. CQ safe during pregnancy. **The CDC considers CQ & mefloquine both safe during pregnancy. For CDC recommendations continue to shrink. See CDC or WHO maps for most current information on CQ resistance.** **Doxy AEs:** photosensitivity, candida vaginitis, gastritis. For Tafenoquine must document on at least 1 occasion during life a quantitative level of >70% normal level of G6PD activity before use. Do not use: screening or qualitative G6PD tests. |
| **For areas with CQ-resistant P. falciparum:** Details on considerations for malaria prophylaxis: N Engl J Med. 2016; 375:247. | Atovaquone 250 mg—Proguanil 100 mg (Malarone) comb. tablet, 1 per day with food 1-2 days prior to, during, & 7 days post-travel. Not in pregnancy. Malarone preferred for trips of a week or less; expense may preclude use for longer trips. Native populations: intermittent pregnancy prophylaxis/treatment programs in a few countries. Fansidar 1 tab po 3 times during pregnancy (Expert Rev Anti Infect Ther 8:589, 2010). | Doxycycline 100 mg po daily for adults & children >8 yrs of age. Take 1-2 days before, during & for 4 wks after travel **OR** TQ 200 mg once daily x 3 days (starting 3 days before travel) then 200 mg once weekly (starting 7 days after last loading regimen dose) then a 200 mg one-time dose (7 days after last dose in malaria area) **OR** Mefloquine (MQ) 250 mg (228 mg base) po once per wk, 1-2 wks before, during, & for 4 wks after travel (see Comment). **Doxy:** 2.2 mg/kg po per day,(max 100 mg/day) **MFQ:** <9 kg: 5 mg/kg weekly (4.6 mg/kg base) 10-19 kg: ¼ adult tab weekly 20-30 kg: ½ tab weekly 31-45 kg: ¾ tab weekly >45 kg: 1 tab weekly **Doxy AEs:** photosensitivity, candida vaginitis, gastritis. | **Pregnancy: CQ current best option.** **Doxycycline and Primaquine:** Insufficient data with Malarone. Avoid **Tafenoquine (TQ), Primaquine: Can cause hemolytic anemia if G6PD deficiency present. For TQ causes benign vortex keratopathy in 21% after 6 months use. MQ not recommended if cardiac conduction abnormalities, seizures, or psychiatric disorders, e.g., depression, psychosis.** If used, can start 3 wks before travel to assure tolerability. Children: Weekly dosing may make MFQ preferable. TQ not licensed in children. If 8 yr or older doxycycline liquid is available. For children under 10 kg, MFQ needs to be compounded but AP pediatric tablets can be cut. TQ option when weekly dosing preferable such as for long-stay trips. TQ not approved for use for >6 months consecutively; use 3-month washout. |

**Treatment of Malaria.** Diagnosis. Blood smear by microscopy. Alternative: rapid antigen detection test (Binax NOW): detects 96-100% of P. falciparum and 50% of other plasmodia (CID 49:908, 2009; CID 54:1637, 2012). Need microscopy to speciate. Can stay positive for over a month after successful treatment.

**Uncomplicated P. falciparum (or species unidentified),** 2015 WHO Guidelines suggest artemisinin combination therapy for adults (except in pregnancy) for all malaria species.

| | | | |
|---|---|---|---|
| Acquired: Cent. Amer., west of Panama Canal; Haiti, Dom. Republic, & most of Mid-East **CQ sensitive** | **Adults: CQ phosphate** 1 gm salt (600 mg base) po, then 0.5 gm in 6 hrs, then 0.5 gm (daily x 2 days. Total: 2500 mg salt. | **Peds: CQ** 10 mg/kg of base po, then 5 mg/kg of base at 6, 24, & 48 hrs. Total: 25 mg/kg base | Other chloroquine salts available in some countries, total dose may differ. **Peds dose should never exceed adult dose. CQ + MQ prolong QTc. Doses >2x recommended may be fatal.** |

* For source of drug, see Table 13D, page 177.

**TABLE 13A (5)**

| INFECTING ORGANISM | SUGGESTED REGIMENS | | COMMENTS |
|---|---|---|---|
| | PRIMARY | ALTERNATIVE | |

**PROTOZOA—EXTRAINTESTINAL/Malaria (Plasmodia species)/Treatment of Malaria** *(continued)*

| INFECTING ORGANISM | PRIMARY | ALTERNATIVE | COMMENTS |
|---|---|---|---|
| **CQ-resistant or unknown resistance.** Note: If >5% parasitemia or Hb <7, treat as severe malaria regardless of clinical findings or lack thereof. Note to reader re: dosing: For Peds, developing world drugs are listed under Primary; drugs of choice are listed under Alternative; Pregnancy alternatives are listed under Comments. | **Adults: Atovaquone-Proguanil** 1 gm-400 mg (4 adult tabs) po 1x/day x 3 days w/ food OR [**QS** 650 mg po tid x 3 days (7 days if SE Asia) + (**Doxy** 100 mg po bid) or (**Tetra** 250 mg po qid) or **Clinda** 20 mg/kg/d divided tid] x 7 days OR **Artemether-Lumefantrine\*** tabs 20/120 mg: 4 tabs po (at 0, 8 hrs) then bid x 2 days (total 6 doses); take with food OR a less desirable adult alternative, **Mefloquine** 750 mg po x 1 dose, then 500 mg po x 1 dose 6-12 hr later. **MQ** is 2nd line alternative due to neuropsychiatric reaction and cannot use in SE Asia due to resistance. Clinda or Tetra only if doxy not available. Other options: Available in Europe and endemic countries, WHO pre-qualified and EMA approved is **Dihydroartemisinin-piperaquine**. Available as PPQ 320 mg/DHA 40 mg (adult tabs) and PPQ 160 mg/DHA 20 mg (pediatric tabs). 5 to <7 kg  PPQ 80 mg/DHA 10 mg po q24h x3 days 7 to <13 kg  PPQ 160 mg/DHA 20 mg po q24h x3 days 13 to <24 kg  PPQ 320 mg/DHA 40 mg po q24h x3 days 24 to <36 kg  PPQ 640 mg/DHA 80 mg po q24h x3 days 36 to <75 kg  PPQ 960 mg/DHA 120 mg po q24h x3 days 75 to 100 kg  PPQ 1280 mg/DHA 160 mg po q24h x3 days >100 kg  no data Available in many endemic countries and WHO pre-qualified and EMA approved ACT is **Pyronaridine/ Artesunate** 2 tablets (180 mg/60 mg) as a single dose each day for 3 days for 24 to >45 kg or 1 tablet if 20 to <24 kg. Pediatric granule formulation for oral suspension • <8 kg 1 sachet Daily for 3 days • 8 - <15 kg 2 sachets Daily for 3 days • 15 - <20 kg 3 sachets Daily for 3 days | **Peds (drugs of choice): QS** 10 mg/kg po tid x 3 days + **Doxy** 2.2 mg/kg/ bid up to 100 mg per dose both x 7 days. AAP now recommends that doxy can safely be administered for durations ≤21 days regardless of age. OR **Atovaquone-Proguanil** (all once daily x 3 d) by weight: • 5-8 kg: 2 peds tabs; • 9-10 kg: 3 peds tabs; • 11-20 kg: 1 adult tab; • 21-30 kg: 2 adult tabs; • 31-40 kg: 3 adult tabs; • >40 kg: 4 adult tabs. OR **MQ Salt:** 15 mg/kg x 1, then 6-12 hrs later, 10 mg/kg ALL po. OR **Artemether-Lumefantrine\*** • 5 kg to <15 kg: 1 tablet (20 mg / 120 mg) as a single dose, then 1 tablet again after 8 hours, then 1 tablet every 12 hours for 2 days • 15 kg to <25 kg: 2 tablets (40 mg / 240 mg) as a single dose, then 2 tablets again after 8 hours, then 2 tablets every 12 hours for 2 days • 25 kg to <35 kg: 3 tablets (60 mg / 360 mg) as a single dose, then 3 tablets again after 8 hours, then 3 tablets every 12 hours for 2 days • ≥35 kg: as per adult dose | **Pregnancy:** • **Artemether-Lumefantrine** 4 tablets (80 mg/ 480 mg) as a single dose, then 4 tablets again after 8 hours, then 4 tablets every 12 hours for 2 days (take with food). Drug of choice in 2nd/3rd trimester. Artemether-Lumefantrine is safer than quinine in the first trimester of pregnancy (*Malar J 13:97, 2014*). Lumefantrine appears safe (*Malar J 14:77, 2015*) and is safer than quinine in the first trimester of pregnancy (*Malar J 13:197, 2014*) and is recommended by experts in the 1st trimester but not yet in official guidelines (*PLoS Med. 2017;14(5):e1002290*). OR • **Quinine sulfate** 10 mg/kg po tid x 3 days (7 days if SE Asia) + **Clindamycin** 20 mg/kg/day divided tid x 7 days • Do not delay therapy if quinine available and Artemether-Lumefantrine is not in U.S., QS is only available as quinine 324 mg capsule, thus hard to use to treat children. **Note: Oral Artemether-Lumefantrine tabs FDA-approved but not widely stocked.** Call 1-800-COARTEM to obtain. |
| **Uncomplicated/P. malariae or P. knowlesi** (*JID 199: 1107 & 1143, 2009*). All regions – always CQ-sensitive | CQ as above: treat adults & peds. In South Pacific, beware of P. malariae; looks like P. malariae, but behaves like P. falciparum (*CID 46:165, 2007*). | **Artemether-Lumefantrine\*** (20/120 mg tab) 4 tabs po x 1 dose, repeat in 8 hrs, then repeat q12h x 2 days (take with food) OR **Atovaquone-Proguanil** (250/100 mg tab) 4 adult tabs po daily x 3 days or **DHA-PPQ** or **Pyronaridine-artesunate** | |

---

\* For source of drug, see *Table 13D, page 177.*

TABLE 13A (6)

| INFECTING ORGANISM | SUGGESTED REGIMENS | | COMMENTS |
|---|---|---|---|
| | PRIMARY | ALTERNATIVE | |

**PROTOZOA—EXTRAINTESTINAL/Malaria (Plasmodium species)/Treatment of Malaria** (continued)

| INFECTING ORGANISM | PRIMARY | ALTERNATIVE | COMMENTS |
|---|---|---|---|
| **Uncomplicated/P. vivax or P. ovale**<br><br>**CQ-sensitive** (except Papua New Guinea, Indonesia which are CQ-resistant–see below) | **Adults:** CQ + **PQ/TQ**. PQ/TQ to start or be given on day 1 or 2 of appropriate blood-stage therapy with CQ (or alternative drug).<br><br>For PQ, 30 mg with food/day x 14 days.<br>Each primaquine phosphate tab is 26.3 mg of salt and 15 mg of base.<br><br>30 mg of base = 2 x 26.3 mg tabs prim. phos. Where available Tafenoquine (TQ) 300 mg single dose preferable to PQ.<br><br>**Peds:** CQ as above + PQ base 0.5 mg po once daily x 14 days. | **Artemether-Lumefantrine or DHA-PPQ or Pyronaridine-artesunate** as above + **PQ** base 0.5 mg po once daily x 14 days. Where available TQ 300 mg single dose preferable to PQ; not approved for age ≤ 16 yrs | TQ/PQ added to eradicate latent parasites in liver. **Screen for G6PD def.** (must have 70% normal G6PD activity to use TQ) **before dose PQ as QS TQ:** If mildly G6PD deficient (cannot use TQ). **Note: rare severe reactions.** CQ safe in pregnancy. Avoid PQ in pregnancy. If P. vivax or P. ovale during pregnancy, after pregnancy check for G6PD deficiency & give PQ 30 mg daily x 14 days or TQ 300 mg. |
| **Uncomplicated/P. vivax**<br><br>**CQ-resistant:** Papua, New Guinea & Indonesia | **Adults/Peds: QS + (doxy or tetra) + PQ/TQ** as above or **Artemether-Lumefantrine or DHA-PPQ + PQ/TQ** | **Adults: MQ + PQ/TQ** as above. | Rarely acute. Lung injury and other serious complications: LnID 8:449, 2008. If pregnant treat as for uncomplicated P. falciparum. In pregnancy, AAP now recommends that doxy can safely be administered for ≤21 days regardless of age. |
| **Severe malaria,** i.e., impaired consciousness, severe anemia, renal failure, pulmonary edema, ARDS, DIC, jaundice, acidosis, seizures, parasitemia >5%.<br>One or more of latter.<br>**Almost always P. falciparum.**<br>Ref.: AnIM 358:1829, 2008; Science 320-30, 20:58.<br>All regions<br>Note:<br>• IV Artesunate is drug of choice but not FDA-approved. Available from CDC Drug Service under specific conditions, need to state quinidine not available or not tolerated.<br>• Possible emergency availability from Eli Lilly. | **Adults:** Quinidine gluconate in normal saline: 10 mg/kg (salt) IV over 1 hr then 0.02 mg/kg/min by constant infusion OR 24 mg/kg IV over 4 hrs & then 12 mg/kg over 4 hrs q8h. Continue until parasite density <1% & can take po QS. **QS** 650 mg po tid x 3 days (7 days if SE Asia) + **[(Doxy** 100 mg IV q12h x 7 days) OR **Artesunate** 2.4 mg/kg IV at 0, 12, 24, 48 hrs, and **Doxy** 100 mg IV q12h x 7days).<br>IV quinidine dihydrochloride still available in many endemic countries; but second line to be used if no IV artemisinin is available. Dosing is complicated and don't think we need to include. | **Peds:** Quinidine gluconate IV—same mg/kg dose as for adults<br>**PLUS**<br>(**Doxy:** if <45 kg, 4 mg per kg IV q12h; if ≥45 kg, dose as for adults)<br>**Pregnancy: Clindamycin** 10 mg/kg IV loading dose, then 5 mg/kg IV or po (as tolerated) q8h x 7 days<br>Follow **IV Artesunate** with a complete oral course of one of: **Atovaquone/Proguanil**, **Artemether/Lumefantrine or Dihydroartemisinin/piperaquine** (not available in US) **Doxy** 100 mg po q12h is less preferred alternative | During quinidine IV: monitor BP, EKG (prolongation of QTc), & blood glucose (hypoglycemia).<br>Exchange transfusion no longer recommended. Switch to QS po + Doxy when patient able to take oral drugs. AAP now recommends that doxy can be used for ≤21 days regardless of age. **Steroids not recommended for cerebral malaria.**<br>IV Artesunate from CDC (8 hr transport time post-approval), see Table 13D (Ref: CID 44:1067 & 1075, 2007). Can cause non-life threatening, late transfusion requiring, hemolytic anemia up to 15 days post-therapy (AnIM 163:498, 2015). |
| **Malaria—self-initiated treatment:** Only for people at high risk. Carry a reliable supply of recommended antimalarials (worried about counterfeit meds). Use only if malaria is lab-diagnosed and no available reliable meds. | **Artemether-Lumefantrine** (20/120 mg tab) 4 tabs po x 1 dose, repeat in 8 hrs, then repeat q12h x 2 days OR **Atovaquone-Proguanil (AP)** 4 adult tabs (1 gm/400 mg) po daily x 3 days | **Peds:** Using adult **AP** tabs for 3 consecutive days: 11-20 kg, 1 tab; 21-30 kg, 2 tabs; 31-40 kg, 3 tabs; >41 kg, 4 tabs. For Peds dosing of Artemether-Lumefantrine, see Uncomplicated/P. falciparum, page 163. | Do not use for renal insufficiency pts. Do not use if weight <11 kg, pregnant, or breast-feeding. **Artemether-Lumefantrine:** sold as Riamet (EU) and Coartem (US & elsewhere). |

* For source of drug, see Table 13D, page 177.

**TABLE 13A (7)**

| INFECTING ORGANISM | SUGGESTED REGIMENS | | COMMENTS |
|---|---|---|---|
| | PRIMARY | ALTERNATIVE | |
| **PROTOZOA—EXTRAINTESTINAL** (continued) | | | |
| **Toxoplasma gondii (Toxoplasmosis)** (Reference: *Ln 363:1965, 2004*) | | | |
| *Immunologically normal patients (For pediatric doses, see reference)* | | | |
| Acute illness w/ lymphadenopathy | No specific rx unless severe/persistent symptoms or evidence of vital organ damage. | | |
| Acq. via transfusion (lab accident) | Treat as for active chorioretinitis. | | |
| **Active chorioretinitis; meningitis;** lowered resistance due to steroids or cytotoxic drugs | [**Pyrimethamine** (pyri) 200 mg x 1 po once on 1st day, then 50-75 mg q24h] + [**Sulfadiazine** (see *footnote*) S 1-1.5 gm po qid] + [**Leucovorin (folinic acid)** 5-20 mg 3x/wk]—see *Comment*. Treat 1-2 wks beyond resolution of signs/symptoms; continue leucovorin 1 wk after stopping pyri. | | For congenital Toxo, Toxo meningitis in adults, & chorioretinitis, **add prednisone 1 mg/kg/day in 2 div. doses** until CSF protein conc. falls or vision-threatening inflammation subsides. Adjust folinic acid dose by following CBC results. |
| Acute in pregnant women. Ref: *CID 47:554, 2008.* | If <18 wks gestation at diagnosis: **Spiramycin**[1] 1 gm po q8h until 16-18 wks; dc if amniotic fluid PCR is negative. Positive PCR: treat as below. If >18 wks gestation & documented fetal infection by positive amniotic fluid PCR: (**Pyrimethamine** 50 mg q12h x 2 days, then 50 mg/kg q12h (max 4 gm/day) + **Sulfadiazine** 75 mg/kg po x 1 dose, then 50 mg/kg q12h for minimum of 4 wks or for duration of pregnancy. **Folinic acid** 10-20 mg po daily) | | Screen patients with IgG/IgM serology at commercial lab. IgG+/IgM+ = remote past infection; IgG+/IgM+ = seroconversion. For pregnant patients, consult with Palo Alto Medical Foundation Toxoplasma Serology Lab: 650-853-4828 or toxlab@pamf.org. Details in *Ln 363:1965, 2004.* **Consultation advisable.** |
| Fetal/congenital | Mgmt complex. Combo rx with pyrimethamine + sulfadiazine + leucovorin—See *Comment* | | |
| **AIDS** | | | |
| **Cerebral toxoplasmosis** Ref: *MMWR 58(RR-4) 1, 2009.* | [**Pyrimethamine** (pyri) 200 mg x 1 po, then 75 mg/day po] + (**Sulfadiazine** [Wt based dose: 1 gm if <60 kg, 1.5 gm if ≥60 kg] po q6h) + **Folinic acid** 10-25 mg/day po for minimum of 6 wks after resolution of signs/ symptoms, and then suppressive rx (see *below*) OR **TMP-SMX**, 10/50 mg/kg per day po or IV q12h x 30 days (*AAC 42:1346, 1998*) | [**Pyri + Folinic acid** (as in primary regimen)] + 1 of the following: (1) **Clinda** 600 mg po/IV q6h or (2) **TMP-SMX** 5/25 mg/kg/day po or IV bid or (3) **Atovaquone** 750 mg po q6h. Treat 4-6 wks after resolution of signs/symptoms, then suppression. | Use alternative regimen for pts with severe sulfa allergy. If multiple ring-enhancing brain lesions (CT or MRI), >85% of pts respond to 7-10 days of empiric rx. If no response, suggest brain biopsy. Pyri penetrates brain even if no inflammation; folinic acid prevents pyrimethamine hematologic toxicity. |
| **Primary prophylaxis.** AIDS pts—IgG Toxo antibody + CD4 count <100 per mcL | **TMP-SMX-DS,** 1 tab po q24h or 3x/wk) or (**TMP-SMX-SS,** 1 tab po q24h) | (**Dapsone** 50 mg po q24h) + (**Pyri** 50 mg po q wk) + (**Folinic acid** 25 mg po q wk) OR **Atovaquone** 1500 mg po q24h | Prophylaxis for pneumocystis also effective vs Toxo. Ref: *MMWR 58(RR-4):1, 2009.* **Another alternative:** (Dapsone 200 mg po + pyrimethamine 75 mg q24h + folinic acid 25 mg po) once weekly. |
| **Suppression after rx of cerebral Toxo** | (**Sulfadiazine** 2-4 gm po divided in 2-4 doses/day) + (**Pyri** 25-50 mg po q24h) + **Folinic acid** 10-25 mg po q24h). DC if CD4 count >200 x 3 mos | ((**Clinda** 600 mg po q8h) + (**Pyri** 25-50 mg po q24h)) + (**Folinic acid** 10-25 mg po q24h) OR **Atovaquone** 750 mg po q6-12h | (Pyri + sulfa) prevents PCP and Toxo; (clinda + pyri) prevents Toxo only. Additional drug needed to prevent PCP. |
| **Trichomonas vaginalis** | See *Vaginitis, Table 1, page 28* | | |

[1] Sulfonamides for Toxo. Sulfadiazine now commercially available. Sulfisoxazole much less effective.

* For source of drug, see *Table 13D, page 177.*

**TABLE 13A (8)**

See Table 13D, page 177, for source information.

| INFECTING ORGANISM | SUGGESTED REGIMENS | | COMMENTS |
|---|---|---|---|
| | **PRIMARY** | **ALTERNATIVE** | |

**PROTOZOA—EXTRAINTESTINAL** (continued)

**Trypanosomiasis. Ref.:** Ln 362:1469, 2003. **Note: Drugs for African trypanosomiasis may be obtained free from WHO or CDC.** See Table 13D, page 177, for source information. Fexinidazole, a completely oral regimen effective against both stages of disease in both species of African trypanosomiasis is in advanced pipeline, very promising. Lancet. 2018; 391:144.

**West African sleeping sickness (T. brucei gambiense)**

| Early: Blood/lymphatic—CNS OK | **Pentamidine** 4 mg/kg IV/IM daily x 7–10 days | In US, free from CDC drug service: **Suramin***  100 mg IV (test dose), then 1 gm IV on days 1, 3, 7, 14, & 21. Peds dose is 20 mg/kg. | Suramin effective but avoid if possible due to possible co-infection with T. volvulus in W. Africa. |
| Late: Encephalitis | Combination of IV **Eflornithine***, 400 mg/kg/day divided q12h x 7 days, plus **Nifurtimox***, 15 mg/kg/day po, divided q8h x 10 days (abbreviated NECT) now WHO standard of care (Lancet 374:56, 2009; CID 56:195 2013). | **Melarsoprol*** 2.2 mg/kg/day IV x 10 days; toxic arsenical now superseded by NECT | Fexinidazole 4 mg/kg/day IV/IM x 1–2 doses. |

**East African sleeping sickness (T. brucei rhodesiense)**

| Early: Blood/lymphatic. Clinical series in Travelers Int J Infect Dis (2018): https://doi.org/10.1016/j.ijid.2018.08.012 | **Suramin***  100 mg IV (test dose), then 1 gm IV on days 1, 3, 7, 14, & 21 | Peds: **Suramin***  2 mg/kg test dose, then 20 mg/kg on days 1, 3, 7, 14 & 21 | Suramin & Melarsoprol: CDC Drug Service or WHO (at no charge) (see Table 13D) |
| Late: Encephalitis (prednisolone may prevent encephalitis). Pre-treatment with Suramin advised by some. | **Melarsoprol*** 2.2 mg/kg/day IV x 10 days (PLOS NTD 6:e1695, 2012) | | Early illness: patient waiting for Suramin, use pentamidine 4 mg/kg IV/IM x 1–2 doses. Does not enter CSF. |

**T. cruzi–Chagas disease** or acute American trypanosomiasis
Ref: NEJM 373:456, 2015.
For chronic disease: no benefit in established cardiomyopathy (NEJM 373:1295, 2015)
US batch reviewed PLoS Negl Trop Dis 2016;10:e0005033.

| *Adult (Age ≥12 years):* **Benznidazole** 5–7 mg/kg/day in 2 doses (q12h) x 60 days *Pediatric (Age <12 years):* **Benznidazole***  7.5 mg/kg/day in 2 doses (q12h) x 60 days. South American pediatric tablet formulation (LAFEPE and ELEA) not widely available. U.S.: available from Exeltis, Inc., Tel: +1 877-303-7181; www.benznidazoletablets.com. **Benznidazole** 12.5 & 100 mg approved tabs for 2–12 yr olds. CDC advocates off-label use in adults. | **Nifurtimox***  8–10 mg/kg per day po div. 4x/day after meals x 120 days. Ages 1–6 yrs: 12.5–15 mg/kg per day div. qid x 90 days. Children <1yrs: 15–20 mg/kg per day div. qid x 90 days. For AEs: Table 13B Ref: CID 2016;63:1056 | Due to adverse effects may give Benznidazole 300 mg per day x 60 days, regardless of body weight OR up to 80 days to prolong treatment to complete the total dose corresponding to 5 mg/kg per day for 60 days. N Engl J Med 373-456, 2015. Immunosuppression can reactivate chronic Chagas disease. Can transmit by organ/transfusions. Do not use benznidazole in pregnancy. |

**NEMATODES—INTESTINAL (Roundworms). Eosinophilia?** Think Strongyloides, toxocariasis and filariasis: CID 34-407, 2005; 42:1781 & 1655, 2006— See Table 13C

| Anisakis simplex (**anisakiasis**) Anisakidosis (fermented from Anisakidosis (CID 51:806, 2010). Other: A. pegreffii, A physeteris), Pseudoterranova decipiens. | Physical removal: endoscope or surgery. Simplex may help diagnosis. No antimicrobial therapy. | Anecdotal reports of possible treatment benefit from albendazole (Ln 360:54, 2002; CID 41:1825, 2005) | Anisakiasis acquired by eating raw fish: herring, salmon, mackerel, cod, squid. Similar illness due to Pseudoterranova species acquired from cod, halibut, red snapper. |
| Ascaris lumbricoides (**ascariasis**) Ln 367:1521, 2006 | **Albendazole** 400 mg po x 1 dose OR **Mebendazole** 100 mg po bid x 3 days or 500 mg po x 1 dose | **Ivermectin** 150–200 mcg/kg po x 1 dose | Review of efficacy of single dose: JAMA 299:1937, 2008. Mebendazole 500 mg tabs not widely available. |
| Capillaria philippinensis (**capillariasis**) | **Albendazole** 400 mg po bid x 10 days | **Mebendazole** 500 mg po daily x 20 days | Albendazole preferred. |
| Enterobius vermicularis (**pinworm**) | **Mebendazole** 500 mg po x 1 dose, repeat in 2 weeks OR **Pyrantel pamoate** 11 mg/kg base (to max. dose of 1 gm) po x 1 dose; repeat in 2 wks | **Albendazole** 400 mg po x 1 dose, repeat in 2 wks. | Side-effects in Table 13B, page 175. Treat whole household. |
| **Gongylonemiasis** (adult worms in oral mucosa) | Surgical removal | **Albendazole** 400 mg/day po x 3 days | Ref: CID 32:1378, 2001; J Helminth 80:425, 2006. |

* For source of drug, see Table 13D, page 177.

**TABLE 13A (9)**

| INFECTING ORGANISM | SUGGESTED REGIMENS | | COMMENTS |
|---|---|---|---|
| | PRIMARY | ALTERNATIVE | |
| **NEMATODES—INTESTINAL (Roundworms)** *(continued)* | | | |
| **Hookworm** (Necator americanus and Ancylostoma duodenale) | Albendazole 400 mg po daily x 3 days | **Mebendazole** 500 mg po daily x 3 days **OR Pyrantel pamoate** 11 mg/kg (to max. dose of 1 gm) po daily x 3 days | **NOTE:** Ivermectin not effective. Single dose therapy as used in public health programs has lower cure rates and 3-day albendazole superior to 1-day mebendazole. *PLoS One 6:e25003, 2011.* |
| **Strongyloides stercoralis (strongyloidiasis)** *(Hyperinfection, See Comment)* | Ivermectin 200 mcg/kg per day po x 2 days | Albendazole 400 mg po bid x 7 days ; less effective | For disseminated disease with larvae in stool and sputum, repeat treatment every 15 days while stools positive and then 1 more treatment cycle. For hyperinfection with sepsis, treat daily for at least 10 days or until larvae undetectable. For hyperinfection: veterinary ivermectin given subcutaneously or rectally *(CID 49:1411, 2009).* |
| **Trichostrongylus orientalis, T. colubriformis** | **Pyrantel pamoate** 11 mg/kg (maximum 1 gm) po x 1 dose **OR** Albendazole 400 mg po daily x 10 doses **OR** Mebendazole 500 mg po qd x 10 days | Albendazole 400 mg po x 1 dose | |
| **Trichuris trichiura** (whipworm) *NEJM 370:610, 2014; PLoS One 6:e25003, 2011* | Mebendazole 100 mg po twice daily x 3 days. Low cure rates with either mebendazole or albendazole | Albendazole 400 mg po qd x 3 days or **Ivermectin** 200 mcg/kg po x 3 days | Mebendazole clearly superior for trichuris *(PLoS One 6:e25003, 2011; N Engl J Med 370:610, 2014).* Single dose Mebendazole 500 mg tab significantly less effective than 3 days (the references currently support this). |
| **NEMATODES—EXTRAINTESTINAL (Roundworms)** | | | |
| Ancylostoma braziliense & caninum: causes **cutaneous larva migrans** | Albendazole 400 mg po bid x 3-7 days *(Ln ID 8-302, 2008).* | Ivermectin 200 mcg/kg po x 1 dose/day x 1-2 days (not in children wt <15 kg) | Also called "creeping eruption." dog and cat hookworm. Ivermectin cure rate 81-100% (1 dose) to 97% (2-3 doses) *(CID 37:493, 2000).* |
| **Angiostrongylus cantonensis (Angiostrongyliasis)**; causes eosinophilic meningitis | Mild/moderate disease: Analgesics, serial LPs (if necessary). Prednisone 60 mg/day x 14 days reduces headache & need for LPs. | Adding **Albendazole** 15 mg/kg/day to prednisone 60 mg/day both for 14 days may reduce duration of headaches and need for repeat LPs. | **Do not use Albendazole without prednisone,** see *TRSMH 102:990, 2008.* Gnathostoma and Baylisascaris also cause eosinophilic meningitis. |
| **Baylisascariasis** (Raccoon roundworm); eosinophilic meningitis | No drug proven efficacious. Try **Albendazole,** Peds: 25-50 mg/kg/day po, Adults: 400 mg po bid with corticosteroids. Treat for one month. | | *Clin Microbiol Rev. 29:375, 2016.* Other causes of eosinophilic meningitis: Gnathostoma & Angiostrongylus. |
| **Dracunculus medinensis, Guinea worm** Dog reservoir found in 3 countries hampering eradication. *Am J Trop Med Hyg. 2018; 99:388* | Slow extraction of pre-emergent worm over several days | No drugs effective. Oral analgesics, anti-inflammatory drugs, topical antiseptics/antibiotic ointments to alleviate symptoms and facilitate worm removal by gentle manual traction over several days. | |

* For source of drug, see *Table 13D, page 177.*

**TABLE 13A (10)**

| INFECTING ORGANISM | SUGGESTED REGIMENS | | COMMENTS |
|---|---|---|---|
| | PRIMARY | ALTERNATIVE | |
| **NEMATODES—EXTRAINTESTINAL (Roundworms)** (continued) | | | |
| **Filariasis: Determine if co-infection with either Loa loa or Onchocerca** | | | |
| Lymphatic filariasis (Elephantiasis): Etiologies: Wuchereria bancrofti Brugia malayi, Brugia timori | *Mono-infection:* **Diethylcarbamazine⁴ (DEC)⁴** 6 mg/kg/day po in 3 divided doses x 12 days + **Doxy** 200 mg/day po x 6 wks | *Dual infection with Onchocerciasis:* Treat Lymphatic filariasis first: **Ivermectin** 150 mcg/kg po x 1 dose, wait 1 month, then start **DEC** as for mono-infection *Dual infection with Loa Loa:* DEC drug of choice for both but can cause severe encephalopathy if >2500 Loa Loa microfilaria/mL in blood. Refer to expert center for apheresis pre-DEC or prednisone + small doses of DEC. If <2500 microfilaria/mL, start regular dose of **DEC** | Doxy x 6 wks may improve microfilaremia/moderate lymphedema independent of parasite infection (CID 55:621, 2012). **Note: DEC can cause irreversible eye damage if concomitant Onchocerciasis.** |
| **Loiasis, Loa loa,** eye worm disease: Look for dual infection with either Onchocerciasis or Lymphatic filariasis. Moxidectin pivotal study *Lancet. 2018 Jan 17. pii: S0140-6736(17)32844-1* | *Mono-infection with <2500 L. loa microfilaria/mL:* **DEC** 8-10 mg/kg/day po in 3 divided doses x 21 days *Mono-infection with >2500 L. loa microfilaria/mL:* Refer to expert center for apheresis prior to DEC therapy; alternatively: **Albendazole** 200 mg po bid x 21 days | *Dual infection with Lymphatic filariasis:* See Lymphatic filariasis, above *Dual infection with Onchocerciasis:* Treat Onchocerciasis first with **Ivermectin**, then treat L. loa with **DEC** | If >5000 L. loa microfilaria/mL in blood & given Ivermectin for Onchocerciasis, can facilitate entry of L. loa into CNS with severe encephalopathy. May require multiple 21 day courses of DEC to clear mono-infection |
| **Onchocerca volvulus (Onchocerciasis),** river blindness: Look for dual infection with either Loa loa or Lymphatic filariasis | *Mono-infection:* **Ivermectin** 150 mcg/kg x 1 dose, then repeat every 3-6 months until asymptomatic + **Doxy** 200 mg/day x 6 wks. No accepted alternative therapy. **Moxidectin** 8 mg po (age 12 or over) to be used instead of ivermectin but not widely available | *Dual infection with Lymphatic filariasis:* See Lymphatic filariasis, above *Dual infection with L. loa:* Treat Onchocerciasis first with **Ivermectin**, then treat L. loa with **DEC**. If >5000 L. Loa microfilaria/mL in blood. Refer to expert center for apheresis before starting DEC | Onchocerciasis and Loa loa are mildly co-endemic in West and Central Africa. |
| Body cavity | | | |
| Mansonella perstans | In randomized trial, **Doxy** 200 mg po once daily x 6 weeks cleared microfilaria from blood in 67 of 69 patients. (NEJM 361:1448, 2009). Doxy may not work outside Mali and Cameroon due to strain variation. **Ivermectin** 150 μg/kg x 1 dose. | **Albendazole** in high dose x 3 weeks. Doxy may not work outside Mali and Cameroon due to strain variation. | Efficacy of doxy believed to be due to inhibition of endosymbiont wolbachia; ivermectin has no activity. Ref: Trans R Soc Trop Med Hyg 100:458, 2006. |
| Mansonella streptocerca | **Diethylcarbamazine** 6 mg/kg x 12 days kills microfilaria in adults but causes transient exacerbation of clinical symptoms and may cause vision loss and hypotension if co-infected with O. volvulus. | | May need antihistamine or corticosteroid for allergic reaction from disintegrating organisms. Chronic pruritic hypopigmented lesions that may be confused with leprosy. Can be asymptomatic. |
| Mansonella ozzardi | **Ivermectin** 200 μ/kg x 1 dose likely effective. Am J Trop Med Hyg 90:1170, 2014; Am J Trop Med Hyg. 2018; 98: 786 | | Usually asymptomatic. Articular pain, pruritus, lymphadenopathy reported. May have allergic reaction from dying organisms. |
| **Dirofilariasis: Heartworms** | | | |
| D. immitis, dog heartworm | No effective drugs; surgical removal only option | | Can lodge in pulmonary artery → coin lesion. Eosinophilia rare. |

⁴ May need antihistamine or corticosteroid for allergic reaction from disintegrating organisms.

* For source of drug, see *Table 13D, page 177.*

**TABLE 13A (11)**

| INFECTING ORGANISM | SUGGESTED REGIMENS | | COMMENTS |
|---|---|---|---|
| | PRIMARY | ALTERNATIVE | |
| **NEMATODES—EXTRAINTESTINAL (Roundworms)/Filariasis/Dirofilariasis: Heartworms** (continued) | | | |
| D. tenuis (raccoon), D. ursi (bear), D. repens (dogs, cats) | No effective drugs | Worms migrate to conjunctivae, subcutaneous tissue including face, scrotum, breasts, extremities. D. repens emerging throughout Europe Clin Microbiol Rev 25:507, 2012 | |
| **Gnathostoma sp ** | | | |
| Cutaneous larva migrans | Albendazole 400 mg po q24h or bid times 21 days | Ivermectin 200 μg/kg/day po x 2 days. | Other etiology of larva migrans: Ancylostoma sp, see page 168 |
| Eosinophilic meningitis | Supportive care; monitor for cerebral hemorrhage | Case reports of steroid use: both benefit and harm from Albendazole or Ivermectin (EID 17:1174, 2011). | Other causes of eosinophilic meningitis: **Angiostrongylus** (see page 168) & **Baylisascaris** (see page 168) |
| **Toxocariasis** (Lancet Infect Dis, 2018, ;18:e14) | Rx directed at relief of symptoms as infection self-limited, e.g., steroids & antihistamines; use of anthelmintics controversial. | | |
| Visceral larval migrans | Albendazole 400 mg po bid x 5 days ± Prednisone 60 mg/day | Mebendazole 100–200 mg po bid times 5 days | Severe lung, heart or CNS disease may warrant steroids (Clin Micro Rev 16:265, 2003). Differential dx of larval migrans syndromes: Toxocara canis & catis, Ancylostoma spp., Gnathostoma spp., Spirometra spp.. |
| Ocular larval migrans | First 4 wks of illness: (Oral **Prednisone** 30–60 mg po q24h + subtenon **Triamcinolone** 40 mg/wk) x 2 wks (Surgery is sometimes necessary) | | No added benefit of anthelmintic drugs. Rx of little effect after 4 wks. Some use steroids (Clin Micro Rev 16:265, 2003) |
| Trichinella spiralis (**Trichinellosis**) — muscle infection (Review: Clin Micro Rev 22:127, 2009). | Albendazole 400 mg po bid x 8–14 days | Mebendazole 500 mg po tid x 10 days (still with concomitant prednisone). | Use albendazole/mebendazole with caution during pregnancy. ↑ IgE, ↑ CPK, ESR 0, massive eosinophilia: >5000/uL. |
| | Concomitant **prednisone** 40–60 mg po q24h | | |
| **TREMATODES (Flukes) – Liver, Lung, Intestinal.** All flukes have snail intermediate hosts; transmitted by ingestion of metacercariae on plants, fish or crustaceans. | | | |
| Liver flukes. Clonorchis sinensis, Metorchis conjunctus, Opisthorchis viverrini | Praziquantel 25 mg/kg po tid x 2 days | | |
| Fasciola hepatica (sheep liver fluke), Fasciola gigantica | Triclabendazole* once, may repeat after 12–24 hrs. 10 mg/kg po x 1 dose. Single 20 mg/kg po dose effective in treatment failures. | | |
| Intestinal flukes: Fasciola buski Heterophyes heterophyes; Metagonimus yokogawai; Nanophyetus salmincola | Praziquantel 25 mg/kg po tid x 1 days | | Same dose in children |
| Lung fluke: Paragonimus sp. | Praziquantel 25 mg/kg po tid x 2 days | Triclabendazole* 10 mg/kg po x 2 doses over 12–24 hrs. | Same dose in children |
| **Schistosoma sp.** | • Travelers and temporary residents lightly infected with no chronic disease.<br>  ○ Light infection detected by serology; eggs not usually present in stool or urine.<br>  ○ Uncommon CNS involvement including spinal cord.<br>  ○ Almost all travel related cases are from Africa. | | |
| **Schistosoma haematobium; GU bilhariziasis** | Praziquantel 40 mg/kg po on the same day (one dose of 40 mg/kg or two doses of 20 mg/kg) | | Same dose in children, (this applies to all schisto species) Some clinicians use 60 mg/kg praziquantel for all species for travelers and temporary residents not expecting re-exposure. |
| Schistosoma intercalatum | Praziquantel 20 mg/kg po on the same day in 1 or 2 doses | | Same dose in children. |
| **Schistosoma japonicum; Oriental schisto.** | Praziquantel 60 mg/kg po on the same day (3 doses of 20 mg/kg). | | Same dose in children. Cures 60–90% pts. |

* For source of drug, see Table 13D, page 177.

## TABLE 13A (12)

| INFECTING ORGANISM | SUGGESTED REGIMENS | | COMMENTS |
|---|---|---|---|
| | PRIMARY | ALTERNATIVE | |

**TREMATODES (Flukes)** (continued)

| INFECTING ORGANISM | PRIMARY | ALTERNATIVE | COMMENTS |
|---|---|---|---|
| Schistosoma mansoni (intestinal bilharziasis) | Praziquantel 40 mg/kg po on the same day in (one dose of 40 mg/kg or two doses of 20 mg/kg) | | Praziquantel: Same dose for children and adults. Cures 60–90% pts. No advantage to splitting dose in 2 Cochrane Database Syst Rev, 8:CD000053, 2014. |
| Schistosoma mekongi | Praziquantel 60 mg per kg po on the same day (3 doses of 20 mg/kg) | | Same dose for children |
| Toxic schisto; Katayama fever | Praziquantel 20 mg per kg po bid with short course of high dose prednisone. Repeat Praziquantel in 4–6 wks (Clin Micro Rev 16:225, 2010). | | Reaction to onset of egg laying 4–6 wks after infection exposure in fresh water. |

**CESTODES (Tapeworms)**

| INFECTING ORGANISM | PRIMARY | ALTERNATIVE | COMMENTS |
|---|---|---|---|
| Echinococcus granulosus (hydatid disease) (LnID 12:871, 2012; BMC Infect Dis 2018; 18:306). Dead or calcified cysts as determined by experienced radiologist require no therapy. | Liver cysts: Meta-analysis supports percutaneous aspiration-injection-reaspiration (PAIR) + albendazole for uncomplicated single liver cysts. Before & after drainage: **albendazole** ≥60 kg, 400 mg po bid or <60 kg, 15 mg/kg per day div, bid, (with meals). After 1-2 days puncture (P) & needle aspirate (A) cyst content. Instill (I) hypertonic saline (15–30%) or absolute alcohol, wait 20–30 min, then re-aspirate (R) with final irrigation. **Continue albendazole for at least 30 days.** Cure in 96% as comp to 90% pts with surgical resection. Albendazole ref: Acta Tropica 114:1, 2010. Complicated or multi vesicular cysts almost always require surgical intervention. Consider watch and wait for asymptomatic or non-compromising cysts | | Niclosamide from Expert Compounding Pharm, see Table 13D. |
| Lung cysts | Surgical resection. Avoid pre-operative Albendazole. May give Albendazole 400 mg po bid x at least 28 days post-operatively. Ruptured or complicated cysts may require longer therapy. **Note:** Brain, cardiac, splenic, renal, bone locations uncommonly occur requiring surgical intervention. Metastatic spread into body cavities with spontaneous or iatrogenic (during surgery) cyst rupture require Albendazole 400 mg po bid indefinitely until clinical response with periodic surgical debulking if feasible. | | |
| Echinococcus multilocularis (alveolar cyst disease) (CID 16:437, 2003) | **Albendazole** efficacy not clearly demonstrated, can try in dosages used for hydatid disease. Wide surgical resection only reliable rx; technique evolving. Post-surgical resection or if inoperable: Albendazole for several years (Acta Tropic 114:1, 2010). | | |

**Intestinal tapeworms**

| INFECTING ORGANISM | PRIMARY | ALTERNATIVE | COMMENTS |
|---|---|---|---|
| Diphyllobothrium latum (fish), Dipylidium caninum (dog), Taenia saginata (beef), & Taenia solium (pork). | Praziquantel 5–10 mg/kg po x 1 dose for children and adults. | Niclosamide* 2 gm po x 1 dose | |
| Hymenolepis diminuta (rats) and nana (humans) | Praziquantel 25 mg/kg po x 1 dose for children and adults. | Niclosamide* 2 gm po daily x 7 days | |

**New cysticercosis (NCC)**
New review, Curr Opin Infect Dis. 2018; 31:377
Larval form of T. solium
IDSA treatment guidelines.
CID 2018;66:1759

| INFECTING ORGANISM | PRIMARY | ALTERNATIVE | COMMENTS |
|---|---|---|---|
| | **NOTE: Treat concomitant T. solium intestinal tapeworms,** if present, with **praziquantel** 5–10 mg/kg po x 1 dose after starting steroid. Both CT and MRI should be performed. Immunoblot preferred; ELISA lacks specificity. Serology insensitive for single lesions, calcified lesions. For multiple parenchymal lesions, subarachnoid NCC, intraventricular NCC, serology almost 100% sensitive; CSF testing no advantage over serum testing. Parenchymal scolex on imaging is diagnostic, serology not necessary. In non-endemic areas, check stools of household contacts of confirmed cases for tapeworm eggs. | | |

| INFECTING ORGANISM | PRIMARY | ALTERNATIVE | COMMENTS |
|---|---|---|---|
| Parenchymal NCC 1–20 "Viable" or degenerating cysts by CT/MRI. Meta-analysis: Treatment assoc with cyst resolution, ↓ seizures, and ↓ seizure recurrence. | Albendazole 15 mg/kg/d (max 800 mg/d) + Praziquantel 50 mg/kg/d po + Dexamethasone 0.1 mg/kg po. Start steroid 1 day before antiparasitics. Treat for 10 days. Continue seizure meds for 1 yr. Slow steroid taper after 10 days increasing back if seizures develop. Albendazole alone adequate if only 1-2 cysts on an MRI. | Albendazole alone 800 mg/day plus Dexamethasone 0.1 mg/kg per day x Anti-seizure medication). See Comment. Limited data indicates that increasing dexamethasone to 8 mg/day X 28 days with 2-week taper decreases seizures but prolongs steroid exposure. Epilepsia 55:1452, 2014 | Retreat after 6 months if any viable cysts remain. Methotrexate at ≤20 mg/wk allows a reduction in steroid use (CID 44:449, 2007). Some recommend longer courses of albendazole (even >30 days) if large number of parenchymal cysts(erci). |
| Dead calcified cysts | No treatment indicated | | |

* For source of drug, see Table 13D, page 177.

**TABLE 13A (13)**

| INFECTING ORGANISM | SUGGESTED REGIMENS | | COMMENTS |
|---|---|---|---|
| | PRIMARY | ALTERNATIVE | |

**CESTODES (Tapeworms)/Neurocysticercosis** (continued)

| INFECTING ORGANISM | PRIMARY | ALTERNATIVE | COMMENTS |
|---|---|---|---|
| **Subarachnoid NCC** | Albendazole 15 mg/kg per day (max. 1200 mg/day) + Dexamethasone (doses as above with very slow taper) + v-p shunt prior to therapy. 30 day course, may need to repeat multiple times or give continuously for months according to clinical and MRI evolution (Expert Rev Inf Ther 9:123, 2011); continue until radiologic resolution. Intracranial pressure must be monitored and managed by an experienced clinician. If diffuse cerebral edema or raised ICP, control with steroids or shunting prior to anti-parasitic therapy. | Long courses of combination therapy with Albendazole/praziquantel combination therapy for refractory disease. | |
| **Intraventricular NCC** | Neuroendoscopic removal is treatment of choice with or without obstruction. If surgery not possible, **Albendazole + Dexamethasone; observe closely for evidence of obstruction of flow of CSF.** | **Albendazole + Dexamethasone** (as above); place v-p shunt prior to therapy when no access to neuroendoscopy. | |
| Sparganosis (Spirometra mansonoides) Larval cysts; source—frogs/snakes | Surgical resection. No antiparasitic therapy. Can inject alcohol into subcutaneous masses. | | |

**ECTOPARASITES.** Ref: CID 36:1355, 2003; Ln 363-889, 2004. **NOTE: Due to potential neurotoxicity and risk of aplastic anemia, lindane not recommended.**

| DISEASE | INFECTING ORGANISM | PRIMARY | ALTERNATIVE | COMMENTS |
|---|---|---|---|---|
| **Head lice** Med Lett 54:61, 2012. | Pediculus humanus, var. capitis. Re-treatment often necessary as current drugs do not kill eggs. | **Permethrin** 1% lotion: Apply to shampooed dried hair for 10 min, repeat in 9-10 days. **OR Malathion** 0.5% lotion (Ovide): Apply to dry hair for 8-12 hrs, then shampoo. 2 doses 7-9 days apart. **OR Spinosad** 0.9% suspension; wash off after 10 min (85% effective). Repeat in 7 days, if needed. Use nit comb initially & repeat in 7-10 days. | **Ivermectin** 200-400 µg/kg po once; 3 doses at 7 day intervals effective in 95% (JID 193:474, 2006). Topical ivermectin 0.5% lotion, 75% effective. **Malathion:** Report that 1-2 20-min. applications 98% effective (Ped Derm 21:670, 2004). In alcohol—potentially flammable. **Benzyl alcohol:** 76% effective. | **Permethrin** success in 78%. Resistance increasing. No advantage to 5% permethrin. **Spinosad** is effective, but expensive. Wash hats, scarves, coats & bedding in hot water, then dry in hot dryer for 20+ minutes. |
| **Pubic lice (crabs)** | Phthirus pubis | **Pubic hair: Permethrin OR Malathion** as for head lice. Shave pubic hair. | **Eyelids:** Petroleum jelly applied qid x 10 days OR **yellow oxide of mercury** 1% qid x 14 days | **Do not use lindane.** Treat sex partners of the last 30 days. |
| **Body lice** | Pediculus humanus, var. corporis | No drugs for the patient. Organism lives in & deposits eggs in seams of clothing. Discard clothing; if not possible, treat clothing with 1% malathion powder or 0.5% permethrin powder. Success with ivermectin in homeless shelter. 12 mg po on days 0, 7, & 14 (JID 193:474, 2006) | | |
| **Myiasis** Due to larvae of flies | | Usually cutaneous/subcutaneous nodule with central punctum. Treatment: Occlude punctum to prevent gas exchange with petrolatum, fingernail polish, makeup cream or bacon. When larva migrates, manually remove. Ref: Clin Microbiol Rev 25:79, 2012. | | |
| **Scabies** **Immunocompetent patients** Refs: MMWR 64(RR-3):1, 2015; NEJM 362:717, 2010. | Sarcoptes scabiei | **Permethrin** 5% cream (ELIMITE) under nails (finger and toe). Apply entire skin from chin down to and including under fingernails and toenails. Leave on 8-14 hrs. Repeat in 1-2 wks. Safe for children age ≥2 mos. | **Ivermectin** 200 µg/kg po with food x 1, then second dose in 2 wks. **Less effective: Crotamiton** 10% cream, apply x 24 hr, rinse off, then reapply x 24 hr. | Trim fingernails. Reapply cream to hands after handwashing. Treat close contacts; wash and heat dry linens. Pruritus may persist times 2 wks after mites gone. |
| **AIDS and HTLV-infected patients** (>104 or >150 per mm³), debilitated or developmentally disabled patients **(Norwegian scabies—see Comments)** | | For Norwegian crusted scabies: **Permethrin** 5% cream daily x 7 days, then twice weekly until cured. Add **ivermectin** po (dose in Alternative) | **Ivermectin** 200 mcg/kg po on days 1, 2, 8, 9 & 15+ daily x 7 days. May need addt'l doses of ivermectin on days 22 & 29. | **Norwegian scabies** in AIDS: Extensive, crusted. Can mimic psoriasis. Not pruritic. Highly contagious—Isolate! |

---

* For source of drug, see Table 13D, page 177.

## TABLE 13B - DOSAGE AND SELECTED ADVERSE EFFECTS OF ANTIPARASITIC DRUGS

Doses vary with indication. For convenience, drugs divided by type of parasite; some drugs used for multiple types of parasites, e.g., albendazole.

| CLASS, AGENT, GENERIC NAME (TRADE NAME) | USUAL ADULT DOSAGE | ADVERSE REACTIONS/COMMENTS |
|---|---|---|
| **Antiprotozoan Drugs** | | |
| *Intestinal Parasites* | | |
| Diloxanide furoate[NUS] (Furamide) | 500 mg po tid x 10 days | Source: *See Table 13D, page 177.* Flatulence, N/V, diarrhea. |
| Iodoquinol (Yodoxin) | Adults: 650 mg po tid or 30-40 mg/kg/day div. tid); children; 40 mg/kg per day div. tid. | Rarely causes nausea, abdominal cramps, rash, acne. **Contraindicated if iodine intolerance** (contains 64% bound iodine). Can cause iododerma (papular or pustular rash) and/or thyroid enlargement. |
| Metronidazole | Side-effects similar for all. *See metronidazole in Table 10B, page 126, & Table 10A, page 123* | Abdominal pain 7.8%, diarrhea 2.1%. Rev.: *CID 40:1173, 2005; Expert Opin Pharmacother 7:953, 2006.* |
| Nitazoxanide (Alinia) | Adults: 500 mg po q12h. Children 4-11: 200 mg susp. po q12h. Take with food. Expensive. | Headaches; rarely yellow sclera (resolves after treatment). |
| Paromomycin (Humatin) | 15-35 mg/kg/day po in 3 divided doses x 5-10 days (250 mg tabs). Source: *See Table 13D.* | **Aminoglycoside similar to neomycin**; if absorbed due to concomitant inflammatory bowel disease can result in oto/nephrotoxicity. Doses >3 gm daily are associated with nausea, abdominal cramps, diarrhea. |
| Quinacrine | 100 mg po tid x 5 days. *www.expertpharmacy.com* | **Contraindicated for pts with history of psychosis or psoriasis. Yellow staining of skin.** Dizziness, headache, vomiting, toxic psychosis (1.5%), hemolytic anemia, leukopenia, thrombocytopenia, urticaria, rash, fever, minor disulfiram-like reactions. |
| Tinidazole (Tindamax) | 250-500 mg tabs, with food. Regimen varies with indication. | Chemical structure similar to metronidazole but better tolerated. Seizures/peripheral neuropathy reported. **Adverse effects:** Metallic taste 4-6%, nausea 3-5%, anorexia 2-3%. |
| **Antiprotozoan Drugs: Non-Intestinal Protozoa** | | |
| *Extraintestinal Parasites* | | |
| Antimony compounds[NUS] Stibogluconate sodium (Pentostam) from CDC or Meglumine antimoniate (Glucantim)—French trade name | For IV use: vials with 100 mg antimony/mL. Dilute selected dose in 50 mL of D5W shortly before use. Infuse over at least 10 minutes. Intralesional injection used in many countries: 20 mg/kg qwk X 5-10 weeks. | **AEs in 1st day:** headache, fatigue, elevated lipase/amylase, clinical pancreatitis. After 10 days: elevated AST/ALT/ALK/PHOS, CBC, biochemistry weekly, EKG q2 weeks if prolonged therapy. **NOTE:** Reversible T wave changes in 30-60%. Risk of QTc prolongation. Renal excretion; modify dose if renal insufficiency. Metabolized in liver; lower dose if hepatic insufficiency. Generic drug may have increased toxicity due to antimony complex formation. |
| Artemether-Lumefantrine, po (Coartem), FDA-approved) | 4 (20 mg Artemether and 120 mg Lumefantrine) combination tabs X 6 doses over 3 days for adults. Take with food. Can be crushed and mixed with a few teaspoons of water | **Can prolong QTc**; avoid in patients with congenital long QTc, family history of sudden death or long QTc, or need for drugs known to prolong QTc *(see list under fluoroquinolones, Table 10A, page 120).* Artemether induces CYP3A4 and both Artemether & Lumefantrine are metabolized by CYP3A4 *(see drug interactions, Table 22A, page 256).* Adverse effects experienced in >30% of adults: headache, anorexia, dizziness, arthralgia and myalgia. Non-life threatening, but transfusion requiring, hemolytic anemia can occur up to 15 days post-therapy *(AnIM 163:498, 2015).* |
| Artesunate, IV Ref: NEJM 358:1829, 2008 | Available from CDC Malaria Branch. 2.4 mg/kg IV at 0, 12, 24, & 48 hrs | **More effective than quinine & safer than quinidine.** Contact CDC at 770-488-7758 or 770-488-7100 after hours. No dosage adjustment for hepatic or renal insufficiency. No known drug interactions. |
| Atovaquone (Mepron) Ref: AAC 46:1163, 2002 | Suspension: 1 tsp (750 mg) po bid 750 mg/5 mL | No. pts stopping rx due to side-effects was 9%; rash 22%, GI 20%, headache 16%, insomnia 10%, fever 14% |
| Atovaquone and Proguanil (Malarone) For prophylaxis of P. falciparum; little data on P. vivax. Generic available in US. | Prophylaxis: 1 tab po (250 mg + 100 mg) q24h with food Treatment: 4 tabs po (1000 mg + 400 mg) once daily with food x 3 days. Adult tab: 250/100 mg. Peds tab 62.5/25 mg. *Treatment see comment, page 164.* | Adverse effects in rx trials: Adults—abd. pain 17%, N/V 12%, headache 10%, dizziness 5%, Rx stopped in 1%. Asymptomatic mild ↑ in ALT/AST. Children—cough, headache, anorexia, vomiting, abd. pain. *See drug interactions, Table 22A.* Safe in G6PD-deficient pts. Can crush tabs for children and give with milk or other liquid nutrients. Renal insufficiency: contraindicated if CrCl <30 mL per min. |

173

---

* For source of drug, see *Table 13D, page 177.*

**TABLE 13B (2)**

| CLASS, AGENT, GENERIC NAME (TRADE NAME) | USUAL ADULT DOSAGE | ADVERSE REACTIONS/COMMENTS |
|---|---|---|
| **Antiprotozoan Drugs: Non-Intestinal Protozoa/Extraintestinal Parasites** *(continued)* | | |
| **Benznidazole\*** Benznidazole 12.5 & 100 mg approved tabs for 2-12 yr olds. CDC advocates off-label use in adults *(www.benznidazoletablets.com)* | 5 mg/kg per day po. 100 mg tabs. May use 300 mg per day for 60 days, regardless of body weight; OR give 300 mg per day but prolong treatment to complete the total dose corresponding to 5 mg/kg per day for 60 days. | **Photosensitivity in 50% of pts.** GI: abdominal pain, nausea/vomiting/anorexia. Dermatitis including Stevens-Johnson. CNS: disorientation, insomnia, twitching/seizures, paresthesias, polyneuritis. Discontinue if leucopenia or thrombocytopenia. **Contraindicated in pregnancy.** Recommended dose range 5-7.5 mg/kg/day but more than 5 mg/kg has unacceptable side effects in adults, higher doses better tolerated in children. |
| **Chloroquine phosphate (Aralen)** | Dose varies—see *Malaria Prophylaxis and rx, pages 163-163.* | Minor: anorexia/nausea/vomiting, headache, dizziness, blurred vision, pruritus in dark-skinned pts. Major: protracted rx in rheumatoid arthritis can lead to retinopathy, psoriasis. Can exacerbate psoriasis. Can block response to intradermally administered rabies vaccine. **Contraindicated in pts with epilepsy.** |
| **Dapsone** *See Comment re methemoglobinemia* | 100 mg po q24h | Usually tolerated by pts with rash after TMP-SMX. **Dapsone is common etiology of acquired methemoglobinemia** *(WER 64:1964-967, 2011).* Metabolite of dapsone converts some iron to + 3 charge (no O2 transport) from normal +2. Normal blood level 1%; cyanosis at 10%; headache, fatigue, tachycardia, dizziness at 30-40%; acidosis & coma at 60%; death at 70-80%. Low G6PD is a risk factor. Treatment: methylene blue 1-2 mg/kg IV over 5 min x 1 dose. |
| **Eflornithine (Ornidyl)** (WHO or CDC drug service) | 400 mg/kg/day IV divided q12h x 7 days in combination with Nifurtimox for West African Trypanosomiasis | Diarrhea in ⅓ pts, vomiting, abdominal pain, anemia/leukopenia in ½ pts, seizures, alopecia, jaundice, ↓ hearing. Contraindicated in pregnancy. |
| **Fumagillin** | Eyedrops + po. 20 mg po tid. Leiter's: 800-292-6772. | Adverse events: Neutropenia & thrombocytopenia |
| **Mefloquine** | One 250 mg tab/wk for malaria prophylaxis; for rx, 1250 mg x 1 or 750 mg & then 500 mg in 6-8 hrs. In U.S.: 250 mg tab = 228 mg base; outside U.S.: 275 mg tab = 250 mg base | Side-effects in roughly 3%. Minor: headache, irritability, insomnia, weakness, diarrhea. **Toxic psychosis, seizures can occur.** Do not use with quinine, quinidine, or halofantrine. Rare! Prolonged QT interval and toxic epidermal necrolysis *(Ln 349:101, 1997)*. **Not used for self-rx due to neuropsychiatric side-effects.** FDA black box for possible prolonged side-effects. Avoid if pre-existing overlay of depression or other psychiatric disorders. |
| **Melarsoprol (Mel B, Arsobal) (CDC)** | 2.2 mg/kg/day IV x 10 days | Post-rx encephalopathy (2-10%) with 50% mortality overall, risk of death 2° to rx 8-14%. Prednisolone 1 mg per kg per day po may ↓ encephalopathy. Other: Heart damage, albuminuria, abdominal pain, vomiting, peripheral neuropathy, Herxheimer-like reaction, pruritus. ○ Prednisone may prevent/attenuate encephalopathy. ○ Pretreatment with Suramin (dose as above) is often used in late-stage East African trypanosomiasis to clear the hemolymphatic system of trypanosomes before administration of melarsoprol. |
| **Miltefosine (Impavido)** No longer available from CDC, purchase from www.impavido.com | 50 mg po bid (wt 33-44 kg); 50 mg po tid (wt ≥45 kg) (max 150 mg/d). Treat for 28 days | **Pregnancy—No:** teratogenic. Side-effects vary: kala-azar pts, vomiting in up to 40%, diarrhea in 17%, motion sickness†, headache & increased creatinine. Metabolized by liver; virtually no urinary excretion. |
| **Nifurtimox (Lampit) (CDC)** (Manufactured in Germany by Bayer) | 8-10 mg/kg per day po div. 4 x per day for 90-120 days for Chaga's. 15 mg/kg po, divided q8h x 10 days for West African trypanosomiasis | Side-effects in 40-70% of pts. GI: abdominal pain, nausea/vomiting. CNS: polyneuritis (1/3), disorientation, insomnia, twitching, seizures. Skin rash. Hemolysis with G6PD deficiency. Monitor CBC, biochemistry after 4-6 weeks. Monitor frequently for neuropathy. Ref: *CID 2015;63:1056.* |
| **Pentamidine** | 4 mg/kg IV or IM daily x 7-10 days for African Trypanosomiasis. 300 mg via aerosol q month. | Hypotension, hypocalcemia, hypoglycemia followed by hyperglycemia, pancreatitis. Neutropenia (15%), thrombocytopenia. Nephrotoxicity. Others: nausea/vomiting, ↑ liver tests, rash. |
| **Primaquine phosphate** | 26.3 mg (=15 mg base). Adult dose is 30 mg of base po daily. | **In G6PD def. pts, can cause hemolytic anemia with hemoglobinuria, esp. African, Asian peoples.** Methemoglobinemia. Rapid G6PD screening tests now readily available. Nausea/abdominal pain if pt. fasting. *(CID 39:1336, 2004).* **Pregnancy: No.** |

\* For source of drug, see *Table 13D, page 177.*

**TABLE 13B (3)**

| CLASS, AGENT, GENERIC NAME (TRADE NAME) | USUAL ADULT DOSAGE | ADVERSE REACTIONS/COMMENTS |
|---|---|---|
| **Antiprotozoan Drugs: Non-Intestinal Protozoa/Extraintestinal Parasites** (continued) | | |
| **Pyrimethamine** (Daraprim, Malocide). Also combined with Sulfadoxine as **Fansidar** (25–500 mg) | 100 mg, then 25 mg/day. **Very expensive:** $75,000 for 100 tabs (25 mg). Financial assistance may be available by calling 1-877-258-8033. Consider compounding pharmacy (imprimusrx.com). | **Major problem is hematologic:** megaloblastic anemia, ↓ WBC, ↓ platelets. Can give 5 mg folinic acid per day to ↓ bone marrow depression and not interfere with antitoxoplasmosis effect. If high-dose pyrimethamine, ↑ folinic acid to 10–50 mg/day. Pyrimethamine + sulfadoxine can cause mental changes due to carnitine deficiency (AJM 95:112, 1993). Other: Rash, vomiting, diarrhea, xerostomia. |
| **Quinidine gluconate** Cardiotoxicity ref: LnID 7:549, 2007 | Loading dose of 10 mg (equiv to 6.2 mg of quinidine base)/kg IV over 1–2 hr, then constant infusion of 0.02 mg of quinidine gluconate / kg per minute. May be available for compassionate use from Lilly. | **Adverse reactions of quinidine/quinine similar:** (1) IV bolus injection can cause fatal hypotension, (2) hyperinsulinemic hypoglycemia, esp. in pregnancy, (3) ↑ rate of infusion of IV quinidine if QT interval ↑ 25% of baseline, (4) reduce dose 30–50% after day 3 due to ↓ renal clearance and ↓ vol. of distribution. |
| **Quinine sulfate** (Qualaquin) | 324 mg tabs. No IV prep. in US. Oral rx of chloroquine-resistant falciparum malaria. 624 mg po tid x 3 days, then (tetracycline 250 mg po qid or doxy 100 mg bid) x 7 days | Cinchonism; tinnitus, headache, nausea, abdominal pain, blurred vision. Rarely, blood dyscrasias, drug fever, asthma, hypoglycemia. Transient blindness in <1% of 500 pts (AnIM 136:339, 2002). **Contraindicated if prolonged QTc, myasthenia gravis, optic neuritis or G6PD deficiency.** |
| **Spiramycin** (Rovamycine) | 1 gm po q8h (see Comment). | GI and allergic reactions have occurred. Available at no cost after consultation with Palo Alto Medical Foundation Toxoplasma Serology Lab: 650-853-4828 or from U.S. FDA 301-796-1600. |
| **Sulfadiazine** | 1–1.5 gm po q6h. | See Table 10A, page 123, for sulfonamide side-effects. |
| **Sulfadoxine & Pyrimethamine combination (Fansidar)** | Contains 500 mg Sulfadoxine & 25 mg Pyrimethamine | Long half-life of both drugs: Sulfadoxine 169 hrs, pyrimethamine 111 hrs allows weekly dosage. In African, used empirically as intermittent preventative treatment (ITPp) against malaria: dosing at 3 set times during pregnancy. Reduces material and fetal mortality if HIV+. See Expert Rev Anti Infect Ther 8:589, 2010. **Fatalities reported due to Stevens-Johnson syndrome and toxic epidermal necrolysis.** |
| **DRUGS USED TO TREAT NEMATODES, TREMATODES, AND CESTODES** | | |
| **Tafenoquine** (Arakoda, Krintafel) (for P. vivax malaria, age ≥ 16 yrs, ≥ 18 yrs for prophylaxis) Arakoda: 100 mg tab Krintafel: 150 mg tab | Radical cure (prevention of relapse): 300 mg singl dose on day 1 or 2 of appropriate blood-stage therapy. Prophylaxis: 200 mg x 3 days (starting 3 days before travel), then 200 mg qwk maintenance starting 7 days after last loading dose, then after leaving endemic area, 200 mg once, 7 days after last maintenance dose | Test for G6PD deficiency before use. **Must have TQ normal G6PD activity on quantitative testing to use TQ:** do not use screening tests or qualitative tests. AEs: hemolytic anemia (G6PD deficiency), methemoglobinemia, psychiatric effects only if previous psychosis, hypersensitivity. Renal excretion—caution if renal impairment. |
| **Albendazole** (Albenza) | Doses vary with indication. Take with food; fatty meal increases absorption. See Table 13D for US availability | FDA Pregnancy Category C due to lack of data but available evidence suggests: no difference in congenital abnormalities. WHO allows use of albendazole in 2nd and 3rd trimesters. CDC suggests consideration in 3rd trimester if infection is compromising the pregnancy. Abdominal pain (with prolonged courses), nausea/vomiting, alopecia, ↑ serum transaminase. Rare leukopenia. |
| **Diethylcarbamazine** (CDC) | Dose varies with species of filaria. | Headache, dizziness, nausea, fever. In Onchocerciasis, host may experience inflammatory reaction to death of microfilariae: Fever, urticaria, asthma, GI upset **(Mazzotti reaction). Pregnancy—No.** |
| **Ivermectin** (Stromectol, Mectizan) (3 mg tab & topical 0.5% lotion for head lice). Take on empty stomach. | Strongyloidiasis dose: 200 µg/kg/day po x 2 days Onchocerciasis: 150 µg/kg x 1 po Scabies: 200 µg/kg po x 1; if AIDS, wait 14 days & repeat | Mild side-effects: Fever, pruritus, rash. In rx of onchocerciasis, can see tender lymphadenopathy, headache, limb/joint pain. |
| **Mebendazole** (Vermox) | In developing world chewable tablet, 500 mg po once in public health campaigns. 100 mg po twice/day for 3 days is optimal for most intestinal nematodes. 100 mg single dose adequate for pinworm. See Table 13D for US availability | Rarely causes abdominal pain, nausea, diarrhea. FDA Pregnancy Category C due to lack of data but available evidence suggests: no difference in congenital abnormalities. WHO allows use of mebendazole in 2nd and 3rd trimesters. CDC suggests consideration in 3rd trimester if infection is compromising the pregnancy. |

\* For source of drug, see Table 13D, page 177.

**TABLE 13B (4)**

| CLASS, AGENT, GENERIC NAME (TRADE NAME) | USUAL ADULT DOSAGE | ADVERSE REACTIONS/COMMENTS |
|---|---|---|
| **DRUGS USED TO TREAT NEMATODES, TREMATODES, AND CESTODES** *(continued)* | | |
| Praziquantel (Biltricide) | Doses vary with parasite; see *Table 13A.* | Mild: dizziness/drowsiness; N/V, rash, fever. **Only contraindication is ocular cysticercosis.** Potential exacerbation of neurocysticercosis. Metab-induced by anticonvulsants and steroids; can negate effect with cimetidine 400 mg po tid. Reduce dose if advanced liver disease. Praziquantel is pregnancy category B. Available evidence suggests no difference in adverse birth outcomes. WHO encourages the use of praziquantel in any stage of pregnancy. CDC advises individual risk-benefit assessment according to clinical disease in the mother. |
| Pyrantel pamoate (over-the-counter) | Oral suspension. Dose for all ages: 11 mg/kg (to max. of 1 gm) x 1 dose | Rare GI upset, headache, dizziness, rash |
| Suramin (Germanin) *(CDC)* | Drug powder mixed to 10% solution with 5 mL water and used within 30 min. First give test dose of 0.1 gm IV. Try to avoid during pregnancy. | Does not cross blood-brain barrier; no effect on CNS infection. Side-effects: vomiting, pruritus, urticaria, fever, paresthesias, albuminuria (discontinue drug if casts appear). Do not use if renal/liver disease present. Deaths from vascular collapse reported. |
| Triclabendazole (Egaten) *(CDC)* | Used for fasciola hepatica liver fluke infection: 10 mg/kg po x 1 dose. May repeat in 12-24 hrs. 250 mg tabs | AEs ≥10%: sweating and abdominal pain. AEs 1-10%: weakness, chest pain, fever, anorexia, nausea, vomiting. **Note: use with caution if G6PD def. or impaired liver function.** |

**TABLE 13C - PARASITES THAT CAUSE EOSINOPHILIA (EOSINOPHILIA IN TRAVELERS)**

| Frequent and Intense (>5000 eos/mcL) | Moderate to Marked Early Infections | During Larval Migration; Absent or Mild During Chronic Infections | Other |
|---|---|---|---|
| Strongyloides (absent in comprimised hosts); Lymphatic Filariasis; Toxocara (cutaneous larva migrans); Trichinella | Ascaris; Hookworm; Clonorchis; Paragonimus; Fasciola | Opisthorchis; Baylisascaris | Schistosomiasis; Cysticercosis; Trichuris; Angiostrongylus; Onchocerciasis; echinococcus | Non-lymphatic filariasis; Gnathostoma; Capillaria; Trichostrongylus |

* For source of drug, see *Table 13D, page 177.*

## TABLE 13D – SOURCES FOR HARD-TO-FIND ANTIPARASITIC DRUGS

| Source | Drugs Available | Contact Information |
|---|---|---|
| **CDC Drug Service** | Artesunate, Diethylcarbamazine (DEC), Eflornithine, Melarsoprol, Nifurtimox, Sodium stibogluconate, Suramin, Triclabendazole | www.cdc.gov/laboratory/drugservice/index.html (+1) 404-639-3670 or drugservice@cdc.gov |
| **WHO** | Drugs for treatment of African trypanosomiasis | priottog@who.int; (+41) 794-682-726; (+41) 227-911-345 francoi@who.int; (+41) 796-198-535; (+41) 227-913-313 |
| **Compounding Pharmacies, Specialty Distributors, Others** | | |
| Expert Compounding Pharmacy | Albendazole, Furazolidone, Iodoquinol, Mebendazole (100 mg tabs), Niclosamide, Paromomycin (oral), Praziquantel, Pyrantel pamoate, Quinacrine, Thiabendazole, Tinidazole | www.expertpharmacy.org 1-800-247-9767; (+1) 818-988-7979 |
| Exeltis, Inc. / Benznidazole | Commercial FDA approved tab for child age 2-12 yrs, may use off-label in adults (www.benznidazoletablets.com) | +1 800-964-9650 |
| Leiter's Pharmacy | Fumagillin | www.leiterrx.com 1-800-292-6772; +1-408-292-6772 |
| Profounda, Inc. | Miltefosine (leishmaniasis or free-living ameba) | www.impavido.com; +1 407-270-7790 |
| Victoria Apotheke Zurich will ship worldwide if sent physicians prescription. | Paromomycin (oral and topical), Triclabendazole. Other hard to find anti-parasitic drugs | www.pharmaworld.com (+41) 43-344-6060 |
| Palo Alto Medical Foundation, Toxoplasma Serology Lab | Spiramycin (consultation required for release) | (+1) 650-853-4828; toxlab@pamf.org |
| Imprimis (compounding pharmacy) | Pyrimethamine | +1 844-446-6979; www.imprimisrx.com |

Note: In the U.S. FDA-approved generic Albendazole (Albenza) or FDA-approved generic Mebendazole marketed by Amedra is very costly and is difficult for retail pharmacies to access. Vermox brand mebendazole 500 mg tablets is FDA-approved but for donation only and not sold in the U.S.

**TABLE 14A – ANTIVIRAL THERAPY[a]**

For HIV, see Table 14C, for Hepatitis, see Table 14C and Table 14E and Table 14F. For Antiviral Activity Spectra, see Table 4C, page 87

| VIRUS/DISEASE | DRUG/DOSAGE | SIDE EFFECTS/COMMENTS |
|---|---|---|
| **Adenovirus:** Cause of RTIs including fatal pneumonia in children & young adults and 60% mortality in transplant pts (*CID 43:331, 2006*). Frequent cause of cystitis in transplant patients. Adenovirus 14 associated with severe pneumonia in otherwise healthy young adults (*MMWR 56(45):1181, 2007*). **Findings include:** Fever, ↑ liver enzymes, leukopenia, thrombocytopenia, diarrhea, pneumonia, or hemorrhagic cystitis. Ref: *Infect Dis Clin N Amer 2017:21:455.* | In severe cases of pneumonia or post HSCT: **Cidofovir**<br>• 5 mg/kg/wk × 2 wks, then q 2 wks + **Probenecid** 1.25 gm/M² given 3 hrs before cidofovir and 3 & 9 hrs after each infusion.<br>• Or 1 mg/kg IV 3x/wk.<br>For adenovirus cystitis (*CID 40:199, 2005; Transplantation 2006; 81:1398*): Intravesical **Cidofovir** (5 mg/kg in 100 mL saline instilled into bladder). | Routine monitoring with HAdV viral load recommended 1-2 times/wk in high-risk patients; Allo-HSCT with haploidentical donor or unrelated cord blood graft; Severe GVHD; Severe lymphopenia; and/or Rx with alemtuzumab. Monitoring should continue until immune reconstitution. Those with at least 1 risk factor and viremia should be Rx'd with cidofovir.<br>Ribavirin not recommended. Vidarabine and Ganciclovir have in vitro activity against adenovirus; little to no clinical data. **Brincidofovir** (CMX001-Chimerix) oral lipid complex cidofovir prodrug shows no evidence of efficacy in Phase III study. Donor specific T-cells should be reserved for those who have failed antiviral therapy and administered as part of a clinical trial. |
| **Bunyaviridae:** Severe fever with thrombocytopenia syndrome virus (SFTSV)<br>Possibly transmitted by *Haemaphysalis longicornis* and *Amblyomma americanum* (lone star) ticks. | No rx recommended. Ribavirin ineffective. Clinical symptoms: Fever, weakness, myalgias, GI symptoms | Lab: Elevated LDH (>1200) and CPK (>800) associated with higher mortality rates. Initially thought to be an anaplasma infection, but serology showed a new virus. |
| **Coronavirus–**<br>**SARS-CoV:** Severe acute respiratory syndrome (*NEJM 348:1953 & 1967, 2003*)<br>**MERS-CoV:** Middle East respiratory syndrome (*NEJM 2017;376:584*) | **SARS:**<br>• Ribavirin—ineffective.<br>• Interferon alfa ± steroids—small case series.<br>• Pegylated IFN-α effective in monkeys.<br>• Low dose steroids alone successful in one Beijing hospital. High dose steroids ? serious fungal infections.<br>• Inhaled nitric oxide improved oxygenation & improved chest x-ray (*CID 39:1531, 2004*).<br>**MERS:** Increased 14 day survival with **Ribavirin** po + **PEG-IFN** 180 mcg/kg sc x 2 wks (*LnID 14:1090, 2014*). Other therapies: *LnID 14:1136, 2014.* | **SARS: Transmission by close contact:** effective infection control practices (**mask changed frequently**), eye protection, gown, gloves) key to stopping transmission.<br>**MERS:** Suspected reservoirs are camels and perhaps other animals. Review: *Clin Micro Rev. 28:465, 2015.* Korean guidelines recommend IFN + lopinavir/ritonavir + ribavirin (though no clinical trials) (*Korean J Intern Med. 2018 Mar; 33(2): 233-246*). |
| **Enterovirus–Meningitis:** most common cause of aseptic meningitis.<br>Rapid CSF PCR test is accurate; reduces costs and hospital stay for infants (*Peds 120:489, 2007*) | **No rx currently recommended.** | No clinical benefit from Pleconaril. Up to 1/3rd of adults have neutrophilic pleocytosis in CSF. Reviewed (*J Clin Virology, 104, 56-60, 2018*). |
| **Hemorrhagic Fever Virus Infections:** Review: *LnID 6-203, 2006.* | | |
| **Congo-Crimean Hemorrhagic Fever (HF)**<br>Tick-borne; symptoms include N/V, fever, headache, myalgias, & stupor (1/3). Signs: *conjunctival injection, hepatomegaly, petechiae (1/3), Lab ↓ platelets, ↓ WBC,↑ ALT, AST, LDH & CPK (100%).* | RBV 30 mg/kg/day po loading dose, then 15 mg/kg q6h × 4 days, then 7.5 mg/kg q8h × 6 days (WHO recommendation) (*see Comment*). Reviewed *Antiviral Res 78:125, 2008.* | 3/3 healthcare workers in Pakistan had complete recovery (*Ln 346:472, 1995*) & 61/69 (89%) with confirmed CCHF rx with ribavirin survived in Iran (*CID 36:1613, 2003*). Shorter time of hospitalization among ribavirin treated pts (7.7 vs. 10.3 days), but no difference in mortality or transfusion needs in study done in Turkey (*J Infection 52: 207-215, 2006*). Suggested benefit from ribavirin & dexamethasone (281 pts) (*CID 57:1270, 2013*). |

[1] HSCT = Hematopoietic stem cell transplant

[a] See page 2 for abbreviations. *NOTE: All dosage recommendations are for adults (unless otherwise indicated) and assume normal renal function.*

**TABLE 14A (2)**

| VIRUS/DISEASE | DRUG/DOSAGE | SIDE EFFECTS/COMMENTS |
|---|---|---|
| **Hemorrhagic Fever Virus Infections** (continued) | | |
| **Ebola/Marburg HF (Central Africa)**<br>Largest ever documented outbreak of Ebola virus (EVD), West Africa, 2014. Diagnostic testing at U.S. CDC. Within a few days of symptom onset, diagnosis is most commonly made by antigen-capture enzyme linked immunosorbent assay (ELISA), IgM antibody ELISA, NAAT or viral culture.<br>Updated in: http://emergency.cdc.gov/han/<br>han02365.asp<br>See also: http://www.bt.cdc.gov/han/han02364.asp<br>Review: PLOS Neglect Trop Dis 2017<br>https://doi.org/10.1371/journal.pntd.0005700 | **No effective antiviral rx** (J Virol 77: 9733, 2003). Investigational antibody treatment "ZMapp" used as compassionate use in a few selected patients (Mapp Biopharma; http://mappbio.com/). ZMapp is a 3 monoclonal antibody preparation derived from mice exposed to small fragments of Ebola virus. Use of convalescent serum from pts who have recovered is approved for use in newly infected pts by NIH. (BMJ 349:g5539, 2014). GS-5734 (Gilead) active in animal models. BCX-4430 (Biocryst) is under evaluation by the NIH. | **Abrupt onset of symptoms typically 8–10 days after exposure (range 2–21 days).** Nonspecific fever, chills, myalgias, and malaise. Fever, anorexia, asthenia / weakness are the most common signs and symptoms. Patients may develop a diffuse erythematous maculopapular rash (days 5–7) (usually involving the face, neck, trunk, and arms) that can desquamate. EVD **can often be confused with** other more common infectious diseases such as malaria, typhoid fever, meningococcemia, and other bacterial infections (e.g., pneumonia). **Gastrointestinal symptoms:** severe watery diarrhea, nausea, vomiting and abdominal pain. **Other:** chest pain, shortness of breath, headache or confusion, may also develop. Patients often have conjunctival injection. Hiccups reported. Seizures may occur, and cerebral edema reported. Bleeding is not universally present but can manifest later in the course as petechiae, ecchymosis/bruising, or oozing from venipuncture sites and mucosal hemorrhage. Frank hemorrhage is less common. Pregnant women may experience spontaneous miscarriages. |
| **With pulmonary syndrome: Hantavirus pulmonary syndrome, "sin nombre virus"** | **No benefit from RBV demonstrated** (CID 39:1307, 2004). Early recognition of disease and supportive (usually ICU) care is key to successful outcome. | Acute onset of fever, headache, myalgias, non-productive cough, thrombocytopenia, increased PT and non-cardiogenic pulmonary edema with respiratory insufficiency following exposure to droppings of infected rodents. |
| **With renal syndrome:** Lassa, Venezuelan, Korean, HF, Sabia, Argentinian HF, Bolivian HF, Junin, Machupo (>90% occur in China CID 59:1040, 2014) | **RBV** 30 mg/kg/day no loading dose, then 15 mg/kg q6h x 4 days, then 7.5 mg/kg x 6 days (WHO recommendation) (see Comment). | Toxicity low, hemolysis reported but recovery when treatment stopped. No significant changes in WBC, platelets, hepatic or renal function. See CID 36:1254, 2003. ARF in Lassa associated with 15-fold higher mortality (Lancet ID 18, (6): 684-695, 2018). |
| **Dengue and dengue hemorrhagic fever (DHF)**<br>www.cdc.gov/ncidod/dvbid/dengue/dengue-hcp.htm<br>Think of diagnosis in traveler to tropics (incubation period usually 4-7 days) with fever, bleeding, thrombocytopenia, or hemoconcentration with shock. Dx by viral isolation or serology; serum to CDC (telephone 787-706-2399). | **No data on antiviral rx.** Fluid replacement with careful hemodynamic monitoring critical. Review of treatment: Current Treatment Opinion ID 9:185-93, 2017. | Diagnosis: ELISA detects IgM antibody. Has some cross-reactivity with West Nile Virus infection. Should only be used in pts with symptoms c/w Dengue Fever. Many candidate antiviral drugs in development; non effective yet. |
| **West Nile virus** (JAMA 310:308, 2013)<br>A flavivirus transmitted by mosquitoes, blood transfusions, transplanted organs & breast-feeding. Birds (>200 species) are main host with humans & horses incidental hosts. The US epidemic continues. | **No proven rx.** Supportive care (See www.cdc.gov/westnile/healthcareproviders). RCT of IVIG of no benefit (BMC Infect Dis 2014;14-248). | Usually nonspecific febrile disease but 1/150 cases develops meningoencephalitis, aseptic meningitis or polio-like paralysis (NEJM 2017:377:1878). Long-term sequelae (neuromuscular weakness & psychiatric impairment). Diagnosis: increased IgM antibody in serum & CSF or CSF PCR (contact State Health Dept./CDC). Blood supply now tested in U.S. |
| **Yellow fever** | **No data on antiviral therapy.**<br>Guidelines for use of preventative vaccine: (http://www.cdc.gov/mmwr/preview/mmwrhtml/mm6643a5_w)<br>Fluids, analgesics, and anti-pyretics (NEJM 371:885, 2014). | Reemergence in Africa & S. Amer. due to urbanization of susceptible population (https://www.nejm.org/doi/full/10.1056/NEJMp1702172). Vaccination Diagnosis: increased IgM antibody safe and effective in HIV patients, especially in those with increased CD4 counts (CID 48:659, 2009). A purified whole-virus, inactivated, cell-culture-derived vaccine (XRX-001) using the 17D strain proven safe and resulted in neutralizing antibodies after 2 doses in a de-escalation, phase I study. (N Engl J Med 2011 Apr 7; 364:1326). |
| **Chikungunya fever:** brake bone fever<br>A self-limited arbovirus illness spread by Aedes mosquito. High epidemic potential (Caribbean). | | Clinical presentation: high fever, severe myalgias & headache, morbilliform rash with occ. thrombocytopenia. Rarely hemorrhagic complications. Dx mostly clinical; definitive diagnosis by PCR (NEJM 372:1231, 2015; JCI 27: 737, 2017). |
| **SFTSV** (Severe fever with thrombocytopenia syndrome virus) | **See Bunyaviridae, page 178** | |

*See page 2 for abbreviations. NOTE: All dosage recommendations are for adults (unless otherwise indicated) and assume normal renal function.*

**TABLE 14A (3)**

| VIRUS/DISEASE | DRUG/DOSAGE | SIDE EFFECTS/COMMENTS |
|---|---|---|
| **Hepatitis Viral Infections** | See Table 14E (Hepatitis A & B), Table 14F (Hepatitis C) | |
| **Herpesvirus Infections** | | |
| **Cytomegalovirus (CMV)** At risk: HIV/AIDS, cancer chemotherapy, post-transplant. Solid Organ Treatment Guidelines (*Transplantation 102:900-31, 2018*) | **Primary prophylaxis** not generally recommended except in certain transplant populations (see *Table 15E*). Preemptive therapy in pts with ↑ CMV DNA plasma VL & CD4 <100/mm³. If used: **valganciclovir** 900 mg po q12h (*CID 32:783, 2001*). Primary prophylaxis may be dc if response to ART with ↑ CD4 >100 for 6 mos. (*MMWR53:96, 2004*). | Risk for developing CMV disease correlates with quantity of CMV DNA in plasma: each log₁₀ ↑ associated with 3.1-fold ↑ in disease (*CID 28:758, 1999*). Antimicrob Chemother associated in 5% of transplant recipients receiving primary prophylaxis (*J Antimicrob Chemother 65:2628, 2010*). Brincidofovir not effective against CMV in transplant patients. Letermovir effective as primary preventative therapy. |
| **CMV: Colitis, Esophagitis, Gastritis** Symptoms relate to site of disease | **Mild: Valganciclovir** 900 mg po bid with food x 14-21 days. **Severe: Ganciclovir** 5 mg/kg IV q12h x 14-21 days OR **Foscarnet** (60 mg/kg IV q8h or 90 mg/kg q12h) x 14-21 days *Post-treatment suppression:* **Valganciclovir** 900 mg po once daily until CD4 >100 x 6 mos. | Diagnosis: Elevated whole blood quantitative PCR & histopathology. Severe bouts of Inflammatory Bowel Disease (IBD) colitis may be complicated by CMV: Rx of CMV in this setting is recommended (*European J Clin Micro & Inf Dis 34:73, 2015*). Rx of CMV in less severe bouts of IBD colitis is unclear. |
| **CMV: Neurologic disease, Encephalitis** Myelitis, polyradiculopathy, peripheral neuropathy Symptoms relate to site of disease | Treat as for colitis, esophagitis, gastritis above | Diagnosis: Elevated whole blood and/or CSF quantitative PCR. NOTE: **Severe or fatal IRIS** has occurred in AIDS pts; suggest delay starting ART for 2 wks after initiation of CMV therapy. |
| **CMV: Pneumonia** At risk: 1st 6 months post-transplant & 3 months post-stopping prophylaxis Require evidence of invasive disease. Diagnosis: prefer whole blood quantitative PCR and/or transplantation lung biopsy pathology Ref: *Transplantation 96:333, 2013; Am J Transplant 13(Suppl 4):93, 2013* | **Viremic but no/mild symptoms: Valganciclovir** 900 mg po bid (*Am J Transplant 7:2106, 2007*). **Severe in lung transplant or AIDS pts: Ganciclovir** 5 mg/kg IV q12h (adjust for renal failure). Treat until clinical resolution & neg blood PCR; min duration: 2 wks **Ganciclovir-resistant: Foscarnet** (60 mg/kg q8h or 90 mg/kg q12h) IV (adjust for renal insufficiency). Try to reduce immunosuppression. | *Post-treatment suppression:* Valganciclovir 900 mg once daily x 1-3 months if high risk of relapse. Suspect resistant CMV if treatment failure or relapse. Do genotype resistance testing (*CID 56:1018, 2013*). IVIG or CMV specific immunoglobulin did not improve overall or attributable mortality in retrospective study of 421 bone marrow transplant pts (*CID 61:31, 2015*). |
| **CMV: Retinitis** Most common ocular complication of HIV/AIDS, Rare in pts on ART with CD4 >200. If not on ART, wait to start until after 2 wks of CMV therapy. **CMV immune recovery retinitis:** new retinitis after starting ART: Do not stop ART or Valganciclovir. No steroids. | **Not sight-threatening: Valganciclovir** 900 mg po bid with food x 14-21 days, then 900 mg po once daily until CD4 >100 x 6 mos. **Sight-threatening** (*see Comment*): **Valganciclovir +** intravitreal **Ganciclovir** 2 mg (1-4 doses over 7-10 days). | Sight-threatening: <1500 microns from fovea or next to head of optic nerve. If can't use Valganciclovir, Ganciclovir 5 mg/kg IV q12h x 14-21 days, then 5 mg/kg IV q12h x 14-21 days, then 5 mg/kg q8h or 90 mg/kg q12h) x 14-21 days once daily. If suspect Ganciclovir resistance: Foscarnet (60 gm/kg q8h or 90 mg/kg q12h) x 14-21 days. Ganciclovir ocular implants no longer available. |
| **CMV in Transplant patients:** See Table 15E for CMV prophylaxis. | **Ganciclovir** 5 mg/kg IV q12h OR **Valganciclovir** 900 mg po q12h (*Am J Transplant 7:2106, 2007*) are effective with or without end-organ disease. **Guidelines for CMV therapy** (*Transplantation 102:900-31, 2018*). **Ganciclovir** 5 mg/kg IV q12h OR **Valganciclovir** 900 mg po q12h (*Am J Transplant 7:2106, 2007*) are effective treatment until (1) CMV PCR or antigenemia has become undetectable, (2) clinical evidence of disease has resolved, and (3) at least 2-3 weeks of treatment (*Am J Transplant 13(Suppl 4):93, 2013; Brincidofovir 43:77, 2009*). Secondary prophylaxis (Valganciclovir 900 mg daily) for a 1-3 month course in patients recently treated with high-dose immunosuppression such as lymphocyte depleting antibodies, those with severe CMV disease, or those with >1 episode of CMV disease. In HSCT recipients, secondary prophylaxis should be considered in similar cases balancing the risk of recurrent infection with drug toxicity. Brincidofovir not effective against CMV in transplant patients. | |
| **CMV in pregnancy:** Hyperimmune globulin 200 IU/kg maternal weight as single dose during pregnancy (early), administered IV reduced complications of CMV in infant at one year of life. (*NEJM 372:933, 2012*). | | |
| **CMV: Congenital/Neonatal** Symptomatic | **Valganciclovir** 16 mg/kg po bid x 6 mos | Better outcome after 6 wks compared to 6 wks with no difference in AEs (*NEJM 372:933, 2015*). Monitor for neutropenia. |

\* *See page 2 for abbreviations. NOTE: All dosage recommendations are for adults (unless otherwise indicated) and assume normal renal function.*

**TABLE 14A (4)**

| VIRUS/DISEASE | DRUG/DOSAGE | SIDE EFFECTS/COMMENTS |
|---|---|---|
| **Herpesvirus Infections** (*continued*) | | |
| **Epstein Barr Virus (EBV) — Mononucleosis** | **No treatment.** Corticosteroids for tonsillar obstruction, CNS complications, or threat of splenic rupture. | Potential therapies reviewed (*Cancers 10: 192, 2018*). **Diff dx of atypical lymphocytes:** EBV, CMV, Hep A, Hep B, Toxo, measles, mumps, drugs, HHV6, HHV7, HIV & others. |
| **HHV-6**—Cause of roseola (exanthem subitum) & other febrile illness of childhood (*NEJM 352:768, 2005*). Fever & rash in transplant pts (*JID 179:311, 1999*). Reactivation in 47% of 110 U.S. hematopoietic stem cell transplant pts (*CID 40:932, 2005*). Associated with meningoencephalitis, infectious mono & DRESS syndrome in immunocompetent adults (*NEJM 2018;379:775*). Diagnosis made by pos. PCR in CSF & compatible clinical syndrome. CSF film array PCR, 15 pos. for HHV-5, only 1 of 15 with compatible clin. illness (*CID 67:1125, 2018*). RX; **Ganciclovir** is primary regimen. | | |
| **HHV-7**—Ubiquitous virus (>90% of the population is infected by age 3 yrs). No relationship to human disease. Infects CD4 receptor; transmitted via saliva. | | |
| **HHV-8**—The agent of Kaposi's sarcoma, Castleman's disease, & body cavity lymphoma. Associated with diabetes in sub-Saharan Africa (*JAMA 299:2770, 2008*). | **No antiviral treatment.** Effective anti-HIV therapy may help. | Localized lesions: radiotherapy, laser surgery or intralesional chemotherapy. Systemic: chemotherapy. Castleman's disease responded to ganciclovir (*Blood 103:1632, 2004*) & valganciclovir (*JID 2006*). |
| **Herpes simplex virus (HSV Types 1 & 2)** | | |
| **Bell's palsy** H. simplex most implicated etiology. Other etiologic considerations: VZV, HHV-6, Lyme disease. | As soon as possible after onset of palsy: **Valacyclovir** 500 mg bid x first 5 days + **Prednisone** 1 mg/kg po divided bid x 5 days then taper to 5 mg bid over the next 5 days (total of 10 days Prednisone). | Cochrane Review (*2015*)(*JAMA 2016;316:874*) "compared with oral corticosteroids alone, addition of valacyclovir or famciclovir associated with greater number of recoveries at 3-12 mos". |
| **Encephalitis** Review: *Clin ID Reports 19:13, 2017* HSV-1 is most common cause of sporadic encephalitis. Survival & recovery from neurological sequelae are related to mental status at time of initiation of rx. **Early dx and rx imperative.** *NEJM 371:68, 2014.* | **Acyclovir** 10 mg/kg IV (infuse over 1 hr) q8h x 14-21 days. 20 mg/kg q8h in children <12 yrs. Dose calculation in obese patients: use actual body weight. To lessen risk of nephrotoxicity with large volume & ideal body weight (IBW) calc, infuse each dose over more than 1 hour. In morbid obesity, use actual body weight; in morbid obesity, use "adjusted" body weight. Adjusted BW = ideal BW + 0.4 (actual BW- ideal BW). | Mortality rate reduced from >70% to 19% with acyclovir rx. PCR analysis of CSF for HSV-1 DNA is 100% specific & 75-98% sensitive. 8/33 (25%) CSF samples drawn before day 3 were neg. by PCR; Hep A. PCR assoc. with ↓ protein & <10 WBC per mm³ in CSF (*CID 36:1335, 2003*). All were + after 3 days. Relapse after successful rx reported in 7/27 (27%) children. Relapse was associated with lower total dose of initial acyclovir rx (285 ± 82 mg per kg in relapse group vs. 462 ± 149 mg per kg, p <0.03). (*CID 30:185, 2000*). Series in 106 adults *J Clin Virol 60:112, 2014* |
| **Genital Herpes:** *Sexually Transmitted Treatment Guidelines MMWR 64(RR-3):1, 2015; NEJM 2016;375:666.* | | |
| **Primary (initial episode)** | **Acyclovir** (Zovirax or generic) 400 mg po tid x 7-10 days | ↓ by 2 days time to resolution of signs & symptoms, ↓ by 4 days time to healing of lesions, ↓ by 7 days duration of viral shedding. Does not prevent recurrences. For severe cases only: 5 mg per kg IV q8h times 5-7 days. |
| | **Valacyclovir** (Valtrex) 1000 mg po bid x 7-10 days **Famciclovir** (Famvir) 250 mg po bid or tid x 7-10 days | An ester of acyclovir, which is well absorbed, bioavailability 3-5 times greater than acyclovir. Metabolized to penciclovir, which is active component. Side effects and activity similar to acyclovir. **Famciclovir** 250 mg po tid **equal to acyclovir** 200 mg 5 times per day. |
| **Episodic recurrences** | **Acyclovir** 800 mg po tid **x 2 days** or 400 mg po tid **x 5 days** or **Famciclovir** 1000 mg po bid **x 1 day**, 250 mg po bid x 2 days or 125 mg po bid **x 5 days** **Valacyclovir** 500 mg po bid **x 3 days** or 1 gm po once daily **x 5 days** Valacyclovir more effective overall (*Meta-analysis in J Oral Path Med 46:561, 2017*). For HIV patients, see *Comment* | For episodic recurrences in **HIV patients**: **Acyclovir** 400 mg po tid x 5-10 days or **Famciclovir** 500 mg po bid x 5-10 days or **Valacyclovir** 1 gm po bid x 5-10 days |

*See page 2 for abbreviations.   NOTE: All dosage recommendations are for adults (unless otherwise indicated) and assume normal renal function.*

**TABLE 14A (5)**

| VIRUS/DISEASE | DRUG/DOSAGE | SIDE EFFECTS/COMMENTS |
|---|---|---|
| **Herpesvirus Infections/Herpes Simplex virus (HSV Types 1 & 2) (continued)** | | |
| Chronic daily suppression | Suppressive therapy reduces the frequency of genital herpes recurrences in pts who have frequent recurrences (i.e., >6 recurrences per yr) & many report no symptomatic outbreaks. **Acyclovir** 400 mg po bid, **or Famciclovir** 250 mg po bid, or **Valacyclovir** 1 gm po q24h; pts with <9 recurrences per yr could use 500 mg po q24h and then use **Valacyclovir** 1 gm po q24h if breakthrough at 500 mg. For HIV patients, see Comment. | For chronic suppression in HIV patients: (all regimens equally efficacious: *Cochrane Database System Rev 8:CD009036, 2014)* **Acyclovir** 400-800 mg po bid or tid or **Famciclovir** 500 mg po bid or **Valacyclovir** 500 mg po bid |
| **Genital, immunocompetent** | | |
| Gingivostomatitis, primary (children) | **Acyclovir** 15 mg/kg po 5x/day x 7 days | Efficacy in randomized double-blind placebo-controlled trial *(BMJ 314:1800, 1997).* |
| Keratoconjunctivitis and recurrent epithelial keratitis | **Trifluridine** (Viroptic) 1 drop 1% solution q2h (max. 9 drops per day) for max. of 21 days *(see Table 1, page 15)* | In controlled trials, response % > Idoxuridine. Suppressive rx with acyclovir (400 mg bid) reduced recurrences of ocular HSV from 32% to 19% *(NEJM 339:300, 1998).* |
| Mollaret's recurrent "aseptic" meningitis (usually HSV-2) *(Ln 363:1772, 2004)* | No controlled trials of antiviral rx & resolves spontaneously. If therapy is to be given, **Acyclovir** (15–30 mg/kg/ day IV) or **Valacyclovir** 1-2 gm po qid should be used. | Pos. PCR for HSV in CSF confirms dx *(EJCMID 23:560, 2004).* In randomized controlled trial, no benefit from valacyclovir suppressive rx *(CID 2012;54:1304).* |
| **Mucocutaneous** *(for Genital see page 181)* | | |
| **Oral labial, "fever blisters":** | | |
| Normal host<br>*See Ann Pharmacotherapy 38:705, 2004;<br>JAC 53:703, 2004* | Start rx with prodrome symptoms (tingling/burning) before lesions show.<br><br>**Oral:** Valacyclovir, Famciclovir[2], Acyclovir[2][3][4][a]<br>**Topical:** Penciclovir 1% cream, Acyclovir 5% cream[3]<br>*See Table 1, page 29* | Penciclovir *(AAC 46: 2848, 2002).* Oral acyclovir 5% cream *(AAC 46:2238, 2002).* Oral famciclovir *(JID 179:303, 1999).* Topical fluocinonide (0.05% Lidex gel) 5 times daily in combination with famciclovir ↓ lesion size and pain when compared to famciclovir alone *(JID 181:1906, 2000).* Acyclovir 5% cream + 1% hydrocortisone (Xerese) superior to acyclovir alone *(AAC 53:1273, 2014).* |
| Herpes Whitlow | | |
| **Oral labial or genital: Immunocompromised** | | |
| (includes pts with AIDS) and critically ill pts in ICU setting/large necrotic ulcers in perineum or face. (See Comment)<br><br>Primary HSV in pregnancy: increased risk of dissemination, including severe hepatitis. Risk greatest in 3rd trimester *(NEJM 370:2211, 2014).* | **Acyclovir** 5 mg per kg IV (infused over 1 hr) q8h times 7 days (250 mg per M[2]) or 400 mg po 5 times per day times 14–21 days. (See Comment if acyclovir-resistant) **OR Famciclovir:** In HIV infected, 500 mg po bid for 7 days for recurrent episodes of genital herpes **OR Valacyclovir[4][a]:** In HIV-infected, 500 mg po bid for 5–10 days for recurrent episodes of genital herpes or 500 mg po bid for chronic suppressive rx. | **Acyclovir-resistant HSV: IV foscarnet** 90 mg/kg IV q12h x 7 days. Suppressive therapy with famciclovir (500 mg po bid), valacyclovir (500 mg po bid) or acyclovir (400-800 mg po bid) reduces viral shedding and clinical recurrences. |

Start rx with prodrome symptoms (tingling/burning) before lesions show.

| Drug | Dose | Sx Decrease |
|---|---|---|
| **Oral:** Valacyclovir | 2 gm po q12h x 1 day | ↓ 1 day |
| Famciclovir[2] | 500 mg po bid x 7 days | ↓ 2 days |
| Acyclovir[2][3][4][a] | 400 mg po 5 x per day (q4h while awake) x 5 days) | ↓ ½ day |
| **Topical:** Penciclovir 1% cream | q2h during day x 4 days | ↓ 1 day |
| Acyclovir 5% cream[3] | 6x/day x 7 days | ↓ ½ day |

---

[2] FDA approved only for HIV pts
[3] Approved for immunocompromised pts

[a] See page 2 for abbreviations.   *NOTE: All dosage recommendations are for adults (unless otherwise indicated) and assume normal renal function.*

**TABLE 14A (6)**

| VIRUS/DISEASE | DRUG/DOSAGE | SIDE EFFECTS/COMMENTS |
|---|---|---|
| **Herpesvirus Infections/Herpes simplex virus (HSV 1 & 2)/Mucocutaneous** (*continued*) | | |
| Pregnancy and genital H. simplex | Acyclovir safe even in first trimester. No proof that acyclovir at delivery reduces risk/severity of neonatal infection. In contrast, C-section in women with active lesions reduces risk of transmission. Ref. *Obstet Gyn 106:845, 2006.* | |
| **Herpes simiae** (Herpes B virus): **Monkey bite** *CID 35:1191, 2002* | **Postexposure prophylaxis: Valacyclovir** 1 gm po q8h times 14 days or acyclovir 800 mg po 5 times per day times 14 days. **Treatment of disease:** (1) CNS symptoms absent: **Acyclovir** 12.5-15 mg per kg IV q8h or ganciclovir 5 mg per kg IV q12h. (2) CNS symptoms present: **Ganciclovir** 5 mg per kg IV q12h. | Fatal human cases of myelitis and hemorrhagic encephalitis have been reported following bites, scratches, or eye inoculation of saliva from monkeys. Initial sx include fever, headache, myalgias and diffuse adenopathy. Incubation period of 2-14 days (*EID 9:246, 2003*). In vitro ACV and ganciclovir less active than other nucleosides (penciclovir or 5-ethyldeoxyuridine may be more active, clinical data needed) (*AAC 57:2028, 2007*). |
| **Varicella-Zoster Virus (VZV)** **Varicella:** Diagnosis (*JEADV 31:20, 2017*) and treatment (*JEADV 31:9, 2017*). Immunization: *www.cdc.gov/vaccines/schedules/hcp/imz/child-adolescent* or *Med Lett 2018;60:73.* | | |
| Normal host (chickenpox) Child (2–12 years) | **In general, treatment not recommended.** Might use oral **acyclovir** for healthy persons at ↑ risk for moderate to severe varicella, i.e., >12 yrs of age; chronic cutaneous or pulmonary diseases; chronic salicylate rx (↑ risk of Reye syndrome). **Acyclovir** dose: 20 mg/kg po qid x 5 days (start within 24 hrs of rash) or **Valacyclovir** 20 mg/kg/day x 5 days. | Acyclovir slowed development and ↓ number of new lesions and ↓ duration of disease in children: 9 to 7.6 days (*PIDJ 21:739, 2002*). Oral dose of acyclovir in children should not exceed 80 mg per kg per day or 3200 mg per day. |
| Adolescents, young adults | Start within 24 hrs of rash: **Valacyclovir** 1000 mg tid x 7 days or **Famciclovir** 500 mg po tid x 7 days (probably effective, but data lacking). | ↓ duration of fever, time to healing, and symptoms. |
| Pneumonia or chickenpox in 3rd trimester of pregnancy | **Acyclovir** 800 mg po 5 times per day or 10 mg per kg IV q8h times 5 days. Risks and benefits to fetus and mother still unknown. Many experts recommend rx, especially in 3rd trimester. Some would add VZIG (varicella-zoster immune globulin). | Varicella pneumonia associated with 41% mortality in pregnancy. Acyclovir ↓ incidence and severity (*JID 185:422, 2002*). If varicella-susceptible mother exposed and respiratory symptoms develop within 10 days after exposure, start acyclovir |
| Immunocompromised host | **Acyclovir** 10-12 mg per kg (500 mg per M²) IV (infused over 1 hr) q8h times 7 days | Disseminated 1° varicella infection reported during infliximab rx of rheumatoid arthritis (*J Rheum 31:2517, 2004*). Continuous infusion of high-dose acyclovir (2 mg per kg per hr) successful in 1 pt with severe hemorrhagic varicella (*NEJM 336:732, 1997*). |
| **Prevention—Postexposure prophylaxis** Varicella deaths still occur in unvaccinated persons (*MMWR 56 (RR-4):1-40, 2007*) | **CDC Recommendations for Prevention:** Since <5% of cases of varicella but >50% of varicella-related deaths occur in adults >20 yrs of age, the CDC recommends a more aggressive approach in this age group: **1st, varicella-zoster immune globulin** (VZIG) (125 units/10 kg (22 lbs) body weight IM up to a max. of 625 units; minimum dose is 125 units) is recommended for postexposure prophylaxis in susceptible persons at greater risk for complications (immunocompromised such as HIV, transplant, pregnancy, and steroid therapy) as soon as possible after exposure (<96 hrs). If varicella develops, initiate treatment quickly (<24 hrs of rash) with **Acyclovir** as below. Some would rx presumptively with acyclovir in high-risk pts. **2nd,** susceptible adults should be vaccinated. Check antibody in adults with negative or uncertain history of varicella (10–30% will be AB-neg.) and vaccinate those who are Ab-neg. **3rd,** susceptible children should receive vaccination. Recommended before age 12–18 mos. but OK at any age. | |

\* *See page 2 for abbreviations.*   NOTE: *All dosage recommendations are for adults (unless otherwise indicated) and assume normal renal function.*

**TABLE 14A (7)**

| VIRUS/DISEASE | DRUG/DOSAGE | SIDE EFFECTS/COMMENTS |
|---|---|---|
| **Herpesvirus Infections** *(continued)* | | |
| **Herpes zoster (shingles)** *(See NEJM 369:255, 2013)* | | |
| **Normal host** — Effective therapy most evident in pts age >50 yrs. *(For treatment of post-herpetic neuralgia, see CID 36: 877, 2003; Ln 374:1252, 2009)* Herpes zoster subunit vaccine (Shingrix) preferred for immunocompetent adults age 50 yrs or older *(NEJM 2016;375:1019)* Analgesics for acute pain associated with Herpes zoster *(NEJM 369:255, 2013)* | [NOTE: Trials showing benefit of therapy: only in pts treated within 3 days of onset of rash] <br><br>**Valacyclovir** 1000 mg po tid times 7 days (adjust dose for renal failure) *(See Table 17A)* <br><br>**OR** <br>**Famciclovir** 500 mg tid x 7 days. Adjust for renal failure *(see Table 17A)* <br><br>**OR** <br>**Acyclovir** 800 mg po 5 times per day times 7 days <br><br>Add **Prednisone** in pts over 50 yrs old to decrease discomfort during acute phase of zoster. Does not decrease incidence of post-herpetic neuralgia. Dose: 30 mg po bid days 1–7, 15 mg bid days 8–14 and 7.5 mg bid days 15–21. | Increasing recognition of risk of stroke during 3 mos. after episode of Shingles. Oral antivirals during clinical H. zoster infection may have protective effect *(CID 58:1497, 1504, 2014)*. VZV found in wall of cerebral and temporal arteries of pts with giant cell arteritis. *(Neurology 84:1948, 2015; JID 51:537, 2015)*. <br><br>Time to healing more rapid. Reduced incidence of post-herpetic neuralgia (PHN) vs placebo in pts >50 yrs of age. Famciclovir similar to acyclovir in reduction of acute pain and incidence of PHN *(J Micro Immunol Inf 37:75, 2004)*. <br><br>A meta-analysis of 4 placebo-controlled trials (691 pts): acyclovir accelerated by approx. 2-fold pain resolution and reduced incidence of post-herpetic neuralgia at 3 & 6 mos. *(CID 22:341, 1996)*; med. time to resolution of pain 41 days vs 101 days in those >50 yrs. In post-herpetic neuralgia, controlled trials demonstrated effectiveness of **gabapentin**, the **lidocaine patch** (5%), & **opioid analgesic** in controlling pain *(Drugs 64:937, 2004; J Clin Virol 29:248, 2004)*. **Nortriptyline** & **amitriptyline** are equally effective but nortriptyline is better tolerated *(CID 36:877, 2003)*. Role of antiviral drugs in rx of PHN unproven *(Neurol 64:21, 2005)* but 8 of 15 pt improved with IV acyclovir 10 mg/kg q 8 hrs x 14 days followed by oral valacyclovir 1 gm 3x a day for 1 month *(Arch Neurol 63:940, 2006)*. Review: NEJM 371:1526, 2014; Expert Opin Pharmacotherapy 15:61, 2014 |
| **Immunocompromised host** | | |
| Not severe | **Acyclovir** 800 mg po 5 times per day times 7 days. <br>**(Options: Famciclovir** 750 mg po q24h or 500 mg bid or 250 mg 3 times per day times 7 days **OR Valacyclovir** 1000 mg po tid times 7 days, though both are not FDA-approved for this indication)) | If progression, switch to IV. <br>RA pts on TNF-alpha inhibitors at high risk for VZV. Zoster more severe, but less post-herpetic neuralgia *(JAMA 301:737, 2009)*. |
| Severe: >1 dermatome, trigeminal nerve or disseminated | **Acyclovir** 10–12 mg per kg IV (infusion over 1 hr) q8h times 7 days. In older pts, ↓ to 7.5 mg per kg. If nephrotoxicity and pt improving, ↓ to 5 mg per kg q8h. | A common manifestation of immune reconstitution following HAART in HIV-infected children *(J All Clin Immun 113:742, 2004)*. <br>Rx must be begun in 72 hrs. For Acyclovir-resistant VZV in HIV+ pts previously treated with acyclovir: **Foscarnet** (40 mg per kg IV q8h for 14–26 days). |
| Progressive Outer Retinal Necrosis (PORN) Reviewed *(Ophthalmology 24(3): 382–392, 2017)* | **Ganciclovir** 5 mg/kg and/or **Foscarnet** 90 mg/kg IV q12h + **Ganciclovir** 2 mg/0.05 mL and/or **Foscarnet** 1.2 mg/0.05 mL intravitreal twice weekly. | Expert consultation with an ophthalmologist. NB: **Ganciclovir** ocular implants no longer manufactured. If HIV pt, optimize ARV therapy. |
| **Human T-cell Leukotrophic Virus-1 (HTLV-1)** Causes infection in only 5% of infected persons. Two are associated with HTLV-1: Adult T-cell leukemia/ lymphoma *(NEJM 367:552, 2012)* and HTLV-1-associated myelopathy (HAM), also known as tropical spastic paraparesis (TSP). | No proven therapy. Some nucleoside antiretroviral therapies used with limited success. Mogamulizumab (anti-CCR4) antibody being evaluated for refractory T-cell cutaneous lymphoma *(Blood: https://doi.org/10.1182/blood-2018-02-835991)*. | Laboratory diagnosis is by blood and CSF. Anti-HTLV-1 antibodies are detected by ELISA antibody testing; Western Blot is used for confirmation *(Focus Diagnostics or Quest Diagnostics)*. HTLV DNA can be detected by PCR in circulating CD4 cells. One tube multiplex qPCR highly specific / sensitive *(Retrovirology 11(Suppl): P105, 2014)*. |

\* See page 2 for abbreviations.   NOTE: All dosage recommendations are for adults (unless otherwise indicated) and assume normal renal function.

**TABLE 14A (8)**

**Influenza A & B and novel influenza viruses** Refs: *http://www.cdc.gov/flu/professionals/antivirals/index.htm; http://www.cdc.gov/flu/weekly; NEJM 370:789, 2014.*

**Vaccine info** (*http://www.cdc.gov/flu/professionals/acip/index.htm*); *Med Lett 56:92, 2014; MMWR 63:691, 2014.*

- **Oseltamivir and zanamivir are recommended drugs.** Amantadine and rimantadine should not be used because of widespread resistance.
- Novel H1N1 (referred to as pandemic H1N1, pH1N1, H1N1pdm and formerly swine flu) emerged in 2009 and now is the dominant H1N1 strain worldwide. Old distinction from seasonal H1N1 is still sometimes used but not relevant.
- Rapid influenza tests can be falsely negative in 20-50%, PCR is gold standard test.
- Initiate therapy as close to the onset of symptoms as possible, and certainly within 48 hrs of onset of symptoms. Starting therapy after 48 hours of onset of symptoms is associated with reduced therapeutic benefit. However, starting therapy up to 5 days after onset in patients who are hospitalized is associated with improved survival (*Clin Infect Dis 55:1198, 2012*).
- Empiric therapy should be started for all patients who are hospitalized, have severe or progressive influenza or are at higher risk of complications due to age or underlying medical conditions.
- Look for concomitant bacterial pneumonia.
- Other important influenza viruses causing human disease
  - **H3N2v influenza:** 159 cases of influenza A/H3N2v reported over the summer of 2012. Most of the cases of influenza A/H3N2v occurred in children under the age of 10 with direct contact with pigs. This variant is susceptible to the neuraminidase inhibitors, oseltamivir and zanamivir. *See MMWR 61:619, 2012.*
  - **Avian influenza H5N1:** Re-emerged in Asia in 2003 and human cases detected in 15 countries mostly in Asia as well as Egypt, Nigeria and Djibouti. Circulation associated with massive poultry die off. Imported cases rare. As of 2012, total of 622 human cases confirmed and 384 deaths (59%). Human infection associated with poultry; very limited human to human transmission. Mortality associated with high viral load, disseminated virus and high cytokine activity (*Nature Medicine 12:1203-1207 2006*). Use oseltamivir and consider IV zanamivir (*NEJM 353:267-272 2005*).
  - **Avian influenza H7N9:** Emerged in Eastern China in March 2013 and 132 cases documented during Spring 2013 with 44 deaths (33%). Cases appeared again in early winter 2013-2014 and continue to increase. Infection associated with close contact with live bird markets; extremely limited human to human transmission to date. Mortality highest among older persons and those with medical conditions. Oseltamivir active against most but not all strains. No zanamivir resistance documented to date.

| Virus/Disease | Susceptible to (Recommended Drug/Dosage): | Resistant to: | Alternatives/Side Effects/Comments |
|---|---|---|---|
| **A/H1N1 (current seasonal resembles pandemic H1N1)**<br>Influenza B<br>Influenza A (A/H3N2, A/H3N2v** A/H5N1, A/H7N9***) | **Oseltamivir**<br>Adult - Oseltamivir 75 mg po bid x 5 days<br>Pediatric: (child age 1-12 years):<br>Infant 2 wks-11 months: 3 mg/kg bid x 5 days<br>≤15 kg: 30 mg bid x 5 days<br>>15 kg to 23 kg: 45 mg bid x 5 days<br>>23 kg to 40 kg: 60 mg bid x 5 days<br>>40 kg: 75 mg bid x 5 days<br>or<br>**Zanamivir** 2 inhalations (5 mg each) bid x 5 days or<br>**Baloxavir** 40 mg po single dose if >12 years (80 mg if > 80 kg) or<br>**Peramivir** 600 mg IV once daily x 5-10 days<br>For IV Zanamivir, see Comment<br><br>**Laninamivir** (approved in Japan):<br>Age < 10yrs: 20 mg once daily by inhalation<br>Age > 10 yrs: 40 mg once daily by inhalation | Amantadine and rimantadine (100%)<br>* A/H3N2v strain are susceptible<br>** A/H7N9 resistant to oseltamivir (rarely) | • **A/H1N1:** Higher dose (150 mg bid) **not** more effective for H1N1<br>• **Zanamivir** not recommended for children <7 years or those with reactive airway disease<br>• **IV zanamivir** is available under compassionate use IND and clinical trials for hospitalized influenza patients with suspected or known gastric stasis, gastric malabsorption, gastrointestinal bleeding, or for patients suspected or confirmed with oseltamivir-resistant influenza virus infection. For compassionate use, contact GlaxoSmithKline at (+1) 919-315-5215 or email: gskclinicalsupportHD@GSK.com.<br>• **Influenza B:** Baloxavir was more effective than oseltamivir in one trial (*IDWeek 2008 LB*). One study suggested virologic benefit to higher dose oseltamivir for critically ill patients with influenza B.<br>• **A/H5N1:** Given high mortality, consider obtaining investigational drug, Zanamivir retains activity against most oseltamivir resistant H5N1<br>• Association between corticosteroid rx & increased mortality (*JID 212:183, 2015*). For now, avoid steroids unless indicated for another reason. |

* See page 2 for abbreviations.   NOTE: All dosage recommendations are for adults (unless otherwise indicated) and assume normal renal function.

**TABLE 14A (9)**

| VIRUS/DISEASE | DRUG/DOSAGE | SIDE EFFECTS/COMMENTS |
|---|---|---|
| **Measles** Increasing reports of measles in unvaccinated children and adults *(MMWR 63:781, 2014; NEJM 371:358, 2014).* | | |
| Children | No therapy or **vitamin A** 200,000 units po daily times 2 days | Vitamin A may ↓ severity of measles. |
| Adults | No rx or **ribavirin** IV: 20–35 mg per kg per day times 7 days | ↓ severity of illness in adults. |
| **Metapneumovirus (HMPV)** A paramyxovirus isolated from pts of all ages, with mild bronchiolitis/bronchospasm to pneumonia. Review: *Infect Dis Clin N Amer 2017;31:455.* | **No proven antiviral therapy** (intravenous ribavirin used anecdotally with variable results) Investigational Agents Reviewed *(Clin Vaccine Immunol 22:8 & 858, 2015)* | Human metapneumovirus isolated from 6-21% of children with RTIs *(NEJM 350:443, 2004)*. Dual infection with RSV assoc. with severe bronchiolitis *(JID 191:382, 2005)*. Clinical picture in elderly *(JID 2018;218:1268-1869)*. Aerosolized ribavirin not reviewed. |
| **Monkeypox** (orthopox virus) *(See LnID 4:17, 2004)* Outbreak from contact with ill prairie dogs. Source likely imported Gambian giant rats *(CID 58:260, 2014).* | **No proven antiviral therapy. Tecovirimat** (Tpoxx) 600 mg (three 200 mg capsules) twice daily x 14 days (active in monkey models; likely effective in humans. Not an FDA approved indication) Cidofovir is active in vitro & in mouse model. | Incubation period of 12 days, then fever, headache, cough, adenopathy, & a vesicular papular rash that pustulates, umbilicates, & crusts on the head, trunk, & extremities. Transmission in healthcare setting rare. |
| **Norovirus** (Norwalk-like virus, or NLV) Vast majority of outbreaks of non-bacterial gastroenteritis *(JID 213(Suppl 1):1, 2016).* | **No antiviral therapy.** Replete volume. Transmission by contaminated food, fecal-oral contact with contaminated surfaces, or fomites. | Sudden onset of nausea, vomiting, and/or watery diarrhea lasting 12-60 hours. Ethanol-based hand rubs effective *(J Hosp Inf 60:144, 2005).* |
| **Papillomaviruses: Warts** | | |
| **External Genital Warts** Also look for warts in anal canal *(MMWR 64(3):1, 2015)* | **Patient applied: Podofilox** (0.5% solution or gel): apply 2x/day x 3 days, 4th day no therapy, repeat cycle 4x; OR **Imiquimod** 5% cream: apply once daily hs 3x/wk for up to 16 wks. **Sinecatechins:** Apply to external genital warts only 3x/day until effect or adverse effect. **Provider administered: Cryotherapy** with liquid nitrogen; repeat q1-2 wks; OR **Trichloroacetic acid** (TCA): repeat weekly as needed; OR surgical removal. | **Podofilox:** Inexpensive and safe (pregnancy safety not established). Mild irritation. **Imiquimod:** Mild to moderate redness & irritation. Topical imiquimod effective for treatment of vulvar intraepithelial neoplasms *(NEJM 358:1465, 2008)*. Safety in pregnancy not established. **Sinecatechins:** Local irritation, redness, pain, and itching **Cryotherapy:** Blistering and skin necrosis common. **Podophyllin resin:** No longer recommended as other less toxic regimens available. **TCA:** Caustic. Can cause severe pain on adjacent normal skin. Neutralize with soap or sodium bicarbonate. |
| Warts on cervix | Need evaluation for evolving neoplasia | Gynecological consult advised. |
| Vaginal warts | Cryotherapy with liquid nitrogen or **TCA** | |
| Urethral warts | Cryotherapy with liquid nitrogen. | |
| Anal warts | Cryotherapy with liquid nitrogen or **TCA** or surgical removal | Advise anoscopy to look for rectal warts. |
| Skin papillomas | Topical **α-lactalbumin. Oleic acid** (from human milk) applied 1x/day for 3 wks | ↓ lesion size & recurrence vs placebo (p <0.001) *(NEJM 350:2663, 2004)*. Further studies warranted. |

\* See page 2 for abbreviations.    NOTE: All dosage recommendations are for adults (unless otherwise indicated) and assume normal renal function.

## TABLE 14A (10)

| VIRUS/DISEASE | DRUG/DOSAGE | SIDE EFFECTS/COMMENTS |
|---|---|---|
| **Parvo B19 Virus (Erythema infectiosum)**, *Review: NEJM 350:586, 2004. Wide range of manifestation.* **Treatment options for common symptomatic infections:** | | |
| Erythema infectiosum<br>Arthritis/arthralgia<br>Transient aplastic crisis<br>Fetal hydrops<br>Chronic infection with anemia<br>Chronic infection without anemia | Symptomatic treatment only<br>Nonsteroidal anti-inflammatory drugs (NSAID)<br>Transfusions and oxygen<br>Intrauterine blood transfusion<br>IVIG and transfusion (*CID 56:968, 2013*) For dose, see *Comment*<br>Perhaps **IVIG** | Diagnostic tools: IgM and Igb antibody titers. Perhaps better: blood parvovirus P.<br>Dose of IVIG not standardized; suggest 400 mg/kg IV of commercial IVIG for 5 or 10 days or 1000 mg/kg IV for 3 days.<br>Most dramatic anemias in pts with pre-existing hemolytic anemia.<br>Bone marrow shows erythrocyte maturation arrest with giant pronormoblasts (*Rev Med Virol 25:224, 2015*). |
| **Papovavirus/Polyomavirus** | | |
| **Progressive multifocal leukoencephalopathy (PML).** Serious demyelinating disease due to JC virus in immunocompromised pts. | No specific therapy for JC virus. Two general approaches:<br>1. In HIV pts: HAART. Cidofovir may be effective.<br>2. Stop or decrease immunosuppressive therapy. | Failure of treatment with interferon alfa-2b, cytarabine and topotecan. Immunosuppressive **Natalizumab** temporarily removed from market due to reported associations with PML. Mixed reports on **cidofovir**. Most likely effective in ART-experienced pts. **Watch for IRIS when starting ARV Rx.** |
| **BK virus induced nephropathy in immunocompromised pts and hemorrhagic cystitis** | Decrease immunosuppression if possible. Suggested antiviral therapy based on anecdotal data. If progressive renal dysfunction:<br>1. **Fluoroquinolone** first;<br>2. **IVIG** 500 mg/kg IV;<br>3. **Leflunomide** 100 mg po daily x 3 days, then 10-20 mg po daily;<br>4. **Cidofovir** only if refractory to all of the above (*see Table 14B for dose*). | Use PCR to monitor viral "load" in urine and/or plasma. Report of cidofovir as potentially effective for BK hemorrhagic cystitis (*CID 49:233, 2009*). Adoptive immunotransfer of BKV specific T-cell being explored to treat hemorrhagic cystitis (*E J Haematology 98:632, 2017*). |
| **Rabies** (*see Table 20B, page 254; diagnosis and management*) | | |
| Rabid dogs account for 50,000 cases per yr worldwide. Most cases in the U.S. are cryptic, 70% with no bat species (*EID 9:151, 2003*).<br>An organ donor with early rabies infected 4 recipients (2 kidneys, liver & artery) and died avg. 13 days after transplant (*NEJM 352:1103, 2005*). | **Mortality 100% with only survivors those who receive rabies vaccine before the onset of illness/symptoms** (*CID 36:61, 2003*). | Corticosteroids ↑ mortality rate and ↓ incubation time in mice. Therapies that have failed after symptoms develop include: vaccine, rabies immunoglobulin, rabies virus neutralizing antibody, ribavirin, alfa interferon, induced coma & ketamine. For post-exposure prophylaxis, *see Table 20B, page 254*. |
| **Respiratory Syncytial Virus (RSV)**<br>Major cause of morbidity in neonates/infants.<br>Diagnosis: airway swab for RSV PCR<br>Review: *Infect Dis Clin N Amer 2017;31:455.* | *All ages:* Hydration, O₂ as needed. If wheezing, trial of beta-agonist.<br>*Corticosteroids:* children-no; adults-maybe<br>Nebulized Ribavirin: for severe RSV in children, adults (*CID 57:1731, 2013*).<br>Nebulized Ribavirin + RSV immune globulin: immunocompromised adults (HSCT) (*CID 56:258, 2013*). Oral ribavirin may be as effective as aerosolized, and much less expensive, in immunocompromised patients (*Transplant ID 20:e12844, 2018*). | In adults, RSV accounted for 10.6% of hospitalizations for pneumonia, 11.4% of AECB, 7.2% for asthma & 5.4% for CHF in pts ≥65 yrs of age (*NEJM 352:1749, 2005*). RSV caused 11% of clinically important respiratory illnesses in military recruits (*CID 41:311, 2005*). |
| **Prevention of RSV in:**<br>(1) Children <24 mos. old with chronic lung disease of prematurity (formerly broncho-pulmonary dysplasia) requiring supplemental O₂ or<br>(2) Premature infants (<32 wks gestation) and <6 mos. old at start of RSV season or<br>(3) Children with selected congenital heart diseases | **Palivizumab** (Synagis) 15 mg per kg IM q month Nov-Apr.<br>See *Pediatrics 126:e16, 2010.* | Expense argues against its use. Guidance from the Academy of Pediatrics recommends use of Palivizumab only in newborn infants born at 29 weeks gestation (or earlier) and in special populations (e.g., infants with significant heart disease) (*Pediatrics 2014;134:415–420*). |

* See page 2 for abbreviations. NOTE: All dosage recommendations are for adults (unless otherwise indicated) and assume normal renal function.

**TABLE 14A (11)**

| VIRUS/DISEASE | DRUG/DOSAGE | SIDE EFFECTS/COMMENTS |
|---|---|---|
| **Respiratory Syncytial Virus (RSV)** *(continued)* | | |
| **Rhinovirus (Colds)**<br>*See Infect Dis Clin N Amer 2017;31:455; Chest 2017;152:1021.*<br>Found in 1/2 of children with community-acquired pneumonia; role in pathogenesis unclear *(CID 39:681, 2004).*<br>High rate of rhinovirus identified in children with significant lower resp tract infections *(Ped Inf Dis 28:337, 2009).* | No antiviral rx indicated *(Ped Ann 34:53, 2005).*<br>Symptomatic rx:<br>• **Ipratropium bromide** nasal (2 sprays per nostril tid)<br>• **Clemastine** 1.34 mg 1–2 tab po bid-tid (OTC).<br>• Oral zinc preparations reduce duration of symptoms by ~1 day; does not reduce severity of symptoms *(JAMA 31:1440, 2014).*<br><br>Avoid intranasal zinc products *(see Comment).* | Sx relief: ipratropium nasal spray ↓ rhinorrhea and sneezing vs placebo *(AnIM 125:89, 1996).* Clemastine (an antihistamine) ↓ sneezing, rhinorrhea but associated with dry nose, mouth & throat in 6–19% *(CID 22:656, 1996).* **Echinacea** didn't work *(CID 38:1367, 2004 & 4:807, 2005),* put it to rest!<br>Public health advisory advising that three over-the-counter cold remedy products containing **zinc** (e.g., Zicam) should not be used because of multiple reports of permanent anosmia *(www.fda.gov/Safety/MedWatch/SafetyInformation/SafetyAlertsforHumanMedicalProducts/ucm166996.htm).* |
| **Rotavirus:** Leading recognized cause of diarrhea-related illness among infants and children world-wide and kills ½ million children annually. | **No antiviral rx available;** oral hydration life-saving. | **Two live-attenuated vaccines highly effective (85 and 98%)** and safe in preventing rotavirus diarrhea and hospitalization *(NEJM 354:1 & 23, 2006).* ACIP recommends either of the two vaccines, RV1 or RV5, for infants *(MMWR 58(RR02):1, 2009).* |
| **Smallpox** *(NEJM 346:1300, 2002)* | Smallpox vaccine (if within 4 days of exposure) + **Tecovirimat** (Tpoxx) 600 mg (three 200 mg capsules) po bid x 14 days OR **cidofovir** (dosage uncertain but likely similar to CMV) 5 mg/kg IV once weekly for 2 weeks followed by once weekly dosing. Must be used with hydration and Probenecid; contact CDC: 770-488-7100. | |
| **Contact vaccinia** *(JAMA 288:1901, 2002)* | From vaccination: Progressive vaccinia—vaccinia immune globulin may be of benefit. To obtain immune globulin, contact CDC: 770-488-7100. *(CID 39:759, 819, 2004)* | |
| **West Nile virus:** *See page 179* | | |
| **Zika Virus:** Mosquito (Aedes sp.) transmitted flavivirus<br>CDC updates at: *http://www.cdc.gov/zika/index.html* | No treatment available. Symptomatic support (avoid aspirin, NSAIDs until Dengue ruled out.<br>Most serious manifestation of infection is **congenital birth defect(s):** microcephaly and fetal demise.<br>Sexual transmission occurs. For preconception counseling and prevention, see *MMWR 65(39):1077, 2016.* | 3-7 day incubation. Asymptomatic infection most often; when symptoms occur, usually consists of low grade fever, arthralgias, morbilliform rash, and / or conjunctival redness (non-purulent conjunctivitis). Duration of symptoms ranges from a few days to one week. Rare Guillain-Barré syndrome. Hospitalization is infrequent, fatalities are very rare. |

* *See page 2 for abbreviations.   NOTE: All dosage recommendations are for adults (unless otherwise indicated) and assume normal renal function.*

# TABLE 14B - ANTIVIRAL DRUGS (NON-HIV)

| DRUG NAME(S) GENERIC (TRADE) | DOSAGE/ROUTE IN ADULTS* | COMMENTS/ADVERSE EFFECTS |
|---|---|---|
| **CMV** | | |
| Cidofovir (Vistide) | 5 mg per kg IV once weekly for 2 weeks, then once every other week. **Properly timed IV prehydration with normal saline & Probenecid must be used with each cidofovir infusion:** 2 gm in 3 hrs before each dose and further 1 gm in doses 2 & 8 hrs after completion of the cidofovir infusion. Renal function (serum creatinine and urine protein) must be monitored prior to each dose (see *pkg insert for details*). Contraindicated (cases of renal failure & fatality) if CrCl ≤55 mL/min or urine protein ≥100 mg/dL. | **Adverse effects: Nephrotoxicity:** dose-dependent proximal tubular injury (Fanconi-like syndrome): proteinuria, glycosuria, bicarbonaturia, phosphaturia, polyuria (nephrogenic diabetic insipidus, ↑ creatinine. Concomitant saline prehydration, probenecid, extended dosing intervals allow use but still highly nephrotoxic. Other major toxicities: neutropenia (give G-CSF as needed); eye: monthly intra-ocular pressure. Dc cidofovir if pressure decreases 50% or uveitis occurs. **Black Box warning.** Renal impairment: can occur after ≤2 doses. Contraindicated in pts receiving concomitant nephrotoxic agents. Monitor for CMV retinitis in HIV pts. Carcinogenic/teratogenic (causes ↓ in sperm and ↓ fertility). Indicated for only CMV retinitis in HIV pts. **Comment:** Dose must be reduced or discontinued if changes in renal function occur during rx. For ↑ of ↑ of 0.3-0.4 mg per dL in serum creatinine, cidofovir dose must be ↓ from 5 to 3 mg per kg; discontinue cidofovir if ↑ of 0.5 mg per dL above baseline or 3+ proteinuria develops (for 2+ proteinuria, observe pts carefully and consider discontinuation). |
| Foscarnet (Foscavir) | Induction: 90 mg per kg IV, over 1.5-2 hours, q12h OR 60 mg per kg, over 1 hour, q8h Maintenance: 90 –120 mg per kg IV, over 2 hours, q24h Dosage adjustment with renal dysfunction (See *Table 17A*). | Use infusion pump to control rate of administration. **Adverse effects: Major toxicity is renal impairment (1/3 of patients).** Can cause infusion-related ionized hypocalcemia: manifests as arrhythmia, paresthesia, changes in mental status. Slow infusion rate and avoid drugs that lower Ca++, e.g., pentamidine. →↑ creatinine, proteinuria, nephrogenic diabetes insipidus, ↓K+, ↓Ca++, ↓ Mg++. Adequate hydration may ↓ toxicity. Other: headache, mild (100%); fatigue (100%), nausea (30%), fever (25%). CNS: seizures. Hemato: ↓ WBC, ↓ Hgb. Hepatic: liver function tests ↑. Neuropathy. Penile and oral ulcers. |
| Ganciclovir (Cytovene) | IV: 5 mg per kg q12h times 14 days (induction) 5 mg per kg IV q24h or 6 mg per kg 5 times per wk (maintenance) Dosage adjust. with renal dysfunction (See *Table 17A*). | **Adverse effects: Black Box warnings:** cytopenias, carcinogenicity/teratogenicity & aspermia in animals. Absolute neutrophil count dropped below 500 per mm³ in 15%, thrombocytopenia 21%, anemia 6%. Fever 48%. GI 50%: nausea, vomiting, diarrhea, abdominal pain 19%; rash 10%. Confusion, headache, psychiatric disturbances and seizures. Neutropenia may respond to granulocyte colony stimulating factor (G-CSF) or ↓ in dose. Severe myelosuppression may be ↑ with co-administration of zidovudine or azathioprine. 32% dc/interrupt therapy due to toxicity, principally for neutropenia. Avoid extravasation. |
| Letermovir (Prevymis) | 480 mg po/IV once daily starting between days 0-28 post-transplant & continuing to day 100 | **Adverse effects:** N/V, diarrhea, peripheral edema, cough, headache, abdominal pain **Drug interactions:** if concomitant cyclosporine, reduce dose to 240 mg once daily. Avoid if severe hepatic impairment. |
| Valganciclovir (Valcyte) | 450 mg tablets; take with food. Oral solution: 50 mg/mL. Adult dose 900 mg. Treatment (induction): 900 mg po q12h with food; Prophylaxis (maintenance): 900 mg po q24h. Dosage adjustment for renal dysfunction (See *Table 17A*). | A prodrug of ganciclovir with better bioavailability than oral ganciclovir: 60% with food. Preg cat: C (may be teratogenic, contraceptive precaution for females). **Adverse effects:** Similar to ganciclovir. May cause dose limiting neutropenia, anemia, thrombocytopenia. Acute renal failure may occur. Diarrhea (16-41%), nausea (8-30%), vomiting (3-21%). CMV retinitis (sight-threatening lesions): 900 mg po q12h + intravitreal Ganciclovir: 900 mg po q12h x 14-21 days, then 900 mg po q24h for maintenance. |
| **Herpesvirus** | | |
| Acyclovir (Zovirax or generic) | Doses: see *Table 14A* for various indications 400 mg or 800 mg tab 200 mg cap Suspension 200 mg per 5 mL Ointment or cream 5% IV injection Dosage adjustment for renal dysfunction (See *Table 17A*). | **po:** Generally well-tolerated with occ. diarrhea, vertigo, arthralgia. Less frequent rash, fatigue, insomnia, fever, menstrual abnormalities, acne, sore throat, muscle cramps, lymphadenopathy. **IV:** Phlebitis, caustic with vesicular lesions with IV infiltration. **IV or po:** Renal (5%): ↑ creatinine, hematuria. With high doses may crystallize in renal tubules → obstructive uropathy (rapid infusion, dehydration, renal insufficiency and ↑ dose ↑ risk). Adequate pre-hydration may prevent such nephrotoxicity. Hepatic: ↑ ALT, AST. Uncommon: neutropenia, rash, diaphoresis, hypotension, headache, nausea. **Neurotoxic:** hallucination, death delusions, involuntary movements. To avoid, lower dose if renal impairment (AJM 128:692, 2015). |

*See page 2 for abbreviations.     NOTE: All dosage recommendations are for adults (unless otherwise indicated) and assume normal renal function.

**TABLE 14B (2)**

| DRUG NAME(S) GENERIC (TRADE)* | DOSAGE/ROUTE IN ADULTS* | COMMENTS/ADVERSE EFFECTS |
|---|---|---|
| **Herpesvirus** *(contin'ued)* | | |
| Famciclovir (Famvir) | 125 mg, 250 mg, 500 mg tabs. Dosage depends on indication. *(See label and Table 14A.)* | Metabolized to penciclovir. **Adverse effects:** similar to acyclovir; included headache, nausea, diarrhea, and dizziness but incidence does not differ from placebo. May be taken without regard to meals. Dose should be reduced if CrCl <60 mL per min *(see package insert & Table 14A, page 181 & Table 17A, page 246)*. May be taken with or without food. |
| Penciclovir (Denavir) | Topical 1% cream | Apply to area of recurrence of herpes labialis with start of sx, then q2h while awake times 4 days. Well tolerated. |
| Trifluridine (Viroptic) | Topical 1% solution 1 drop q2h (max. 9 drops/day) until corneal re-epithelialization, then dose is ↓ to 1 drop q4h for at least 5 drops/day), not to exceed 21 days, total rx. | Mild burning (5%), palpebral edema (3%), punctate keratopathy, stromal edema. For HSV keratoconjunctivitis or recurrent epithelial keratitis. |
| Valacyclovir (Valtrex) | 500 mg, 1 gm tabs. Dosage depends on indication and renal function *(see label, Table 14A & Table 17A)*. | An ester pro-drug of acyclovir that is well-absorbed, bioavailability 3–5 times greater than acyclovir. **Adverse effects** similar to acyclovir. Thrombotic thrombocytopenic purpura/hemolytic uremic syndrome reported in pts with advanced HIV disease and transplant recipients participating in clinical trials at doses of 8 gm per day. Death delusion with high serum levels. |
| Valganciclovir (Valcyte) | 450 mg tablets; take with food. Oral solution: 50 mg/mL. Adult dose 900 mg. Treatment (induction): 900 mg po q12h with food; Prophylaxis (maintenance): 900 mg po q24h. Dosage adjustment for renal dysfunction *(See Table 17A)*. | A prodrug of ganciclovir with better bioavailability than oral ganciclovir; 60% with food. Preg cat: C (may be teratogenic, contraceptive precaution for females). **Adverse effects:** Similar to ganciclovir. May cause dose limiting neutropenia, anemia, thrombocytopenia. Acute renal failure may occur. Diarrhea (16–41%), nausea (8–30%), vomiting (3-21%). CMV retinitis (sight-threatening lesions): 900 mg po q12h + intravitreal Ganciclovir: 900 mg po q12h x 14-21 days, then 900 mg po q24h for maintenance. |
| **Hepatitis B** | | |
| Adefovir dipivoxil (Hepsera) | 10 mg po q24h (with normal CrCl) 10 mg tab | It is an acyclic nucleotide analog with activity against hepatitis B (HBV) at 0.2–2.5 mM (IC$_{50}$). *See Table 9* for Cmax & T½. Active against lamivudine-resistant HBV strains and in vitro vs. entecavir- resistant strains. To minimize resistance, use in combination with lamivudine for lamivudine-resistant virus; consider alternative therapy if viral load remains >1,000 copies/mL with treatment. Primarily renal excretion—adjust dose. No food interactions. Generally few side effects, but **Black Box warning** regarding lactic acidosis/hepatic steatosis with nucleoside analogs. At 10 mg per day potential for delayed nephrotoxicity. Monitor renal function, esp. with pre-existing or other risks for renal impairment. Pregnancy Category C. **Hepatitis may exacerbate when treatment discontinued;** Up to 25% of pts developed ALT ↑ 10 times normal within 12 wks; usually responds to re-treatment or self-limited, but hepatic decompensation has occurred. **Do not use adefovir in HIV infected patients.** |
| Entecavir (Baraclude) | 0.5 mg q24h, if refractory or resistant to lamivudine or telbivudine: 1 mg per day Tabs: 0.5 mg & 1 mg. Oral solution: 0.05 mg/mL. Administer on an empty stomach. | A nucleoside analog active against HBV including lamivudine-resistant mutants. Minimal adverse effects reported; headache, fatigue, dizziness, & nausea reported in 22% of pts. Alopecia, anaphylactoid reactions reported. Potential for lactic acidosis and exacerbation of hepB at discontinuation **(Black Box warning)**. Do not use as single anti-retroviral agent in HIV co-infected pts; M134 mutation can emerge *(NEJM 356-2674, 2007)*. Adjust dosage in renal impairment *(see Table 17A, page 244)*. |
| Lamivudine (3TC) (Epivir-HBV) | **HBV dose:** 100 mg po q24h Dosage adjustment with renal dysfunction *(see label)*. Tabs 100 mg and oral solution 5 mg/mL. | **Black Box warnings:** caution; lactic acidosis/hepatic steatosis; severe exacerbation of liver disease can occur on or dc. YMDD-mutants resistant to lamivudine may emerge on treatment. Dose is lower than HIV dose, so must exclude co-infection with HIV before using this formulation; lactic acidosis/hepatic steatosis. **Adverse effects:** See Table 14D. |

*See page 2 for abbreviations.  NOTE: All dosage recommendations are for adults (unless otherwise indicated) and assume normal renal function.

**TABLE 14B (3)**

| DRUG NAME(S) GENERIC (TRADE) | DOSAGE/ROUTE IN ADULTS* | COMMENTS/ADVERSE EFFECTS |
|---|---|---|
| **Hepatitis B** (continued) | | |
| Telbivudine (Tyzeka) | **HBV:** 600 mg orally q24h, without regard to food. Dosage adjustment with renal dysfunction, Ccr <50 mL/min (see label). 600 mg tabs; 100 mg per 5 mL. solution. | An oral nucleoside analog approved for Rx of Hep B. It has ↑ rates of response and superior viral suppression than lamivudine (NEJM 357:2576, 2007). **Black Box warnings** regarding lactic acidosis/hepatic steatosis with nucleosides and potential for severe exacerbation of HepB on dc. Generally well-tolerated with a mitochondrial toxicity observed (Medical Letter 49:11, 2007). Myalgias, abdominal pain, increased CK with occasional myopathy and rhabdomyolysis reported. Peripheral neuropathy. Genotypic resistance rate was 4.4% by one yr, ↑ to 21.9% by 2 yrs of rx of eAg+ pts. Selects for YMDD mutation like lamivudine. Combination with lamivudine was inferior to monotherapy (Hepatology 45:507, 2007). |
| Tenofovir (TDF/TAF) | See page 208 | |
| **Hepatitis C** - (For all HCV direct acting agents (DAA) a **Black Box warning** exists regarding potential flare of HBV in those coinfected with HBV and HCV.) | | |
| **Direct Acting Agents:** | | |
| Daclatasvir (Daklinza) | 60 mg 1 tab po once daily (dose adjustment when used with CYP 3A4 inhibitors / inducers) | Contraindicated with strong CYP3A inducers, e.g., phenytoin, carbamazepine, Rifampin, St. John's wort. Most common AEs: headache and fatigue. Bradycardia when administered in combination with Sofosbuvir and Amiodarone. **Co-administration with Amiodarone not recommended.** If used, cardiac monitoring advised. |
| Elbasvir + Grazoprevir (Zepatier) | Combination formulation (Elbasvir 50 mg + Grazoprevir 100 mg) 1 tab po once daily | NS5A and NS3-4a PI inhibitors with activity against genotypes 1 and 4. Contraindicated in patients with moderate or severe hepatic impairment (Child-Pugh Class B or C). Also contraindicated with concomitant use of organic ion transporter polypeptide 1B (OATP1B) inhibitors, strong inducers of cytochrome P450 3A (CYP3A), and efavirenz. |
| Glecaprevir + Pibrentasvir (Mavyret) | Combination formulation (Glecaprevir 100 mg + Pibrentasvir 40 mg) 3 tabs po once daily with food | Contraindicated if severe hepatic impairment (Child-Pugh C). **Do not co-administer with Atazanavir or Rifampin.** Most common AEs: headache and fatigue. |
| Ledipasvir + Sofosbuvir (Harvoni); Velpatasvir + Sofosbuvir (Epclusa); Voxilaprevir + Velpatasvir + Sofosbuvir (Vosevi) | Combination formulations: (Ledipasvir 90 mg + Sofosbuvir 400 mg) 1 tab po once daily; (Velpatasvir 100 mg + Sofosbuvir 400 mg) 1 tab po daily; (Velpatasvir 100 mg + Voxilaprevir 100 mg + Sofosbuvir 400 mg) 1 tab po once daily with food | NS5A/NS5B inhibitor combination for Genotype 1 HCV. First agent for HCV treatment without Ribavirin or Interferon. No dose adjustment for mild/moderate renal or hepatic impairment. Most common AEs: fatigue (16%), headache (14%), nausea (7%), diarrhea (3%), insomnia (5%). Antacids and H2 blockers interfere with absorption of ledipasvir. The drug solubility decreases as pH increases. Recommended to separate administration of ledipasvir and antacid Rx by at least 4 hours. |
| Paritaprevir + Ritonavir + Dasabuvir + Ombitasvir (ProD) (Viekira Pak); Paritaprevir + Ritonavir + Ombitasvir (Technivie) | Ombitasvir 12.5 mg, Paritaprevir 75 mg, and Ritonavir 50 mg co-packaged with tablets of Dasabuvir 250 mg (Viekira Pak) or without Dasabuvir (Technivie) | Do not co-administer with drugs that are highly dependent on CYP3A for clearance; strong inducers of CYP3A and CYP2C8; and strong inhibitors of CYP2C8. Do not use if known hypersensitivity to Ritonavir (e.g., toxic epidermal necrolysis, Stevens-Johnson syndrome). If used with Ribavirin: fatigue, nausea, pruritus, other skin reactions, insomnia and asthenia. When used without Ribavirin: nausea, pruritus and insomnia. **Warning: Hepatic decompensation and hepatic failure, including liver transplantation or fatal outcomes, have been reported mostly in patients with advanced cirrhosis.** |
| Simeprevir (Olysio) | 150 mg 1 cap po once daily with food + both Ribavirin and Interferon | NS3/4A inhibitor. Need to screen patients with HCV genotype 1a for the Q80K polymorphism; if present consider alternative therapy. Contraindicated in pregnancy and in men whose female partners are pregnant (risk category C); concern is combination with ribavirin (risk category X). No dose adjustment required in patients with mild, moderate or severe renal impairment; no dose adjustment for mild hepatic impairment. Most common AEs (in combination with Ribavirin, Interferon): rash, pruritus, nausea. CYP3A inhibitors affect plasma concentration of Simeprevir. |
| Sofosbuvir (Sovaldi) | 400 mg 1 tab po once daily with food + both Pegylated Interferon and Ribavirin. For combination formulation, see Led/pasvir. | NS5B inhibitor for Genotypes 1, 2, 3, 4 HCV. Efficacy established in patients awaiting liver transplant and in patients with HIV-1/HCV co-infection. No adjustment needed for mild to moderate renal impairment. No dose adjustment for mild, moderate, or severe hepatic impairment. Most common AEs (in combination with interferon and ribavirin): fatigue, headache, nausea, insomnia, anemia. Rifampin and St. John's wort may alter concentrations of Sofosbuvir. |

\* See page 2 for abbreviations.

*NOTE: All dosage recommendations are for adults (unless otherwise indicated) and assume normal renal function.*

TABLE 14B (4)

| DRUG NAME(S) GENERIC (TRADE) | DOSAGE/ROUTE IN ADULTS* | COMMENTS/ADVERSE EFFECTS |
|---|---|---|
| **Hepatitis C** (continued) | | |
| **Other:** | | |
| **Interferon alfa is available as alfa-2a and alfa-2b** (Roferon-A), **alfa-2b** (Intron-A). | For HCV combination therapy, usual Roferon-A and Intron-A doses are 3 million international units 3x weekly subQ. | Depending on agent, available in pre-filled syringes, vials of solution, or powder. **Black Box warnings:** can cause/aggravate psychiatric illness, autoimmune disorders, ischemic events, infection. Withdraw therapy if any of these suspected. |
| **PEG interferon alfa-2b** (PEG-Intron) | 0.5–1.5 mcg/kg subQ q wk | **Adverse effects: Flu-like syndrome** is common, esp. during 1st wk of rx: fever 98%, fatigue 89%, myalgia 73%, headache 71%. **Gi:** anorexia 46%, diarrhea 29%, dizziness 21%. **CNS:** dizziness 21%. Hemorrhagic or ischemic stroke. Rash 18% may progress to Stevens Johnson or exfoliative dermatitis. Alopecia. ↑ TSH, autoimmune thyroid disorders with ↓ or ↑ thyroidism. **Hemat:** ↓ WBC 49%, ↓ Hgb 27%, ↓ platelets 35%. Post-marketing reports of antibody-mediated pure red cell aplasia in patients receiving interferon/ribavirin with erythropoiesis-stimulating agents. |
| **Pegylated-40k interferon alfa-2a** (Pegasys) | 180 mcg subQ q wk | Acute reversible hearing loss &/or tinnitus in up to 1/3 (Ln 343/134, 1994). Optic neuropathy (retinal hemorrhage, cotton wool spots, ↓ in color vision) reported (AIDS 18/1805, 2004). Doses may require adjustment (or ↓) based on individual response or adverse events, and can vary by product. Indication (eg, HCV or HBV) and mode of use (mono- or combination-rx). (Refer to labels of individual products and to ribavirin if used in combination for details of use.) |
| **Ribavirin** (Rebetol, Copegus) | For use with an interferon for hepatitis C. Available as 200 mg caps and 40 mg/mL oral solution (Rebetol) or 200 mg and 400 mg tabs (Copegus) (See Comments regarding dosage). | **Black Box warnings:** ribavirin monotherapy of HCV is ineffective; hemolytic anemia may precipitate cardiac events; teratogenic/ embryocidal. (**Preg Category X**). Drug may persist for 6 mos, avoid pregnancy for at least 6 mos after end of rx of women & **their partners.** Only approved for pts with Ccr >50 mL/min. Do not use in pts with severe heart disease or hemoglobinopathies. ARDS reported (Chest 124:406, 2003). **Adverse effects:** hemolytic anemia (may require dose reduction or ↓). Additive cardiac/periodontal disorders, and all adverse effects of concomitant interferon used (see above). Postmarketing: retinal detachment, ↓ hearing, hypersensitivity reactions. See Table 14A for specific regimens, but dosing depends on: interferon used, weight, HCV genotype, and is modified (↓) or based on side effects (especially degree of hemolysis), with different criteria in those with/without cardiac disease). **Initial Rebetol dose with Intron A (interferon alfa-2b) is wt-based:** 400 mg am & 600 mg pm for wt ≤75 kg, and 600 mg am & 600 mg pm for wt >75 kg, but with Pegintron approved dose is 400 mg am & 400 mg pm with meals. Doses and duration of Copegus with peg-interferon alfa-2a are less in pts with genotype 2 or 3 (800 mg per day divided into 2 doses, for 24 wks) than with genotypes 1 or 4 (1000 mg per day divided into 2 doses for wt ≤75 kg and 1200 mg per day divided into 2 doses for >75 kg for 48 wks); in HIV/HCV co-infected pts, dose is 800 mg per day regardless of genotype. (See individual labels for details, including initial dosing and criteria for dose modification in those with/without cardiac disease.) |
| **Influenza A** | | |
| **Amantadine** (Symmetrel) or **Rimantadine** (Flumadine) Influenza A is intrinsically resistant and most circulating Influenza A is resistant. | **Amantadine** 100 mg caps, tabs; 50 mg/mL oral solution & syrup. Treatment or prophylaxis: 100 mg bid; or 100 mg daily if age ≥65 y; dose reductions with CrCl starting at ≤50 mL/min. **Rimantadine** 100 mg tabs, 50 mg/5 mL syrup. Treatment or prophylaxis: 100 mg bid or 100 mg daily in elderly nursing home pts, or severe hepatic disease, or CrCl <10 mL/min. For children, rimantadine only approved for prophylaxis. | **Side-effects/toxicity: CNS** (can be mild: nervousness, anxiety, difficulty concentrating, and lightheadedness). Serious: delirium, hallucinations, and seizures—are associated with high plasma drug levels resulting from renal insufficiency, esp. in older pts, those with prior seizure disorders, or psychiatric disorders. |

* See page 2 for abbreviations.  NOTE: All dosage recommendations are for adults (unless otherwise indicated) and assume normal renal function.

**TABLE 14B (5)**

| DRUG NAME(S) GENERIC (TRADE) | DOSAGE/ROUTE IN ADULTS* | COMMENTS/ADVERSE EFFECTS |
|---|---|---|
| **Influenza A and B—For both drugs, initiate within 48 hrs of symptom onset** | | |
| Baloxavir marboxil (Xofluza) | For age ≥12 yrs & within 48 hr of symptoms onset.<br>Wt 40-80 kg: 40 mg po x 1 dose<br>Wt ≥80 kg: 80 mg po x 1 dose | FDA indicated for uncomplicated influenza. One trial demonstrated efficacy in high risk patients with similar efficacy against flu A and superior activity against flu B. Active against oseltamivir-resistant influenza. Compared to oseltamivir, faster reduction in viral load in airway and, if Influenza B, faster clinical recovery.<br>Distinct mechanism of action: inhibits viral endonuclease. Cost: $150 per dose compared to $50 for 5 days of oseltamivir.<br>**AEs:** diarrhea (3%) headache (1%), nausea (1%) |
| Zanamivir (Relenza)<br>For pts ≥ 7 yrs of age (treatment) or<br>≥5 yrs (prophylaxis) | Powder is inhaled by specially designed inhalation device. Each blister contains 5 mg zanamivir. **Treatment:** oral inhalation of 2 blisters (10 mg) bid for 5 days. **Prophylaxis:** oral inhalation of 2 blisters (10 mg) once daily for 10 days (household outbreak) to 28 days (community outbreak). | Active by inhalation against neuraminidase of both influenza A and B and inhibits release of virus from epithelial cells of respiratory tract. Approx. 4–17% of inhaled dose absorbed into plasma. Excreted by kidney but with low absorption, dose reduction not necessary in renal impairment. Minimal side-effects: <3% cough, sinusitis, diarrhea, nausea and vomiting. **Reports of respiratory adverse events in pts with or without h/o airways disease, should be avoided in pts with underlying respiratory disease.** Allergic reactions and neuropsychiatric events have been reported.<br>**Caution: do not reconstitute zanamivir powder for use in nebulizers or mechanical ventilators** (MedWatch report of death). **Zanamivir for IV** administration is available for compassionate use through an emergency IND application.<br>Contact GSK: (999-375-5215) for forms, then contact FDA: (301-796-1500 or 301-796-9900). |
| Oseltamivir (Tamiflu)<br>For pts ≥1 yr (treatment or prophylaxis) | For adults: **Treatment,** 75 mg po bid for 5 days; 150 mg po bid has been used for morbidly obese patients but this dose is not FDA-approved. **Prophylaxis,** 75 mg po once daily for 10 days to 6 wks. (See label for pediatric weight-based dosing.) Adjust doses for CrCl ≤30 mL/min. 30 mg, 45 mg, 75 mg caps; powder for oral suspension. | Well absorbed (80% bioavailable) after po dose as ethyl ester of active compound GS 4071. T½ 6–10 hrs; excreted unchanged by kidney. Adverse effects include diarrhea, nausea, vomiting, headache. Nausea ↓ with food. Rarely, severe skin reactions (toxic epidermal necrolysis, Stevens-Johnson syndrome, erythema multiforme). **Delirium & abnormal behavior reported** (CID 48:1003, 2009). No benefit from higher dose in non- critically ill; not recommended (CID 57:1511, 2013). |
| Peramivir (Rapivab) | 600 mg IV single dose<br>(acute uncomplicated influenza) | FDA indication is for single dose use in acute uncomplicated influenza. No approved dose for hospitalized patients or patients on mechanical ventilators. Dose used for hospitalized patients 200–400 mg IV daily for 5 days used in trial. Flu with H275Y oseltamivir resistance has moderate resistance to peramivir. |
| **Pox viruses (Smallpox, Monkeypox)** | | |
| Tecovirimat (Tpoxx) | 600 mg (three 200 mg caps) po bid x 14 days | Inhibitor of the orthopoxvirus VP37 envelope wrapping protein. **No Clinical Trial data in humans** (approval by FDA for smallpox based on animal treatment studies). |
| **Respiratory Syncytial Virus (RSV) monoclonal antibody** | | |
| Palivizumab (Synagis)<br>Used for prevention of RSV infection in high-risk children | 15 mg per kg IM a month throughout RSV season<br>Single dose 100 mg vial | A monoclonal antibody directed against the surface F glycoprotein; **AEs:** uncommon, occ. ↑ ALT. Anaphylaxis <1/7,000 pts; acute hypersensitivity reaction <1/1000. Postmarketing reports: URI, otitis media, fever, ↓ plts, injection site reactions. Preferred over polyclonal immune globulin in high risk infants & children. |
| **Warts Regimens are from drug labels specific for indications, regimens, age limits.** | | |
| Interferon alfa-2b (IntronA) | Injection of 1 million international units into base of lesion, thrice weekly on alternate days for up to 3 wks. Maximum 5 lesions per course. | Interferons may cause "flu-like" illness and other systemic effects. 88% had at least one adverse event.<br>**Black box warning:** alpha interferons may cause or aggravate neuropsychiatric, autoimmune, ischemic or infectious disorders. |
| Interferon alfa-N3 (Alferon N) | Injection of 0.05 mL into base of each wart, up to 0.5 mL total per session, twice weekly for up to 8 weeks. | Flu-like syndrome and hypersensitivity reactions. Contraindicated with allergy to mouse IgG, egg proteins, or neomycin. |
| Imiquimod (Aldara) | 5% cream. Thin layer applied at bedtime, washing off after 6-10 hr, thrice weekly to maximum of 16 wks; 3.75% cream apply qd. | Erythema, itching & burning, erosions. Flu-like syndrome, increased susceptibility to sunburn (avoid UV). |

\* See page 2 for abbreviations.    NOTE: All dosage recommendations are for adults (unless otherwise indicated) and assume normal renal function.

**TABLE 14B (6)**

| DRUG NAME(S) GENERIC (TRADE) | DOSAGE/ROUTE IN ADULTS* | COMMENTS/ADVERSE EFFECTS |
|---|---|---|
| **Warts** *continued* | | |
| Podofilox (Condylox) | 0.5% gel or solution twice daily for 3 days, no therapy for 4 days; can use up to 4 such cycles. | Local reactions—pain, burning, inflammation in 50%. Can ulcerate. Limit surface area treated as per label. |
| Sinecatechins (Veregen) | 15% ointment. Apply 0.5 cm strand to each wart three times per day until healing but not more than 16 weeks. | Application site reactions, which may result in ulcerations, phimosis, meatal stenosis, superinfection. |

# TABLE 14C – ANTIRETROVIRAL THERAPY (ART) IN TREATMENT-NAÏVE ADULTS (HIV/AIDS)

## Overview

- Human immunodeficiency virus (HIV)
- Antiretroviral therapy (ART) in **treatment-naïve adults** (*aidsinfo.nih.gov/guidelines/html/1/adult-and-adolescent-treatment-guidelines/0*)
- Guidelines: *www.aidsinfo.nih.gov; iasusa.org; JAMA 2018; 320-379*

## When to Start ART

- **All patients with HIV regardless of CD4 count** (*NEJM 373-795, 2015; NEJM 373-808, 2015*)
- Only exceptions are:
  - Patient is not ready to start (for personal reasons or lack of commitment to take medications)
  - Patient is an "Elite Controller", i.e., HIV RNA undetectable for extended period without ART. Controversy exists about treating such patients, though many experts suggest ART owing to inflammation resulting from ongoing de novo HIV replication.
  - Many clinics are adopting a "treat now" policy whereby the ARV regimen is started on the first encounter with the clinic. In such instances, resistance tests are obtained and the regimen(s) adjusted as indicated once the resistance test data return.

## What Regimen to Start

- Design a regimen consisting of:

| Dual nucleoside / nucleotide reverse transcriptase inhibitor (**NRTI component**) PLUS either a | Non-nucleoside reverse transcriptase inhibitor (**NNRTI**) OR<br>Protease Inhibitor (**PI**) OR<br>Integrase strand-transfer inhibitor (**INSTI**) |
| --- | --- |

*Note*: Prefer combination that includes Tenofovir-AF over original Tenofovir-DF

**NRTI:** e.g. Tenofovir (TAF or TDF), Abacavir (ABC), Emtricitabine (FTC), or Lamivudine (3TC)
**NNRTI:** e.g., Efavirenz (EFV), Rilpivirine (RPV), or Etravirine (ETV)
**PI:** e.g., Darunavir (DRV) or Atazanavir (ATV) [both boosted with either Ritonavir (*r*) or Cobicistat (Cobi)]
**INSTI:** e.g., Bictegravir (BIC), Dolutegravir (DTG), Elvitegravir (ETG), or Raltegravir (RAL)

- Selection of components is influenced by many factors, including:
  - Results of viral resistance testing
  - **Pregnancy:** EFV is now permitted for use in pregnancy; DTG and TAF not recommended yet for pregnant women owing to higher drug levels in fetus and reports of higher than expected neural tube defects in newborn with dolutegravir (DOI: 10.1056/NEJMc1807653, 2018)
  - Potential drug interactions or adverse drug effects; special focus on tolerability (even low grade side effects can profoundly affect adherence)
  - Co-morbidities (e.g., lipid effects of PIs, liver or renal disease, cardiovascular disease risk, chemical dependency, psychiatric disease)
  - Convenience of dosing. Co-formulations increase convenience, but sometimes prescribing the two constituents individually is preferred, as when dose-adjustments are needed for renal disease
  - HLA-B5701 testing required prior to using ABC

TABLE 14C (2)

## RECOMMENDED AND ALTERNATIVE TREATMENT REGIMENS FOR HIV INFECTED ADULTS

| | Frequency & Formulation | Drug/Dose | Components | Comments |
|---|---|---|---|---|
| Recommended | Once daily, single tablet | **Biktarvy** 1 tablet once daily | Bictegravir (BIC) + FTC + TAF | |
| | | **Triumeq** 1 tablet once daily | ABC + 3TC + DTV | Only if HLA-B* 5701 neg (See Warnings) |
| | Once daily, separate tablets | **Descovy + Dolutegravir** 1 tablet each once daily | (FTC + TAF) + DTV | |
| Alternative | Once daily, single tablet combinations | **Atripla** 1 tablet once daily ghs | TDF + FTC + EFV | |
| | | **Complera/Eviplera** 1 tablet once daily with food | FTC + TDF + RPV | Avoid when VL >100,000 cells/mL |
| | | **Delstrigo** 1 tablet once daily | Doravirine (DOR) + 3TC + TDF | |
| | | **Genvoya** 1 tablet once daily | EVG + Cobi + FTC + TAF | |
| | | **Odefsey** 1 tablet once daily | FTC + TAF + RPV | |
| | | **Stribild** 1 tablet once daily | EVG + Cobi + FTC + TDF | |
| | | **Symtuza** 1 tablet once daily | DRV + Cobi + FTC + TAF | |
| Alternative | NNRTI-based, multi-tablet | **Efavirenz** (EFV) 1 tablet once daily + (**Descovy** or **Truvada** or **Epzicom/Kivexa**) 1 tablet once daily | **Descovy:** FTC + TAF; **Truvada:** FTC + TDF; **Epzicom/Kivexa:** ABC + 3TC; **Evotaz:** ATV + Cobi; /r: Ritonavir boosted; **Prezcobix:** DRV + Cobi | Epzicom/Kivexa: take ghs. Avoid when VL >100,000 cells/mL. Use only if HLA-B* 5701 neg; see Warnings. Rilpivirine-based regimens should not be used in patients with VL > 100,000 c/mL (except if RPV is used with DTG) |
| | | **Rilpivirine** (RPV) 1 tablet once daily + (**Descovy** or **Truvada** or **Epzicom/Kivexa**) 1 tablet once daily | | |
| | | **Doravirine** 1 tablet once daily + (**Descovy** or **Truvada** or **Epzicom/Kivexa**) 1 tablet once daily | | |
| | PI-based (boosted), multi-tablet | **Evotaz** 1 tablet once daily + (**Descovy** or **Truvada** or **Epzicom/Kivexa**) 1 tablet once daily | | |
| | | **Atazanavir/r** 1 tablet once daily + (**Descovy** or **Truvada** or **Epzicom/Kivexa**) 1 tablet once daily | | |
| | | **Prezcobix** 1 tablet once daily + (**Descovy** or **Truvada** or **Epzicom/Kivexa**) 1 tablet once daily | | |
| | | **Darunavir/r** 1 tablet once daily + (**Descovy** or **Truvada** or **Epzicom/Kivexa**) 1 tablet once daily | | |
| | INSTI-based, multi-tablet | **Descovy** 1 tablet once daily + **Raltegravir** (RAL) 600 mg 2 tablets once daily | | |
| | | **Truvada + Dolutegravir** (DTG) 1 tablet each once daily | | |
| | | **Epzicom/Kivexa + DTG** 1 tablet each once daily | | |
| | Dual therapy | **DTG + (3TC** or **FTC)** 1 tablet each once daily | | |
| | | **DTG + RPV** 1 tablet each once daily | | |

## TABLE 14C (3)

### Legend, Warnings and Notes Regarding Regimens

- Legend
  - **NNRTI** = Non-nucleoside reverse transcriptase inhibitor
  - **PI** = Protease inhibitor
  - **INSTI** = Integrase strand-transfer inhibitor
- Warnings
  - Epzicom/Kivexa (ABC/3TC) containing regimens: Use only in patients who are HLA-B5701 negative.
  - Use ABC with caution in those with HIV RNA > 100,000 c/mL at baseline (this does not apply when DTG is the anchor drug of the regimen).
- Notes
  - Co-formulations increase convenience, but sometimes prescribing the components individually is preferred, e.g., when dose adjustments are needed for renal impairment.
  - Rilpivirine (RPV) with 2 nucleosides should be used only in patients with a baseline HIV RNA level < 100,000 c/mL. However, RPV can be used in combination with DTG in those with > 100,000 c/mL.
  - Higher rates of renal dysfunction occur when TDF is combined with boosted PIs; TAF is the preferred drug in this setting. Conversely, TDF does not have nearly as much renal toxicity when paired with non-boosted PI drugs.
  - RAL reformulated as 600 mg tablet. Preferred dose is 2 tablets (1200 mg) once daily.

### Other drugs that may be used in selected populations (typically not used as initial therapy)

- FDC DTG/RPV can be used to simplify 3-drug regimen to 2-drugs when initial regimen successful (< 50c/ml for > 6 months), no baseline pre-Rx resistance mutations, and no virologic failure.
- ETV and RPV are options for some patients who have NNRTI resistance mutations, e.g., K103N, at baseline. Expert consultation is recommended.
- Boosted PIs can be administered once or twice daily.
- Both Ritonavir and Cobicistat are available as PI-boosting agents.
- Non-boosted PIs are no longer recommended.

### Pregnancy Considerations

- Timing of initiation of therapy and drug choice must be individualized.
- Viral resistance testing should be performed.
- Long-term effects of agents is unknown.
- Efavirenz is a permitted alternative in pregnancy.
- DTG, BIC, Cobi, and TAF based regimens should NOT be used in pregnancy until further data are available.
- If recommended drugs are not available, remember that certain drugs are contraindicated, e.g., Didanosine plus Stavudine.

### Other Special Populations

- Primary (acute) HIV (INSTI preferred).
- Hepatitis B/C co-infection (See Table 14E & 14F) (Should always use a TDF or TAF-based regimen).
- Opportunistic infection (Treat early in course of Rx or OI; use DTG or BIC if possible owing to fewer drug-drug interactions).

## TABLE 14C (4)

### Selected Characteristics of Antiretroviral Drugs (*CPE = CSF penetration effectiveness; 1-4)

1. **Selected Characteristics of Nucleoside or Nucleotide Reverse Transcriptase Inhibitors (NRTIs)**

All agents have Black Box warning: Risk of lactic acidosis/hepatic steatosis. Also, risk of fat redistribution/accumulation. For combinations, *see warnings for component agents.*

\* **CPE (CNS Penetration Effectiveness) value:** 1= Low Penetration; 2 - 3 = Intermediate Penetration; 4 = Highest Penetration into CNS (*AIDS 25:357, 2011*)

| Generic/ Trade Name | Pharmaceutical Prep. | Usual Adult Dosage & Food Effect | % Absorbed, po | Serum T½ hrs | Intracellular T½ hrs | CPE* | Elimination | Major Adverse Events/Comments (See *Table 14D*) |
|---|---|---|---|---|---|---|---|---|
| **Abacavir** (ABC, Ziagen) | 300 mg tabs or 20 mg/mL oral solution | 300 mg po bid or 600 mg po q24h. Food OK | 83 | 1.5 | 20 | 1 | Liver metab., renal excretion of metabolites, 82% | **Hypersensitivity reaction:** fever, rash, N/V, malaise, diarrhea, abdominal pain, respiratory symptoms. (Severe reactions may be ↑ with 600 mg dose.) **Do not rechallenge!** Report to 800-270-0425. **Test HLA-B*5701 before use.** See **Comment Table 14D.** Studies raise concerns re ABC/3TC regimens in pts with VL ≥ 100,000 (*www.niaid.nih.gov/news/newsreleases/2008/actg5202bulletin.htm*). Controversy re increased CV events with use of ABC. Large meta-analysis shows no increased risk (*AIDS 61, 441, 2012*) |
| **Abacavir** (ABC)/**lamivudine** (Epzicom or Kivexa) | Film coated tabs: ABC 600 mg + 3TC 300 mg | 1 tab once daily (not recommended) | | | | | | (See *for individual components*). **Black Box warning**— limited data for VL >100,000 copies/mL. Not recommended as initial therapy because of inferior virologic efficacy. |
| **Abacavir** (ABC)/ **lamivudine** (3TC)/ **dolutegravir** (DTV) (**Triumeq**) | Film coated tabs: ABC 600 mg + 3TC 300 mg + DTV 50 mg | 1 tab po once daily | | | | | | (See individual components) |
| **Abacavir** (ABC)/ **lamivudine** (3TC)/ **zidovudine** (AZT) (**Trizivir**) | Film-coated tabs: ABC 300 mg + 3TC 150 mg + ZDV 300 mg | 1 tab po bid (not recommended for wt <40 kg or CrCl <50 mL/min or impaired hepatic function) | | | | | | |
| **Didanosine** (ddI; Videx or Videx EC) | 125, 200, 250, 400 enteric-coated caps; 100, 167, 250 mg powder for oral solution) | ≥60 kg Usually 400 mg enteric-coated po q24h. 0.5 hr before or 2 hrs after meal. Do not crush; <60 kg: 250 mg EC po q24h. Food ↓ levels. See **Comment** | 30–40 | 1.6 | 25–40 | 2 | Renal excretion, 50% | **Pancreatitis**, peripheral neuropathy, lactic acidosis & hepatic steatosis (rare but life-threatening, esp. combined with stavudine in pregnancy). Retinal, optic nerve changes. **The combination ddI + TDF is generally avoided, but if used, reduce dose of ddI-EC from 400 mg to 250 mg EC q24h (or from 250 mg EC 200 mg) to 125 mg) EC q24h. Monitor for ↑ toxicity & possible ↓ in efficacy of this combination; may result in ↓ CD4.** |
| **Dolutegravir** (DTV)/ **Rilpivirine** (RPV) (Juluca) | Film-coated tabs: DTV 50 mg + RPV 25 mg | 1 tab once daily with meal | | | | | | Contraindicated if prior hypersensitivity reaction to DTV or RPV; do not co-administer with dofetilide or with drugs that significantly decrease RPV plasma concentrations. Warnings: Severe skin and hypersensitivity reactions (rash) and sometimes liver injury reported with DTV and RPV. **Common AEs:** diarrhea and headache. |

**TABLE 14C (5)**

Selected Characteristics of Antiretroviral Drugs (*CPE = CSF penetration effectiveness: 1-4)

1. Selected Characteristics of Nucleoside or Nucleotide Reverse Transcriptase Inhibitors (NRTIs) *(continued)*

| Generic/ Trade Name | Pharmaceutical Prep. | Usual Adult Dosage & Food Effect | % Absorbed, po | Serum T½ hrs | Intracellular T½ hrs | CPE* | Elimination | Major Adverse Events/Comments (See Table 14D) |
|---|---|---|---|---|---|---|---|---|
| Emtricitabine (FTC, Emtriva) | 200 mg caps; 10 mg per mL oral solution. | 200 mg po q24h. Food OK | 93 (caps), 75 (oral soln) | Approx. 10 | 39 | 3 | Renal excretion 86% | Well tolerated; headache, nausea, vomiting & diarrhea occasionally. Skin rash rarely. Skin hyperpigmentation. Differs only slightly in structure from lamivudine (5-fluoro substitution). **Exacerbation of Hep B reported in pts after stopping FTC.** Monitor at least several months after stopping FTC. In Hep B pts; some may need anti-HBV therapy. |
| Emtricitabine/ tenofovir disoproxil fumarate (Truvada) | Film-coated tabs: FTC 200 mg + TDF 300 mg | 1 tab po q24h for CrCl ≥50 mL/min. Food OK | 92/25 | 10/17 | — | *(See Individual components)* | Primarily renal/renal | *See Comments for individual agents* **Black Box warning—Exacerbation of HepB after stopping FTC;** but preferred therapy for those with Hep B/HIV co-infection. |
| Emtricitabine/ Tenofovir/Efavirenz (Atripla) | Film-coated tabs: FTC 200 mg + TDF 300 mg + Efavirenz 600 mg | 1 tab po q24h on an empty stomach, preferably at bedtime. Do not use if CrCl <50 mL/min | | | *(See individual components)* | | | Not recommended for pts <18 yrs. *(See warnings for individual components)* **Exacerbation of Hep B** reported in pts discontinuing component drugs; some need anti-HBV therapy (tenofovir preferred). **Pregnancy category D**- Efavirenz may cause fetal harm. Avoid in pregnancy or in women who may become pregnant. |
| Emtricitabine/ Tenofovir/ Rilpivirine (Complera/Eviplera) | Film-coated tabs: FTC 200 mg + TDF 300 mg + RPL 25 mg | 1 tab po q24h with food | | | *(See individual components)* | | | *See individual components.* Preferred use in pts with HIV RNA level <100,000 c/mL. Should not be used with PPI agents. |
| Lamivudine (3TC, Epivir) | 150, 300 mg tabs; 10 mg/mL oral solution | 150 mg po bid or 300 mg po q24h. Food OK | 86 | 5–7 | 18 | 2 | Renal excretion, minimal metabolism | **Use HIV dose, not Hep B dose.** Usually well-tolerated. **Risk of exacerbation of Hep B after stopping 3TC.** Monitor at least several months after stopping 3TC in Hep B pts; some may need anti-HBV therapy. |
| Lamivudine/ abacavir (Epzicom) | Film-coated tabs: 3TC 300 mg + abacavir 600 mg | 1 tab po q24h. Food OK Not recommended for CrCl <50 mL/min or impaired hepatic function | 86/86 | 5–7/1.5 | 16/20 | *(See individual components)* | Primarily renal/ metabolism | *See Comments for individual agents.* Note abacavir **hypersensitivity Black Box warnings** (severe reactions may be frequent, more frequent with 600 mg dose) and 3TC Hep B warnings. Test HLA-B*5701 before use. |
| Lamivudine/ zidovudine (Combivir) | Film-coated tabs: 3TC 150 mg + ZDV 300 mg | 1 tab po bid. Not recommended for CrCl <50 mL/min or impaired hepatic function Food OK | 86/64 | 5–7/0.5–3 | — | *(See individual components)* | Primarily renal/ metabolism with renal excretion of glucuronide | *See Comments for individual agents.* **Black Box warning**—exacerbation of Hep B in pts stopping 3TC |

**TABLE 14C (6)**

**Selected Characteristics of Antiretroviral Drugs** (*CPE = CSF penetration effectiveness: 1-4)

| Generic/ Trade Name | Pharmaceutical Prep. | Usual Adult Dosage & Food Effect | % Absorbed, po | Serum T½ hrs | Intracellular T½ hrs | CPE* | Elimination | Major Adverse Events/Comments (See Table 14D) |
|---|---|---|---|---|---|---|---|---|
| **1. Selected Characteristics of Nucleoside or Nucleotide Reverse Transcriptase Inhibitors (NRTIs)** (continued) | | | | | | | | |
| Stavudine (d4T; Zerit) | 15, 20, 30, 40 mg capsules; 1 mg per mL oral solution | ≥60 kg: 40 mg po bid <60 kg: 30 mg po bid Food OK | 86 | 1.2-1.6 | 3.5 | 2 | Renal excretion, 40% | Not recommended by DHHS as initial therapy because of adverse reactions. **Highest incidence of lipoatrophy, hyperlipidemia, & lactic acidosis of all NRTIs.** Pancreatitis. Peripheral neuropathy. (See Didanosine comments.) |
| Tenofovir disoproxil fumarate (TDF; Viread)— a nucleotide | 300 mg | CrCl ≥50 mL/min: 300 mg po q24h. Food OK; high-fat meal ↑ absorption — — — — — — — — — CrCl >30 mL/min Food OK; high-fat meal ↑ absorption | 39 (with food) 25 (fasted) | 17 | >60 | 1 | Renal excretion | Headache, N/V. **Cases of renal dysfunction reported:** check renal function before using (dose reductions necessary if CrCl <50 cc/min); avoid concomitant nephrotoxic agents. One study found ↑ renal function at 48-wks in pts receiving TDF with a PI (mostly lopinavir/ritonavir) than with a NNRTI (JID 197:102, 2008). Avoid concomitant ddl. Atazanavir & lopinavir/ritonavir ↑ tenofovir concentrations: monitor for adverse effects. **Black Box warning—exacerbations of Hep B reported after stopping tenofovir.** Monitor liver enzymes if TDF stopped on HBV pts. |
| Tenofovir alafenamide (TAF) | 25 mg (10 mg when used with Cobi or RTV) | | | | | | | |
| Zidovudine (ZDV, AZT, Retrovir) | 100 mg caps, 300 mg tabs; 10 mg per mL IV solution; 10 mg/mL oral syrup | 300 mg po q12h. Food OK | 64 | 1.1 | 11 | 4 | Metabolized to glucuronide & excreted in urine | Bone marrow suppression, GI intolerance, headache, insomnia, malaise, myopathy. |
| **2. Selected Characteristics of Non-Nucleoside Reverse Transcriptase Inhibitors (NNRTIs)** | | | | | | | | |
| Delavirdine (Rescriptor) | 100, 200 mg tabs | 400 mg po three times daily. Food OK | 85 | 5.8 | 3 | ND | Cytochrome P450 (3A inhibitor) 51% excreted in urine (<5% unchanged) | Rash severe enough to stop drug in 4.3%. ↑ AST/ALT, headaches. **Use of this agent is not recommended.** |
| Doravirine (Pifeltro) | 100 mg tabs | 100 mg po q24h. Food OK. | 64 | 20 | ND | ND | Metabolism; 6% excreted in urine unchanged | GI, dizziness, headache, fatigue, abnormal dreams. **Co-administration with strong CYP3A4 inducers is contraindicated.** No issues with acid-suppressing agents. Retains activity against viruses containing many common NNRTI resistance mutations. Also available in combination with TDF and 3TC as Delstrigo. |

**TABLE 14C (7)**

Selected Characteristics of Antiretroviral Drugs (*CPE = CSF penetration effectiveness: 1-4)

2. **Selected Characteristics of Non-Nucleoside Reverse Transcriptase Inhibitors (NNRTIs)** *(continued)*

| Generic/ Trade Name | Pharmaceutical Prep. | Usual Adult Dosage & Food Effect | % Absorbed, po | Serum T½, hrs | Intracellular T½, hrs | CPE | Elimination | Major Adverse Events/Comments *(See Table 14D)* |
|---|---|---|---|---|---|---|---|---|
| **Efavirenz** (Sustiva) New Guidelines indicate is OK to use in pregnant women (WHO Guidelines) or continue EFV in women identified as pregnant (HHS Guidelines). | 50, 100, 200 mg capsules; 600 mg tablet | 600 mg po q24h at bedtime, without food. Food may ↑ serum conc, which can lead to ↑ in risk of adverse events. | 42 | 40-55 See Comment | 3 | | Cytochrome P450 286 (3A mixed inducer/ inhibitor). 14-34% excreted in urine as glucuroni-dated metabolites, 16-61% in feces | Severe rash in 1.7%. High frequency of CNS AEs: somnolence, dreams, confusion, agitation. Serious psychiatric symptoms. Certain CYP2B6 poly-morphisms may predict exceptionally high plasma levels with standard doses (CID 45:1230, 2007). False-pos. cannabinoid screen. Very long tissue T½; **If rx to be discontinued, stop Efavirenz 1-2 wks before stopping companion drugs.** Otherwise, risk of developing Efavirenz resistance, as after 1-2 days only Efavirenz in blood &/or tissue. Some bridge this gap by adding a PI to the NRTI backbone after Efavirenz is discontinued. (CID 42:401, 2006) |
| **Etravirine** (Intelence) | 100 mg tabs 200 mg tabs | 200 mg twice daily after a meal. May also be given as 400 mg once daily | Unknown (↓ systemic exposure if taken fasting) | 41 | 2 | | Metabolized by CYP 3A4 (inducer) & 2C9, 2C19 (inhibitor). Fecal extraction. | For pts with HIV-1 resistant to NNRTIs & others. Active in vitro against most such isolates. Rash common, but rarely can be severe. Potential for multiple drug interactions. Generally, multiple mutations are required for high-level resistance. *See Table 14D, page 208 for specific mutations and effects.* Because of interactions, do not use with boosted atazanavir, boosted tipranavir, unboosted PIs, or other NNRTIs. |
| **Nevirapine** (Viramune) Viramune XR | 200 mg tabs; 50 mg per 5 mL oral suspension; XR 400 mg tabs | 200 mg po q24h x 14 days & then 200 mg po bid (see comments) & **Black Box warning**. Food OK. **If using Viramune XR, Still need the lead in dosing of 200 mg q24h prior to using 400 mg/d** | >90 | 25-30 | 4 | | Cytochrome P450 (3A4, 2C9) excreted 80% excreted in urine as glucuronid-ed metaboli-tes, 10% in feces | **Black Box warning—fatal hepatotoxicity.** Women with CD4 >250 esp. vulnerable, inc. pregnant women. Avoid in this group unless benefits clearly > risks (www.fda.gov/cder/drug/advisory/nevirapine.htm). Intensive monitoring for liver toxicity required. Men with CD4 >400 also at ↑ risk. Severe rash in 7%. **severe or life-threatening skin reactions** in 2%. Do not restart if any suspicion of such reactions. Because of long T½, consider continuing companion agents for several days if nevirapine is discontinued. |

TABLE 14C (8)

| Generic/Trade Name | Pharmaceutical Prep. | Usual Adult Dosage & Food Effect | % Absorbed, po | Intracellular T½, hrs | Serum T½, hrs | CPE | Elimination | Major Adverse Events/Comments (See Table 14D) |
|---|---|---|---|---|---|---|---|---|

**Selected Characteristics of Antiretroviral Drugs** (°CPE = CSF penetration effectiveness: 1-4)

**2. Selected Characteristics of Non-Nucleoside Reverse Transcriptase Inhibitors (NNRTIs)** *(continued)*

| Generic/Trade Name | Pharmaceutical Prep. | Usual Adult Dosage & Food Effect | % Absorbed, po | Intracellular T½, hrs | Serum T½, hrs | CPE | Elimination | Major Adverse Events/Comments (See Table 14D) |
|---|---|---|---|---|---|---|---|---|
| Rilpivirine (Edurant) | 25 mg tabs | 25 mg daily with food | absolute bioavailability unknown; 40% lower Cmax in fasted state | unknown | 50 | | Metabolized by Cyp3A4 in liver, 25% excreted unchanged in feces. | QTc prolongation with doses higher than 50 mg per day. Common AEs: depression, insomnia, headache, and rash. Do not co-administer with carbamazepine, oxcarbazepine, phenobarbital, phenytoin, rifabutin, rifampin, rifapentine, proton pump inhibitors, or multiple doses of dexamethasone. A fixed dose combination of rilpivirine + TDF/FTC (Complera/Eviplera) is approved. **Needs stomach acid for absorption. Do not administer with PPI.** |

**3. Selected Characteristics of Protease Inhibitors (PIs)**

All PIs: Glucose metabolism: new diabetes mellitus or deterioration of glucose control; fat redistribution; possible hyperlipidemia bleeding; hypertriglyceridemia or hypercholesterolemia. Exercise caution re: potential drug interactions & contraindications. QTc prolongation has been reported in a few pts taking PIs; some PIs can block hERG channels in vitro (*Lancet 365:682, 2005*).

| Generic/Trade Name | Pharmaceutical Prep. | Usual Adult Dosage & Food Effect | % Absorbed, po | Serum T½, hrs | CPE* | Elimination | Major Adverse Events/Comments (See Table 14D) |
|---|---|---|---|---|---|---|---|
| Atazanavir (Reyataz) | 100, 150, 200, 300 mg capsules | 400 mg po q24h with food. Ritonavir-boosted dose (atazanavir 300 mg po q24h + ritonavir 100 mg po q24h), with food, is recommended for ART-experienced pts. Use boosted dose when combined with either Efavirenz 600 mg po q24h or TDF 300 mg po q24h. If used with buffered ddl, take with food 2 hrs pre or 1 hr post ddl. | Good oral bioavailability; food enhances bioavailability & ↓ pharmacokinetic variability. Absorption ↓ by antacids, H₂-blockers, proton pump inhibitors. Avoid unboosted drug with PPIs/H2-blockers. Boosted drug can be used with or >10 hr after H2-blockers or >12 hr after a PPI, if limited doses of the acid agents are used. | Approx. 7 | 2 | Cytochrome P450 (3A4, 1A2 & 2C9 inhibitor) & UGT1A1 inhibitor, 13% excreted in urine (7% unchanged), 79% excreted in feces (20% unchanged) | Lower potential for ↑ lipids. Asymptomatic unconjugated hyperbilirubinemia common; jaundice especially likely in Gilbert's syndrome (*JID 192:1381, 2005*). Headache, rash, GI symptoms. Prolongation of PR interval (1st degree AV block) reported. Caution in pre-existing conduction system disease. Efavirenz & Tenofovir ↓ atazanavir exposure: use atazanavir/ritonavir regimen; also, atazanavir ↑ tenofovir concentrations—watch for adverse events. In rx-experienced pts taking TDF and needing H2 blockers, atazanavir 400 mg with ritonavir 100 mg can be given; do not use PPIs. Rare reports of renal stones. |
| Darunavir (Prezista) | 400, 600 mg, 800 mg tablets | [600 mg darunavir + 100 mg ritonavir] po bid, with food or [800 mg darunavir (two 400 mg tabs or one 800 mg tab) + 100 mg ritonavir] po once daily with food (Preferred regimen in ART naive pts) | 82% absorbed (taken with ritonavir). Food ↑ absorption. | Approx 15 hr (with ritonavir) | 3 | Metabolized by CYP3A and is a CYP3A inhibitor | Contains sulfa moiety. Rash, nausea, headaches seen. Coadmin of certain drugs cleared by CYP3A is contraindicated (see below). Use with caution in about occasional hepatic dysfunction early in the course of treatment). Monitor carefully, esp. first several months and with pre-existing liver disease. May cause hormonal contraception failure. |

TABLE 14C (9)

Selected Characteristics of Antiretroviral Drugs (*CPE = CSF penetration effectiveness: 1-4)

3. **Selected Characteristics of Protease Inhibitors (PIs)** (continued)

| Generic/ Trade Name | Pharmaceutical Prep. | Usual Adult Dosage & Food Effect | % Absorbed, po | Serum T½, hrs | CPE* | Elimination | Major Adverse Events/Comments (See Table 14D) |
|---|---|---|---|---|---|---|---|
| Fosamprenavir (Lexiva) | 700 mg tablet, 50 mg/mL oral suspension | 1400 mg tablet po bid OR [1400 mg fosamprenavir (2 tabs) + ritonavir 100 mg or 200 mg] po q24h OR [700 mg fosamprenavir (1 tab) + ritonavir 100 mg] po bid | Bioavailability not established. Food OK | Amprenavir 7.7 | 3 | Hydrolyzed to amprenavir, then acts as cytochrome P450 (3A4 substrate, inhibitor, inducer) | Amprenavir prodrug. Contains sulfa moiety. Potential for serious drug interactions (see label). Rash, including Stevens-Johnson syndrome. Once daily regimens: (1) not recommended for PI-experienced pts, (2) additional ritonavir needed if given with Efavirenz (see label). Boosted twice daily regimen is recommended for PI-experienced pts. Potential for PI cross-resistance with darunavir. |
| Indinavir (Crixivan) | 100, 200, 400 mg capsules Store in original container with desiccant | Two 400 mg caps (800 mg) po q8h, without food or with light meal. Can take with enteric-coated Videx. [If taken with ritonavir (e.g., 800 mg indinavir + 100 mg ritonavir po q12h), no food restrictions] | 65 | 1.2-2 | 4 | Cytochrome P450 (3A4 inhibitor) | Maintain hydration. Nephrolithiasis, nausea, inconsequential ↑ of indirect bilirubin (jaundice in Gilbert syndrome), ↑ AST/ALT, headache, asthenia, blurred vision, metallic taste, hemolysis. ↑ urine WBC (>100/hpf) has been assoc. with nephritis/medullary calcification, cortical atrophy. |
| Lopinavir + ritonavir (Kaletra) | (200 mg lopinavir + 50 mg ritonavir), and (100 mg lopinavir + 25 mg ritonavir) tablets. Tabs do not need refrigeration. Oral solution: (80 mg lopinavir + 20 mg ritonavir) per mL. Refrigerate, but can be kept at room temp. (<77°F) x 2 mos. | (400 mg lopinavir + 100 mg ritonavir)—2 tabs po bid. Higher dose may be needed in non-rx-naive pts when used with Efavirenz, nevirapine, or unboosted fosamprenavir. [Dose adjustment in concomitant drugs may be necessary; see Table 22B. | No food effect with tablets. | ≠ 5-6 | 3 | Cytochrome P450 (3A4 inhibitor) | Nausea/vomiting/diarrhea (worse when administered with zidovudine), ↑ AST/ ALT, pancreatitis. Oral solution 42% alcohol. Lopinavir + ritonavir can be taken as a single daily dose of 4 tabs (total 800 mg lopinavir + 200 mg ritonavir), except in treatment-experienced pts or those taking concomitant Efavirenz, nevirapine, amprenavir, or nelfinavir. Possible PR and QT prolongation. Use with caution in those with cardiac conduction abnormalities or when used with drugs with similar effects. |
| Nelfinavir (Viracept) | 625, 250 mg tabs; 50 mg/gm oral powder | Two 625 mg tabs (1250 mg) po bid, with food | 20-80 Food ↑ exposure & ↓ variability | 3.5-5 | 1 | Cytochrome P450 (3A4 inhibitor) | Diarrhea. Coadministration of drugs with life-threatening toxicities & which are cleared by CYP3A4 is contraindicated. Not recommended in initial regimens because of inferior efficacy; prior concerns about EMS now resolved. **Acceptable choice in pregnant women although it has inferior virologic efficacy than most other ARV anchor drugs.** |

**TABLE 14C (10)**

### 3. Selected Characteristics of Antiretroviral Drugs (*CPE = CSF penetration effectiveness: 1-4)

#### Selected Characteristics of Protease Inhibitors (PIs). (continued)

| Generic/Trade Name | Pharmaceutical Prep. | Usual Adult Dosage & Food Effect | % Absorbed, po | Serum T½ hrs | CPE | Elimination | Major Adverse Events/Comments (See Table 14D) |
|---|---|---|---|---|---|---|---|
| Ritonavir (Norvir) | 100 mg capsules; 600 mg per 7.5 mL solution. Refrigerate caps but not solution. Room temperature for 1 mo. is OK. | Full dose not recommended (see comments). With rare exceptions, used exclusively to enhance pharmacokinetics of other PIs, using lower ritonavir doses. | Food ↑ absorption | 3–5 | 1 | Cytochrome P450; Potent 3A4 & 2d6 inhibitor | Nausea/vomiting/diarrhea, extremity & circumoral paresthesias, hepatitis, pancreatitis, taste perversion. ↑ CPK & uric acid. **Black Box warning—potentially fatal drug interactions. Many drug interactions— see Table 22A–Table 22B.** |
| **Saquinavir** (Invirase—hard gel caps or tabs) **+ ritonavir** | Saquinavir 200 mg caps, 500 mg film-coated tabs; ritonavir 100 mg caps | [2 tabs saquinavir (1000 mg) + 1 cap ritonavir (100 mg)] po bid with food | Erratic, 4 (Saquinavir alone). Much more reliably absorbed when boosted with ritonavir. | 1–2 | 1 | Cytochrome P450 (3A4 inhibitor) | Nausea, diarrhea, headache, ↑ AST/ALT. Avoid rifampin with saquinavir + ritonavir: ↑ hepatitis risk. **Black Box warning—Invirase to be used only with ritonavir.** Possible QT prolongation. Use with caution in those with cardiac conduction abnormalities or when used with drugs with similar effects. |
| Tipranavir (Aptivus) | 250 mg caps. Refrigerate unopened bottles. Use opened bottles within 2 mo. 100 mg/mL solution | [500 mg (two 250 mg caps) + ritonavir 200 mg] po bid with food. | Absorption low, ↑ with high fat meal, ↓ with Al⁺⁺⁺ & Mg⁺⁺ antacids. | 5.5–6 | 1 | Cytochrome 3A4 but with ritonavir, most of drug is eliminated in feces. | Contains sulfa moiety. **Black Box warning—reports of fatal/nonfatal intracranial hemorrhage, hepatitis, fatal/nonfatal hepatic failure.** Use cautiously in liver disease, esp. hepB, hepC. Contraindicated in Child-Pugh class B-C. Monitor LFTs. Coadministration of certain drugs contraindicated (see label). **For highly ART-experienced pts or for multiple-PI resistant virus.** Do not use tipranavir and etravirine together owing to 76% reduction in etravirine levels. |

### 4. Selected Characteristics of Fusion Inhibitors

| Generic/Trade Name | Pharmaceutical Prep. | Usual Adult Dosage | % Absorbed | Serum T½ hrs | CPE* | Elimination | Major Adverse Events/Comments (See Table 14D) |
|---|---|---|---|---|---|---|---|
| Enfuvirtide (T20, Fuzeon) | Single-use vials of 90 mg/mL when reconstituted. Vials should be stored at room temperature. Reconstituted vials can be refrigerated for 24 hrs only. | 90 mg (1 mL) subcut. bid. Rotate injection sites, avoiding those currently inflamed. | 84 | 3.8 | 1 | Catabolism to its constituent amino acids with subsequent recycling of the amino acids in the body pool. Elimination pathway(s) have not been performed in humans. Does not use the metabolism of CYP3A4, CYP2 d6, CYP1A2, CYP2C19 or CYP2E1 substrates. | Local reaction site reactions 98%, 4% discontinue; erythema/induration ~80–90%, nodules/cysts ~60%. **Hypersensitivity reactions reported** (fever, rash, chills, N/V, ↓ BP, δ/or ↑ AST/ALT)—do not restart if these occur. Including background regimens, peripheral neuropathy 8.9%, insomnia 11.3%, ↓ appetite 6.3%, myalgia 5%, lymphadenopathy 2.5%, eosinophilia ~10%, ↑ incidence of bacterial pneumonias. |

**TABLE 14C (11)**

**Selected Characteristics of Antiretroviral Drugs** (°CPE = CSF penetration effectiveness: 1-4)

5. **Selected Characteristics of CCR-5 Co-receptor Antagonists**

| Generic/ Trade Name | Pharmaceutical Prep. | Usual Adult Dosage & Food Effect | % Absorbed | Serum T½ hrs | CPE | Elimination | Major Adverse Events/Comments (See Table 14D) |
|---|---|---|---|---|---|---|---|
| Maraviroc (Selzentry) | 150 mg, 300 mg film-coated tabs | Without regard to food: -150 mg bid if concomitant meds include CYP3A inhibitors including PIs (except tipranavir/ritonavir) and delavirdine (with/ without CYP3A inducers) -300 mg bid without significantly interacting meds including NRTIs, tipranavir/ritonavir, nevaprine -600 mg bid if concomitant meds include CYP3A inducers, including Efavirenz (without strong CYP3A inhibitors) | Est. 33% with 300 mg dosage | 14-18 | 3 | CYP3A and P-glycoprotein substrate. Metabolites (via CYP3A) excreted feces > urine | **Black Box Warning-Hepatotoxicity,** may be preceded by rash, ↑ eos or IgE: no hepatotoxicity was noted in MVC trials. Black box inserted owing to concern about potential CCR5 class effect. Data lacking in hepatic/renal insufficiency; ↑ concern with either could ↑ risk of UBP. Currently for treatment-experienced patients with multi-resistant strains. **Document CCR-5-tropic virus before use, as treatment failures assoc. with appearance of CXCR-4 or mixed-tropic virus.** |

6. **Selected Characteristics of Integrase Strand Transfer Inhibitors (INSTI)**

| Generic/ Trade Name | Pharmaceutical Prep. | Usual Adult Dosage & Food Effect | % Absorbed | Serum T½ hrs | CPE | Elimination | Major Adverse Events/Comments (See Table 14D) |
|---|---|---|---|---|---|---|---|
| Raltegravir (Isentress) | 600 mg film-coated tabs | 600 mg bid without regard to food | Unknown | ~ 9 | 3 | Glucuronidation via UGT1A1, with excretion into feces and urine. (Therefore does NOT require ritonavir boosting). | For naïve patients and treatment experienced pts with multiply-resistant virus. Well-tolerated. Nausea, diarrhea, headache, fever similar to placebo. CK↑ & rhabdomyolysis reported; unclear relationship. Increased depression in those with a history of depression. Low genetic barrier to resistance. Increase in CPK, myositis, rhabdomyolysis have been reported. Rare Stevens Johnson Syndrome. Better oral absorption if chewed (CID 57:490, 2013). |
| Bictegravir (part of Biktarvy) | 50 mg (per Biktarvy tab) | 50 mg once daily with or without food | No data | 17.3 | No data | Mainly metabolized by CYP3A enzymes; also glucuronidated by UGT1A1. | Indicated (as Biktarvy) for treatment naïve pts and as replacement for prior or existing therapy. Generally well tolerated. Expect increased serum creatinine by 0.1-0.15 mg/dL due to inhibition of proximal tubular secretion; does not reflect a reduced GFR. **Black box warning: possible acute exacerbation of hep B** in co-infected patients who discontinue Biktarvy. |

**TABLE 14C (12)**

### 6. Selected Characteristics of Strand Transfer Integrase Inhibitors *(continued)*

| Generic/ Trade Name | Pharmaceutical Prep. | Usual Adult Dosage & Food Effect | % Absorbed | Serum T½ hrs | CPE | Elimination | Major Adverse Events/Comments *(See Table 14D)* |
|---|---|---|---|---|---|---|---|
| **Elvitegravir/ cobicistat** (Stribild) | 150 mg - 150 mg | 150 mg-150 mg once daily with or without food | <10% | 12.9 (CobI), 3.5 (ELV) | Un-known | The majority of **elvitegravir** metabolism is mediated by CYP3A enzymes. Elvitegravir also undergoes glucuronidation via UGT1A1/3 enzymes. **Cobicistat** is metabolized by CYP3A and to a minor extent by CYP2D6 | For both treatment naïve patients and treatment experienced pts with multiply-resistant virus. Generally well-tolerated. Use of cobicistat increases serum creatinine by ~ 0.1 mg/dl via inhibition of proximal tubular enzyme; this does not result in reduction in true GFR but will result in erroneous apparent reduction in eGFR by MDRD or Cockcroft Gault calculations. Usual AEs are similar to those observed with ritonavir (cobi) and tenofovir/FTC. |
| **Dolutegravir** (Tivicay) | 50 mg | 50 mg po once daily 50 mg po bid (if STII resistance present or if co-admin with EFV, FOS, TIP, or RIF | Unknown | 14 | 4 | Glucuronidation via UGT1A1 (therefore does not require ritonavir or cobicistat boosting) | Hypersensitivity (rare). Most common: insomnia (3%) headache (2%), N/V (1%), rash (<1%). Watch for IRIS; Watch for elevated LFTs in those with HCV |

### Other Considerations in Selection of Therapy

Caution: Initiation of ART may result in immune reconstitution syndrome with significant clinical consequences. *See Table 11B, of Sanford Guide to HIV/AIDS Therapy (AIDS Reader 16:199, 2006).*

1. Resistance testing: Given current rates of resistance, resistance testing is recommended in all patients prior to initiation of therapy, including those with acute infection syndrome (may initiate therapy while waiting for test results and adjusting Rx once results return), at time of change of therapy owing to antiretroviral failure, when suboptimal virologic response is observed, and in pregnant women. **Resistance testing NOT recommended if pt is off ART for >4 weeks or if HIV RNA is <1000 c/mL.** *See Table 6F of Sanford Guide to HIV/AIDS Therapy.*

2. Drug-induced disturbances of glucose & lipid metabolism *(see Table 14D)*
3. Drug-induced lactic acidosis & other FDA "box warnings" *(see Table 14D)*
4. Drug-drug interactions *(see Table 22B)*
5. Risk in pregnancy *(see Table 8)*
6. Use in women & children *(see Table 14C)*
7. Dosing in patients with renal or hepatic dysfunction *(see Table 17A & Table 17B)*

* **CPE (CNS Penetration Effectiveness) value:** 1= Low Penetration; 2 - 3 = Intermediate Penetration; 4 = Highest Penetration into CNS *(AIDS 25:357, 2011)*

## TABLE 14D - ANTIRETROVIRAL DRUGS & ADVERSE EFFECTS
### (www.aidsinfo.nih.gov)

| DRUG NAME(S): GENERIC (TRADE) | MOST COMMON ADVERSE EFFECTS | MOST SIGNIFICANT ADVERSE EFFECTS |
|---|---|---|
| **Nucleoside Reverse Transcriptase Inhibitors (NRT)** Black Box warning for all nucleoside/nucleotide RTIs: lactic acidosis/hepatic steatosis, potentially fatal. Also carry Warnings that fat redistribution and immune reconstitution syndromes (including autoimmune syndromes with delayed onset) have been observed | | |
| Abacavir (Ziagen) | Headache 7-13%, nausea 7-19%, diarrhea 7%, malaise 7-12% | **Black Box warning—Hypersensitivity reaction (HR)** in 8% with malaise, fever, GI upset, rash, lethargy & respiratory symptoms most commonly reported; myalgia, arthralgia, edema, paresthesia less common. **Discontinue immediately if HR suspected. Rechallenge contraindicated; may be life-threatening.** Severe HR may be more common with once-daily dosing. **HLA-B*5701 allele** predicts ↑ risk of HR in Caucasian pop.; excluding pts with B*5701 markedly ↓d HR incidence (NEJM 358:568, 2008; CID 46:1111-1118, 2008). DHHS guidelines recommend testing for B*5701 and use of abacavir-containing regimens only if HLA-B*5701 negative. Vigilance essential in all groups. Possible increased risk of MI with use of abacavir has been suggested (JID 201:318, 2010). Other studies found no increased risk of MI (CID 52: 929, 2011). A meta-analysis of randomized trials by FDA did not show increased risk of MI (www.fda.gov/drugs/drugsafety/ucm245164.htm). Nevertheless, care is advised to optimize potentially modifiable risk factors when abacavir is used. |
| Didanosine (ddI) (Videx) | Diarrhea 28%, nausea 6%, rash 9%, headache 7%, fever 12%, hyperuricemia 2% | **Pancreatitis 1-9%. Black Box warning—Cases of fatal & nonfatal pancreatitis** have occurred in pts receiving ddI, especially when used in combination with d4T or d4T + hydroxyurea. Fatal lactic acidosis in pregnancy with ddI + d4T. Peripheral neuropathy in 20%, 12% required dose reduction. ↑ toxicity if used with ribavirin. Use with TDF generally avoided (but would require dose reduction of ddI) because of ↑ toxicity and possible ↓ efficacy; may result in ↓ CD4. Rarely, retinal changes or optic neuropathy. Diabetes mellitus and rhabdomyolysis reported in post-marketing surveillance. Possible increased risk of MI under study (www.fda.gov/CDER/JID 201:318, 2010). Non-cirrhotic portal hypertension with ascites, varices, splenomegaly reported in post-marketing surveillance. See also Clin Infect Dis. 49:626, 2009; Amer J Gastroenterol 102:2536, 2009. |
| Emtricitabine (FTC) (Emtriva) | Well tolerated. Headache, diarrhea, nausea, rash, skin hyperpigmentation | Potential for lactic acidosis (as with other NRTIs). Also in **Black Box—severe exacerbation of hepatitis B on stopping drug in pts infected w/hep B. Monitor clinically/lab for several months after stopping in pts with hepB.** Anti-HBV rx may be warranted if FTC stopped. |
| Lamivudine (3TC) (Epivir) | Well tolerated. Headache 35%, nausea 33%, diarrhea 18%, abdominal pain 9%, insomnia 11% (all in combination with ZDV). Pancreatitis more common in pediatrics. | **Black Box warning. Make sure to use HIV dosage, not Hep B dosage. Exacerbation of hepatitis B on stopping drug. Patients with hepB who stop lamivudine require close clinical/lab monitoring for several months.** Anti-HBV rx may be warranted if 3TC stopped. |
| Stavudine (d4T) (Zerit) | Diarrhea, nausea, vomiting, headache | **Peripheral neuropathy** 15-20%. Pancreatitis 1%. Appears to produce lactic acidosis, hepatic steatosis and lipoatrophy/lipodystrophy more commonly than other NRTIs. **Black Box warning—Fatal & nonfatal pancreatitis with d4T + ddI.** Use with TDF generally avoided (but would require dose reduction of ddI) because of ↑ toxicity and possible ↓ efficacy; may result in ↓ CD4. Rarely, retinal changes or optic neuropathy. Diabetes mellitus and rhabdomyolysis reported in post-marketing surveillance. **Fatal lactic acidosis/steatosis in pregnant women receiving d4T + ddI.** Fatal and non-fatal lactic acidosis and severe hepatic steatosis can occur in others receiving d4T with particular caution in patients with risk factors for liver disease, but lactic acidosis can occur even in those without known risk factors. Possible ↑ toxicity if used with ribavirin. Motor weakness in the setting of lactic acidosis mimicking the clinical presentation of Guillain-Barré syndrome (including respiratory failure) (rare). |
| Zidovudine (ZDV, AZT) (Retrovir) | Nausea 50%, anorexia 20%, vomiting 17%, headache 62%. Also reported: asthenia, insomnia, myalgias, nail pigmentation. Macrocytosis expected with all dosage regimens. | **Black Box warning—hematologic toxicity, myopathy. Anemia** (<8 gm, 1%), granulocytopenia (<750, 1.8%). Anemia may respond to erythropoietin if endogenous serum erythropoietin levels are ≤500 milliUnits/mL. Possible ↑ toxicity if used with ribavirin and co-administration with ribavirin not advised. Hepatic decompensation may occur in HIV/HCV co-infected patients receiving zidovudine with interferon alfa ± ribavirin. |

TABLE 14D (2)

| DRUG NAME(S): GENERIC (TRADE) | MOST COMMON ADVERSE EFFECTS | MOST SIGNIFICANT ADVERSE EFFECTS |
|---|---|---|
| **Nucleotide Reverse Transcriptase Inhibitor (NRTI)** Black Box warning for all nucleoside/nucleotide RTIs: lactic acidosis/hepatic steatosis, potentially fatal. Also carry Warnings that fat redistribution and immune reconstitution syndromes (including autoimmune syndromes with delayed onset) have been observed *(continued)* | | |
| Tenofovir disoproxil fumarate (TDF) (Viread); Tenofovir alafenamide (TAF) | Diarrhea 11%, nausea 8%, vomiting 5%, flatulence 4% (generally well tolerated) | **Black Box Warning—Severe exacerbations of hepatitis B reported in pts who stop tenofovir.** Monitor carefully if drug is stopped; anti-HBV rx may be warranted if TDF stopped. Reports of renal injury from TDF, including Fanconi syndrome *(CID 37:e174, 2003; J AIDS 35:269,204; CID 42:283, 2006)*. Fanconi syndrome and diabetes insipidus reported with TDF + ddI *(AIDS Reader 17:90-92, 2007)*. Modest decline in renal function appears greater with TDF than with TAF *(Lancet 385:2606-2615, 2010)* or TAF, and may be greater in those receiving TDF with a PI instead of an NNRTI *(JID 197:102, 2008; AIDS 26:567, 2012)*. In a VA study that followed >10,000 HIV-infected individuals, TDF exposure was significantly associated with increased risk of proteinuria, a more rapid decline in renal function and chronic kidney disease *(AIDS 26:862, 2012)*. Monitor Ccr, serum phosphate and urinalysis, especially carefully in those with pre-existing renal dysfunction or nephrotoxic medications. TDF, but not TAF, also appears to be associated with increased risk of bone loss. In a subgroup of an ACTG comparative treatment trial, those randomized to TDF-FTC experienced greater decreases in spine and hip bone mineral density (BMD) at 96 weeks compared with those treated with ABC-3TC *(JID 203:1791, 2011)*. Consider monitoring BMD in those with history of pathologic fractures, or who have risks for osteoporosis or bone loss. |
| **Non-Nucleoside Reverse Transcriptase Inhibitors (NNRTI).** Labels caution that fat redistribution and immune reconstitution can occur with ART. | | |
| Delavirdine (Rescriptor) | **Skin rash** has occurred in 18%; can continue or restart drug in most cases. Stevens-Johnson syndrome & erythema multiforme have been reported rarely. ↑ in liver enzymes in <5% of patients. | |
| Doravirine (Pifeltro) | Nausea (5-7%), diarrhea (3-5%), abdominal pain (1-5%), headache (4-6%), fatigue (4-6%), rash (2%). Dizziness: 9% (37% with Atripla). Sleep disturbances: 12% (26% with Atripla). Better lipid profile than efavirenz- or PI-based regimens. | Co-administration with drugs that are strong CYP3A inducers will significantly decrease Doravirine plasma concentrations. Monitor for IRIS during initiation of therapy. |
| Efavirenz (Sustiva) | **CNS side effects 52%** symptoms include dizziness, insomnia, somnolence, impaired concentration, psychiatric sx, & abnormal dreams; symptoms are worse after 1st or 2nd dose & improve over 2-4 weeks; discontinuation rate 2.6%. Rash 26% (vs. 17% in comparators); often improves with oral antihistamines; discontinuation rate 1.7%. Can cause false-positive urine test results for cannabinoid with CEDIA DAU multi-level THC assay. Metabolite can cause false-positive urine screening test for benzodiazepines *(CID 48:1797, 2009)*. | **Caution:** CNS effects may impair driving and other hazardous activities. Serious neuropsychiatric symptoms reported, including severe depression (2.4%) & suicidal ideation (0.7%). Elevation in liver enzymes. Fulminant hepatic failure has been reported *(see FDA label)*. **Teratogenicity reported in primates; pregnancy category D—may cause fetal harm, avoid in pregnant women or those who might become pregnant.** NOTE: No single method of contraception is 100% reliable. Barrier + 2nd method of contraception advised, continued 12 weeks after stopping efavirenz. Contraindicated with certain drugs metabolized by CYP3A4. Slow metabolism in those homozygous for the CYP-2B6 G516T allele can result in exaggerated toxicity and intolerance; this allele much more common in blacks and women *(CID 42:408, 2006)*. Stevens-Johnson syndrome and erythema multiforme reported in post-marketing surveillance. |
| Etravirine (Intelence) | Rash 9%, generally mild to moderate and spontaneously resolving; in 2% of clinical trials for rash. More common in women. Nausea 5%. | Severe rash (erythema multiforme, toxic epidermal necrolysis, Stevens-Johnson syndrome) has been reported. Hypersensitivity reactions can occur with rash, constitutional symptoms and organ dysfunction, including hepatic failure *(see FDA label)*. Potential for CYP450-mediated drug interactions. Rhabdomyolysis has been reported in post-marketing surveillance. |

**TABLE 14D (3)**

| DRUG NAME(S): GENERIC (TRADE) | MOST COMMON ADVERSE EFFECTS | MOST SIGNIFICANT ADVERSE EFFECTS |
|---|---|---|
| **Non-Nucleoside Reverse Transcriptase Inhibitors (NNRTI)** *(continued)* | | |
| Nevirapine (Viramune) | Rash 37% usually occurs during 1st 4 wks of therapy. Follow recommendations for 14-day lead-in period to ↓ risk of rash (see *Table 14C*). Women experience 7-fold ↑ in risk of severe rash (CID 32:124, 2001). 50% resolve within 2 wks of dc drug & 80% by 1 month. 6.7% discontinuation rate. | **Black Box warning—Severe life-threatening skin reactions reported:** Stevens-Johnson syndrome, toxic epidermal necrolysis, & hypersensitivity reactions (may be associated with hepatic necrosis & systemic sx (DRESS)) (AIDS 161:2501, 2001). For severe rashes, dc drug immediately & do not restart. In a clinical trial, the use of prednisone 2/3 during the first 12 wks of rx. Overall 1% develops hepatitis. Pts with pre-existing ↑ in ALT or AST &/or history of chronic Hep B or C ↑ susceptible (Hepatol 35:182, 2002). Women with CD4 >250, including pregnant women, at ↑ risk. Avoid in this group unless no other option. Men with CD4 >400 also at ↑ risk. Monitor pts intensively (clinical & LFTs), esp. during the first 12 wks of rx. If clinical hepatotoxicity, severe skin or hypersensitivity reactions occur, dc drug & never rechallenge. |
| Rilpivirine (Edurant) | Headache (3%), rash (3% led to discontinuation in 0.1%), insomnia (3%), depressive disorders (4%). Psychiatric disorders led to discontinuation in 1%. Increased liver enzymes observed. | Drugs that induce CYP3A or increase gastric pH may decrease plasma concentration of rilpivirine and co-administration with rilpivirine should be avoided. Among these are certain anticonvulsants, rifamycins, PPIs, dexamethasone and St. John's wort. At supra-therapeutic doses, rilpivirine can increase QTc interval; use with caution with other drugs known to increase QTc. May cause depressive disorder, including suicide attempts or suicidal ideation. Overall, appears to cause fewer neuropsychiatric side effects than Efavirenz (AIDS 60:33, 2012). |
| **Protease inhibitors (PI)** | | |
| Diarrhea is common AE (crofelemer 125 mg bid may help, but expensive). Abnormalities in glucose metabolism, dyslipidemias, fat redistribution syndromes are potential problems. Pts taking PI may be at increased risk for developing osteoporosis. Spontaneous bleeding episodes have been reported in HIV+ pts with hemophilia being treated with PI. Rheumatoid complications have been reported (An Rheum Dis 61:82, 2002). Potential for QTc prolongation. **Caution for all PIs**—Coadministration with drugs dependent on CYP3A or other enzymes for elimination & for which ↑ levels can cause serious toxicity may be contraindicated. ART may result in immune reconstitution syndrome, which may include early or late presentations of autoimmune syndromes. Increased premature births among women receiving ritonavir-boosted PIs as compared with those not receiving other antiretroviral therapy, even after accounting for other potential risk factors (CID 54: 1348, 2012). | | |
| Atazanavir (Reyataz) | Asymptomatic unconjugated hyperbilirubinemia in up to 60% of pts, jaundice in 7–9% [especially with Gilbert syndrome (CID 192: 1381, 2005)]. Moderate to severe events: Diarrhea 1–3%, nausea 6–14%, abdominal pain 4%, headache 6%, rash 20%. | Prolongation of PR interval (1st degree AV block, QTc increase and torsades reported (CID 44:e62, 2007). Acute interstitial nephritis (Am J Kid Dis 44:E81, 2004) and urolithiasis (atazanavir stones) reported (AIDS 20:2131, 2006; NEJM 355:2158, 2006). Potential ↑ transaminases in pts co-infected with HBV or HCV. Severe skin eruptions (Stevens-Johnson syndrome, erythema multiforme, and toxic eruptions, or DRESS syndrome) have been reported. |
| Darunavir (Prezista) | With background regimens, headache 15%, nausea 18%, diarrhea 20%, ↑ amylase 17%. Rash in 10% of treated; 0.5% discontinuation. | Hepatitis in 0.5%, some with fatal outcome. Use caution in pts with HBV or HCV co-infections or other hepatic dysfunction. Monitor for clinical symptoms and LFTs. Stevens-Johnson syndrome, toxic epidermal necrolysis, erythema multiforme. Contains sulfa moiety. Potential for major drug interactions. May cause failure of hormonal contraceptives. |
| Fosamprenavir (Lexiva) | Skin rash ~ 20% (moderate or worse in 3–8%), nausea, headache, diarrhea. | Rarely Stevens-Johnson syndrome, hemolytic anemia. Pro-drug of amprenavir. Contains sulfa moiety. Angioedema and nephrolithiasis reported in post-marketing experience. Potential for increased risk of MI (see FDA label). Angioedema, oral paresthesias, myocardial infarction and nephrolithiasis reported in post-marketing experience. Elevated LFTs seen with higher than recommended doses; increased risk in those with pre-existing liver abnormalities. Acute hemolytic anemia reported with amprenavir. |
| Indinavir (Crixivan) | ↑ in indirect bilirubin 10–15% (≥2.5 mg/dl, with overt jaundice especially likely in those with Gilbert syndrome (CID 192: 1381, 2005). Nausea 12%, vomiting 4%, diarrhea 5%. Metallic taste. Paronychia and ingrown toenails reported (CID 32:140, 2001). | Kidney stones. Due to indinavir crystals in collecting system. Nephrolithiasis in 12% of adults, higher in pediatrics. Minimize risk with good hydration (at least 48 oz. water/day) (AAC 42:332, 1998). Tubulointerstitial nephritis/renal cortical atrophy reported in association with asymptomatic ↑ urine WBC. Severe hepatitis reported in 3 cases (Ln 349:924, 1997). Hemolytic anemia reported. |

**TABLE 14D (4)**

| DRUG NAME(S): GENERIC (TRADE) | MOST COMMON ADVERSE EFFECTS | MOST SIGNIFICANT ADVERSE EFFECTS |
|---|---|---|
| **Protease inhibitors (PI)** (continued) | | |
| Lopinavir/Ritonavir (Kaletra) | GI: **diarrhea** 14–24%, nausea 2–16%. More diarrhea with q24h dosing. | Lipid abnormalities in up to 20–40%. Possible increased risk of MI with cumulative exposure (JID 201:318, 2010). ↑ PR interval, 2° or 3° heart block described. Post-marketing reports of ↑ QTc and torsades; avoid use in circumstances that prolong QTc or increase susceptibility to torsades. Pancreatitis. Hepatitis, with hepatic decompensation; caution especially in those with pre-existing liver disease. Inflammatory edema of legs (AIDS 16:673, 2002). Stevens-Johnson syndrome & erythema multiforme reported. Note high drug concentration of oral solution. Toxic potential of oral solution (contains ethanol and propylene glycol) in neonates. |
| Nelfinavir (Viracept) | Mild to moderate **diarrhea** 20%. Oat bran tabs, calcium, or oral anti-diarrheal agents (e.g., loperamide, diphenoxylate/atropine sulfate) can be used to manage diarrhea. | Potential for drug interactions. Powder contains phenylalanine. |
| Ritonavir (Norvir)<br>(Currently, primary use is to enhance levels of other anti-retrovirals, because of ↑ toxicity/ interactions with full-dose ritonavir) | GI: bitter aftertaste ↓ by taking whole chocolate milk, Ensure, or Advera; nausea 23%, ↓ by initial dose esc (titration) regimen; vomiting 13%; diarrhea 15%. Circumoral paresthesias 5–6%. Dose >100 mg bid assoc. with ↑ GI side effects & ↑ in lipid abnormalities. | **Black Box warning** relates to many important drug-drug interactions—inhibits P450 CYP3A & CYP2 D6 system—may be life-threatening (see Table 22A). Several cases of iatrogenic Cushing's syndrome reported with concomitant use of ritonavir and corticosteroids, including dosing of the latter by inhalation, epidural injection or a single IM injection. Rarely Stevens-Johnson syndrome, toxic epidermal necrolysis anaphylaxis. Primary A-V block (and higher) and pancreatitis have been reported. Hepatic reactions, including fatalities. Monitor LFTs carefully during therapy, especially in those with pre-existing liver disease, including HBV and HCV. |
| Saquinavir (Invirase: hard cap, tablet) | **Diarrhea**, abdominal discomfort, nausea, headache | **Warning—Use Invirase only with ritonavir.** Avoid garlic capsules (may reduce SQV levels) and use cautiously with proton-pump inhibitors (increased SQV levels). Use of saquinavir/ritonavir can prolong QTc interval or may rarely cause 2° or 3° heart block; torsades reported. Contraindicated in patients with prolonged QTc or those taking drugs or who have other conditions (e.g., low K+ or Mg++) that pose a risk with prolonged QTc. (http://www.fda.gov/drugs/drugsafety/ucm230916.htm accessed May 25, 2011). Contraindicated in patients with complete AV block, or those at risk, who do not have pacemaker. Hepatic toxicity encountered in patients with pre-existing liver disease or in individuals receiving concomitant rifampin. Rarely, Stevens Johnson syndrome. |
| Tipranavir (Aptivus) | Nausea & vomiting, diarrhea, abdominal pain. Rash in 8–14%, more common in women, & 33% in women taking ethinyl estradiol. Major lipid effects. | **Black Box Warning—associated with hepatitis & fatal hepatic failure.** Risk of hepatotoxicity increased in hepB or hepC co-infection. Possible photosensitivity skin reactions. Contraindicated in Child-Pugh Class B or C hepatic impairment. **Associated with fatal/nonfatal intracranial hemorrhage (can inhibit platelet aggregation).** Caution in those with bleeding risks. Potential for major drug interactions. Contains sulfa moiety and vitamin E. |
| **Fusion Inhibitor** | | |
| Enfuvirtide (T20, Fuzeon) | Local injection site reactions (98% have at least 1 local ISR, 4% dc because of ISR) (pain & discomfort, induration, erythema, nodules & cysts, pruritus, & ecchymosis). Diarrhea 32%, nausea 23%. | Rate of bacterial pneumonia (3.2 pneumonia events/100 pt. yrs). **hypersensitivity reactions** ≤1% (rash, fever, nausea & vomiting, chills, rigors, hypotension, & ↑ serum liver transaminases); can occur with reexposure. Cutaneous amyloid deposits containing enfuvirtide peptide reported in skin plaques persisting after discontinuation of drug (J Cutan Pathol 39:220, 2012). |
| **CCR5 Co-receptor Antagonists** | | |
| Maraviroc (Selzentry) | With ARV background: Cough 13%, fever 12%, rash 10%, abdominal pain 8%. Also, dizziness, myalgia, arthralgias. ↑ Risk of URI, HSV infection. | **Black box warning-Hepatotoxicity.** May be preceded by allergic features (rash, ↑eosinophils or ↑IgE levels). Use with caution in patients with HepB or C. Cardiac ischemia/infarction in 1.3%. May cause ↓BP, orthostatic syncope, especially in patients with renal dysfunction. Significant interactions with CYP3A inducers/inhibitors. Long-term risk of malignancy unknown. Stevens-Johnson syndrome reported post-marketing. Generally favorable safety profile during trial of ART-naive individuals (JID 201: 803, 2010). |

**TABLE 14D (5)**

| DRUG NAME(S): GENERIC (TRADE) | MOST COMMON ADVERSE EFFECTS | MOST SIGNIFICANT ADVERSE EFFECTS |
|---|---|---|
| **Integrase Inhibitors** | | |
| Bictegravir (part of Biktarvy) | Reported in at least 5% of patients: nausea, diarrhea, headache. May increase serum creatinine 0.1-0.15 mg/dL due to inhibition of proximal tubular secretion of creatinine (does not reflect a decrease in GFR). | **Black Box Warning:** possible severe hepatitis B exacerbation in co-infected patients who discontinue therapy. Monitor for IRIS if treating an ARV-naive patient with a lower CD4 cell count (<150/microliter). |
| Dolutegravir (Tivicay) | Insomnia and headache (2-4%) | Rash, liver injury reported. Increased ALT/AST in 203%. Competition with creatinine for tubular secretion increased serum creatinine by a mean of 0.1 mg/dL with no change in GFR. |
| Elvitegravir+ Cobicistat (Stribild), Elvitegravir (Vitekta) | Nausea and diarrhea are the two most common AEs. Increased serum creatinine 0.1-0.15 mg/dL due to inhibition of prox. tubular enzymes by cobicistat with no decrease in GFR. | **Same Black Box warnings as ritonavir and tenofovir (TDF and TAF).** Rare lactic acidosis syndrome. Owing to renal toxicity, should not initiate Rx when pre-Rx eGFR is <70 cc/min. Follow serial serum creatinine and urinary protein and glucose. Discontinue drug if serum Cr rises >0.4 mg/dl above baseline value. |
| Raltegravir (Isentress) | Diarrhea, headache, insomnia, nausea. LFT ↑ may be more common in pts co-infected with HBV or HCV. | Hypersensitivity reactions can occur. Rash, Stevens-Johnson syndrome, toxic epidermal necrolysis reported. Hepatic failure reported. ↑CK, myopathy and rhabdomyolysis reported (AIDS 22:1382, 2008). ↑ of preexisting depression reported in 4 pts; all could continue raltegravir after adjustment of psych. meds (AIDS 22:1890, 2008). Chewable tablets contain phenylalanine. |

**TABLE 14E – HEPATITIS A & HBV TREATMENT**
For HBV Activity Spectra, *see Table 4C, page 87*

**Hepatitis A Virus (HAV)**

1. Outbreaks in homeless populations. Vaccination is primary defense *(https://emergency.cdc.gov/han/han00412.asp)*.

2. **Drug/Dosage:** No therapy recommended. If within 2 wks of exposure, prophylactic IVIG 0.02 mL per kg IM times 1 protective. Hep A vaccine equally effective as IVIG in randomized trial and is emerging as preferred Rx *(NEJM 357:1685, 2007)*.

3. **HAV Superinfection:** 40% of pts with chronic Hepatitis C virus (HCV) infection who developed superinfection with HAV developed fulminant hepatic failure *(NEJM 338:286, 1998)*. Similar data in pts with chronic Hepatitis B virus (HBV) infection that suffer acute HAV *(Ann Trop Med Parasitol 93:745, 1999)*. **Hence, need to vaccinate all HBV and HCV pts with HAV vaccine.**

**Hepatitis B Virus (HBV): Treatment**

| | ALT | HBV DNA | HBe Ag | Recommendation |
|---|---|---|---|---|
| Immune-Tolerant Phase | Normal | >1x106 IU/mL | Positive | **Monitor:** ALT levels be tested at least every 6 months for adults with immune tolerant CHB to monitor for potential transition to immune-active or - inactive CHB.<br>**NB:** For those over 40 years of age + liver fibrosis, TREAT as Immune Active (below) |
| HBeAg+ Immune Active Phase | Elevated | >20,000 IU/mL | Positive | **TREAT (Duration of therapy+):**<br>Tenofovir (indefinitely; esp. if fibrosis) OR Entecavir (indefinitely; esp. if fibrosis) OR Peg-IFN++ (48 weeks of Rx ) |
| Inactive CHB Phase | Normal | <2,000 IU/mL | Negative | **Monitor:** ALT levels at least once / year |
| HBeAg-neg Immune Reactivation Phase | Elevated | >2,000 IU/mL | Negative | **TREAT (Duration of therapy+):**<br>Tenofovir (indefinitely; esp. if fibrosis) OR Entecavir (indefinitely; esp. if fibrosis) OR Peg-IFN++ (48 weeks of Rx) |

+ Duration of therapy largely unknown; most experts favor indefinite Rx, esp. among those with moderate to advanced fibrosis or inflammation (liver biopsy). Ref: *JAMA 2018,319:1802.*
++ Peg-INF contraindicated in patients with decompensated cirrhosis, autoimmune disease, uncontrolled psychiatric disease, cytopenias, severe cardiac disease, and uncontrolled seizures

For details of therapy, especially in special populations (e.g., pregnant women, children) *see updated AASLD Guidelines (Hepatology, 2015 Nov 13. doi: 10.1002/hep.2)*

**HBV Treatment Regimens. Single drug therapy is usually sufficient; combination therapy recommended for HIV co-infection.**

| | Drug/Dose | Comments |
|---|---|---|
| **Preferred Regimens** | **Pegylated-Interferon-alpha 2a** 180 µg sc once weekly OR<br>**Entecavir** 0.5 mg po once daily OR<br>**Tenofovir alafenamide (TAF/Vemlidy)** 25 mg po once daily | PEG-IFN: Treat for 48 weeks<br>Entecavir: Do not use Entecavir if Lamivudine resistance present.<br>Entecavir/Tenofovir: Treat for at least 24-48 weeks after seroconversion from HBeAg to anti-HBe (if no mod-adv fibrosis present). Indefinite chronic therapy for HBeAg negative patients. Renal impairment dose adjustments necessary. |
| **Alternative Regimens** | **Lamivudine** 100 mg po once daily OR<br>**Telbivudine** 600 mg po once daily OR<br>**Emtricitabine** 200 mg po once daily (investigational) OR<br>**Adefovir** 10 mg po once daily OR<br>**Tenofovir disoproxil (TDF)** 300 mg po once daily | These alternative agents are rarely used except in combination. When used, restrict to short term therapy owing to high rates of development of resistance.<br>Not recommended as first-line therapy. Use of Adefovir has mostly been replaced by Tenofovir. |
| **Preferred Regimen for HIV-HBV Co-Infected Patient** | **Truvada** (Tenofovir 300 mg + Emtricitabine 200 mg) po once daily + another anti-HIV drug | ALL patients if possible as part of a fully suppressive anti-HIV/anti-HBV regimen. Continue therapy indefinitely. |

## TABLE 14F – HCV TREATMENT REGIMENS AND RESPONSE
For HCV Activity Spectra, *see Table 4C, page 87*

1. **Indications for Treatment.** Treatment is indicated for **all patients** with chronic HCV. Rx should be initiated urgently for those with more advanced fibrosis (F3 / F4) and those with underlying co-morbid conditions due to HCV. Type and duration of Rx is based on genotype and stage of fibrosis. Pegylated interferon (Peg-IFN) is no longer a recommended regimen; all DAA regimens with or without ribavirin are the preferred choice.

2. **Definitions of Response to Therapy.**

| End of Treatment Response (ETR) | Undetectable at end of treatment. |
|---|---|
| Relapse | Undetectable at end of therapy (ETR) but rebound (detectable) virus within 12 weeks after therapy stopped. |
| Sustained Virologic Response (SVR) | CURE! Still undetectable at end of therapy and beyond 12 weeks after therapy is stopped. |

3. **HCV Treatment Regimens**

   - Biopsy is a 'gold standard' for staging HCV infection and is helpful in some settings to determine the ideal timing of HCV treatment. When bx not obtained, "non-invasive" tests are often employed to assess the relative probability of advanced fibrosis or cirrhosis. Fibroscan (elastography) is now approved in the US and most of the world as a means of assessing liver fibrosis. Elastography values of >10 kPa (Kilopascals) correlates with significant fibrosis (F3 or F4 disease).

   - Resistance tests: Genotypic resistance assays are available that can determine polymorphisms associated with reduction in susceptibility to some DAAs (Direct Acting Agents, e.g., protease inhibitors). **However, resistance tests are recommended only for those who have failed treatment with a prior NS5A or protease inhibitor regimen.**

   - Patients with decompensated cirrhosis should only be treated by hepatologists owing to the risk of rapid clinical deterioration while receiving treatment for HCV.

   - **IMPORTANT NOTE REGARDING TREATMENT DECISION-MAKING:** Newer drugs are in development and options for Rx are changing rapidly (i.e., several times per year). Monitor updates at *webedition.sanfordguide.com* or *hcvguidelines.org*.

   - **Black Box Warning for ALL Direct Acting Agents (DAA):** Cases of HBV reactivation, occasionally fulminant, during or after DAA therapy have been reported in HBV/HCV coinfected patients who were not already on HBV suppressive therapy. *See U.S. FDA Drug Safety Announcement, Oct 4, 2016.* **For HCV/HBV coinfected patients who are HBsAg+ and are not already on HBV suppressive therapy, monitoring HBV DNA levels during and immediately after DAA therapy for HCV is recommended and antiviral therapy for HBV should be given if treatment criteria for HBV are met.** *See HBV treatment.*

### CURRENT DRUGS FOR INITIAL TREATMENT FOR PATIENTS WITH CHRONIC HCV

   - Drugs and regimens are evolving. For updates go to: webedition.sanfordguide.com and www.hcvguidelines.org

| Agents/Abbreviation | Tradename | Formulation/Dosing Specifics |
|---|---|---|
| Daclatasvir (DCV) | Daklinza | 60 mg tab po once daily. Note: decrease dose to 30 mg/d when co-administered with a strong CYP3A inhibitor, e.g., several ARV drugs; increase dose to 90 mg/d when co-administered with a mild-moderate CYP3A inducer. Contraindicated when co-administered with a strong CYP3A inducer. |
| Elbasvir + Grazoprevir | Zepatier | Fixed dose combination (Elbasvir 50 mg + Grazoprevir 100 mg) 1 tab po once daily |
| Glecaprevir + Pibrentasvir | Mavyret | Fixed dose combination (Glecaprevir 100 mg + Pibrentasvir 40 mg) 3 tabs once daily with food |
| Paritaprevir/ritonavir + Ombitasvir (PrO) | Technivie | Fixed dose combination (Paritaprevir 150 mg/ritonavir 100 mg + Ombitasvir 25 mg) 1 tab once daily |
| Paritaprevir/ritonavir + Ombitasvir + Dasabuvir (PrOD) | Viekira Pak | Fixed dose combination [(Paritaprevir 150 mg/ritonavir 100 mg + Ombitasvir 25 mg) 1 tab once daily plus Dasabuvir 250 mg] 1 tab twice daily with food |
| | Viekira XR | Extended release fixed dose combination [(Dasabuvir 200 mg + Paritaprevir 50 mg/ritonavir 33.3 mg + Ombitasvir 8.33 mg) 3 tabs once daily with food |
| Simeprevir (SMV) | Olysio | 150 mg tab po once daily with food |
| Sofosbuvir (SOF) | Solvadi | 400 mg tab po once daily |
| Sofosbuvir + Ledipasvir | Harvoni | Fixed dose combination (Sofosbuvir 400 mg + Ledipasvir 90 mg) 1 tab po once daily |
| Sofosbuvir + Velpatasvir | Epclusa | Fixed dose combination (Sofosbuvir 400 mg + Velpatasvir 100 mg): 1 tab po once daily |
| Sofosbuvir + Velpatasvir + Voxilaprevir | Vosevi | Fixed dose combination (Sofosbuvir 400 mg + Velpatasvir 100 mg + Voxilaprevir 100 mg): 1 tab po once daily with food |
| Ribavirin | Ribavirin, Copegus | Weight-based daily dosing: 1000 mg (Wt <75 kg) or 1200 mg (Wt >75 kg). Low dose: 600 mg/day. Taken with food. |
| Pegylated interferon (alfa 2a) | Roferon, Intron-A, Peg-Intron, Pegasys | 180 mcg sc per week |

TABLE 14F (2)

## HCV RECOMMENDED TREATMENT REGIMENS (P = Primary regimen, A = Alternative regimen, Regimens from prior page)

### HCV Mono Infection

| Genotype | P/A | Regimen | Cirrhosis | Duration | Comments |
|---|---|---|---|---|---|
| 1-6 | P | Epclusa 1 tab po once daily | With or without | 12 weeks | Pan-genotypic DAAs |
| | P | Mavyret 3 tabs po once daily | Without | 8 weeks | |
| | | | With | 12 weeks | |
| 1a | P | Epclusa 1 tab po once daily | With or without | 12 weeks | |
| | P | Harvoni 1 tab po once daily | Without* | 8 weeks | * If patient is non-black, HIV-uninfected, non-cirrhotic, and HCV RNA <6 million c/mL |
| | | | With** | 12 weeks | ** If patient is black, HIV-co-infected, compensated cirrhosis, or HCV RNA >6 million c/mL |
| | P | Mavyret 3 tabs po once daily | Without | 8 weeks | |
| | | | With | 12 weeks | |
| | P | Zepatier 1 tab po once daily | With or without | 12 weeks | If no baseline high-fold NS5A resistance associated mutations |
| | A | Viekira Pak (as directed) + RBV | Without only | 12 weeks | RBV dosing is wt-based |
| | A | (DCV + SOF) po once daily | Without only | 12 weeks | |
| | A | (SOF + SMV ± RBV) po divided twice daily | With or without | 12 weeks | RBV dosing is wt-based |
| 1b | P | Epclusa 1 tab po once daily | With or without | 12 weeks | |
| | P | Harvoni 1 tab po once daily | Without* | 8 weeks | * If patient is non-black, HIV-uninfected, non-cirrhotic, and HCV RNA <6 million c/mL |
| | | | With** | 12 weeks | ** If patient is black, HIV-co-infected, compensated cirrhosis, or HCV RNA >6 million c/mL |
| | P | Mavyret 3 tabs po once daily | Without | 8 weeks | |
| | | | With | 12 weeks | |
| | P | Zepatier 1 tab po once daily | With or without | 12 weeks | |
| | A | Viekira Pak (as directed) | With or without | 12 weeks | |
| | A | (DCV + SOF) po once daily | Without only | 12 weeks | |
| | A | (SOF + SMV ± RBV) po divided twice daily | With or without | 12 weeks | RBV dosing is wt-based |
| 2 | P | Epclusa 1 tab po once daily | With or without | 12 weeks | |
| | P | Mavyret 3 tabs po once daily | Without | 8 weeks | |
| | | | With | 12 weeks | |
| | A | (DCV + SOF) po once daily | Without | 12 weeks | |
| | | | With | 16-24 weeks | |
| 3 | P | Epclusa 1 tab po once daily | With or without | 12 weeks | Do not use in cirrhosis if RAV Y93H is present |
| | P | Mavyret 3 tabs po once daily | Without | 8 weeks | |
| | | | With | 12 weeks | |
| | A | Vosevi 1 tab po once daily | With | 12 weeks | RAS Y93H is present |
| | A | (DCV + SOF) po once daily | Without | 12 weeks | |
| | | | With | 16-24 weeks | |

**TABLE 14F (3)**

## HCV Mono Infection (continued)

| Genotype | P/A | Regimen | Cirrhosis | Duration | Comments |
|---|---|---|---|---|---|
| 4 | P | **Epclusa** 1 tab po once daily | With or without | 12 weeks | |
| | P | **Harvoni** 1 tab po once daily | Without* | 8 weeks | * If patient is non-black, HIV-uninfected, non-cirrhotic, and HCV RNA <6 million c/mL |
| | | | With** | 12 weeks | ** If patient is black, HIV-co-infected, compensated cirrhosis, or HCV RNA >6 million c/mL |
| | P | **Mavyret** 3 tabs po once daily | Without | 8 weeks | |
| | | | With | 12 weeks | |
| | P | **Zepatier** 1 tab po once daily | With or without | 12 weeks | |
| | A | **Technivie** once daily | Without | 12 weeks | |
| | A | **Technivie** once daily + **RBV** twice daily | With | 12 weeks | RBV dosing is wt-based |
| 5 & 6 | P | **Epclusa** 1 tab po once daily | With or without | 12 weeks | |
| | P | **Harvoni** 1 tab po once daily | Without* | 8 weeks | * If patient is non-black, HIV-uninfected, non-cirrhotic, and HCV RNA <6 million c/mL |
| | | | With** | 12 weeks | ** If patient is black, HIV-co-infected, compensated cirrhosis, or HCV RNA >6 million c/mL |
| | P | **Mavyret** 3 tabs po once daily | Without | 8 weeks | |
| | | | With | 12 weeks | |

## HCV+HIV Co-infection

| Genotype | P/A | Regimen | Cirrhosis | Duration | Comments |
|---|---|---|---|---|---|
| 1a & 1b | P/A | Same as for HCV Mono Infection | | 8-12 weeks* | Watch for drug-drug interactions. * 8 weeks ONLY in HCV Rx naive co-infected patients receiving **Mavyret**; otherwise, minimum 12 weeks with any other regimen |
| 2 | P/A | Same as for HCV Mono Infection | | 8-12 weeks* | Watch for drug-drug interactions. * 8 weeks ONLY in HCV Rx naive co-infected patients receiving **Mavyret**; otherwise, minimum 12 weeks with any other regimen |
| 3 | P/A | Same as for HCV Mono Infection | | | Watch for drug-drug interactions. |
| 4, 5, 6 | | Not enough experience; if treatment required, use same as for HCV Mono Infection | | | |

## Decompensated Cirrhosis

| Genotype | P/A | Regimen | Cirrhosis | Duration | Comments |
|---|---|---|---|---|---|
| 1, 4, 5, 6 | P | **Epclusa** 1 tab po once daily + **RBV** | | 12 weeks | RBV dosing is wt-based. If RBV-intolerant, treat without RBV for 24 weeks. If prior SOF or NS5A treatment experience, RBV alone for 24 weeks. |
| | P | **Harvoni** 1 tab po once daily + low dose **RBV** | | 12 weeks | If RBV-intolerant, treat without RBV for 24 weeks. If prior SOF or NS5A treatment experience, RBV alone for 24 weeks. |
| 1, 4 | P | (**DCV + SOF**) po once daily + low dose **RBV** | | 12 weeks | 24 weeks if RBV intolerant |
| 2, 3 | P | **Epclusa** 1 tab po once daily + **RBV** | | 12 weeks | RBV dosing is wt-based. If RBV-intolerant, treat without RBV for 24 weeks. If prior SOF or NS5A treatment experience, RBV alone for 24 weeks. |
| | P | (**DCV + SOF**) po once daily + low dose **RBV** | | 12 weeks | 24 weeks if RBV intolerant |

**TABLE 14F (4)**

| Post-Liver Transplant | | | | | |
|---|---|---|---|---|---|
| Genotype | P/A | Regimen | Cirrhosis | Duration | Comments |
| 1, 4, 5, 6 | P | **Mavyret** 3 tabs po once daily | Without | 12 weeks | Alternative if compensated cirrhosis |
| | P | **Harvoni** 1 tab po once daily + **RBV** | With or without | 12 weeks | RBV dosing is wt-based. Dose as tolerated. |
| | A | (**DCV + SOF**) po once daily + low dose **RBV** | Without | 12 weeks | RBV dosing is wt-based. |
| 1, 4 | A | (**SOF + SMV ± RBV**) po divided twice daily | Without | 12 weeks | Alternative if compensated cirrhosis |
| 2, 3 | P | **Mavyret** 3 tabs po once daily | With | 12 weeks | Compensated or decompensated |
| | P | (**DCV + SOF**) po once daily + low dose **RBV** | With | 12 weeks | Compensated or decompensated. RBV dosing is wt-based |
| | A | **Epclusa** 1 tab po once daily + **RBV** | | 24 weeks | RBV initial dose 600 mg/day, increased monthly by 200 mg/day as tolerated up to max wt-based dose |
| | A | **SOF + RBV** po daily | | | |

## TABLE 15A – ANTIMICROBIAL PROPHYLAXIS FOR SELECTED BACTERIAL INFECTIONS*

| CLASS OF ETIOLOGIC AGENT/DISEASE/CONDITION | PROPHYLAXIS AGENT/DOSE/ROUTE/DURATION | COMMENTS |
|---|---|---|
| **Group B streptococcal disease (GBS), neonatal: Approaches to management** (CDC Guidelines, *MMWR 59 (RR-10):1, 2010; CID 2017;65(S2):S143*) | | |
| **Pregnant women—intrapartum antimicrobial prophylaxis procedures:**<br>1. Screen all pregnant women with vaginal & rectal swab for GBS at 35-37 wks gestation (unless other indications for prophylaxis exist: GBS bacteria during this pregnancy or previously delivered infant with invasive GBS disease; even then cultures may be useful for susceptibility testing). Use transport medium; GBS survive at room temp. up to 96 hrs. **Rx during labor if swab culture positive.**<br>2. Rx during labor if previously delivered infant with invasive GBS infection, or if any GBS bacteriuria during this pregnancy.<br>3. Rx if GBS status unknown but, if any of the following are present: (a) delivery at <37 wks gestation [see *MMWR 59 (RR-10): 1, 2010* algorithms for preterm labor and preterm premature rupture of membranes]; or (b) duration of ruptured membranes ≥18 hrs; or (c) intrapartum temp. ≥100.4ºF (≥38.0ºC). If amnionitis suspected, broad-spectrum antibiotic coverage should include an agent active vs. group B streptococci.<br>4. Rx if positive intra-partum NAAT for GBS.<br>5. Unless other conditions exist, Rx not indicated if: negative vaginal/rectal cultures at 35-37 wks gestation or C-section performed before onset of labor with intact amniotic membranes (use standard surgical prophylaxis). | **Regimens for prophylaxis against early-onset group B streptococcal disease in neonate used during labor:**<br>**Pen G** 5 million Units IV (initial dose) then 2.5 to 3 million Units IV q4h until delivery<br>Alternative: **AMP** 2 gm IV (initial dose) then 1 gm IV q4h until delivery<br>**Penicillin-allergic patients:**<br>• Patient not at high risk for anaphylaxis: **Cefazolin** 2 gm IV (initial dose) then 1 gm IV q8h until delivery<br>• Patient at high risk for anaphylaxis from β-lactams:<br>  ○ If organism is both clindamycin- and erythromycin-susceptible, **or** is erythromycin-resistant, but clindamycin-susceptible confirmed by D-zone test (or equivalent) showing lack of inducible resistance: **Clinda** 900 mg IV q8h until delivery<br>  ○ If susceptibility of organism unknown, lack of inducible resistance to clindamycin has not been excluded, or patient is allergic to clindamycin: **Vanco** 1 gm IV q12h until delivery |
| **Neonate of mother given prophylaxis** | *See detailed algorithm in MMWR 59 (RR-10):1, 2010.* | |
| **Preterm, premature rupture of the membranes: Grp B strep-negative women**<br>Cochrane Database Rev 12:CD001058, 2013; Obstet Gyn 124:515-2014; Am J Ob-Gyn 207:475. 2012. | (**AMP** 2 gm IV q6h + **Erythro** 250 mg IV q6h) x 48 hrs, then (**Amox** 250 mg po q8h + **Erythro base** 333 mg po q8h) x 5 days (*ACOG Practice Bulletin; Obstet Gynecol 127: e39, 2016*). | |
| **Post-splenectomy bacteremia.** Usually encapsulated bacteria: pneumococci, meningococci, H. flu type B; bacteremia: Enterobacter, S. aureus, Capnocytophaga, P. aeruginosa. Also at risk for fatal malaria, severe babesiosis.<br>Asplenia review (*Chest 2016;150:1394*) | Protein conjugate and polysaccharide vaccines at age and timing appropriate intervals (Adults: *www.cdc.gov/vaccines/schedules/downloads/adult/adult-combined-schedule.pdf*. Children: *www.cdc.gov/vaccines/schedules/downloads/child/0-18yrs-child-combined-schedule.pdf*). Daily Prophylaxis in asplenic child (daily until age 5 yrs or minimum of 1 yr rx): **Amox** 125 mg po bid (age 2mo-3yr); **Amox** 250 mg po bid (age >3yr-5 yr). If allergic, e.g. rash only: **Cephalexin** 250 mg po bid. Fever in Children & Adults: **AM-CL** 875/125 po bid (adult), 90 mg/kg po div bid (child); Alternative: (**Levo** 750 mg po or **Moxi** 400 mg po) once daily. Seek immediate medical care. Some recommend **Amox** 2 gm po before sinus or airway procedures. | |

**TABLE 15A (2)**

| CLASS OF ETIOLOGIC AGENT/DISEASE/CONDITION | PROPHYLAXIS AGENT/DOSE/ROUTE/DURATION | COMMENTS |
|---|---|---|
| **Sexual Exposure** | | |
| Sexual assault survivor [likely agents and risks, see CDC Guidelines at *MMWR 64(RR-3):1, 2015*]. For review of overall care: *NEJM 365:834, 2011*. | [**Ceftriaxone** 250 mg IM + **Azithro** 1 gm po once + (**Metro** 2 gm po once or **Tinidazole** 2 gm po once)]. Can delay Metro/Tinidazole if alcohol was recently ingested. | • Obtain expert individualized advice re: forensic exam and specimens, pregnancy (incl. emergency contraception), physical-trauma, psychological support <br> • Test for chlamydia and gonococci at sites of penetration or attempted penetration by NAATs. Obtain molecular tests for trichomonas and check vaginal secretions for BV and candidiasis. <br> • Serological evaluation for syphilis, HIV, HBV, HCV <br> • Initiate post-exposure protocols for HBV vaccine, HIV post-exposure prophylaxis as appropriate <br> • HPV vaccine recommended for females 9-26 or males 9-21, if not already immunized <br> • Follow-up in 1 week to review results, repeat negative tests in 1-2 weeks to detect infections not detected previously, repeat syphilis testing 4-6 weeks and 3 months, repeat HIV testing 6 weeks and 3-6 months. <br> • Check for anogenital warts at 1-2 months. <br> Notes: <br> If ceftriaxone not available, can use cefixime 400 mg po once in its place for prevention of gonorrhea, but the latter is less effective for pharyngeal infection and against strains with reduced susceptibility to cephalosporins. <br> For non-pregnant individuals who cannot receive cephalosporins, treatment with (Gemifloxacin 320 mg po once + azithro 2 gm po once) or (Gentamicin 240 mg IM once + azithro 2 gm po once) can be substituted for ceftriaxone/azithro. |
| Contact with specific sexually transmitted diseases. *See comprehensive guidelines for specific pathogens in MMWR 64(RR-3):1, 2015.* | | |
| Syphilis exposure | | Presumptive rx for exposure within 3 mos., as tests may be negative. *See Table 1, page 24.* If exposure occurred >90 days prior, establish dx or treat empirically. |
| **Sickle-cell disease.** Likely agent: S. pneumoniae (see post-splenectomy, above) Ref.: *NEJM 376: 1561, 2017* | Children <5 yrs: **Pen V** 62.5 to 125 mg po bid ≥5 yrs: **Pen V** 250 mg po bid. (Alternative in children: **Amox** 20 mg/kg/day) | Start prophylaxis by 2 mos. (*Pediatrics 106:367, 2000*); continue until at least age 5. When to d/c must be individualized. Age-appropriate vaccines, including pneumococcal, Hib, influenza, meningococcal. Treating infections, consider possibility of penicillin non-susceptible pneumococci. May need malaria prophylaxis entire life. |

# TABLE 15B – ANTIBIOTIC PROPHYLAXIS TO PREVENT SURGICAL INFECTIONS IN ADULTS*
*2013 Guidelines: Am J Health Syst Pharm 70:195, 2013; Med Lett 58:63, 2016*

**General Comments:**
- To be optimally effective, antibiotics must be started within 60 minutes of the surgical incision. Vancomycin and FQs may require 1-2 hr infusion time, so start dose 2 hrs before the surgical incision.
- Most applications employ a single preoperative dose or continuation for less than 24 hrs.
- For procedures lasting >2 half-lives of prophylactic agent, intraoperative supplementary dose(s) may be required.
- Dose adjustments may be desirable in pts with BMI >30.
- Prophylaxis does carry risk: e.g., C. difficile colitis, allergic reactions
- Active S. aureus screening, decolonization & customized antimicrobial prophylaxis demonstrated efficacious in decreasing infections after hip, knee & cardiac surgery (*JAMA 313:2131 & 2162, 2015*).
- See educational details for prevention of surgical site infections per CDC (*JAMA Surg 152:784, 2017*) and Am Coll Surg/Surg Infect Soc (*J Am Coll Surg 224: 59, 2016*). Both support no further antibiotics once surgical wound is closed, although latter includes possible exceptions: breast reconstruction, joint arthroplasty, and cardiac procedures.

**Use of Vancomycin:**
- For many common prophylaxis indications, vancomycin is considered an alternative to β-lactams in pts allergic to or intolerant of the latter.
- Vancomycin use may be justifiable in centers where rates of post-operative infection with methicillin-resistant staphylococci are high or in pts at high risk for these.
- Unlike β-lactams in common use, vancomycin has no activity against gram-negative organisms. **When gram-negative bacteria are a concern following specific procedures, it may be necessary or desirable to add a second agent with appropriate in vitro activity.** This can be done using cefazolin with vancomycin in the non-allergic pt, or in pts intolerant of β-lactams using vancomycin with another non-negative agent (e.g., aminoglycoside, fluoroquinolone, possibly aztreonam, if pt not allergic, local resistance patterns and pt factors would influence choice).
- Infusion of vancomycin, especially too rapidly, may result in hypotension and other manifestations of histamine release (red person syndrome). Does not indicate an allergy to vancomycin.

| TYPE OF SURGERY | PROPHYLAXIS | COMMENTS |
|---|---|---|
| **Cardiovascular Surgery** | | |
| Antibiotic prophylaxis in cardiovascular surgery has been proven beneficial in the following procedures:<br>- Reconstruction of abdominal aorta<br>- Procedures on the leg that involve a groin incision<br>- Any vascular procedure that inserts prosthesis/foreign body<br>- Lower extremity amputation for ischemia<br>- Cardiac surgery<br>- Heart transplant<br>- Permanent Pacemakers (*Circulation 121:458, 2010*)<br>- Implanted cardiac defibrillators | **Cefazolin** 1-2 gm (Wt <120 kg) or 3 gm (Wt >120 kg) IV as a single dose or q8h for 1-2 days or **Cefuroxime** 1.5 gm IV q12 dose or single dose IV, then q12h x total of 6 gm or **Vanco** 1 gm IV as a single dose or q12h for 1-2 days. For pts weighing >90 kg, use vanco 1.5 gm IV as a single dose or q12h for 1-2 days. Re-dose cefazolin q4h if CrCl>30 mL/min or q8h if CrCl ≤30 mL/min<br>Consider **intranasal Mupirocin** evening before, day of surgery & bid for 5 days post-op in pts with pos. nasal culture for S. aureus. Mupirocin resistance has been encountered. | **Timing & duration:** Single infusion just before surgery as effective as multiple doses, customary to give as multiple doses. For prosthetic heart valves, customary to continue prophylaxis either after removal of retained drainage catheters or for 48 hr after coming off bypass. **Vanco** may be preferable in hospitals with ↑ freq of MRSA. In high-risk pts, those colonized with MRSA or Pen-allergic pt. Clindamycin 900 mg IV is another alternative for Pen-allergic or Vanco-allergic pt. Implanted devices ref: *JAC 70:325, 2015*. For insertion of ventricular assist devices, prophylaxis same as for cardiac surgery (e.g., cefazolin ± vancomycin) (*CID 64: 222, 2017*). |
| **Gastric, Biliary and Colonic Surgery** | | |
| **Gastroduodenal/Biliary** | | |
| Gastroduodenal, includes percutaneous endoscopic gastrostomy (high risk only), pancreatoduodenectomy (Whipple procedure) | **Cefazolin** (1-2 gm IV) or **Cefoxitin** (1-2 gm IV) or **Cefotetan** (1-2 gm IV) or **Ceftriaxone** (2 gm IV) as a single dose (some give additional doses q12h for 2-3 days). *See Comment.* | Gastroduodenal (PEG placement): High-risk is marked obesity, obstruction, ↓ gastric acid or ↓ motility. Re-dose Cefazolin q4h and Cefoxitin q2h if CrCl >30 mL/min; q8h and q4h, respectively, if CrCl ≤30 mL/min. |
| Biliary, includes laparoscopic cholecystectomy | Low risk, laparoscopic: No prophylaxis<br>Open cholecystectomy: **Cefazolin, Cefoxitin, Cefotetan, Ampicillin-sulbactam** | Biliary high-risk or open procedure: age >70, acute cholecystitis, non-functioning gallbladder, obstructive jaundice or common duct stones. With cholangitis, treat as infection, not prophylaxis. |
| Endoscopic retrograde cholangiopancreatography | No rx without obstruction. If obstruction:<br>**CIP** 500-750 mg po or 400 mg IV 2 hrs prior to procedure or **PIP-TZ** 4.5 gm IV 1 hr prior to procedure | Most studies show that achieving adequate drainage will prevent post-procedural cholangitis or sepsis and no further benefit from prophylactic antibiotics; greatest benefit likely when complete drainage cannot be achieved. *See Gastrointest Endosc 81: 81, 2015 for American Society of Gastrointestinal Endoscopy recommendations for ERCP). Gut 58:868, 2009* |

**TABLE 15B (2)**

| TYPE OF SURGERY | PROPHYLAXIS | COMMENTS |
|---|---|---|
| **Gastric, Biliary and Colonic Surgery** (continued) | | |
| **Colorectal**<br>Recommend combination of:<br>• Mechanical bowel prep<br>• po antibiotic (See Comment)<br>• IV antibiotic<br><br>Mechanical bowel prep + po antibiotics recommended for all elective colectomies (J Am Coll Surg 224:59, 2016). | **Parenteral regimens** (emergency or elective):<br>[**Cefazolin** 1-2 gm IV + **Metro** 0.5 gm IV]<br>(see Comment)<br>or<br>**Cefoxitin** or **Cefotetan** 1-2 gm IV (if available)<br>or<br>**Ceftriaxone** 2 gm IV + **Metro** 0.5 gm IV<br>or<br>**ERTA** 1 gm IV<br>Beta-lactam allergy, see Comment | **Oral regimens: Neomycin + Erythro**. Pre-op day: (1) 10 am 4L polyethylene glycol electrolyte solution (Colyte, GoLYTELY) po over 2 hr. (2) Clear liquid diet only. (3) 1 pm, 2 pm & 11 pm, Neomycin 1 gm + Erythro base 1 gm po. (4) NPO after midnight.<br>Alternative regimens (in hospitals where rates have been well studied: GoLYTELY 1–6 pm, then Neomycin 2 gm po + Metronidazole 2 gm po at 7 pm & 11 pm.<br>Oral regimen as effective as parenteral; parenteral in addition to oral not required but often used (Am J Surg 189:395, 2005).<br>Study found **Ertapenem** more effective than cefotetan, but associated with non-significant ↑ risk of C. difficile (NEJM 355:2640, 2006).<br>**Beta lactam allergy: Clinda** 900 mg IV + (**Gent** 5 mg/kg or **Aztreonam** 2 gm IV or **CIP** 400 mg IV). |
| Ruptured viscus: See Peritoneum/Peritonitis, Secondary, Table 1, page 48. | | |
| **Head and Neck Surgery** | **Cefazolin** 2 gm IV (Single dose) (some add **Metro** 500 mg IV) OR **Clinda** 600–900 mg IV (single dose) ± **Gent** 5 mg/kg IV (single dose) (See Table 10D for weight-based dose calculation.) | Antimicrobial prophylaxis in head & neck surg appears efficacious only for procedures involving oral/ pharyngeal mucosa (e.g., laryngeal or pharyngeal tumor) but even with prophylaxis, wound infection rate can be high. **Clean, uncontaminated head & neck surg does not require prophylaxis.** Re-dose cefazolin q4h if CrCl>30 mL/min or q8h if CrCl ≤30 mL/min |
| **Neurosurgical Procedures** | | |
| Clean, non-implant, e.g., elective craniotomy. | **Cefazolin** 1-2 gm IV once. Alternative: **Vanco** 1 gm IV once; for pts weighing >90 kg, use vanco 1.5 gm IV as single dose. | Clindamycin 900 mg IV is alternative for vanco-allergic or beta-lactam allergic pt. Re-dose cefazolin q4h if CrCl>30 mL/min or q8h if CrCl ≤30 mL/min |
| Clean, contaminated (cross sinuses, or naso/oropharynx) | **Clinda** 900 mg IV (single dose) | British recommend Amoxicillin-Clavulanate 1.2 gm IV^NUS or (Cefuroxime 1.5 gm IV + Metronidazole 0.5 gm IV) |
| CSF shunt surgery, intrathecal pumps | **Cefazolin** 1-2 gm IV (Wt <120 kg) or 3 gm (Wt >120 kg) IV once. Alternative: **Vanco** 1 gm IV once; for pts weighing >90 kg, use vanco 1.5 gm IV as single dose OR **Clinda** 900 mg IV. | Randomized study in a hospital with high prevalence of infection due to methicillin-resistant staphylococci showed Vancomycin was more effective than cefazolin in preventing CSF shunt infections (J Hosp Infect 69:337, 2008). Re-dose cefazolin q4h if CrCl >30 mL/min or q8h if CrCl ≤30 mL/min |
| **Obstetric/Gynecologic Surgery** | | |
| Vaginal or abdominal hysterectomy | **Cefazolin** 1-2 gm IV or **Cefoxitin** 1-2 gm or **Cefotetan** 1-2 gm or **AM-SB** 3 gm IV 30 min. before surgery. | Alternative: (**Clinda** 900 mg IV or **Vanco** 1 gm IV) + (**Gent** 5 mg/kg x 1 dose or **Aztreonam** 2 gm IV or **CIP** 400 mg IV) OR (**Metro** 500 mg IV + **CIP** 400 mg IV) |
| Cesarean Section for premature rupture of membranes or active labor | **Cefazolin** 1-2 gm IV x 1 dose.<br>Alternative: **Clinda** 900 mg IV + (**Gent** 5 mg/kg IV or **Tobra** 5 mg/kg IV) x 1 dose.<br>Increased risk of infection vs. cefazolin (Obstet Gyn 2018;132:e49). | Administering prophylaxis before the skin incision reduces surgical site infections.<br>**In non-elective C-section,** addition of **Azithro** 500 mg IV in addition to standard antibiotics significantly reduced endometritis and wound infections (NEJM 375: 1231, 2016).<br>**In obesity,** give standard pre-op prophylaxis, then (Cephalexin 500 mg po q8h + Metro 500 mg po q8h) x 18 hrs. (JAMA 2017;318:1012 & 1026). |
| Surgical Abortion (1st trimester) | 1st trimester: **Doxy** 300 mg po: 100 mg 1 hr before procedure +200 mg post-procedure. | Meta-analysis showed benefit of antibiotic prophylaxis in all risk groups. |
| **Ophthalmic Surgery** | (Neomycin-Gent-Polymyxin B or Gati or Moxi) eye drops, 1 drop q5-15 min x 5 doses | Some add **Cefazolin** 100 mg under conjunctiva at end of surgery. |

TABLE 15B (3)

| TYPE OF SURGERY | PROPHYLAXIS | COMMENTS |
|---|---|---|
| **Orthopedic Surgery** | | |
| Hip arthroplasty, spinal fusion | Same as cardiac surgery | Customarily stopped after "Hemovac" removed, 2013 Guidelines recommend stopping prophylaxis within 24 hrs of surgery. (*Am J Health Syst Pharm 70:195, 2013*) |
| Total joint replacement (other than hip) | **Cefazolin** 1–2 gm IV (or 3 gm if ≥ 120 kg) at 2nd dose, or **Vanco** 1 gm IV. For pts weighing >90 kg, use Vanco 1.5 gm IV as single dose or **Clinda** 900 mg IV. | 2013 Guidelines recommends stopping prophylaxis within 24 hrs of surgery. (*Am J Health Syst Pharm 70:195, 2013*). Usual to administer before tourniquet inflation. Intranasal mupirocin if colonized with S. aureus. |
| Open reduction of closed fracture with internal fixation | **Ceftriaxone** 2 gm IV once | 3.6% (ceftriaxone) vs 8.3% (for placebo) infection found in Dutch trauma trial (*Ln 347:1133, 1996*). Several alternative antimicrobials can ↓ risk of infection (*Cochrane Database Syst Rev 2010: CD 000244*). |
| Prophylaxis to protect prosthetic joints from hematogenous infection related to distant procedures (patients with plates, pins and screws only or are not considered to be at risk) | | • A prospective, case-control study concluded that antibiotic prophylaxis did not decrease the risk of hip or knee prosthesis infection (*Clin Infection Dis 50:8, 2010*).<br>• An expert panel of the American Dental Association concluded that, in general, prophylactic antibiotics are not recommended prior to dental procedures to prevent prosthetic joint infection (*J Amer Dental Assoc 146: 11, 2015*).<br>• Individual circumstances should be considered; when there is a planned manipulation of tissues thought to be actively infected, antimicrobial therapy for the infection is likely to be appropriate. |
| Peritoneal Dialysis Catheter Placement | **Vanco** single 1 gm IV 12 hrs prior to procedure | Effectively reduced peritonitis during 14 days post-placement in 221 pts: Vanco 1%, Cefazolin 7%, placebo 12% (p=0.02) (*Am J Kidney Dis 36:1014, 2000*). |
| **Urologic Surgery/Procedures** | | |
| • See *Best Practice Policy Statement* of Amer. Urological Assoc. (AUA) (*J Urol 179:1379, 2008*) and 2013 Guidelines (*Am J Health Syst Pharm 70:195, 2013*). | | |
| • Selection of agents targeting urinary pathogens should require modification based on local resistance patterns; ↑ TMP-SMX and fluoroquinolone (FQ) resistance among enteric gram-negative bacteria is a concern. | | |
| Cystoscopy | • Prophylaxis generally not necessary if urine is sterile (however, AUA recommends FQ or TMP-SMX for those with several potentially adverse host factors (e.g., advanced age, immunocompromised state, anatomic abnormalities, etc.)<br>• Treat patients with ↑ risk prior to procedure using an antimicrobial active against pathogen isolated | |
| Cystoscopy with manipulation | **CIP** 500 mg po (**TMP-SMX** 1 DS tablet po may be an alternative in populations with low rates of resistance). | Procedures mentioned include ureteroscopy, biopsy, fulguration, TURP, etc. Treat UTI with targeted therapy before procedure if possible. |
| Transrectal prostate biopsy | **CIP** 500 mg po 12 hrs prior to biopsy and repeated 12 hrs after 1st dose. See Comment. | Bacteremia 7% with **CIP** vs 37% with **Gent** (*JAC 39:115, 1997*). Levofloxacin 500 mg 30–60 min before procedure was effective in low risk pts; additional doses were given for ↑ risk (*J Urol 168:1021, 2002*). Serious bacteremias due to FQ-resistant organisms have been encountered in patients receiving FQ prophylaxis. Screening stool cultures pre-procedure for colonization with FQ-resistant organisms is increasingly utilized to inform choice of prophylaxis (*Clin Infect Dis 60: 979, 2015*). One study showed non-significant decrease in risk of infection with culture-directed antimicrobial prophylaxis (*Urology 146: 11, 2015*). Pre-operative prophylaxis should be determined on an institutional basis based on susceptibility profiles of prevailing organisms. Although 2nd or 3rd generation Cephalosporins or addition of single-dose gentamicin has been suggested, infection due to ESBL-producing and gent-resistant organisms have been encountered (*Urol 74:332, 2009*). Meta-analysis found fosfomycin trometamol more effective than FQ in preventing infection after transrectal prostate biopsy (*World J Urol. 36: 323, 2018*). |
| **Other** | | |
| Breast surgery, herniorrhaphy, thoracotomy | **Cefazolin** 1–2 gm IV x 1 dose or **AM-SB** 3 gm IV x 1 dose or **Clinda** 900 mg IV x 1 dose or **Vanco** 1 gm IV x 1 dose (1.5 gm if wt >90 kg). | *Am J Health Syst Pharm 70:195, 2013*. |
| Vascular surgery: aneurysm repair, revascularization | **Cefazolin** 2 gm IV x 1 dose | |

# TABLE 15C – ANTIMICROBIAL PROPHYLAXIS FOR THE PREVENTION OF BACTERIAL ENDOCARDITIS IN PATIENTS WITH UNDERLYING CARDIAC CONDITIONS*

In 2007, the American Heart Association guidelines for the prevention of bacterial endocarditis were updated. The resulting document (*Circulation 2007; 116:1736-1754 and http://circ.ahajournals.org/cgi/reprint/116/15/1736*), which was also endorsed by the Infectious Diseases Society of America, represents a significant departure from earlier recommendations.

- Antibiotic prophylaxis for dental procedures is now directed at those patients who are likely to suffer the most devastating consequences should they develop endocarditis. Prophylaxis to prevent endocarditis is no longer specified for gastrointestinal or genitourinary procedures. The following is adapted from and reflects the new AHA recommendations.
  *See original publication for explanation and precise details.*

| | SELECTION OF PATIENTS FOR ENDOCARDITIS PROPHYLAXIS | | | |
|---|---|---|---|---|
| FOR PATIENTS WITH ANY OF THESE HIGH-RISK CARDIAC CONDITIONS ASSOCIATED WITH ENDOCARDITIS: | WHO UNDERGO DENTAL PROCEDURES INVOLVING: | WHO UNDERGO INVASIVE RESPIRATORY PROCEDURES INVOLVING: | WHO UNDERGO INVASIVE PROCEDURES OF THE GI OR GU TRACTS: | WHO UNDERGO PROCEDURES INVOLVING INFECTED SKIN AND SOFT TISSUES: |
| Prosthetic heart valves<br>Previous infective endocarditis<br>Congenital heart disease with any of the following:<br>• Completely repaired cardiac defect using prosthetic material (Only for 1st 6 months)<br>• Partially corrected but with residual defect near prosthetic material<br>• Uncorrected cyanotic congenital heart disease<br>• Surgically constructed shunts and conduits<br>Valvulopathy following heart transplant [Benefit unclear in pt with VAD (CID 64: 222, 2017).] | Any manipulation of gingival tissue, dental periapical regions, or perforating the oral mucosa.<br>**PROPHYLAXIS RECOMMENDED‡**<br>*(See Dental Procedures Regimens table below)*<br><br>(Prophylaxis is *not* recommended for routine anesthetic injections (unless through infected area), dental x-rays, shedding of primary teeth, adjustment of orthodontic appliances or placement of orthodontic brackets or removable appliances.) | Incision of respiratory tract mucosa<br>**CONSIDER PROPHYLAXIS**<br>*(See Dental Procedures Regimens table)*<br><br>OR<br><br>For treatment of established infection<br>**PROPHYLAXIS RECOMMENDED**<br>*(See Dental Procedures Regimens and Footnote 1 above, but include anti-staphylococcal coverage when S. aureus is of concern)* | PROPHYLAXIS is no longer recommended solely to prevent endocarditis, **but the following approach is reasonable:**<br><br>For patients with enterococcal UTIs<br>• treat before elective GU procedures<br>• include enterococcal coverage in perioperative regimen for non-elective procedures†<br>For patients with existing GU or GI infections or those who receive perioperative antibiotics to prevent surgical site infections or sepsis<br>• it is reasonable to include agents with anti-enterococcal activity in perioperative coverage† | Include coverage against staphylococci and β-hemolytic streptococci in treatment regimens |

† Agents with anti-enterococcal activity include penicillin, ampicillin, amoxicillin, vancomycin and others. Check susceptibility if available. *(See Table 5 for highly resistant organisms.)*

‡ 2008 AHA/ACC focused update of guidelines on valvular heart disease use term "is reasonable" to reflect level of evidence (*Circulation 118:887, 2008*).

| PROPHYLACTIC REGIMENS FOR DENTAL PROCEDURES | | |
|---|---|---|
| SITUATION | AGENT | REGIMEN¹ |
| Usual oral prophylaxis | Amox | Adults 2 gm, children 50 mg per kg; orally, 1 hour before procedure |
| Unable to take oral medications | AMP² | Adults 2 gm, children 50 mg per kg; IV or IM, within 30 min before procedure. |
| Allergic to penicillins | Cephalexin³ OR | Adults 2 gm, children 50 mg per kg; orally, 1 hour before procedure |
| | Clinda OR | Adults 600 mg, children 20 mg per kg; orally, 1 hour before procedure |
| | Azithro or Clarithro | Adults 500 mg, children 15 mg per kg; orally, 1 hour before procedure |
| Allergic to penicillins and unable to take oral medications | Cefazolin³ OR | Adults 1 gm, children 50 mg per kg; IV or IM, within 30 min before procedure |
| | Clinda | Adults 600 mg, children 20 mg per kg; IV or IM, within 30 min before procedure |

¹ Children's dose should not exceed adult dose. AHA document lists all doses at 30-60 min before procedure.

² AHA lists Cefazolin or Ceftriaxone (at appropriate doses) as alternatives here.

³ Cephalosporins should not be used in individuals with immediate-type hypersensitivity reaction (urticaria, angioedema, or anaphylaxis) to penicillins or other β-lactams. AHA proposes ceftriaxone as potential alternative to cefazolin; and either 1st or 2nd generation cephalosporin in equivalent doses as potential alternatives to cephalexin.

## TABLE 15D – MANAGEMENT OF EXPOSURE TO HIV-1 AND HEPATITIS B AND C[a]

**OCCUPATIONAL EXPOSURE TO BLOOD, PENILE/VAGINAL SECRETIONS OR OTHER POTENTIALLY INFECTIOUS BODY FLUIDS OR TISSUES WITH RISK OF TRANSMISSION OF HEPATITIS B/C AND/OR HIV-1 (E.G., NEEDLESTICK INJURY)**

**Free consultation for occupational exposures, call (PEPline) 1-888-448-4911.** *[Information also available at www.aidsinfo.nih.gov]*

**General steps in management:**
1. Wash clean wounds/flush mucous membranes immediately (use of caustic agents or squeezing the wound is discouraged; data lacking regarding antiseptics).
2. (a) Determine if exposed individual is HIV/hepatitis B/C positive; (b) Determine/evaluate source of exposure by medical history, risk behavior, & testing for hepatitis B/C, HIV;
   (c) Evaluate and test exposed individual for hepatitis B/C & HIV.

**Hepatitis B Occupational Exposure Prophylaxis** *(MMWR 62(RR-10):1-19, 2013)*

| Exposed Person Vaccine Status | Exposure Source | | |
|---|---|---|---|
| | HBs Ag+ | HBs Ag– | Status Unknown or Unavailable for Testing[†] |
| Unvaccinated | Give HBIG 0.06 mL per kg IM & initiate HB vaccine | Initiate HB vaccine | Initiate HB vaccine |
| Vaccinated (antibody status unknown) | Do anti-HBs on exposed person: If titer ≥10 milli-international units per mL, no rx If titer <10 milli-international units per mL, give HBIG + 1 dose HB vaccine** | No rx necessary | Do anti-HBs on exposed person: If titer ≥10 milli-international units per mL, no rx § If titer <10 milli-international units per mL, give 1 dose of HB vaccine** |

[§] Persons previously infected with HBV are immune to reinfection and do not require postexposure prophylaxis.

For known vaccine series responder (titer ≥10 milli-international units per mL), monitoring of levels or booster doses not currently recommended. Known non-responder (<10 milli-international units per mL) to 1st vaccine series & exposed to either HBsAg+ source–rx with HBIG & re-initiate vaccine series or give 2 doses HBIG 1 month apart. For non-responders after a 2nd vaccine series, 2 doses HBIG 1 month apart is preferred approach to new exposure.

If known high risk source, treat as if source were HBsAG positive.

** Follow-up to assess vaccine response or address completion of vaccine series.

### Hepatitis B Non-Occupational Exposure & Reactivation of Latent Hepatitis B

**Non-Occupational Exposure** *(MMWR 55(RR-10):1, 2010)*
- Exposure to blood or sexual secretion of HBsAg-positive person
  - o Percutaneous (bite, needlestick)
  - o Sexual assault†
- Initiate immunoprophylaxis within 24 hrs or sexual exposure & no more than 7 days after parenteral exposure
- Use Guidelines for occupational exposure for use of HBIG and HBV vaccine

**Reactivation of Latent HBV** *(AnM 164:30 & 64, 2016)*
- Patients requiring administration of anti-CD 20 monoclonal antibodies as part of treatment selected malignancies, rheumatoid arthritis and vasculitis are at risk for reactivation of latent HBV
- Use of two FDA-approved anti-CD 20 drugs: ofatumumab (Arzerra) & rituximab (Rituxan) put patients at risk
- Prior to starting anti-CD 20 drugs, test for latent HBV with test for HBsAg and Anti IgG HBc core antibody & perhaps HIV PCR. Positive HBsAg and/or Anti IgG HBc AB = occult Hepatitis B
- **If pt has latent (occult) HBV & anti-CD 20 treatment is necessary, treatment should include an effective anti-HBV drug**

### Hepatitis C Exposure

Determine antibody to hepatitis C for both exposed person & source. If source + or unknown and exposed hepatitis C RNA (detectable in blood in 1-3 weeks) and HCV antibody (90% will do so 3 months) is advised. **No experimental prophylaxis;** immune serum globulin not effective. Monitor for early infection, as therapy may ↓ risk of progression to chronic hepatitis. Persons who remain viremic 8-12 weeks after exposure should be treated with a course of pegylated interferon *(Gastro 130:632, 2006 and Hpt 43:923, 2006)*.
*See Table 14F:* Case-control study suggested risk factors for occupational HCV transmission include percutaneous exposure to needle that had been in artery or vein, deep injury, male sex of HCW, & was more likely when source VL >6 log10 copies/mL.

## A. HIV OCCUPATIONAL EXPOSURE

The decision to initiate post-exposure prophylaxis (PEP) is a clinical judgment made in concert with the exposed individual and is based on three factors:

1. Type of exposure

    a. Potentially infectious substances include: blood, unfixed tissues, CSF; semen and vaginal secretions (these have not been implicated in occupational transmission of HIV); synovial, pleural, peritoneal, ascitic, and amniotic fluids; other _visibly_ bloody fluids.

    b. Fluids of low or negligible risk for transmission, unless visibly bloody include: urine, sweat, vomitus, stool, saliva, nasal secretions, tears, and sputum. **PEP is not indicated.**

    c. If the exposure occurred to intact skin, regardless of whether the substance is potentially infectious or not, and regardless of the HIV status of the source patient, **PEP is not indicated.**

    d. If the exposure occurred to mucous membranes (e.g., blood splash to the eye) or non-intact skin (e.g., abraded skin, open wound, dermatitis) or occurred percutaneously as a consequence of a needle stick, scalpel, or other sharps injury or cut, then **PEP may be indicated.** Human bites resulting in a break in the skin could theoretically transmit HIV, particularly if oral blood is present, although these have not been implicated in occupational transmission of HIV.

2. Likelihood that the source patient is HIV infected

    a. If the exposure constitutes a risk of HIV transmission as described above and the source patient is **known positive for HIV**, then **PEP should be instituted** immediately, within hours of exposure (Animal studies show PEP less effective when started >72h post-exposure but interval after which PEP not beneficial is unknown; initiation of PEP after a longer interval may be considered if exposure risk of transmission is extremely high).

    b. If exposure constitutes a risk of HIV transmission, and the HIV status is **unknown**, but patient is **likely to be HIV infected** or there is a **reasonable suspicion** for infection based on HIV risk factors, then **PEP should be initiated pending confirmation of the source patient's HIV status.**

        i. If a rapid HIV test of the source patient can be performed, it is reasonable to withhold therapy pending results of this test and initiating PEP if the test is positive.

        ii. If rapid testing cannot be performed, PEP should be initiated pending results of source patient testing and discontinued if the test returns negative.

        iii. NOTE: Antibody testing is sufficient to rule out HIV infection, unless the source patient has suspected acute retroviral syndrome, in which case HIV viral load testing is recommended.

    c. If the **source is unknown** or the source is known but status and risk cannot be determined, the decision to initiate PEP should be made on a case-by-case basis in **consultation with an expert** (PEPline at _http://www.nccc.ucsf.edu/about_nccc/pepline/_) (1-888-448-4911), guided by the severity of the exposure and epidemiologic likelihood of HIV exposure.

3. Adverse effects and potential for drug interactions with the PEP regimen

    a. Newer agents are better tolerated and should allow a higher proportion of exposed healthcare providers to complete the prescribed four-week course of therapy. Doses of some agents may need to be adjusted based on renal function.

    b. Information about drug interactions is available in Tables 16A and 16B, in the package insert and on-line at _hivinsite.ucsf.edu_

    c. Breast feeding and pregnancy are not contraindications to PEP (efavirenz is contraindicated during pregnancy).

**PEP Algorithm**

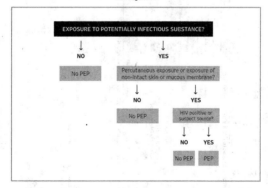

**REGIMENS FOR PEP: a 4-week course of 3 or more drugs now routinely recommended for all PEP**

| Preferred | • **Descovy** (FTC 200 mg + TAF)(but not recommended if CrCl <30 mL/min) po once daily + (**Raltegravir** 1200 mg (two 400 tabs) once daily or **Dolutegravir** 50 mg orally daily) or **Bictegravir** (FTC + TAF fixed dose formulation) one tab once daily<br>• Creatinine clearance < 30 ml/min: [**Tenofovir disoproxil fumarate** (TDF) 300 mg q72-96h + **Emtricitabine** (FTC) 200 mg q72-96h + (**Dolutegravir** 50 mg po once daily OR **Raltegravir** 400 mg po twice daily] |
|---|---|
| Alternative | **Descovy** po once daily + ([DRV 800 mg po once daily + RTV 100 mg po once daily] or [**Prezcobix** (DRV 800 mg + Cobi 150 mg) one tab once daily] |
| | **Descovy** po once daily + **Lopinavir-Ritonavir** 800/200 mg po once daily |
| | Creatinine clearance < 30 ml/min: Renally adjusted doses of **Zidovudine** + **Lamivudine** + **Darunavir** 800 mg po once daily + **Ritonavir** 100 mg po once daily |

1. Abacavir, efavirenz, enfuvirtide, maraviroc should be used only in consultation with an expert.
2. Didanosine, nelfinavir, tipranavir, stavudine (d4T) and nevirapine (contraindicated) are not recommended.
3. If transmission of drug resistant virus is suspected, the regimen should be appropriately modified in consultation with an expert to include agents to which it is likely to be susceptible.
4. **Descovy is the preferred substitute for Truvada** given lower potential for renal injury and osteomalacia for TAF vs. TDF. Note that Descovy is not recommended for CrCl <30 mL/min.
5. Do not use dolutegravir in pregnancy.

**FOLLOW-UP**
1. Complete blood count, renal and hepatic panels recommended at baseline and repeated at 2 weeks with further testing if results are abnormal.
2. HIV antibody testing to monitor seroconversion should be performed at baseline, 6 weeks, 12 weeks, and 6 months post-exposure.
3. If a 4th generation p24 antigen-HIV antibody test is used, testing may be terminated at 4 months.
4. Extended follow-up for 12 months is recommended if HCV conversion occurred upon exposure to an HIV-HCV co-infected patient.

---

**B. HIV NON-OCCUPATIONAL EXPOSURE**
• Risk of transmission of HIV via sexual contact or needle sharing may reach or exceed that of occupational needlestick exposure, thus HIV post-exposure prophylaxis (PEP) not later than 72 hours (and ideally within a few hours) of the exposure is recommended for HIV-negative persons non-occupationally exposed to blood or other potentially infected fluids from an HIV+ source.
• Substantial risk of HIV acquisition from HIV+ source
  o Exposure of vagina, rectum, eye, mouth, mucous membrane, non-intact skin, percutaneous contact
    ○ With blood semen, vaginal secretions, rectal secretions, breast milk, or any body visibly contaminated with blood
• Negligible risk of HIV acquisition regardless of HIV status for any exposure to
  o Urine, nasal secretions, saliva, sweat, or tears if not visibly contaminated with blood
• PEP not effective and not recommended if ≥73 hours after an exposure.
• 4-week course of 3 ARV drugs is recommended for PEP.

**Preferred Regimens**

| Age | Regimen |
|---|---|
| Age ≥13 years (not pregnant women; avoid TAF and dolutegravir with pregnancy. Use TDF 300 mg + FTC 200mg instead of Descovy as part of regimen), CrCl ≥30 ml/min | **Descovy** (Emtricitabine [FTC] 200 mg + Tenofovir alafenamide fumarate [TAF]) + (**Dolutegravir** 50 mg po once daily OR **Raltegravir** 400 mg po twice daily) or **Bictegravir** (FTC + TAF fixed dose formulation) one tab once daily (*See comments*; not recommended if CrCl is <30 ml/min). |
| Age ≥13 years (includes pregnant women), CrCl <30 ml/min | **Tenofovir disoproxil fumarate** (TDF) 300 mg q72-96h + **Emtricitabine** (FTC) 200 mg q72-96h + (**Dolutegravir** 50 mg po once daily OR **Raltegravir** 1200 po once daily) |
| Children aged 2-12 years | **TDF + FTC + Raltegravir**, each dose adjusted for age and weight |
| Children aged 4 weeks to <2 years | **Zidovudine** + **Lamivudine** + (**Raltegravir** OR **Lopinavir-Ritonavir**) each as an oral solution dose adjusted for age and weight |
| Children aged birth to 27 days | Consult a pediatric HIV specialist |

**Alternative Regimens**

| Age | Regimen |
|---|---|
| Age ≥13 years (in pregnancy use TDF 300 mg + FTC 200 mg instead of Descovy), CrCl ≥30 ml/min | **Descovy** (FTC 200 mg + Tenofovir alafenamide fumarate [TAF]) + **Darunavir** 800 mg po once daily + **Ritonavir** 100 mg po once daily (See comments; not recommended if creatinine clearance is <30 ml/min). |
| Age ≥13 years (includes pregnant women), CrCl <30 ml/min | Renally adjusted doses of **Zidovudine** + **Lamivudine** + **Darunavir** 800 mg po once daily + **Ritonavir** 100 mg po once daily |
| Children aged 2-12 years | **Zidovudine** + **Lamivudine** + (**Raltegravir** OR **Lopinavir-Ritonavir**) once daily each dose adjusted for age and weight OR **TDF + FTC +** (**Lopinavir-Ritonavir** OR [**Darunavir** + **Ritonavir**]) each dose adjusted for age and weight |
| Children aged 4 weeks to <2 years | **Zidovudine** + FTC + (**Raltegravir** OR [**Lopinavir-Ritonavir**]) each as an oral solution dose adjusted for age and weight |

## TABLE 15E - PREVENTION OF SELECTED OPPORTUNISTIC INFECTIONS IN HUMAN HEMATOPOIETIC CELL TRANSPLANTATION (HCT) OR SOLID ORGAN TRANSPLANTATION (SOT) IN ADULTS WITH NORMAL RENAL FUNCTION

**General comments:** Medical centers performing transplants will have detailed protocols for the prevention of opportunistic infections which are appropriate to the infections encountered, patients represented and resources available at those sites. Regimens continue to evolve and protocols adopted by an institution may differ from those at other centers. Care of transplant patients should be guided by physicians with expertise in this area.

**References:**

For HCT: Expert guidelines endorsed by the IDSA, updating earlier guidelines *(MMWR 49 (RR-10):1, 2000)* in: *Biol Blood Marrow Transpl 15:1143, 2009*. These guidelines provide recommendations for prevention of additional infections not discussed in this table and provide more detailed information on the infections included here.

For SOT: Recommendations of an expert panel of The Transplantation Society for management of CMV in solid organ transplant recipients in: *Transplantation 89:779, 2010*. Timeline of infections following SOT in: *Amer J Transpl 9 (Suppl 4):S3, 2009*.

| OPPORTUNISTIC INFECTION | TYPE OF TRANSPLANT | PROPHYLACTIC REGIMENS |
|---|---|---|
| **CMV** (Recipient + or Donor +/Recipient −) Ganciclovir resistance: risk, detection, management *(CID 56:1018, 2013)* | SOT | **Prophylaxis: Valganciclovir** 900 mg po q24h<br>Alternatives include **Ganciclovir** 1000 mg po 3 x/day, **Valacyclovir** 2 gm po 4 x/day *(kidney only, see comment)*, CMV IVIG or IVIG.<br>**Also consider preemptive therapy** (monitor weekly for CMV viremia by PCR (or antigenemia) for 3-6 months post transplant. If viremia detected, start Valganciclovir 900 mg po bid or Ganciclovir 5 mg/kg IV q12h until clearance of viremia, but for not less than 2 weeks followed by secondary prophylaxis or preemptive approach. Prophylaxis vs pre-emptive rx compared: *CID 58:785, 2014*. CMV hyper IVIG is as adjunct to prophylaxis in high-risk lung, heart/lung, heart, or pancreas organ transplant recipients. Dosing: 150 mg/kg within 72 hrs. of transplant and at 2, 4, 6, and 8 weeks; then 100 mg/kg at weeks 12 and 16. |
| | HCT | **Preemptive Strategy:** Monitor weekly for CMV viremia by PCR (or antigenemia) for 3-6 months post transplant with consideration for more prolonged monitoring in patients at risk for late-onset CMV disease (chronic GVHD, requiring systemic treatment, patients receiving high-dose steroids, T-cell depleted or cord blood transplant recipients, and CD4 <100 cells/mL). Start treatment with identification of CMV viremia or antigenemia as above. Consider prophylaxis (beginning post-engraftment) with **Valganciclovir** 900 mg po q24h or **Letermovir** 480 mg po/IV once daily. *National Comprehensive Cancer Network Guidelines on Prevention and Treatment of Cancer-Related Infections, Version 1.2013, Blood 113-5711, 2009, and Biol Blood Marrow Transpl 15:1143, 2009.* |
| **Hepatitis B** | SOT | For anti-viral agents with activity against HBV, see Table 14B, page 184. For discussion of prevention of HBV re-infection after transplantation and prevention of donor-derived infection see *Am J Transplant 9: S176, 2013.* |
| | HCT | Patients who are anti-HBC positive and anti-HBs positive, but without evidence of active viral replication, can be monitored for ↑LFTs and presence of +HBV-DNA, and given pre-emptive therapy at that time. Alternatively, prophylactic anti-viral therapy can be given, commencing before transplant. *(See guidelines for other specific situations: Biol Blood Marrow Transpl 15:1143, 2009.)* These guidelines recommend Lamivudine 100 mg po q24h as an anti-viral. |
| **Herpes simplex** | SOT | **Acyclovir** 400 mg po bid, starting early post-transplant *(Clin Microbiol Rev 10:86, 1997).* |
| | HCT | **Acyclovir** 250 mg/m² IV bid **or Acyclovir** 400 mg to 800 mg po bid, from conditioning through engraftment or resolution or mucositis. For those requiring prolonged suppression of HSV, the higher dose (Acyclovir 800 mg po bid) is recommended to minimize the risk of emerging resistance. |

**TABLE 15E (2)**

| OPPORTUNISTIC INFECTION | TYPE OF TRANSPLANT | PROPHYLACTIC REGIMENS |
|---|---|---|
| Aspergillus spp. | SOT | Lung and heart/lung transplant: Inhaled **Ampho B** and/or a mold active oral azole are commonly used, but optimal regimen not defined. Aerosolized **Ampho B** 6 mg q8h (or 25 mg/day) OR aerosolized **LAB** 25 mg/day OR **Vori** 200 mg po bid OR **Itra** 200 mg po bid. 59% centers employ universal prophylaxis in lung transplant recipients with 97% targeting Aspergillus. Most use Voriconazole alone or in combination with inhaled Amphotericin B *(Am J Transplant 11:361, 2011)*. Consider restarting prophylaxis during periods of intensified immune suppression.<br>Liver transplant: Consider only in high-risk, re-transplant and/or those requiring renal-replacement therapy. Recommendations on aspergillus prophylaxis in SOT can be found at *(Am J Transplant 13:228, 2013)*. |
| | HCT/Heme malignancy | For prophylaxis against Aspergillus include AML and MDS with neutropenia and HCT with GVHD. Posaconazole 200 mg po tid approved this indication *(NEJM 356:335, 2007 and NEJM 356:348, 2007)*. Posaconazole ER tablets, also approved for prophylaxis (300 mg po BID x 1 day, then 300 mg BID). Retrospective analysis suggests that Voriconazole would have efficacy in steroid-treated patients with GVHD *(Bone Marrow Transpl 45:662, 2010)*, but is not approved for this indication. Amphotericin B and echinocandins are alternatives as well. |
| Candida spp. | SOT | Consider in select, high risk patients (liver, small bowel, pancreas): Consider in select, high-risk patients (re-transplants, dialysis). **Flu** 400 mg daily for 4 weeks post-transplant *(Amer J Transpl 13:200, 2013)*. |
| | HCT | Recipient with positive serology, no active infection at time of transplant: **Flu** 400 mg once daily x 1 year; then 200 mg once daily indefinitely.<br>Recipient of organ from donor with positive serology, no active infection:<br>○ Lung transplant recipients: **Flu** 400 mg once daily, indefinitely.<br>○ Other organ recipients: **Flu** 400 mg once daily x 1 year; then 200 mg once daily indefinitely.<br>Recipient residing in an endemic area who underwent an organ transplant (primary prevention): **Flu** 200 mg once daily x 6-12 months post transplantation *(Clin Infect Dis 63:e112, 2016)*. |
| Coccidioides immitis | Any | **Flu** 200-400 mg q24h *(Transpl Inf Dis 5:3, 2003; Am J Transpl 6:340, 2006). See COID 21-45, 2008* for approach at one center in endemic area; e.g., for positive serology without evidence of active infection, **Flu** 400 mg q24h for first year post-transplant, then 200 mg q24h thereafter. |
| Pneumocystis jirovecii | SOT | **TMP-SMX** 1 single-strength tab po q24h or 1 double-strength tab po once daily for 3 to 7 days per week. Duration: kidney: 6 mos to 1 year *(Amer J Transpl 9 (Suppl 3): S59, 2009)*; heart, lung, liver: ≥ 1 year to life-long *(Amer J Transpl 4 (Suppl 10): 135, 2004)*. |
| | HCT | **TMP-SMX** 1 single-strength tab po q24h or 1 double-strength tab po once daily or once a day for 3 days per week, from engraftment to ≥ 6 mos post transplant. |
| Toxoplasma gondii | SOT | **TMP-SMX** (1 SS tab po q24h or 1 DS tab po once daily) x 3-7 days/wk for 6 mos post-transplant. *(See Clin Micro Infect 14:1089, 2008)*. |
| | HCT | **TMP-SMX** 1 single-strength tab po q24h or 1 double-strength tab po once daily or once a day for 3 days per week, from engraftment to ≥ 6 mos post transplant for seropositive allogeneic HCT recipients. |
| Trypanosoma cruzi | Heart | May be transmitted from organs or transfusions *(CID 48:1534, 2009)*. Inspect peripheral blood of suspected cases for parasites *(MMWR 55:798, 2006)*. Risk of reactivation during immunosuppression is variable *(JAMA 298:2171, 2007; JAMA 299:1134, 2008; J Cardiac Fail 15:249, 2009)*. If known Chagas disease in donor or recipient, contact CDC for treatment options (phone 770-488-7775 or in emergency 770-488-7100). *Am J Transplant 11:672, 2011*. |

**TABLE 16 – PEDIATRIC DOSING (AGE >28 DAYS)**

**Editorial Note**
There is limited data on when to switch adolescents to adult dosing. In general, pediatric weight based dosing is appropriate through mid puberty (Tanner 3) if no maximum dose is specified. Some change to adult dosing at 40 kg. If in doubt, when treating serious infections in peri-pubertal adolescents with drugs that have large margins of safety (e.g. Beta lactams and carbapenems) it may be safer to err on the side of higher doses.

| DRUG | DOSE (AGE >28 DAYS) (Daily maximum dose shown, when applicable) |
|---|---|
| **ANTIBACTERIALS** | |
| **Aminoglycosides** | |
| Amikacin | 15-20 mg/kg q24h; 5-7.5 mg/kg q8h |
| Gentamicin | 5-7 mg/kg q24h; 2.5 mg/kg q8h |
| Tobramycin | 5-7 mg/kg q24h; 2.5 mg/kg q8h. |
| **Beta-Lactams** | |
| **Carbapenems** | |
| Ertapenem | 30 mg/kg/day (divided q12h). Max per day: 1 gm |
| Imipenem | 60-100 mg/kg/day (divided q6-8h). Max per day: 2-4 gm |
| Meropenem | 60 mg/kg/day (divided q8h); Meningitis: 120 mg/kg/day (divided q8h). Max per day: 2-4 gm |
| **Cephalosporins (po)** | |
| Cefaclor | 20-40 mg/kg/day (divided q8-12h). Max per day: 1 gm |
| Cefadroxil | 30 mg/kg/day (divided q12h). Max per day: 2 gm |
| Cefdinir | 14 mg/kg/day (divided q12-24h) |
| Cefixime | 8 mg/kg/day (divided q12-24h) |
| Cefpodoxime | 10 mg/kg/day (divided q12h). Max per day: 400 mg |
| Cefprozil | 15-30 mg/kg/day (divided q12h) -- use 30 for AOM |
| Ceftibuten | 9 mg/kg/day (divided q12-24h). Max per day: 1 gm |
| Cefuroxime axetil | 20-30 mg/kg/day (divided q12h) -- use 30 for AOM. Max per day: 1 gm |
| Cephalexin | 25-100 mg/kg/day (divided q6h). Max per day: 4 gm |
| Loracarbef | 15-30 mg/kg/day (divided q12h). Max per day: 800 mg |
| **Cephalosporins (IV)** | |
| Cefazolin | 50-150 mg/kg/day (divided q6-8h). Max per day: 6 gm |
| Cefepime (non-Pseudomonal) | 100 mg/kg/day (divided q8h) |
| Cefepime (Pseudomonal) | 150 mg/kg/day (divided q8h) |
| Cefotaxime | 150-200 mg/kg/day (divided q6-8h). Meningitis: 300 mg/kg/day (divided q6h) |
| Cefotetan | 60-100 mg/kg/day (divided q12h). Max per day: 6 gm |
| Cefoxitin | 80-160 mg/kg/day (divided q6-8h) |
| Ceftaroline | 2 mon to <2 yrs: 8 mg/kg q8h<br>≥2 yrs to <18 yrs, ≤33 kg: 12 mg/kg q8h<br>≥2 yrs to <18 yrs, >33 kg: 400 mg q8h or 600 mg q12h |
| Ceftazidime | 150-200 mg/kg/day (divided q8h)<br>CF: 300 mg/kg/day (divided q8h) |
| Ceftizoxime | 150-200 mg/kg/day (divided q6-8h) |
| Ceftriaxone | 50-100 mg/kg q24h; Meningitis: 50 mg/kg q12h |
| Cefuroxime | 150 mg/kg/day (divided q8h); Meningitis: 80 mg/kg q8h |
| **Penicillins** | |
| Amoxicillin | 25-50 mg/kg/day (divided q8h) |
| Amoxicillin (AOM, pneumonia) | 80-100 mg/kg/day (divided q8-12h; q12h for AOM) |
| Amoxicillin-clavulanate 7:1 formulation | 45 mg/kg/day (divided q12h) |
| Amoxicillin-clavulanate 14:1 (AOM) | 90 mg/kg/day (divided q12h) for wt <40 kg |
| Ampicillin (IV) | 200 mg/kg/day (divided q6h); Meningitis: 300-400 mg/kg/day (divided q6h) |
| Ampicillin-sulbactam | 100-300 mg/kg/day (divided q6h) |
| Cloxacillin (po) | If <20 kg: 25-50 mg/kg/day (divided q6h); Otherwise dose as adult |
| Dicloxacillin (mild - moderate) | 12.5-25 mg/kg/day (divided q6h) |
| Dicloxacillin (osteo articular infection) | 100 mg/kg/day (divided q 6h) |
| Flucloxacillin | Age 2-10: 50% of adult dose; Age<2: 25% of adult dose |
| Nafcillin | 150-200 mg/kg/day (divided q6h) |
| Oxacillin | 150-200 mg/kg/day (divided q6h) |
| Penicillin G | 150,000-300,000 units/kg/day (divided q4-6h). Max per day: 12-20 million units |
| Penicillin VK | 25-75 mg/kg/day (divided q6-8h) |
| Piperacillin-tazobactam | 300 mg/kg/day (divided q6h) |
| Temocillin | 25 mg/kg q12h |
| **Fluoroquinolones** ※ Approved only for CF, anthrax, and complicated UTI | |
| Ciprofloxacin (po) | 20-40 mg/kg/day (divided q12h) ※. Max per day: 1.5 gm |
| Ciprofloxacin (IV) | 20-30 mg/kg/day (divided q12h) ※. Max per day: 1.2 gm |
| Levofloxacin (IV/po) | 16-20 mg/kg/day (divided q12h) ※. Max per day: 750 mg |

TABLE 16 (2)                                                                                   229

| DRUG | DOSE (AGE >28 DAYS) (Daily maximum dose shown, when applicable) |
|---|---|
| **ANTIBACTERIALS** *(continued)* | |
| **Lincosamides** | |
| Clindamycin (po) | 30-40 mg/kg/day (divided q6-8h) |
| Clindamycin (IV) | 20-40 mg/kg/day (divided q6-8h) |
| Lincomycin | 10-20 mg/kg/day (divided q8-12h) |
| **Lipopeptides** | |
| Daptomycin, cSSSI (infusion only, up to 14 days) | Age 12-17: 5 mg/kg (over 30 min) q24h<br>Age 7-11: 7 mg/kg (over 30 min) q24h<br>Age 2-6: 9 mg/kg (over 60 min) q24h<br>Age 1 to <2: 10 mg/kg (over 60 min) q24h |
| Daptomycin, S. aureus bacteremia (infusion only, up to 42 days) | Age 12-17: 7 mg/kg (over 30 min) q24h<br>Age 7-11: 9 mg/kg (over 30 min) q24h<br>Age 1-6: 12 mg/kg (over 60 min) q24h |
| **Macrolides** | |
| Azithromycin (po) | 5-12 mg/kg/day (once daily) |
| Azithromycin (IV) | 10 mg/kg/day (once daily) |
| Clarithromycin | 15 mg/kg/day (divided q12h). Max per day: 1 gm |
| Erythromycin (po, IV) | 40-50 mg/kg/day (divided q6h) |
| **Monobactams** | |
| Aztreonam | 90-120 mg/kg/day (divided q8h). Max per day: 8 gm |
| **Tetracyclines** | |
| Doxycycline (po/IV) | 2-4.4 mg/kg/day (divided q12h). Max per day: 200 mg. Max duration: 21 days |
| Minocycline (po, age >8) | 4 mg/kg/day (divided q12h) |
| Sarecycline | Age >9 yrs, Wt 33-54 kg: 60 mg po q24h<br>Age >9 yrs, Wt 55-84 kg: 100 mg po q24h<br>Age >9 yrs, Wt 85-136 kg: 150 mg po q24h |
| Tetracycline | Age >8: 25-50 mg/kg/day (divided q6h). Max per day: 2 gm |
| **Other** | |
| Chloramphenicol (IV) | 50-100 mg/kg/day (divided q6h). Max per day: 2-4 gm |
| Colistin | 2.5-5 mg/kg/day (divided q6-12h) CF: 3-8 mg/kg/day (divided q8h) |
| Fosfomycin (po) | 2 gm once |
| Fusidic acid (po) | Age 1-5: 250 mg q8h Age 6-12: 250-500 mg q8h |
| Linezolid (up to age 12 yrs) | 30 mg/kg/day IV/po (divided q8h) |
| Methenamine hippurate (age 6-12) | 500-1000 mg q12h |
| Methenamine mandelate | Age >2 to 6: 50-75 mg/kg/day (divided q6-8h) Age 6-12: 500 mg q6h |
| Metronidazole (po) | 30-40 mg/kg/day (divided q6h) |
| Metronidazole (IV) | 22.5-40 mg/kg/day (divided q6h) |
| Nitrofurantoin (po Cystitis) | 5-7 mg/kg/day (divided q 6h) |
| Nitrofurantoin (po UTI prophylaxis) | 1-2 mg/kg/day (once daily) |
| Polymyxin B (age 2 and older) | 2.5 mg/kg (load), then 1.5 mg/kg q12h |
| Rifampin (meningococcal prophylaxis) | 10 mg/kg q12h x2 days |
| Tinidazole (age >3 for Giardia, amebiasis) | 50 mg/kg q24h x1-5 days. Max per day: 2 gm |
| Sulfadiazine | 120-150 mg/kg/day (divided q4-6h). Max per day: 6 gm |
| TMP-SMX (UTI and other) | 8-12 mg TMP/kg/day (divided q12h) |
| TMP-SMX (PCP) | 15-20 mg TMP/kg/day (divided q12h) |
| Trimethoprim | 4 mg/kg/day (divided q12h) |
| Vancomycin (IV) | 40-60 mg/kg/day (divided q6-8h) (Use serum concentration to target trough 10-15 mcg/mL; 60 mg/kg/day most likely to achieve target) |
| Vancomycin (po for C. difficile) | 40 mg/kg/day (divided q6h) |
| **ANTIMYCOBACTERIALS** | |
| Capreomycin | 15-30 mg/kg/day (divided q12-24h). Max per day: 1 gm |
| Cycloserine | 10-15 mg/kg/day (divided q12h). Max per day: 1 gm |
| Ethambutol | 15-25 mg/kg/day (once daily). Max per day: 2.5 gm |
| Ethionamide | 15-20 mg/kg/day (divided q12h). Max per day: 1 gm |
| Isoniazid (daily dosing) | 10-15 mg/kg/day (once daily). Max per day: 300 mg |
| Isoniazid (2 x/week) | 20-30 mg/kg twice weekly. Max per day: 900 mg |
| Kanamycin | 15 -30 mg/kg/day (divided q12-24h). Max per day: 1 gm |
| Para-aminosalicylic acid | 200-300 mg/kg/day (divided q6-12h) |
| Pyrazinamide (daily) | 15-30 mg/kg/day (once daily). Max per day: 2 gm |
| Pyrazinamide (2 x/week) | 50 mg/kg/day (2 days/week). Max per day: 2 gm |
| Rifabutin (MAC prophylaxis) | 5 mg/kg/day (once daily). Max per day: 300 mg |
| Rifabutin (active TB) | 10-20 mg/kg/day (once daily). Max per day: 300 mg |

| DRUG | DOSE (AGE >28 DAYS) (Daily maximum dose shown, when applicable) |
|---|---|
| **ANTIMYCOBACTERIALS** *(continued)* | |
| Rifampin | 10-20 mg/kg/day (divided q12-24h). Max per day: 600 mg |
| Streptomycin (age 2 and older) | 20-40 mg/kg/day (once daily). Max per day: 1 gm |
| **ANTIFUNGALS** | |
| Amphotericin B deoxycholate | 0.5-1 mg/kg/day (once daily) |
| Amphotericin B lipid complex | 5 mg/kg/day (once daily) |
| Anidulafungin | 1.5-3 mg/kg loading dose then .75-1.5 mg/kg/day (once daily) |
| Caspofungin | 70 mg/m2 loading dose then 50 mg/m2 (once daily) |
| Fluconazole | 6 mg/kg/day for oral/esophageal Candida; 12 mg/kg/day for invasive disease |
| Griseofulvin | Tinea capitis: micro susp 20-25 mg/kg/day, ultra tab 10-15 mg/kg/day (duration ≥6 weeks, continue until clinically clear)<br>Tinea corporis: micro susp 10-20 mg/kg/day x 2-4 weeks<br>Tinea pedis: micro susp 10-20 mg/kg/day x 4-8 weeks |
| Isavuconazonium sulfate (prodrug of Isavuconazole) | Not known; adult dose 372 mg q8h x 3 doses loading dose then 744 mg/day (divided q12h) |
| Itraconazole | 5-10 mg/kg/day (divided q12h) |
| Ketoconazole | 3.3-6.6 mg/kg/day (once daily) |
| Micafungin | Age >4 mon: 2 mg/kg q24h (max 100 mg) for candidiasis; for EC use 3 mg/kg q24h if <30 kg, 2.5 mg/kg q24h (max 150 mg) if >30 kg |
| Nystatin | Adolescents, children: 500,000 units (5 mL) swish & swallow qid<br>Infants: 200,000 units (2 mL) qid<br>Premature infants: 100,000 units (1 mL) qid |
| Posaconazole | Not known; adult dose 300 mg bid loading dose then 300 mg/day (extended release) |
| Terbinafine | Tinea capitis: 4-6 mg/kg/day (tabs)<br>Wt 10-20 kg: 62.5 mg q24h<br>Wt 20-40 kg: 125 mg q24h<br>Wt >40 kg: 250 mg q24h<br>Duration: 2 wks for T. tonsurans, 4 wks for M. canis |
| Voriconazole | 12-20 mg/kg/day (divided q12h) (Variable bioavailability and metabolism. Adjust to trough level 1-6 mcg/mL) |
| **ANTIRETROVIRALS** | |
| Abacavir (ABC) | Oral soln, age <3 mon: not approved<br>Oral soln, age ≥3 mon:<br>8 mg/kg q12h or 16 mg/kg q24h (start soln q12h)<br>Tabs, wt-based:<br>14 to <20 kg: 150 mg q12h (300 mg q24h also ok)<br>≥20 to <25 kg: 150 mg qAM, 300 mg qPM (450 mg q24h also ok)<br>≥25 kg: 300 mg q12h (600 mg q24h also ok)<br>Adolescent: 300 mg q12h or 600 mg q24h |
| Atazanavir (ATV) | Neonates: not recommended<br>Age ≥3 mon, oral powder:<br>5 to <15 kg: ATV 200 mg + RTV 80 mg q24h<br>(5 to <10 kg, can't tolerate ATV 200 mg, PI naive: ATV 150 mg + RTV 80 mg q24h with close monitoring of VL)<br>15 to <25 kg: ATV 250 mg + RTV 80 mg q24h<br>≥25 kg: ATV 300 mg + RTV 100 mg q24h<br>Age >6 yrs, capsules:<br>15 to <35 kg: ATV 200 mg + RTV 100 mg q24h<br>≥35 kg: ATV 300 mg + RTV 100 mg q24h<br>Adolescents: 400 mg q24h, or ATV 300 mg + RTV 100 mg q24h |
| Darunavir (DRV) | Neonate: not approved<br>Age <3 or wt <10 kg: avoid use<br>Age ≥3 yr, tx naive or exp ± one or more DRV mut:<br>10 to <11 kg: 200 mg (+ RTV 32 mg) q12h<br>11 to <12 kg: 220 mg (+ RTV 32 mg) q12h<br>12 to <13 kg: 240 mg (+ RTV 40 mg) q12h<br>13 to <14 kg: 260 mg (+ RTV 40 mg) q12h<br>14 to <15 kg: 280 mg (+ RTV 48 mg) q12h<br>15 to <30 kg: 375 mg (+ RTV 48 mg) q12h<br>30 to <40 kg: 450 mg (+ RTV 100 mg) q12h<br>≥40 kg: 600 mg (+ RTV 100 mg) q12h<br>Adolescent:<br>≥30 to <40 kg, tx naive/exp ± ≥1 DRV mut: 450 mg (+ RTV 100 mg) q12h<br>≥40 kg, tx naive/exp, no DRV mut: 800 mg (+ RTV 100 mg) q24h<br>≥40 kg, tx exp, ≥1 DRV mut: 600 mg (+ RTV 100 mg) q12h |
| Delavirdine (DLV) | Safety/efficacy in patients ≤16 years not established |
| Didanosine (ddl) | Age 2 wk to 3 mon: 50 mg/m2 q12h<br>Age ≥3 mon to 8 mon: 100 mg/m2 q12h<br>Age >8 mon: 120 mg/m2 q12h<br>(240 mg/m2 q24h if age 3-21 yr and tx naive)<br>EC caps (age 6-18 yr):<br>20 to <25 kg, 200 mg q24h<br>25 to <60 kg, 250 mg q24h<br>≥60 kg, 400 mg q24h |

TABLE 16 (4)                                                                                231

| DRUG | DOSE (AGE >28 DAYS) (Daily maximum dose shown, when applicable) |
|---|---|
| **ANTIRETROVIRALS** *(continued)* | |
| Dolutegravir (DTG) | Wt <30 kg: Clinical trials ongoing<br>Wt 30 to <40 kg: 35 mg q24h<br>Wt ≥40 kg: 50 mg q24h<br>↑ to q12h if given w/EFV, FPV/r, TPV/r, CBZ, rifampin |
| Efavirenz (EFV) | Neonates: not approved for use<br>Age ≥3 yr:<br>10 to <15 kg, 200 mg q24h<br>15 to <20 kg, 250 mg q24h<br>20 to <25 kg, 300 mg q24h<br>25 to <32.5 kg, 350 mg q24h<br>32.5 to <40 kg, 400 mg q24h<br>≥40 kg, 600 mg q24h<br>Age 3 mon to <3 yr, wt ≥3.5 kg: not recommended (variable PK) |
| Elvitegravir (EVG) | As Vitekta, not for use in children age <18 yrs |
| Emtricitabine (FTC) | Oral soln:<br>0 to ≤3 mon, 3 mg/kg q24h<br>3 mon to 17 yr: 6 mg/kg (max 240 mg) q24h<br>≥18 yr, 240 mg q24h<br>Caps, wt >33 kg: 200 mg q24h |
| Enfuvirtide (T-20) | Age <6 yrs: not approved for use<br>Age 6-16 yr: 2 mg/kg (max 90 mg) sc q12h<br>Age >16 yr: 90 mg sc q12h |
| Etravirine (ETR) | Age 6-18 yr:<br>16 to <20 kg, 100 mg q12h<br>20 to <25 kg, 125 mg q12h<br>25 to <30 kg, 150 mg q12h<br>≥30 kg, 200 mg q12h<br>Age <6 yr: not rcommended |
| Fosamprenavir (FPV) | Neonate: use not recommended<br>Age 2-5 yrs (ARV naive): 30 mg/kg q12h (not recommended)<br>Age 6 mon to 18 yrs (ARV naive or experienced):<br><11 kg: 45 mg/kg q12h (+ RTV 7 mg/kg q12h)<br>11 to <15 kg: 30 mg/kg q12h (+ RTV 3 mg/kg q12h)<br>15 to <20 kg: 23 mg/kg q12h (+ RTV3 mg/kg q12h)<br>≥20 kg: 18 mg/kg q12h (+ RTV 3 mg/kg q12h)<br>Adolescent, ARV naive:<br>700 mg q12h (+ RTV 100 mg q12h), or<br>1400 mg q24h (+ RTV 100-200 mg q24h)<br>Adolescent, ARV exp: 700 mg q12h (+ RTV 100 mg q12h) |
| Indinavir (IDV) | Neonate/infant: not approved for use<br>Children: not approved for use<br>Adolescent: 800 mg q12h (+ RTV 100-200 mg q12h) |
| Lamivudine (3TC) | Oral solution:<br>Age 0 to <4 wks: 2 mg/kg q12h<br>Age ≥4 wks to <3 mon: 4 mg/kg q12h<br>Age ≥3 mon to <3 yrs: 5 mg/kg (max 150 mg) q12h<br>Age ≥3 yr: 5 mg/kg (max 150 mg) q12h, OR 10 mg/kg (max 300 mg) q24h<br>Tabs:<br>14 to <20 kg: 75 mg q12h (or 150 mg q24h)<br>≥20 to <25 kg: 75 mg qam + 150 mg qpm (or 225 mg q24h)<br>≥25 kg: 150 mg q12h (or 300 mg q24h) |
| Maraviroc (MVC) | Age ≥2 yrs, w/3A4 inhibitor:<br>10 to <20 kg: 50 mg q12h (tab or soln)<br>20 to <30 kg: 80 mg soln q12h or 75 mg tab q12h<br>30 to <40 kg: 100 mg q12h (tab or soln)<br>≥40 kg, 150 mg q12h (tab or soln)<br>Age ≥2 yrs, no interacting meds:<br><30 kg: not recommended<br>≥30 kg 300 mg q12h (tab or soln)<br>Age ≥2 yrs, w/3A4 inducer: not recommended |
| Nelfinavir (NFV) | Neonate (NICHD/HPTN 040/PACTG 1043):<br>Wt 1.5 to 2 kg: 100 mg q12h<br>Wt >2 to 3 kg: 150 mg q12h<br>Wt >3 kg: 200 mg q12h<br>Age 2-13 yrs: 45-55 mg/kg q12h (8th CROI 2001, #250)<br>Adolescent: 1250 mg q12h |
| Nevirapine (NVP) | Neonate, 34-37 wk EGA: 4 mg/kg q12h (no lead-in); increase to 6 mg/kg q12h<br>after one week<br>Neonate, ≥37 wk EGA to <1 mon: 6 mg/kg q12h (no lead-in)<br>Neo prophylaxis: 2 mg/kg at birth, 48 hr after dose 1, 96 hr after dose 2<br>1 mon to <8 yr: 7 mg/kg or 200 mg/m2 q12h<br>≥8 yr: 4 mg/kg or 120-150 mg/m2 q12h<br>Adolescens: 200 mg q24h x14 days, then 200 mg q12h (or 400 mg XR q24h) |

| DRUG | DOSE (AGE >28 DAYS) (Daily maximum dose shown, when applicable) |
|---|---|
| **ANTIRETROVIRALS** *(continued)* | |
| Raltegravir (RAL) | Film-coated tab:<br>≥40 kg, tx-naive or suppr on 400 mg q12h: 1200 mg q24h<br>≥25 kg: 400 mg q12h<br><25 kg: use chew tabs<br>Chewable tab:<br>11 to <14 kg, 75 mg q12h<br>14 to <20 kg, 100 mg q12h<br>20 to <28 kg, 150 mg q12h<br>28 to <40 kg, 200 mg q12h<br>≥40 kg, 300 mg q12h<br>Oral susp, age ≥4 weeks:<br>3 to <4 kg, 25 mg q12h<br>4 to <6 kg, 30 mg q12h<br>6 to <8 kg, 40 mg q12h<br>8 to <11 kg, 60 mg q12h<br>11 to <14 kg, 80 mg q12h<br>14 to <20 kg, 100 mg q12h<br>Oral susp, neonate, full term, age 1-4 weeks:<br>2 to <3 kg: 8 mg q12h<br>3 to <4 kg: 10 mg q12h<br>4 to <5 kg: 15 mg q12h<br>Oral susp, neonate, full term, age 0-1 week:<br>2 to <3 kg: 4 mg q24h<br>3 to <4 kg: 5 mg q24h<br>4 to <5 kg: 7 mg q24h<br>Preterm or low birth weight: no data |
| Rilpivirine (RPV) | Adolescent ≥12 yrs, ≥35 kg: 25 mg q24h |
| Ritonavir (RTV) | Neonates: dose not established<br>Peds dose: 350-400 mg/m2 q12h (not recommended)<br>Used as pharmacologic enhancer |
| Saquinavir (SQV) | Neonate/infant: not approved for use<br>Age <2 yrs: dose not determined<br>Age ≥2 yrs:<br>Wt 5 to <15 kg: 50 mg/kg q12h (+RTV 3 mg/kg q12h)<br>Wt 15 to <40 kg: 50 mg/kg q12h (+RTV 2.5 mg/kg q12h)<br>Wt ≥40 kg: 50 mg/kg q12h (+RTV 100 mg q12h)<br>Adolescent (age ≥16 yrs): 1gm q12h (+RTV 100 mg q12h) |
| Stavudine (d4T) | Age 0-13 days: 0.5 mg/kg q12h<br>Age ≥14 days, <30 kg: 1 mg/kg q12h<br>≥30 kg: 30 mg q12h |
| Tenofovir alafenamide (TAF) | ≥12 yrs, wt ≥35 kg:<br>10 mg q24h (part of Genvoya)<br>25 mg q24h (part of Descovy, Odefsey)<br>Vemlidy not approved for patients <18 yrs of age |
| Tenofovir (TDF) | Age 2 to <12 yr:<br>8 mg/kg powder (max 300 mg) q24h [1 scoop=40 mg]<br>Tablets, weight-based:<br>17 to <22 kg: 150 mg q24h<br>22 to <28 kg: 200 mg q24h<br>28 to <35 kg: 250 mg q24h<br>≥35 kg: 300 mg q24h |
| Tipranavir (TPV) | Age <2 yrs: use not approved<br>Age ≥2 to 18 yrs:<br>by BSA: 375 mg/m2 q12h (+RTV 150 mg/m2 q12h)<br>by wt: 14 mg/kg q12h (+RTV 6 mg/kg q12h)<br>(not recommended for tx naive pts)<br>Adolescent: 500 mg q12h (+RTV 200 mg q12h)<br>(not recommended for tx naive pts) |
| Zidovudine (ZDV) | Neonate, EGA <30 wks:<br>age 0-4 weeks: 2 mg/kg po q12h or 1.5 mg/kg IV q12h<br>(increase to 3 mg/kg po q12h at age 4 weeks)<br>Neonate, EGA ≥30 to <35 wks:<br>age 0-2 weeks: 2 mg/kg po q12h or 1.5 mg/kg IV q12h<br>(increase to 3 mg/kg po q12h at age 2 weeks)<br>EGA ≥35 wks, age 0-4 wks: 4 mg/kg q12h or 3 mg/kg IV q12h<br>Infant/child (EGA ≥35 wks, age ≥4 wks):<br>4 to <9 kg: 12 mg/kg po q12h<br>9 to <30 kg: 9 mg/kg po q12h<br>≥30 kg: 300 mg po q12h<br>Dosing by BSA: 180-240 mg/m2 po q12h<br>Adolescent: 300 mg po q12h |
| **Antiretroviral combination products** | |
| Atripla (EFV/FTC/TDF) | Age ≥12 yr, wt ≥40 kg: one tab q24h |
| Biktarvy (BIC/FTC/TAF) | Age ≥12 to 18 yr, wt ≥35 kg: 1 tab q24h (investigational dose) |
| Combivir (3TC/AZT) | Age ≥12 yr, wt ≥30 kg: one tab q12h |
| Complera (RPV/FTC/TDF) | Age ≥12 yr, wt ≥35 kg: one tab q24h |
| Descovy (FTC/TAF) | Age ≥12 yr, wt ≥35 kg: one tab q24h |

TABLE 16 (6) 233

| DRUG | DOSE (AGE >28 DAYS) (Daily maximum dose shown, when applicable) |
|---|---|
| **ANTIRETROVIRALS** *(continued)* | |
| **Antiretroviral combination products** *(continued)* | |
| Epzicom (ABC/3TC) | Wt ≥25 kg: one tab q24h |
| Evotaz (ATV/cobi) | Age <18: not recommended |
| Genvoya (EVG/cobi/FTC/TAF) | Age ≥12 yr, wt ≥35 kg: one tab q24h |
| Kaletra (LPV/RTV) | Age <14 days: avoid use. Age 14 days to 12 mon: 300 mg/75 mg per m2 q12h. Age >12 mon to 18 yrs: 300 mg/75 mg per m2 q12h (tx-experienced); 230 mg/57.5 mg per m2 q12h (tx-naive) |
| Odefsey (RPV/FTC/TAF) | Age ≥12 yr, wt ≥35 kg: one tab q24h |
| Prezcobix (DRV/cobi) | Age <18: not recommended |
| Stribild (EVG/cobi/FTC/TDF) | Age ≥12 yr, wt ≥35 kg: one tab q24h |
| Triumeq (DTG/ABC/3TC) | Wt ≥40 kg: one tab q24h |
| Trizivir (ABC/3TC/ZDV) | Wt ≥40 kg: one tab q12h |
| Truvada (FTC/TDF) | Wt 17 to <22 kg: 100 mg/150 mg q24h; Wt 22 to <28 kg: 133 mg/200 mg q24h; Wt 28 to <35 kg: 167 mg/250 mg q24h; Wt ≥35 kg: 200 mg/300 mg q24h |
| **ANTIVIRALS** | |
| Acyclovir (IV) neonatal herpes simplex | 60 mg/kg/day (divided q8h) |
| Acyclovir (IV) HSV encephalitis >3 months | 30-45 mg/kg/day (divided q8h) |
| Acyclovir (IV) varicella immunocompromised | <1 year: 30 mg/kg/day (divided q8h); >1 year: 30 mg/kg/day or 1500 mg/m2/day (divided q8h) |
| Acyclovir (IV) HSV immunocompromised | 30 mg/kg/day (divided q8h) |
| Cidofovir | Induction 5 mg/kg once weekly. Suppressive therapy 3 mg/kg once weekly (all with hydration + probenecid) |
| Entecavir (treatment-naive) | Wt 10-11 kg, 0.15 mg q24h; >11 to 14 kg, 0.2 mg q24h; >14 to 17 kg, 0.25 mg q24h; >17 to 20 kg, 0.3 mg q24h; >20 to 23 kg, 0.35 mg q24h; >23 to 26 kg, 0.4 mg q24h; >26 to 30 kg, 0.45 mg q24h; >30 kg, 0.5 mg q24h |
| Entecavir (lamivudine-experienced) | Wt 10-11 kg, 0.3 mg q24h; >11 to 14 kg, 0.4 mg q24h; >14 to 17 kg, 0.5 mg q24h; >17 to 20 kg, 0.6 mg q24h; >20 to 23 kg, 0.7 mg q24h; >23 to 26 kg, 0.8 mg q24h; >26 to 30 kg, 0.9 mg q24h; >30 kg, 1 mg q24h |
| Foscarnet | 120-180 mg/kg/day (divided q8-12h) |
| Ganciclovir | Symptomatic congenital CMV 12 mg/kg/day (divided q12h). CMV tx or first 2 weeks after SOT: 10 mg/kg/day (divided q12h). Suppressive tx or prophylaxis 5 mg/kg/day (divided q24h) |
| Glecaprevir/pibrentasvir (Mavyret) | Age <18: safety and effectiveness not established |
| Laninamivir | Treatment or prophylaxis, age <10 yrs: 20 mg inhaled x1 Treatment or prophylaxis, age ≥10 yrs: 40 mg inhaled x1 |
| Ledipasvir/sofosbuvir (Harvoni) | Age ≥12 yrs or ≥35 kg: 1 tab q24h; Geno 1, tx-naive, no cirr or comp: 12 wks; Geno 1, tx-exp, no cirr=12 wks; Geno 1, tx-exp with comp=24 wks; Geno 4/5/6, tx-naive/exp, no cirr or comp=12 wks |
| Oseltamivir <1 year old | 6 mg/kg/day (divided q12h) |
| Oseltamivir ≥1 year old | <15 kg: 30 mg bid; >15 to 23 kg: 45 mg bid; >23 to 40 kg: 60 mg bid; >40 kg: 75 mg bid (adult dose) |
| Peramivir | Not studied |
| Ribavirin (with sofosbuvir) | Wt <47 kg: 15 mg/kg/day; 47-49 kg: 600 mg/day; 50-65 kg: 800 mg/day; 66-80 kg: 1000 mg/day; >80 kg: 1200 mg/day (all doses divided bid) |
| Sofosbuvir | Age ≥12 yrs or ≥35 kg: 400 mg (1 tab) q24h; Geno 2, tx-naive/exp, no cirr or comp=12 wks (with ribavirin); Geno 3, tx-naive/exp, no cirr or comp=24 wks (with ribavirin). |
| Tecovirimat | Wt 13 to <25 kg: 200 mg bid x 14 days Wt 25 to <40 kg: 400 mg bid x 14 days Wt ≥40 kg: 600 mg bid x 14 days |
| Valacyclovir (Varicella or Herpes Zoster) | 60 mg/kg/day (divided q8h) |
| Valganciclovir | Symptomatic congenital CMV: 32 mg/kg/day (divided q12h); Prevention of CMV after SOT: 7 mg x BSA x CrCl; (once daily; use Schwartz formula for CrCl). |
| Zanamivir (age >7 years) | 10 mg (two 5-mg inhalations) q12h |

# TABLE 17A – DOSAGE OF ANTIMICROBIAL DRUGS IN ADULT PATIENTS WITH RENAL IMPAIRMENT

- For listing of drugs with NO need for adjustment for renal failure, see Table 17B.
- Adjustments for renal failure are based on an estimate of creatinine clearance (CrCl) which reflects the glomerular filtration rate.
- **Different methods for calculating estimated CrCl are suggested for non-obese and obese patients.**
  - Calculations for ideal body weight (IBW) in kg:
    - Men: 50 kg plus 2.3 kg/inch over 60 inches height.
    - Women: 45 kg plus 2.3 kg/inch over 60 inches height.
  - Obese is defined as 20% over ideal body weight or body mass index (BMI) >30

> **Estimated CrCl is the most common method used for FDA-approved dose adjustments for renal insufficiency.** The bulk of the data in this table are based on calculated estimates of CrCl. **Emerging methods use calculations designed to estimate the glomerular filtration rate (eGFR).** Going forward the FDA may require that renal dosing adjustments be based on estimated CrCl and/or eGFR. See Adv Chronic Kid Dis 2018;25:14.

- Calculations of estimated CrCl (References, see (NEJM 354:2473, 2006 (non-obese), AJM 84:1053, 1988 (obese))
  - **Non-obese patient—**
    - Calculate ideal body weight (IBW) in kg (as above)—
    - Use the following formula to determine the estimated CrCl

$$\frac{(140\ minus\ age) \times (IBW\ in\ kg)}{72 \times serum\ creatinine} = \begin{array}{l} \text{CrCl in mL/min for men.} \\ \text{Multiply answer by 0.85} \\ \text{for women (estimated)} \end{array}$$

  - **Obese patient—**
    - Weight ≥20% over IBW or BMI >30
    - Use the following formulas to determine estimated CrCl

$$\frac{(137\ minus\ age) \times [(0.285 \times wt\ in\ kg) + (12.1 \times ht\ in\ meters^2)]}{51 \times serum\ creatinine} = CrCl\ (obese\ male)$$

$$\frac{(146\ minus\ age) \times [(0.287 \times wt\ in\ kg) + (9.74 \times ht\ in\ meters^2)]}{60 \times serum\ creatinine} = CrCl\ (obese\ female)$$

- If estimated CrCl ≥90 mL/min, see Tables 10A and 10D for dosing.
- What weight should be used to calculate dosage on a mg/kg basis?
  - If less than 20% over IBW, use the patient's actual weight for all drugs.
  - For obese patients ≥20% over IBW (or BMI >30):
    - **Aminoglycosides:** (IBW plus 0.4(actual weight minus IBW) = adjusted weight.
    - **Vancomycin:** actual body weight whether non-obese or obese.
    - **All other drugs:** see Table 17C.

- For slow or sustained extended daily dialysis **(SLEDD)** over 6–12 hours, adjust doses as for CRRT. For details, see CID 49:433, 2009; CCM 39:560, 2011.
- **SLEDD:** Limited data on dose adjustment for sustained low efficiency dialysis (SLEDD)(Can J Kidney Health Dis 2018;5:1).
- General reference: Drug Prescribing in Renal Failure, 5th ed., Aronoff, et al. (eds) (Amer College Physicians, 2007 and drug package inserts).

TABLE 17A (2)

| ANTIMICROBIAL | Half-life, hrs (renal function normal) | Half-life, hrs (ESRD) | Dose (renal function normal) | CrCl >50-90 | CrCl 10-50 | CrCl <10 | Hemodialysis | CAPD | CRRT |
|---|---|---|---|---|---|---|---|---|---|
| **ANTIBACTERIAL ANTIBIOTICS** | | | | | | | | | |
| **AMINOGLYCOSIDES, MDD** | | | | | | | | | |
| Amikacin[a] | 2-3 | 30-70 | 7.5 mg/kg IM/IV q12h (once-daily dosing below) | 7.5 mg/kg IM/IV q12h | 7.5 mg/kg q24h | 7.5 mg/kg q48h | 7.5 mg/kg q48h (+ extra 3.75 mg/kg AD) | 15-20 mg lost per L of dialysate/day | 7.5 mg/kg q24h |
| Plazomicin | 3.5 | No data | 15 mg/kg IV q24h | CrCl ≥60-15 mg/kg q24h | CrCl ≥30 to <60: 10 mg/kg q24h | CrCl ≥15 to <30: 10 mg/kg q48h; CrCl <15: No data | No data | No data | No data |
| Gentamicin, Netilmicin[NUS], Tobramycin[a,b] | 2-3 | 30-70 | 1.7-2.0 mg/kg IM/IV q8h | 1.7-2.0 mg/kg q8h | 1.7-2.0 mg/kg q12-24h | 1.7-2.0 mg/kg q48h | 1.7-2.0 mg/kg q48h (+ extra 0.85-1.0 mg/kg AD) | 3-4 mg lost per L of dialysate/day | 1.7-2.0 mg/kg q24h |
| **AMINOGLYCOSIDES, ODD** (see *Table 10D*) | | | | | | | | | |
| | | | **Dose for CrCl >80 (mg/kg q24h)** | **CrCl 60-80 (mg/kg q24h)** | **CrCl 40-60 (mg/kg q24h)** | **CrCl 30-40 (mg/kg q24h)** | **CrCl 20-30 (mg/kg q48h)** | **CrCl 10-20 (mg/kg q48h)** | **CrCl 0-10 (mg/kg q72h and AD)** |
| Gentamicin, Tobramycin | 2-3 | 30-70 | 5.1 | 4 | 3.5 | 2.5 | 4 | 3 | 2 |
| Amikacin, Kanamycin, Streptomycin | 2-3 | 30-70 | 15 | 12 | 7.5 | 4 | 7.5 | 4 | 3 |
| Isepamicin[NUS] | 2-3 | 30-70 | 8 | 8 | 8 | 8 mg/kg q48h | 8 | 8 mg/kg q72h | 8 mg/kg q96h |
| Netilmicin[NUS] | 2-3 | 30-70 | 6.5 | 5 | 4 | 2 | 3 | 2.5 | 2 |
| **BETA-LACTAMS** | | | | | | | | | |
| **Carbapenems** | | | | | | | | | |
| Doripenem | 1 | 18 | 500 mg IV q8h | 500 mg q8h | CrCl 30-50: 250 mg q8h; CrCl 10-30: 250 mg q12h | No data | No data | No data | 500 mg q8h (*JAC 69:2508, 2014*) |
| Ertapenem | 4 | >4 | 1 gm IV q24h | 1 gm q24h | CrCl <30: 0.5 gm q24h | 0.5 gm q24h | 0.5 gm q24h (+ 150 mg AD if given within 6 hr prior to HD) | 0.5 gm q24h | 0.5-1 gm q24h |
| Imipenem | 1 | 4 | 500 mg IV q6h | 250-500 mg q6-8h | 250 mg q8-12h | 125-250 mg q12h | 125-250 mg q12h (give one of the dialysis day doses AD) | 125-250 mg q12h | 0.5-1 gm q12h (*AAC 49:2421, 2005*) |
| Meropenem | 1 | 10 | 1 gm IV q8h | 1 gm q8h | CrCl 25-50: 1 gm q12h; CrCl 10-25: 0.5 gm q12h | 0.5 gm q24h | 0.5 gm q24h (give dialysis day dose AD) | 0.5 gm q24h | 1 gm q12h |

**TABLE 17A (3)**

| ANTIMICROBIAL | Half-life, hrs (renal function normal) | Half-life, hrs (ESRD) | Dose (renal function normal) | CrCl >50-90 | CrCl 10-50 | CrCl <10 | Hemodialysis | CAPD | CRRT |
|---|---|---|---|---|---|---|---|---|---|
| **Carbapenems** (continued) | | | | | | | | | |
| Meropenem-vaborbactam | Mer 1.2 Vab 1.7 | Mer 10 Vab ND | 2 gm/2 gm IV q8h | eGFR ≥50: 2 gm/2 gm q8h | eGFR 30-49: 1 gm/1 gm q8h; 15-29: 1 gm/1 gm q12h | eGFR <15: 0.5 gm/0.5 gm q12h | 0.5 gm/0.5 gm q12h (AD) | No data | No data |
| **Cephalosporins, IV, 1ˢᵗ gen** | | | | | | | | | |
| Cefazolin | 1.9 | 40-70 | 1-2 gm IV q8h | 1-2 gm q8h | 1-2 q12h | 1-2 gm q24-48h | 1-2 gm q24-48h (+ extra 0.5-1 gm AD) | 0.5 gm IV q12h | 1-2 gm q12h |
| **Cephalosporins, IV, 2ⁿᵈ gen** | | | | | | | | | |
| Cefotetan | 4 | 13-25 | 1-2 gm IV q12h | 1-2 gm q12h | 1-2 gm q24h | 2 gm q24h | 1-2 gm q24h (+ extra 1 gm AD) | 1 gm q24h | 750 mg q12h |
| Cefoxitin⁴ | 0.8 | 13-23 | 2 gm IV q8h | 2 gm q8h | 2 gm q8-12h | 2 gm q24-48h | 2 gm q24-48h (+ extra 1 gm AD) | 1 gm q24h | 2 gm q8-12h |
| Cefuroxime | 1.5 | 17 | 0.75-1.5 gm IV q8h | 0.75-1.5 gm q8h | 0.75-1.5 gm q8-12h | 0.75-1.5 gm q24h | 0.75-1.5 gm q24h (give dialysis day dose AD) | 0.75-1.5 gm q24h | 0.75-1.5 gm q8-12h |
| **Cephalosporins, IV, 3ʳᵈ gen, non-antipseudomonal** | | | | | | | | | |
| Cefotaxime⁵ | 1.5 | 15-35 | 2 gm IV q8h | 2 gm q8-12h | 2 gm q12-24h | 2 gm q24h | 2 gm q24h (+ extra 1 gm AD) | 0.5-1 gm q24h | 2 gm q12-24h |
| Ceftizoxime⁵ | 1.7 | 15-35 | 2 gm IV q8h | 2 gm q8-12h | 2 gm q12-24h | 2 gm q24h | 2 gm q24h (+ extra 1 gm AD) | 0.5-1 gm q24h | 2 gm q12-24h |
| Ceftriaxone⁵ | 8 | Unchanged | 1-2 gm IV q12-24h | 1-2 gm q12-24h | 1-2 gm q12-24h | 1-2 gm q12-24h | 1-2 gm q12-24h | 1-2 gm q12-24h | 1-2 gm q12-24h |
| **Cephalosporins, IV, antipseudomonal** | | | | | | | | | |
| Cefepime | 2 | 18 | 2 gm IV q8h | >60: 2 gm q8-12h | 30-60: 2 gm q12h; 11-29: 2 gm q24h | 1 gm q24h | 1 gm q24h (+ extra 1 gm AD) | 1-2 gm q48h | 2 gm q12-24h |
| Ceftazidime | 1.9 | 13-25 | 2 gm IV q8h | 2 gm q8-12h | 2 gm q12-24h | 2 gm q24-48h | 2 gm q24-48h (+ extra 1 gm AD) | No data | 1-2 gm q12-24h (depends on flow rate) |
| Ceftazidime/avibactam | ceftaz 2.8, avi 2.7 | ceftaz 13-25 | 2.5 gm IV q8h | 2.5 gm q8h | 30-50: 1.25 gm q8h; 10-30: 0.94 gm q12h | 0.94 gm q48h | 0.94 gm q48h (give dialysis day dose AD) | No data | 1.25 gm q8h (AAC 2017;61:e00464-17) |
| Ceftolozane/tazobactam | ceftolozane 3.1 | ceftolozane 40 | 1.5 gm IV q8h | 1.5 gm q8h | 30-50: 750 mg q8h 15-30: 375 mg q8h | <15: see HD | 750 mg x1, then 150 mg q8h (give dialysis day doses AD) | No data | No data |
| **Cephalosporins, IV, anti-MRSA** | | | | | | | | | |
| Ceftaroline | 2.7 | No data | 600 mg (over 5-60 min) IV q12h | 600 mg q12h | 30-50: 400 mg q12h; 15-30: 300 mg q12h | <15: 200 mg q12h | 200 mg q12h | No data | No data |

**TABLE 17A (4)**

| ANTIMICROBIAL | Half-life, hrs (renal function normal) | Half-life, hrs (ESRD) | Dose (renal function normal) | CrCl >50-90 | CrCl 10-50 | CrCl <10 | Hemodialysis | CAPD | CRRT |
|---|---|---|---|---|---|---|---|---|---|
| **Cephalosporins, IV, anti-MRSA** *(continued)* | | | | | | | | | |
| Ceftobiprole^NUS | 2.9-3.3 | 21 | 500 mg IV q8-12h | 500 mg q8h | 30-50: 500 mg q12h over 2 hr; 10-30: 250 mg q12h over 2 hr | No data | No data | No data | No data |
| **Cephalosporins, oral, 1st gen** | | | | | | | | | |
| Cefadroxil | 1.5 | 20 | 1 gm q12h | 1 gm q12h | 1 gm, then 500 mg q12-24h | 1 gm, then 500 mg q36h | 1 gm, then 1 gm AD | 500 mg q24h | No data |
| Cephalexin | 1 | 20 | 500 mg po q6h | 500 mg po q6h | 500 mg q12h | 250 mg q12h | 250 mg q12h (give one of the dialysis day doses AD) | 500 mg q12h | No data |
| **Cephalosporins, oral, 2nd gen** | | | | | | | | | |
| Cefaclor | 0.8 | 3 | 500 mg po q8h | 500 mg q8h | 500 mg q8h | 500 mg q12h | 500 mg q12h (give one of the dialysis day doses AD) | 500 mg q12h | No data |
| Cefprozil | 1.5 | 5-6 | 500 mg po q12h | 500 mg q12h | 500 mg q24h | 250 mg q12h | 250 mg q12h (give one of the dialysis day doses AD) | 250 mg q24h | No data |
| Cefuroxime axetil | 1.5 | 17 | 500 mg po q8h | 500 mg q8h | 500 mg q12h | 500 mg q24h | 500 mg q24h (give extra 250 mg AD) | 500 mg q24h | No data |
| **Cephalosporins, oral, 3rd gen** | | | | | | | | | |
| Cefdinir | 1.7 | 16 | 300 mg po q12h | 30-49: 300 mg q12h 11-29: 300 mg q24h | 300 mg q12h | 300 mg q24h | 300 mg q24h (dose AD on dialysis days) | 300 mg q24h | No data |
| Cefditoren pivoxil | 1.6 | 5 | 400 mg po q12h | 400 mg q12h | 200 mg q12h | 200 mg 24h | 200 mg q24h (dose AD on dialysis days) | 200 mg q24h | No data |
| Cefixime | 3 | 12 | 400 mg po q24h | 400 mg q24h | 300 mg q24h | 200 mg q24h | 200 mg q24h (dose AD on dialysis days) | 200 mg q24h | No data |
| Cefpodoxime proxetil | 2.3 | 10 | 200 mg po q12h | 200 mg q12h | 200 mg q12h | 200 mg q24h | 200 mg q24h (dose AD on dialysis days) | 200 mg q24h | No data |
| Ceftibuten | 2.5 | 13 | 400 mg po q24h | 400 mg q24h | 200 mg q24h | 100 mg q24h | 100 mg q24h (dose AD on dialysis days) | 100 mg po q24h | No data |
| **Monobactams** | | | | | | | | | |
| Aztreonam | 2 | 6-8 | 2 gm IV q8h | 2 gm q8h | 1-1.5 gm q8h | 500 mg q8h | 500 mg q8h (give additional 250 mg AD) | 500 mg q8h | 1-1.5 gm q8h |

**TABLE 17A (5)**

| ANTIMICROBIAL | Half-life, hrs (renal function normal) | Half-life, hrs (ESRD) | Dose (renal function normal) | CrCl >50-90 | CrCl 10-50 | CrCl <10 | Hemodialysis | CAPD | CRRT |
|---|---|---|---|---|---|---|---|---|---|
| **Penicillins (natural)** | | | | | | | | | |
| Penicillin G | 0.5 | 6-20 | 0.5-4 million U IV q4h | 0.5-4 million U q4h | 0.5-4 million U q8h | 0.5-4 million U q12h | 0.5-4 million U q12h (give one of the dialysis day doses AD) | 0.5-4 million U q12h | 1-4 million U q6-8h |
| Penicillin V | 0.5 | 4.1 | 250-500 mg po q6-8h | 250-500 mg q6-8h | 250-500 mg q6-8h | 250-500 mg q6-8h | 250-500 mg q6-8h (give one or more doses AD) | 250-500 mg q6-8h | No data |
| **Penicillins (amino)** | | | | | | | | | |
| Amoxicillin | 1.2 | 5-20 | 250-500 mg po q8h | 250-500 mg q8h | 250-500 mg q8-12h | 250-500 mg q24h | 250-500 mg q24h (give dialysis dose AD) | 250 mg q12h | 250-500 mg q8-12h |
| Amoxicillin ER | 1.2-1.5 | ? | 775 mg po q24h | 775 mg q24h | 30: No data, avoid usage | No data, avoid usage | No data | No data | No data |
| Amoxicillin/ Clavulanate* | amox 1.4, clav 1 | amox 5-20, clav 4 | 500/125 mg po q8h | 500/125 mg q8h | 250-500 mg (amox component) q12h | 250-500 mg (amox) q24h | 250-500 mg (amox) q24h (give all extra on dialysis days) | No data | No data |
| Ampicillin | 1.2 | 7-20 | 1-2 gm IV q4-6h | 1-2 gm q4-6h | 30-50: 1-2 gm q6-8h; 10-30: 1-2 gm q8-12h | 1-2 gm q12h | 1-2 gm q12h (give one of the dialysis day doses AD) | 500 mg – 1 gm q12h | 1-2 gm q8-12h |
| Ampicillin/Sulbactam | amp 1.4, sulb 1.7 | amp 7-20, sulb 10 | 3 gm IV q6h | >60: 3 gm q6h | 30-60: 3 gm q8h 10-30: 3 gm q12h | 3 gm q24h | 3 gm q24h (give AD on dialysis day) | 3 gm q24h | 3 gm q12h |
| **Penicillins (penicillinase-resistant)** | | | | | | | | | |
| Dicloxacillin | 0.7 | No change | 125-500 mg po q6h | 125-500 mg q6h | 125-500 mg q6h | 125-500 mg q6h | | | |
| Temocillin | 4 | No data | 1-2 gm IV q12h | 1-2 gm q12h | 1-2 gm q24h | 1 gm q48h | 1 gm q48h (give AD on dialysis days) | 1 gm q48h | No data |
| **Penicillins (antipseudomonal)** | | | | | | | | | |
| Piperacillin/ Tazobactam (non-Pseudomonas dose) | pip 1, Tazo 1 | pip 3-5, Tazo 2.8 | 3.375 gm IV q6h (over 30 min) | >40: 3.375 gm q6h | 20-40: 2.25 gm q6h; <20: 2.25 gm q8h | 2.25 gm q8h | 2.25 gm q12h (+ extra 0.75 gm AD) | 2.25 gm q12h | 2.25 gm q8h |
| Piperacillin/ Tazobactam (Pseudomonas dose) | pip 1, Tazo 1 | pip 3-5, Tazo 2.8 | 4.5 gm IV q6h (over 30 min) | >40: 4.5 gm q6h | 20-40: 3.375 gm q6h; <20: 2.25 gm q6h | 2.25 gm q6h | 2.25 gm q8h (+ extra 0.75 gm AD) | 2.25 gm q8h | MIC ≤16: 3.375 gm (over 30 min) q6h; MIC >16 to 64: 4.5 gm (over 4h) q8h (*Pharmacother* 35:600, 2015) |

**TABLE 17A (6)**

| ANTIMICROBIAL | Half-life, hrs (renal function normal) | Half-life, hrs (ESRD) | Dose (renal function normal) | CrCl >50-90 | CrCl 10-50 | CrCl <10 | Hemodialysis | CAPD | CRRT |
|---|---|---|---|---|---|---|---|---|---|
| **FLUOROQUINOLONES** | | | | | | | | | |
| Ciprofloxacin po (not XR) | 4 | 6-9 | 500-750 mg po q12h | 500-750 mg q12h | 250-500 mg q12h | 500 mg q24h | 500 mg q24h (dose AD on dialysis days) | 500 mg q24h | 250-500 mg q12h |
| Ciprofloxacin XR po | 5-7 | 6-9 | 500-1000 mg po q24h | 500-1000 mg q24h | 30-50: 500-1000 mg q24h; 10-30: 500 mg q24h | 500 mg q24h | 500 mg q24h (dose AD on dialysis days) | 500 mg q24h | No data |
| Ciprofloxacin IV | 4 | 6-9 | 400 mg IV q12h | 400 mg q12h | 400 mg q24h | 400 mg q24h | 400 mg q24h (dose AD on dialysis days) | 400 mg q24h | 200-400 mg q12h |
| Delafloxacin IV | 4.2-8.5 | No data | 300 mg IV q12h | 300 mg q12h | eGFR 30-50: 300 mg q12h; 15-29: 200 mg q12h | eGFR<15: No data | No data | No data | No data |
| Delafloxacin po | 4.2-8.5 | No data | 450 mg po q12h | 450 mg q12h | eGFR 15-50: 450 mg q12h | eGFR<15: No data | No data | No data | No data |
| Gatifloxacin^NUS | 7-8 | 11-40 | 400 mg po/IV q24h | 400 mg q24h | 400 mg, then 200 mg q24h | 400 mg, then 200 mg q24h | 200 mg q24h (give dialysis day dose AD) | 200 mg q24h | 400 mg, then 200 mg q24h |
| Gemifloxacin | 7 | >7 | 320 mg po q24h | 320 mg q24h | 160 mg q24h | 160 mg q24h | 160 mg q24h (give dialysis day dose AD) | 160 mg q24h | No data |
| Levofloxacin | 7 | 76 | 750 mg po/IV q24h | 750 mg q24h | 20-49: 750 mg q48h | <20: 750 mg x1, then 500 mg q48h | 750 mg x1, then 500 mg q48h | 750 mg x1, then 500 mg q48h | 750 mg x1, then 500 mg q48h |
| Norfloxacin | 3-4 | 8 | 400 mg po q12h | 400 mg q12h | 30-49: 400 mg q12h; 10-30: 400 mg q24h | 400 mg q24h | 400 mg q24h | 400 mg q24h | Not applicable |
| Ofloxacin | 7 | 28-37 | 200-400 mg po q12h | 200-400 mg q12h | 200-400 mg q24h | 200 mg q24h | 200 mg q24h (give dialysis day dose AD) | 200 mg q24h | 200-400 mg q24h |
| Prulifloxacin^NUS | 10.6-12.1 | No data | 600 mg po q24h | No data | No data | No data | No data | No data | No data |

TABLE 17A (7)

| ANTIMICROBIAL | Half-life, hrs (renal function normal) | Half-life, hrs (ESRD) | Dose (renal function normal) | CrCl >50-90 | CrCl 10-50 | CrCl <10 | Hemodialysis | CAPD | CRRT |
|---|---|---|---|---|---|---|---|---|---|
| **GLYCOPEPTIDES, LIPOGLYCOPEPTIDES, LIPOPEPTIDES** | | | | | | | | | |
| Dalbavancin | 147-258 (terminal) | No data | 1 gm IV x1, then 500 mg IV in 7 days | 1 gm x1, then 500 mg in 7 days | 30-49: 1 gm x1, then 500 mg in 7 days; <30, non-regular HD: 750 mg x1, then 375 mg in 7 days | | Regularly scheduled HD: 1 gm x1, then 500 mg in 7 days | No data | No data |
| Daptomycin | 8-9 | 30 | 4-6 mg/kg IV q24h | 4-6 mg/kg q24h | 30-49: 4-6 mg/kg q24h; <30: 6 mg/kg q48h | 6 mg/kg q48h | 6 mg/kg q48h (during or after q48h dialysis); if next planned dialysis is 72 hrs away, give 9 mg/kg (AAC 57:864, 2013; JAC 69-200, 2014) | 6 mg/kg q48h | 6 mg/kg q48h |
| Oritavancin | 245 (terminal) | No data | 1200 mg IV x1 | 1200 mg x1 | <30: No data | No data | Not removed by hemodialysis | No data | No data |
| Teicoplanin[NUS] | 70-100 | up to 230 | 6 mg/kg IV q12h x3 doses (load), then 6 mg/kg q24h | CrCl 30-80: load, then 6 mg/kg q48h | CrCl <30: load, then 6 mg/kg q72h | Load, then 6 mg/kg q72h | Load, then 6 mg/kg q72h. Give AD on dialysis day. | 6 mg/kg q72h | 6 mg/kg q48h |
| Telavancin | 8.1 | 17.9 | 10 mg/kg IV q24h | 10 mg/kg q24h | 30-50: 7.5mg/kg q24h; 10-30: 10 mg/kg q48h | 10 mg/kg q48h | No data* | No data | No data |
| Vancomycin[7] | 4-6 | 200-250 | 15-30 mg/kg IV q12h | 15-30 mg/kg q12h | 15 mg/kg q24-96h | 7.5 mg/kg q2-3 days | For trough conc of 15-20, give 15 mg/kg if next dialysis in 1 day; give 25 mg/kg if next dialysis in 2 days; give 35 mg/kg if next dialysis in 3 days (CID 53:124, 2011) | 7.5 mg/kg q2-3 days | CAVH/CVVH: 500 mg q24-48h |
| **MACROLIDES, AZALIDES, LINCOSAMIDES, KETOLIDES** | | | | | | | | | |
| Azithromycin | 68 | Unchanged | 250-500 mg IV/po q24h | 250-500 mg q24h | 250-500 mg q24h | 250-500 mg q24h | 250-500 mg q24h | 250-500 mg q24h | 250-500 mg q24h |
| Clarithromycin (not ER) | 5-7 | 22 | 500 mg po q12h | 500 mg q12h | 500 mg q12-24h | 500 mg | 500 mg q24h (dose AD on dialysis days) | 500 mg q24h | 500 mg q12-24h |
| Telithromycin[5] | 10 | 15 | 800 mg q24h | 800 mg q24h | 30-50: 800 mg 10-30: 600 mg q24h | 600 mg | 600 mg q24h (give AD on dialysis days) | No data | No data |

TABLE 17A (8)

| ANTIMICROBIAL | Half-life, hrs (renal function normal) | Half-life, hrs (ESRD) | Dose (renal function normal) | CrCl >50-90 | CrCl 10-50 | CrCl <10 | Hemodialysis | CAPD | CRRT |
|---|---|---|---|---|---|---|---|---|---|
| **MISCELLANEOUS ANTIBACTERIALS** | | | | | | | | | |
| Chloramphenicol³ | 4.1 | Unchanged | 50-100 mg/kg/day po/IV (divided q6h) | 50-100 mg/kg/day (divided q6h) | 50-100 mg/kg/day (divided q6h) | 50-100 mg/kg/day (divided q6h) | 50-100 mg/kg/day (divided q6h) | 50-100 mg/kg/day (divided q6h) | 50-100 mg/kg/day (divided q6h) |
| Fosfomycin IV^NUS | 5,7 | 50 | 6 gm IV q6h | 6 gm IV q6h | >40: 6 gm q6h 40-70% of norm 30: 60% of norm 20: 40% of norm (all div q8-12h) | CrCl 10: 20% of norm (div q8-12h) | 2 gm q48h (give AD) | No data | No data |
| Fosfomycin po | 5,7 | 50 | 3 gm po x1 | | | | | | |
| Fusidic acid^NUS,3 | 8.9-11 | 8.9-11 | 250-750 mg po q8-12h | 250-750 mg po q8-12h | 250-750 mg q8-12h | 250-750 mg q8-12h | 250-750 mg q8-12h | 250-750 mg q8-12h | 250-750 mg q8-12h |
| Metronidazole³ | 6-14 | 7-21 | 7.5 mg/kg IV/po q6h | 7.5 mg/kg q6h | 7.5 mg/kg q6h | 7.5 mg/kg q12h | 7.5 mg/kg q12h (give one of the dialysis days doses AD) | 7.5 mg/kg q12h | 7.5 mg/kg q6h |
| Nitrofurantoin | 1 | - | 100 mg po q12h (Macrobid) | 100 mg q12h (Macrobid) | Do not use (low urine concentrations) | Avoid use | Avoid use | Avoid use | Avoid use |
| Tinidazole³ | 13 | No data | 2 gm po q24h x 1-5 days | 2 gm q24h x1-5 days | Avoid use | 2 gm q24h x1-5 days | Avoid use | No data | Avoid use |
| Trimethoprim | 8-15 | 20-49 | 100-200 mg po q12h | 100-200 mg q12h | >30: 100-200 mg q12h; 10-30: 100-200 mg q18h | 100-200 mg q24h | 100-200 mg q24h (+ extra 1 gm AD) | 100-200 mg q24h | 100-200 mg q18h |
| TMP/SMX (treatment) | TMP 8-15, SMX 10 | TMP 20-49, SMX 20-50 | 5-20 mg/kg/day po/IV (div q6-12h) base on TMP | 5-20 mg/kg/day po/IV (div q6-12h) | 30-50: 5-20 mg/kg/day (div q6-12h); 10-29: 5-10 mg/kg/day (div q12h) | Not recommended (but if used: 5-10 mg/kg q24h) | Not recommended (but if used: 5-10 mg/kg q24h, give dialysis day dose AD) | Not recommended (but if used: 5-10 mg/kg q24h) | 5 mg/kg q8h |
| TMP/SMX (prophylaxis) | as above | as above | 1 DS tab q24h or 3x/week | 1 DS tab q24h or 3x/week | 1 DS tab q24h or 3x/week | 1 DS tab q24h or 3x/week | | | |
| **OXAZOLIDINONES** | | | | | | | | | |
| Linezolid | 5 | 6-8 | 600 mg po/IV q12h | 600 mg q12h | 600 mg q12h | 600 mg q12h | 600 mg q12h (give one of the dialysis day doses AD) | 600 mg q12h | 600 mg q12h |
| Tedizolid | 12 | Unchanged | 200 mg po/IV q24h | 200 mg q24h | 200 mg q24h | 200 mg q24h | 200 mg q24h | 200 mg q24h | 200 mg q24h |

**TABLE 17A (9)**

| ANTIMICROBIAL | Half-life, hrs (renal function normal) | Half-life, hrs (ESRD) | Dose (renal function normal) | CrCl >50-90 | CrCl 10-50 | CrCl <10 | Hemodialysis | CAPD | CRRT |
|---|---|---|---|---|---|---|---|---|---|
| **POLYMYXINS** | | | | | | | | | |
| Colistin (polymyxin E) See Table 10A All doses refer to colistin base in mg | 6.3-12 | ≥48 | Load: (4) x (pt wt in kg). Use lower of ideal or actual wt. Load may exceed 300 mg. Start maintenance 12 hrs later. | ≥90, 180 q12h; 80-<90, 170 mg q12h; 70-<80, 150 mg q12h; 60-<70, 137.5 mg q12h; 50-<60, 122.5 mg q12h | 40-<50, 110 mg q12h; 30-<40, 97.5 mg q12h; 20-<30, 87.5 mg q12h; 10-<20, 80 mg q12h | 5-<10, 72.5 mg q12h; <5, 65 mg q12h | On non-HD days, give 65 mg IV q12h. On HD days, add 40-50 mg to the daily dose after a 3-4 hr session. Give this supplement with the next regular dose after the dialysis has ended. | No data | Add 13 mg per hour of CRRT (or SLED) to the baseline dose of 65 mg q12h. |
| **TETRACYCLINES, GLYCYLCYCLINES** | | | | | | | | | |
| Tetracycline | 6-12 | 57-108 | 250-500 mg po q6h | 250-500 mg q8-12h | 250-500 mg q12-24h | 250-500 mg q24h | 250-500 mg q24h | 250-500 mg q24h | 250-500 mg q12-24h |
| **ANTIMETABOLITES** | | | | | | | | | |
| Flucytosine[a] | 3-5 | 75-200 | 25 mg/kg po q6h | 25 mg/kg q6h | 25 mg/kg q12h | 25 mg/kg q24h | 25 mg/kg q24h (give dialysis day dose AD) | 0.5-1 gm q24h | 25 mg/kg q12h |
| **ALLYLAMINES, AZOLES** | | | | | | | | | |
| Fluconazole | 20-50 | 100 | 100-400 mg po/IV q24h | 100-400 mg q24h | 50-200 mg q24h | 50-200 mg q24h | 100-400 mg q24h (give dialysis day dose AD) | 50-200 mg q24h | 200-400 mg q24h |
| Itraconazole (IV)[s] | 35-40 | Unchanged | 200 mg IV q12h | 200 mg q12h | Do not use IV itraconazole if CrCl<30 due to accumulation of cyclodextrin vehicle | | | | |
| Itraconazole (oral solution)[s] | 35-40 | Unchanged | 100-200 mg po q12h | 100-200 mg q12h | 100-200 mg q12h | 50-100 mg q12h | 100 mg q12-24h | 100 mg q12-24h | 100-200 mg q12h |
| Terbinafine | 36 | No data | 250 mg po q24h | 250 mg q24h | Avoid use | Avoid use | Avoid use | Avoid use | Avoid use |
| Voriconazole (IV)[s] | dose-dependent | dose-dependent | 6 mg/kg IV q12h x2 doses, then 4 mg/kg IV q12h | 6 mg/kg q12h x2 doses, then 4 mg/kg q12h | If CrCl<50, IV vehicle (cyclodextrin) accumulates. Use oral or discontinue. | | | | |
| **ANTIMYCOBACTERIALS First line, tuberculosis** | | | | | | | | | |
| Ethambutol[s] | 4 | 7-15 | 15-25 mg/kg po q24h | 15-25 mg/kg q24h | CrCl 30-50: 15-25 mg/kg q24-36h; CrCl 10-30: 15-25 mg/kg q36-48h | 15 mg/kg q48h | 15 mg/kg q48h (administer AD on dialysis days) | 15 mg/kg q48h | 15-25 mg/kg q24h |
| Isoniazid (INH)[s] | 0.7-4 | 8-17 | 5 mg/kg po q24h | 5 mg/kg q24h | 5 mg/kg q24h | 5 mg/kg q24h | 5 mg/kg q24h (administer AD on dialysis days) | 5 mg/kg q24h | 5 mg/kg q24h |

TABLE 17A (10)

| ANTIMICROBIAL | Half-life, hrs (renal function normal) | Half-life, hrs (ESRD) | Dose (renal function normal) | CrCl >90 | CrCl 10-50 | CrCl <10 | Hemodialysis | CAPD | CRRT |
|---|---|---|---|---|---|---|---|---|---|
| **ANTIMYCOBACTERIALS/First line, tuberculosis** *(continued)* | | | | | | | | | |
| Pyrazinamide | 10-16 | 26 | 25 mg/kg (max 2.5 gm) po q24h | 25 mg/kg q24h | CrCl 21-50: 25 mg/kg q24h; CrCl 10-20: 25 mg/kg q48h | 25 mg/kg q48h | 25 mg/kg q48h (administer AD on dialysis days) | 25 mg/kg q24h | 25 mg/kg q24h |
| Rifabutin[5] | 32-67 | Unchanged | 300 mg q24h | 300 mg q24h | 150 mg q24h | 150 mg q24h | No data | No data | No data |
| Rifampin[5] | 1.5-5 | up to 11 | 600 mg po q24h | 600 mg q24h | 300-600 mg q24h | 300-600 mg q24h | 300-600 mg q24h | 300-600 mg q24h | 300-600 mg q24h |
| Rifapentine | 13.2-14.1 | Unchanged | 600 mg po 1-2x/wk | 600 mg 1-2x/wk | 600 mg 1-2x/wk | 600 mg 1-2x/wk | 600 mg 1-2x/wk | 600 mg 1-2x/wk | 600 mg 1-2x/wk |
| Streptomycin[1,2] | 2-3 | 30-70 | 15 mg/kg (max 1 gm) IM q24h | 15 mg/kg q24h | 15 mg/kg q24-72h | 15 mg/kg q72-96h | 15 mg/kg q72-96h (+ extra 7.5 mg/kg AD) | 20-40 mg lost per L of dialysate/day | 15 mg/kg q24-72h |
| **Second line, tuberculosis** | | | | | | | | | |
| Bedaquiline | 24-30 (terminal 4-5 mo) | No data | 400 mg q24h x2 wks, then 200 mg po 3x/wks x22 wks | 400 mg q24h x2 wk, then 200 mg 3x/wks x22 WKS | 400 mg q24h x2 wks, then 200 mg 3x/wks x22 wks | Use with caution | Use with caution | Use with caution | Use with caution |
| Capreomycin | 2-5 | No data | 15 mg/kg IM/IV q24h | 15 mg/kg q24h | 15 mg/kg q24h | 15 mg/kg 3x/wk | 15 mg/kg 3x/wk (give AD on dialysis days) | No data | No data |
| Cycloserine[10] | 10 | No data | 250-500 mg po q12h | 250-500 mg q12h | 250-500 mg q12h-24h (dosing interval poorly defined) | 500 mg q48h (or 3x/wk) | 500 mg 3x/wk (give AD on dialysis days) | No data | No data |
| Ethionamide | 2 | 9 | 500 mg po q12h | 500 mg q12h | 500 mg q12h | 250 mg q12h | 250 mg q12h | 250 mg q12h | 500 mg q12h |
| Kanamycin[1,2] | 2-3 | 30-70 | 7.5 mg/kg IM/IV q12h | 7.5 mg/kg q12h | 7.5 mg/kg q24h | 7.5 mg/kg q48h | 7.5 mg/kg q48h (+ extra 3.25 mg/kg AD) | 15-20 mg lost per L of dialysate/day | 7.5 mg/kg q24h |
| Para-aminosalicylic acid (PAS) | 0.75-1.0 | 23 | 4 gm q12h | 4 gm q12h | 2-3 gm q12h | 2 gm q12h | 2 gm q12h (dose AD on dialysis days) | No data | No data |
| **ANTIPARASITICS: ANTIMALARIALS** | | | | | | | | | |
| Artemether/ lumefantrine (20 mg/120 mg) | art, DHA 1.6-2.2, lum 101-119 | No data | 4 tabs x1, 4 tabs in 8 hr, then 4 tabs q12h x2 days | 4 tabs x1, 4 tabs in 8 hr, then 4 tabs q12h x2 days | 4 tabs x1, 4 tabs in 8 hr, 4 tabs q12h x2 days | 4 tabs x1, 4 tabs in 8 hr, 4 tabs q12h x2 days | No data | No data | No data |
| Atovaquone | 67 | No data | 750 mg po q12h | 750 mg q12h | CrCl 30-50: 750 mg q12h; CrCl 10-30: use with caution | Use with caution | No data | No data | No data |

**TABLE 17A (11)**

| ANTIMICROBIAL | Half-life, hrs (renal function normal) | Half-life, hrs (ESRD) | Dose (renal function normal) | CrCl >50-90 | CrCl 10-50 | CrCl <10 | Hemodialysis | CAPD | CRRT |
|---|---|---|---|---|---|---|---|---|---|
| **ANTIPARASITICS, ANTIMALARIALS** *(continued)* | | | | | | | | | |
| Atovaquone/ Proguanil (250 mg/100 mg) | atov 67, pro 12-21 | No data | 4 tabs po q24h x3 days | 4 tabs q24h x3 days | CrCl <30: use with caution | Use with caution | No data | No data | No data |
| Chloroquine phosphate | 45-55 days (terminal) | No data | 2.5 gm po over 3 days | 2.5 gm over 3 days | 2.5 gm over 3 days | 2.5 gm over 3 days (consider reducing dose 50%) | 2.5 gm over 3 days (consider reducing dose 50%) | No data | No data |
| Mefloquine | 13-24 days | No data | 750 mg po, then 500 mg po in 6-8 hrs | 750 mg, then 500 mg in 6-8 hrs | 750 mg, then 500 mg in 6-8 hrs | 750 mg, then 500 mg in 6-8 hrs | No data | No data | No data |
| Quinine | 9.7-12.5 | up to 16 | 648 mg po q8h | 648 mg q8h | 648 mg q8-12h | 648 mg q24h | 648 mg q24h (give dialysis day dose AD) | 648 mg q24h | 648 mg q8-12h |
| **OTHER** | | | | | | | | | |
| Albendazole | 8-12 | No data | 400 mg po q12-24h | 400 mg q12-24h | 400 mg q12-24h | 400 mg q12-24h | No data | No data | No data |
| Dapsone | 10-50 | No data | 100 mg q24h | No data | No data | No data | No data | No data | No data |
| Ivermectin | 20 | No data | 200 µg/kg/day po x1-2 days | 200 µg/kg/day x1-2 days | 200 µg/kg/day x1-2 days | 200 µg/kg/day x1-2 days | No data | No data | No data |
| Miltefosine | 7-31 days | No data | 50 mg po q8h | No data | No data | No data | No data | No data | No data |
| Nitazoxanide | tizoxanide 1.3-1.8 | No data | 500 mg po q12h | No data | No data | No data | No data | No data | No data |
| Pentamidine | 3-12 | 73-118 | 4 mg/kg IM/IV q24h | 4 mg/kg q24h | 4 mg/kg q24h | 4 mg/kg q24-36h | 4 mg/kg q48h (give dialysis day dose AD) | 4 mg/kg q24-36h | 4 mg/kg q24h |
| **ANTIVIRALS HEPATITIS B** | | | | | | | | | |
| Adefovir | 7.5 | 15 | 10 mg po q24h | 10 mg q24h | 10 mg q48-72h | 10 mg q72h | 10 mg weekly (dose AD on dialysis days) | No data | No data |
| Entecavir | 128-149 | ? | 0.5 mg po q24h | 0.5 mg q24h | 0.15-0.25 mg q24h | 0.05 mg q24h | 0.05 mg q24h (dose AD on dialysis days) | 0.05 mg q24h | No data |
| Telbivudine | 40-49 | No data | 600 mg po q24h | 600 mg q24h | 30-49: 600 mg q48h; 10-30: 600 mg q72h | 600 mg q96h | 600 mg q96h (dose AD on dialysis days) | No data | No data |

**TABLE 17A (12)**

| ANTIMICROBIAL | Half-life, hrs (renal function normal) | Half-life, hrs (ESRD) | Dose (renal function normal) | CrCl >50-90 | CrCl 10-50 | CrCl <10 | Hemodialysis | CAPD | CRRT |
|---|---|---|---|---|---|---|---|---|---|
| **HEPATITIS C (SINGLE AGENTS)** | | | | | | | | | |
| Daclatasvir | 12-15 | No data | 60 mg q24h | 60 mg q24h | 60 mg q24h | 60 mg q24h | No data | No data | No data |
| Ribavirin | 44 | No data | Depends on indication | No dosage adjustment | Use with caution | Use with caution | No data | No data | No data |
| Simeprevir | 41 | Unchanged | 150 mg q24h | 150 mg q24h | Use with caution (no data for use in patients with CrCl<30) | Use with caution (no data for use in patients with CrCl<30) | No data | No data | No data |
| Sofosbuvir | sofosbuvir 0.5-0.75 | Unchanged | 400 mg q24h | 400 mg q24h | Use with caution (no data for use in patients with CrCl<30) | Use with caution (no data for use in patients with CrCl<30) | No data | No data | No data |
| **HEPATITIS C (FIXED-DOSE COMBINATIONS)** | | | | | | | | | |
| Epclusa (Velpatasvir, Sofosbuvir) | velpat 15, sofos 0.5 | No data | 1 tab po q24h | 1 tab q24h | Use with caution (no data for use in patients with CrCl<30) | | No data | No data | No data |
| Harvoni (Ledipasvir, Sofosbuvir) | ledipasvir 47 | No data | 1 tab po q24h | 1 tab q24h | Use with caution (no data for use in patients with CrCl<30) | | No data | No data | No data |
| Technivie (Ombitasvir, Paritaprevir, RTV) | ombit 28-34, parita 5.8 | No data | 2 tabs q24h | 2 tabs q24h | 2 tabs q24h | 2 tabs q24h | No data | No data | No data |
| Viekira Pak (Dasabuvir, Ombitasvir, Paritaprevir, RTV) | dasabuvir 5-8 | No data | 2 Ombit/Parita/RTV tabs q24h, Dasa 250 mg q12h | 2 Ombit/Parita/RTV tabs q24h, Dasa 250 mg q12h | 2 Ombit/Parita/RTV tabs q24h, Dasa 250 mg q12h | 2 Ombit/Parita/RTV tabs q24h, Dasa 250 mg q12h | No data | No data | No data |
| Zepatier (Elbasvir, Grazoprevir) | elba 24, grazo 31 | No data | 1 tab po q24h | 1 tab po q24h | 1 tab po q24h | 1 tab po q24h | 1 tab po q24h | No data | No data |
| **HERPESVIRUS** | | | | | | | | | |
| Acyclovir (IV)¹ | 2.5-3.5 | 20 | 5-12.5 mg/kg IV q8h | 5-12.5 mg/kg q8h | 5-12.5 mg/kg q12-24h | 2.5-6.25 mg/kg q24h | 2.5-6.25 mg/kg q24h (dose AD on dialysis days) | 2.5-6.25 mg/kg q24h | 5-10 mg/kg q24h |
| Acyclovir (po) | 2.5-3.5 | 20 | 800 mg po q4h (5x/day) | 800 mg q4h (5x/day) | CrCl >25: 800 mg q4h (5x/day); 10-25: 800 mg q8h | 800 mg q12h | 800 mg q12h (give extra dose AD) | 800 mg q12h | No data |
| Cidofovir (induction) | 2.6 | No data | 5 mg/kg IV q-week x2 weeks | CrCl>55: 5 mg/kg q-week x2 weeks | Contraindicated in patients with CrCl of 55 mL/min or less | Contraindicated in patients with CrCl of 55 mL/min or less | Contraindicated | Contraindicated | Contraindicated |
| Cidofovir (maintenance) | 2.6 | No data | 5 mg/kg IV every 2 weeks | CrCl>55: 5 mg/kg every 2 weeks | Contraindicated in patients with CrCl of 55 mL/min or less | Contraindicated in patients with CrCl of 55 mL/min or less | Contraindicated | Contraindicated | Contraindicated |

## TABLE 17A (13)

| ANTIMICROBIAL | Half-life, hrs (renal function normal) | Half-life, hrs (ESRD) | Dose (renal function normal) | CrCl >50-90 | CrCl 10-50 | CrCl <10 | Hemodialysis | CAPD | CRRT |
|---|---|---|---|---|---|---|---|---|---|
| **HERPESVIRUS** *(continued)* | | | | | | | | | |
| Famciclovir | penciclovir 2-3 | 10-22 | 500 mg po q8h (VZV) | 500 mg q8h | 500 mg q12-24h | 250 mg q24h | 250 mg q24h (dose AD on dialysis days) | No data | No data |
| Ganciclovir (IV induction) | 3.5 | 30 | 5 mg/kg IV q12h | CrCl 70-90, 5 mg/kg q12h; CrCl 50-69, 2.5 mg/kg q12h | CrCl 25-49, 2.5 mg/kg q24h; CrCl 10-24, 1.25 mg/kg q24h | 1.25 mg/kg 3x/week | 1.25 mg/kg 3x/week (dose AD on dialysis days) | 1.25 mg/kg 3x/week | CVVHF: 2.5 mg/kg q24h (AAC 58:94, 2014) |
| Ganciclovir (IV maintenance) | 3.5 | 30 | 5 mg/kg IV q24h | 2.5-5 mg/kg q24h | 0.625-1.25 mg/kg q24h | 0.625 mg/kg 3x/week | 0.625 mg/kg 3x/week (dose AD on dialysis days) | 0.625 mg/kg 3x/week | No data |
| Ganciclovir (oral) | 3.5 | 30 | 1 gm po q8h | 0.5-1 gm q8h | 0.5-1 gm q24h | 0.5 gm 3x/week | 0.5 gm 3x/week (dose AD on dialysis days) | No data | No data |
| Letermovir | 12 | ND | 480 mg po/IV q24h | 480 mg q24h | 480 mg q24h | No data | No data | No data | No data |
| Valacyclovir | 3 | 14 | 1 gm po q8h (VZV) | 1 gm q8h | 1 gm q12-24h | 0.5 gm q24h | 0.5 gm q24h (dose AD on dialysis days) | 0.5 gm q24h | 1 gm q12-24h |
| Valganciclovir | ganciclovir 4 | ganciclovir 67 | 900 mg po q12h | 900 mg q24h | 450 mg q24-48h | Do not use | *See prescribing information* | No data | No data |
| Foscarnet (induction) special dosing scale | 3 (terminal 18-88) | Very long | **CrCl above 1.4 mL/min/kg (foscarnet only)** | **CrCl >1 to 1.4 mL/min/kg (foscarnet only)** | **CrCl >0.8 to 1.0 mL/min/kg (foscarnet only)** | **CrCl >0.6 to 0.8 mL/min/kg (foscarnet only)** | **CrCl >0.5 to 0.6 mL/min/kg (foscarnet only)** | **CrCl 0.4 to 0.5 mL/min/kg (foscarnet only)** | **CrCl <0.4 mL/min/kg (foscarnet only)** |
| | | | 60 mg/kg IV q8h | 45 mg/kg q8h | 50 mg/kg q12h | 40 mg/kg q12h | 60 mg/kg q48h | 50 mg/kg q24h | Not recommended |
| Foscarnet (maintenance) special dosing scale | 3 (terminal 18-88) | Very long | 90-120 mg/kg IV q24h | 70-90 mg/kg q24h | 50-65 mg/kg q24h | 80-105 mg/kg q48h | 60-80 mg/kg q48h | 50-65 mg/kg q48h | Not recommended |
| **INFLUENZA** | | | | | | | | | |
| Amantadine | 14.8 | 500 | 100 mg q12h | 100 mg q12h | 100 mg q24-48h | 100 mg weekly | 100 mg weekly (give 100 mg AD on dialysis days) | 100 mg weekly | 100 mg q24-48h |
| Oseltamivir | carboxylate 6-10 | carboxylate >20 | 75 mg po q12h | CrCl >60: 75 mg q12h | CrCl 31-60: 30 mg q12h; CrCl 10-30: 30 mg q24h | No recommendation unless HD | 30 mg after each dialysis, no drug on non-HD days (see comments) | 30 mg after a dialysis exchange | No data |
| Peramivir | 20 | No data | 600 mg IV q24h | 600 mg q24h | CrCl 31-49: 200 mg q24h; CrCl 10-30: 100 mg q24h | 100 mg x1, then 15 mg q24h | 100 mg x1, then 100 mg 2 hrs AD on dialysis days only | No data | No data |
| Rimantadine[s] | 24-36 | prolonged | 100 mg q12h | 100 mg q12h | 100 mg q12-24h | 100 mg q24h | No data | No data | Use with caution |

TABLE 17A (14)

| ANTIMICROBIAL | Half-life, hrs (renal function normal) | Half-life, hrs (ESRD) | Dose (renal function normal) | CrCl >50-90 | CrCl 10-50 | CrCl <10 | Hemodialysis | CAPD | CRRT |
|---|---|---|---|---|---|---|---|---|---|
| **ANTIRETROVIRALS (NRTIs)** | | | | | | | | | |
| Abacavir (ABC)ᵃ | 1.5 | No data | 600 mg po q24h | 600 mg q24h | 600 mg q24h | 600 mg q24h | No data | No data | No data |
| Didanosine enteric coated (ddI) | 1.6 | 4.5 | 400 mg EC po q24h | 400 mg EC q24h | 125-200 mg EC q24h | Do not use | No data | No data | No data |
| Emtricitabine capsules (FTC) | 10 | >10 | 200 mg po q24h | 200 mg q24h | CrCl 30-49: 200 mg q48h; CrCl 15-29: 200 mg q72h | CrCl <15: 200 mg q96h | 200 mg q96h | No data | No data |
| Emtricitabine oral solution (FTC) | 10 | >10 | 240 mg po q24h | 240 mg q24h | CrCl 30-49: 120 mg q24h; CrCl 15-29: 80 mg q24h | CrCl <15: 60 mg q24h | 60 mg q24h | No data | No data |
| Lamivudine (3TC) | 5-7 | 15-35 | 300 mg po q24h (HIV dose) | 300 mg q24h (HIV) | 50-150 mg q24h (HIV) | 25-50 mg q24h (HIV) | 25-50 mg q24h (dose AD on dialysis days) (HIV) | 25-50 mg q24h (HIV) | 100 mg first day, then 50 mg q24h (HIV) |
| Stavudine (d4T) | 1.2-1.6 | 5.5-8 | 30-40 mg po q12h | 30-40 mg q12h | 15-20 mg q12h | ≥60 kg: 20 mg q24h; <60 kg: 15 mg q24h | ≥60 kg: 20 mg q24h; <60 kg: 15 mg q24h (dose AD on dialysis days) | No data | 30-40 mg q12h |
| Tenofovir (TDF) | 17 | Prolonged | 300 mg po q24h | 300 mg q24h | CrCl 30-49: 300 mg q48h; CrCl 10-29: 300 mg q72-96h | No data | 300 mg after every 3rd dialysis, or q7 days if no dialysis | No data | No data |
| Zidovudine (ZDV) | 0.5-3 | 1.3-3 | 300 mg po q12h | 300 mg q12h | 300 mg q12h | 100 mg q8h | 100 mg q8h (dose AD on dialysis days) | No data | 300 mg q12h |
| **FUSION/ENTRY INHIBITORS** | | | | | | | | | |
| Enfuvirtide (ENF, T20)ᵇ | 3.8 | Unchanged | 90 mg sc q12h | 90 mg q12h | Not studied in patients with CrCl<35; DO NOT USE | | | Avoid use | Avoid use | Avoid use |
| Maraviroc (MVC) | 14-18 | No data | 300 mg po q12h | 300 mg q12h | No data | No data | No data | No data | No data |
| **FIXED-DOSE COMBINATIONS** | | | | | | | | | |
| Atripla (EFV/FTC/TDF) | *See components* | *See components* | 1 tab po q24h | 1 tab q24h | Do not use | Do not use | Do not use | Do not use | Do not use |
| Biktarvy (BIC-FTC-TAF) | *See components* | *See components* | 1 tab po q24h | 1 tab q24h | CrCl 30-49: 1 tab q24h; do not use if CrCl <30 | Do not use | Do not use | Do not use | Do not use |
| Cimduo (3TC-TDF) | *See components* | *See components* | 1 tab po q24h | 1 tab q24h | Do not use | Do not use | Do not use | Do not use | Do not use |

**TABLE 17A (15)**

**FIXED-DOSE COMBINATIONS** *(continued)*

| ANTIMICROBIAL | Half-life, hrs (renal function normal) | Half-life, hrs (ESRD) | Dose (renal function normal) | CrCl >50-90 | CrCl 10-50 | CrCl <10 | Hemodialysis | CAPD | CRRT |
|---|---|---|---|---|---|---|---|---|---|
| Combivir (3TC/ZDV) | *See components* | *See components* | 1 tab po q12h | 1 tab q12h | Do not use | Do not use | Do not use | Do not use | Do not use |
| Complera, Eviplera (RPV/FTC/TDF) | *See components* | *See components* | 1 tab po q24h | 1 tab q24h | Do not use | Do not use | Do not use | Do not use | Do not use |
| Descovy (FTC-TAF) | *See components* | *See components* | 1 tab po q24h | 1 tab q24h | CrCl 30-49: 1 tab q24h; not use if CrCl <30 | Do not use | Do not use | Do not use | Do not use |
| Dutrebis (3TC/RAL) | *See components* | *See components* | 1 tab po q12h | 1 tab q12h | Do not use | Do not use | Do not use | Do not use | Do not use |
| Epzicom, Kivexa (ABC/3TC) | *See components* | *See components* | 1 tab po q24h | 1 tab q24h | Do not use | Do not use | Do not use | Do not use | Do not use |
| Evotaz (ATV/cobi)[12] | *See components* | *See components* | 1 tab po q24h | 1 tab q24h | 1 tab q24h | 1 tab q24h | Do not use | No data | No data |
| Genvoya (EVG/FTC/TAF/cobi) | *See components* | *See components* | 1 tab po q24h | 1 tab po q24h | CrCl 30-49: 1 tab po q24h; do not use if CrCl <30 | Do not use | Do not use | Do not use | Do not use |
| Juluca (DTG-RPV) | *See components* | *See components* | 1 tab po q24h | 1 tab q24h | 1 tab q24h | 1 tab q24h | No data | No data | No data |
| Odefsey (RPV-FTC-TAF) | *See components* | *See components* | 1 tab po q24h | 1 tab q24h | CrCl 30-49: 1 tab q24h; do not use if CrCl <30 | Do not use | Do not use | Do not use | Do not use |
| Prezcobix (DRV/cobi)[12] | *See components* | *See components* | 1 tab po q24h | 1 tab q24h | 1 tab q24h | 1 tab q24h | 1 tab q24h | 1 tab q24h | 1 tab q24h |
| Symfi, Symfi Lo (EFV-3TC-TDF) | *See components* | *See components* | 1 tab po q24h | Do not use if CrCl <70 | Do not use | Do not use | Do not use | Do not use | Do not use |
| Stribild (EVG/FTC/TDF/cobi) | *See components* | *See components* | 1 tab po q24h | 1 tab q24h | Do not use | Do not use | Do not use | Do not use | Do not use |
| Symtuza (DRV-cobi-FTC-TAF) | *See components* | *See components* | 1 tab po q24h | 1 tab q24h | CrCl 30-49: 1 tab q24h; do not use if CrCl <30 | Do not use | Do not use | Do not use | Do not use |
| Triumeq (DTG/ABC/3TC) | *See components* | *See components* | 1 tab po q24h | 1 tab q24h | Do not use | Do not use | Do not use | Do not use | Do not use |
| Trizivir (ABC/3TC/ZDV) | *See components* | *See components* | 1 tab po q12h | 1 tab q12h | Do not use | Do not use | Do not use | Do not use | Do not use |

**TABLE 17A (16)**

| ANTIMICROBIAL | Half-life, hrs (renal function normal) | Half-life, hrs (ESRD) | Dose (renal function normal) | CrCl >50-90 | CrCl 10-50 | CrCl <10 | Hemodialysis | CAPD | CRRT |
|---|---|---|---|---|---|---|---|---|---|
| **FIXED-DOSE COMBINATIONS** *(continued)* | | | | | | | | | |
| Truvada (FTC/TDF) | *See components* | *See components* | 1 tab po q24h | 1 tab q24h | CrCl 30-49: 1 tab q48h; do not use if CrCl <30 | Do not use | Do not use | Do not use | Do not use |

[1] High flux HD membranes lead to unpredictable drug Cl; measure post-dialysis drug levels.
[2] Check levels with CAPD. PK highly variable. Usual method w/CAPD: 2L dialysis fluid replaced qid (Example amikacin: give 8L x 20 mg lost/L = 160 mg amikacin IV supplement daily).
[3] Gentamicin SLEDD dose: 6 mg/kg IV q48h beginning 30 min before start of SLEDD (AAC 54:3635, 2010).
[4] May falsely increase Scr by interference with assay.
[5] Dosage adjustment may be required in hepatic disease.
[6] Clav cleared by liver; thus, as dose of combination is decreased, a clav deficiency may occur (JAMA 285:386, 2001). If CrCl≤30, do not use 875/125 or 1000/62.5.
[7] New hemodialysis membranes increase Vancomycin clearance; check levels.
[8] Monitor serum concentrations if possible in dialysis patients.
[9] Goal peak serum concentration: 25-100 µg/mL.
[10] Goal peak serum concentration: 20-35 µg/mL.
[11] Rapid infusion can increase Scr.
[12] Do not use with Tenofovir if CrCl <70.

**TABLE 17B – NO DOSAGE ADJUSTMENT WITH RENAL INSUFFICIENCY BY CATEGORY**

| Antibacterials | | Antifungals | Anti-TBc | Antivirals | | Antiparasitics |
|---|---|---|---|---|---|---|
| Azithromycin | Minocycline | Amphotericin B | Bedaquiline | Abacavir | Mavyret | Albendazole |
| Ceftriaxone | Moxifloxacin | Anidulafungin | Ethionamide | Atazanavir | Nelfinavir | Artesunate |
| Chloramphenicol | Nafcillin | Caspofungin | Isoniazid | Daclatasvir | Nevirapine | Ivermectin |
| Clindamycin | Oritavancin | Isavuconazonium | Rifampin | Darunavir | Raltegravir | Mefloquine |
| Dicloxacillin | Polymyxin B | sulfate | Rifabutin | Delavirdine | Ribavirin | Praziquantel |
| Doxycycline | Rifaximin | Itraconazole oral | Rifapentine | Dolutegravir | Rilpivirine | Primaquine |
| Eravacycline | Secnidazole | solution | | Efavirenz | Ritonavir | Pyrimethamine |
| Fidaxomicin | Tedizolid | Ketoconazole | | Elvitegravir | Saquinavir | |
| Fusidic acid | Tigecycline | Micafungin | | Enfuvirtide[1] | Simeprevir[2] | |
| Linezolid[3] | | Posaconazole, | | Epclusa[2] | Sofosbuvir[2] | |
| Quinupristin- | | **po only** | | Etravirine | Technivie | |
| Dalfopristin | | Voriconazole, | | Fosamprenavir | Tecoviromat | |
| | | **po only** | | Harvoni[2] | Tipranavir | |
| | | | | Ibalizumab-uiyk | Viekira Pak | |
| | | | | Indinavir | Viekira XR | |
| | | | | Letermovir | Zepatier | |
| | | | | Lopinavir | | |

[1] Enfuvirtide: Not studied in patients with CrCl <35 mL/min. DO NOT USE.
[2] No data for CrCl <30 mL/min
[3] Increased risk of bone marrow toxicity

**TABLE 17C – ANTIMICROBIAL DOSING IN OBESITY**

The number of obese patients is increasing. Intuitively, the standard doses of some drugs may not achieve effective serum concentrations. Pertinent data on anti-infective dosing in the obese patient is gradually emerging. Though some of the data needs further validation, the following table reflects what is currently known. **Obesity is defined as ≥20% over Ideal Body Weight (Ideal BW) or Body Mass Index (BMI) >30. Dose** = suggested body weight (BW) for dose calculation in obese patient, or specific dose if applicable. In general, the absence of a drug in the table indicates a lack of pertinent information in the published literature.

| Drug | Dose | Comments |
|---|---|---|
| Acyclovir | Use **Adjusted BW** (see Comments) Example: for HSV encephalitis, give 10 mg/kg of Adjusted BW q8h | Unpublished data from 7 obese volunteers (Davis, et al., ICAAC abstract, 1991) suggested ideal BW, but newer and more convincing PK data suggest that adjusted BW better approximates drug exposure in normals (AAC 60:1830, 2016). |
| Aminoglycosides | Use **Adjusted BW** Example: Critically ill patient, Gent or Tobra (not Amikacin) 7 mg/kg of Adjusted BW IV q24h (see Comments) | Adjusted BW = Ideal BW + 0.4(Actual BW – Ideal BW). Ref: Pharmacother 27:1081, 2007. Follow levels so as to lower dose once hemodynamics stabilize. |
| Anidulafungin | Consider dose increase if wt > 140 kg | PK modeling suggests a 25% increase in load and maintenance dose in pts > 140 kg results in exposure similar to non-obese pts receiving usual dose (AAC 62:e00063-18, 2018). |
| Cefazolin (surgical prophylaxis) | No dose adjustment may be required: 2 gm x 1 dose (repeat in 3 hours?) (see Comments) | Conflicting data; unclear whether dose should be repeated, or if an even higher dose is required. Patients with BMI 40-80 studied. PK: 2-4 gm given to obese pts before c-section yielded inadequate conc in myometrium and subcutaneous adipose tissue despite adequate plasma conc. Refs: Surg 136:738, 2004; Eur J Clin Pharmacol 67:985, 2011; Surg Infect 13:33, 2012; Pharmacother 37:1415, 2017. |
| Cefepime | Modest dose increase: 2 gm IV q8h instead of the usual q12h | Data from 10 patients (mean BMI 48) undergoing bariatric surgery; regimen yields free T > MIC of 60% for MIC of 8 µg/mL. Ref: Obes Surg 22:465, 2012. |
| Cefotetan | No dose adjustment may be required. (see Comments) | No difference in surg wound infection rates between 2 and 3 gm prophylaxis doses in patients ≥120 kg, median BMI 42 kg/m² (Surg Infect 19:504, 2018). |
| Cefoxitin | Larger dose possibly required but data insufficient for a firm recommendation (see Comments) | Single 40 mg/kg pre-op dose in obese pts (based on actual BW; range 4-7.5 gm) resulted in suboptimal achievement of pharmacodynamic targets in serum and tissue, although performance was better than a simulated 2 gm dose (AAC 60:5885, 2016). |
| Clindamycin | Possibly use **Actual BW** (see Comments) | Combined PK modeling data from three prospective trials in children suggests actual BW to be most appropriate; no clinical outcome data available (AAC 61:e02014, 2016). |
| Daptomycin | Use **Actual BW** Example: 4-12 mg/kg of Actual BW IV q24h | Data from a single-dose PK study in 7 obese volunteers. Ref: Antimicrob Ag Chemother 51:2741, 2007. New data suggest similar outcomes with ideal BW and actual BW (AAC 58:88, 2014). Fixed, non-weight-based dosing in morbid obesity also suggested by a recent PK study (Pharmacother 2018 June 15 [Epub ahead of print]). |
| Fluconazole | Larger dose possibly required but data insufficient for a firm recommendation (see Comments) | Case reports suggest larger dose required in critically ill obese pts. Recent paper suggests that wt-based dosing (12 mg/kg load then 6 mg/kg/day using total BW) reaches desired PK/PD targets more reliably than fixed dosing; clinical validation required (Pharmacother 17:1023, 1997; AAC 60:6550, 2016). |

| Drug | Dose | Comments |
|------|------|----------|
| Flucytosine | Use **Ideal BW**<br>Example: Crypto meningitis, give 25 mg/kg of Ideal BW po q6h | Date from one obese patient with cryptococcal disease. Ref: *Pharmacother 15:251, 1995.* |
| Levofloxacin | **No dose adjustment may be required**<br>Example: 750 mg po/IV q24h<br>(see Comments) | Data from 13 obese patients; variability in study findings renders conclusion uncertain. Refs: *AAC 55:3240, 2011; JAC 66:1653, 2011.* A recent PK study (requiring clinical validation) in patients with BMI of 40 or more suggests that higher doses may be necessary to achieve adequate drug exposure (*Clin Pharmacokin 53:753, 2014*). |
| Linezolid | **No dose adjustment may be required**<br>Example: 600 mg po/IV q12h<br>(see Comments) | Data from 20 obese volunteers up to 150 kg body weight suggest standard doses provide AUC values similar to nonobese subjects. In a recent case report, standard dosing in a 265 kg male with MRSA pneumonia seemed to have reduced clinical effectiveness. Refs: *Antimicrob Ag Chemother 57:1144, 2013; Ann Pharmacother 47: e25, 2013.* |
| Micafungin | Higher dose may be required.<br>(see Comments) | PK/PD study suggests 100 mg q24h inadequate. 150 mg q24h adequate for C. albicans in pts ≤115 kg, 200 mg q24h in pts >115 kg. 200 mg q24h adequate for C. glabrata in pts <115 kg (*Crit Care 2018;22(1): 94*). |
| Oseltamivir | **No dose adjustment may be required**<br>Example: 75 mg po q12h<br>(see Comments) | Data from 10 obese volunteers, unclear if applicable to patients >250 kg (OK to give 150 mg po q12h). Ref: *J Antimicrob Chemother 66:2083, 2011.* Newer data consistent (*AAC 58:1616, 2014*). |
| Piperacillin-tazobactam | 6.75 gm IV over 4 hours and dosed every 8 hours. No data for pt with impaired renal function | Data need confirmation. Based on 14 obese patients with actual BW >130 kg and BMI >40 kg/m². Ref: *Int J Antimicrob Ag 41:52, 2013.* High dose required to ensure adequate conc of both pip and tazo for pathogens with MIC ≤16 mcg/mL, but enhanced bleeding risk is a concern particularly in renal dysfunction. |
| Telavancin | If weight is 30% or more over ideal BW, dose using adjusted BW as for aminoglycosides. | The correct dosing weight to use for Telavancin is unclear. Actual BW may overdose and increase nephrotoxicity, ideal BW may underdose (*JAC 67:723, 2012; JAC 67:1300, 2012*). Problematic because serum levels are not routinely available. |
| Vancomycin | Use **Actual BW**<br>Example: in critically ill patient give 25-30 mg/kg of Actual BW IV load, then 15-20 mg/kg of Actual BW IV q8h-12h (infuse over 1.5-2 hr). No single dose over 2 gm. Check trough levels. | Data from 24 obese patients; Vancomycin half-life appears to decrease with little change in Vd. Ref: *Eur J Clin Pharmacol 54:621, 1998.* |
| Voriconazole po | **No dose adjustment** required (use **Ideal BW**) *See Comments*<br>Example: 400 mg po q12h x2 doses then 200 mg po q12h. Check trough concentrations (underdosing common with Voriconazole). | Data from a 2-way crossover study of oral Voriconazole in 8 volunteers suggest no adjustment required, but other data support use of adjusted BW. Best for now to use ideal BW and check serum concentrations (*AAC 55:2601, 2011; CID 53:745, 2011; CID 63:286, 2016*). |

### TABLE 17D – NO DOSING ADJUSTMENT REQUIRED IN OBESITY

The pharmacokinetics of antibacterials in obese patients is emerging, but only selected drugs have been evaluated. Those drugs where data justifies a dose adjustment are summarized in *Table 17C*. Those drugs where data indicates **NO NEED** for dose adjustment are listed below.

| Drug | Drug |
|------|------|
| Ceftaroline | Imipenem/cilastatin |
| Ceftazidime/avibactam | Meropenem |
| Ceftolozane/tazobactam | Moxifloxacin |
| Dalbavancin | Oritavancin |
| Doripenem | Tedizolid |
| Ertapenem | Tigecycline |

Ref: *Pharmacotherapy 37:1415, 2017*

### TABLE 18 – ANTIMICROBIALS AND HEPATIC DISEASE: DOSAGE ADJUSTMENT*

The following alphabetical list indicates antibacterials excreted/metabolized by the liver **wherein a dosage adjustment may be indicated** in the presence of hepatic disease. Space precludes details; consult the PDR or package inserts for details. List is **not** all-inclusive:

| Antibacterials | | Antifungals | Antiparasitics | Antivirals§ | |
|----------------|---|-------------|----------------|-------------|---|
| Ceftriaxone | Nafcillin | Caspofungin | Antimony, pentavalent | Abacavir | Indinavir |
| Chloramphenicol | Rifabutin | Itraconazole | Benznidazole | Atazanavir | Lopinavir/Ritonavir |
| Clindamycin | Rifampin | Voriconazole | Nifurtimox | Darunavir | Nelfinavir |
| Eravacycline | Synercid** | | Praziquantel | Delavirdine | Nevirapine |
| Fusidic acid | Telithromycin** | | | Efavirenz | Ritonavir |
| Isoniazid | Tigecycline | | | Enfuvirtide | |
| Metronidazole | Tinidazole | | | Fosamprenavir | |

§ Ref. on antiretrovirals: *CID 40:174, 2005*   ** Quinupristin-Dalfopristin   ** Telithro: reduce dose in renal & hepatic failure

**TABLE 19 – TREATMENT OF CAPD PERITONITIS IN ADULTS**
(Adapted from Guidelines – Int'l Soc Peritoneal Dialysis, *Periton Dialysis Intl 2016, 36:481*)

**Principles: Empiric antibiotic therapy**

- Initiate antibiotics asap after collection of peritoneal fluid & blood for culture
- Empiric regimens must be guided by local susceptibilities
  - Possible gram-positive infection: suggest either Cefazolin or Vanco
  - Possible gram-negative infection: suggest either Cefepime or aminoglycoside, e.g. Gentamicin
- No need to adjust intraperitoneal (IP) dose for residual renal function
- Can treat by IP route or systemic IV therapy, but Guidelines favor IP therapy

**Intraperitoneal (IP) therapy**

- Can be either continuous (drugs in each exchange) or intermittent (once daily)
- If intermittent, need antibiotic-containing dialysis fluid to dwell for minimum 6 hrs
- Vanco, aminoglycosides, cephalosporins can be combined in same dialysis bag; penicillins and aminoglycosides **cannot** be combined

**Specific recommendations**

| IP Antibiotic Dosing Recommendations for Treatment of Peritonitis | | |
|---|---|---|
| | **Intermittent** (1 exchange daily) | **Continuous** (all exchanges) |
| **Aminoglycosides:** | | |
| Amikacin | 2 mg/kg daily | LD 25 mg/L, MD 12 mg/L |
| Gentamicin | 0.6 mg/kg daily | LD 8 mg/L, MD 4 mg/L |
| Tobramycin | 0.6 mg/kg daily | LD 3 mg/kg, MD 0.3 mg/kg |
| **Cephalosporins:** | | |
| Cefazolin | 15-20 mg/kg daily | LD 500 mg/L, MD 125 mg/L |
| Cefepime | 1000 mg daily | LD 250-500 mg/L, MD 100-125 mg/L |
| Ceftazidime | 1000-1500 mg daily | LD 500 mg/L, MD 125 mg/L |
| Ceftriaxone | 1000 mg daily | No data |
| **Penicillins:** | | |
| Penicillin G | No data | LD 50,000 unit/L, MD 25,000 unit/L |
| Amoxicillin | No data | MD 150 mg/L |
| Ampicillin | No data | MD 125 mg/L |
| Amp/sulb | 2 gm/1 gm q12h | LD 750-100 mg/L, MD 100 mg/L |
| Pip/tazo | No data | LD 4 gm/0.5 gm, MD 1 gm/0.125 gm |
| **Others:** | | |
| Aztreonam | 2 gm daily | LD 1000 mg/L, MD 250 mg/L |
| Ciprofloxacin | No data | MD 50 mg/L |
| Clindamycin | No data | MD 600 mg/bag |
| Daptomycin | No data | LD 100 mg/L, MD 20 mg/L |
| Imipenem | 500 mg in alternate exch | LD 250 mg/L, MD 50 mg/L |
| Polymyxin B | No data | MD 300,000 unit (30 mg)/bag |
| Meropenem | 1 gm daily | No data |
| Teicoplanin | 15 mg/kg every 5 days | LD 400 mg/bag, MD 20 mg/bag |
| Vancomycin | 15-30 mg/kg every 5-7 days | LD 30 mg/kg, MD 1.5 mg/kg/bag |
| **Antifungals:** | | |
| Fluconazole | IP 200 mg q24-48 hrs | No data |
| Voriconazole | IP 2.5 mg/kg daily | No data |

LD = loading dose in mg; MD = maintenance dose in mg; IP = intraperitoneal
Ref: *Periton Dialysis Intl 2016;36:481*

**Systemic dosing recommendations** for treatment of CAPD peritonitis

- In general, IP dosing leads to high IP drug levels and, hence, IP is preferable to IV antibiotic administration
- See individual systemic drugs for dose recommendations for patients with end stage renal disease (ESRD)
- Do not co-administer the same drug IP and systemically (either po or IV)

**Indications for removal of CAPD catheter**

- Relapse with same organism within one month
- No clinical response within 5 days (failure)
- Infection at catheter exit site and/or catheter subcutaneous tunnel
- Fungal peritonitis
- Fecal flora peritonitis; sign of bowel wall erosion & perforation

**TABLE 20A – ANTI-TETANUS PROPHYLAXIS, WOUND CLASSIFICATION, IMMUNIZATION**

| WOUND CLASSIFICATION | | |
|---|---|---|
| Clinical Features | Tetanus Prone | Non-Tetanus Prone |
| Age of wound | >6 hours | ≤6 hours |
| Configuration | Stellate, avulsion | Linear |
| Depth | >1 cm | ≤1 cm |
| Mechanism of injury | Missile, crush, burn, frostbite | Sharp surface (glass, knife) |
| Devitalized tissue | Present | Absent |
| Contaminants (dirt, saliva, etc.) | Present | Absent |

| IMMUNIZATION SCHEDULE | | | | |
|---|---|---|---|---|
| History of Tetanus Immunization | Dirty, Tetanus-Prone Wound | | Clean, non-Tetanus-Prone Wound | |
| | Td[1,2] | Tetanus Immune Globulin | Td[1,2] | Tetanus Immune Globulin |
| Unknown or <3 doses[3] | Yes | Yes | Yes | No |
| 3 or more doses | No[4] | No | No[5] | No |

Ref: *MMWR 60:13, 2011; MMWR 61:468, 2012; MMWR 62:131, 2013 (pregnancy)*

[1] Td = Tetanus & diphtheria toxoids, adsorbed (adult). For adult who has not received Tdap previously, substitute one dose of Tdap for Td when immunization is indicated (*MMWR 61:468, 2012*).
[2] For children <7 years, use DTaP unless contraindicated; for persons ≥7 years, Td is preferred to tetanus toxoid alone, but single dose of Tdap can be used if required for catch-up series.
[3] Individuals who have not completed vaccine series should do so.
[4] Yes, if >5 years since last booster.
[5] Yes, if >10 years since last booster.

**TABLE 20B – RABIES POSTEXPOSURE PROPHYLAXIS**
**All wounds should be cleaned immediately & thoroughly with soap & water.**
**This has been shown to protect 90% of experimental animals![1]**

Exposure to animal saliva or nervous system tissue through a bite, scratch, or contamination of open wounds or mucous membranes *(www.cdc.gov/rabies/exposure/type.html)* or when such exposure cannot be reliably excluded (e.g., bat found in room of sleeping person).

| Animal Type | Evaluation & Disposition of Animal | Recommendations for Prophylaxis |
|---|---|---|
| Dogs, cats, ferrets | Healthy & available for 10-day observation | Don't start unless animal develops sx, then immediately begin HRIG + vaccine |
| | Rabid or suspected rabid | Immediate HRIG + vaccine |
| | Unknown (escaped) | Consult public health officials |
| Skunks, raccoons, *bats, foxes, coyotes, most carnivores | Regard as rabid | Immediate prophylaxis unless brain of animal tests negative for rabies virus |
| Livestock, horses, rodents, rabbits; includes hares, squirrels, hamsters, guinea pigs, gerbils, chipmunks, rats, mice, woodchucks | Consider case-by-case | Consult public health officials. Bites of squirrels, hamsters, guinea pigs, gerbils, chipmunks, rats, mice, other small rodents, rabbits, and hares **almost never** require rabies post-exposure prophylaxis. |

* Most recent cases of human rabies in U.S. due to contact (not bites) with silver-haired bats or rarely big brown bats but risk of acquiring rabies from non-contact bat exposure is exceedingly low *(CID 48:1493, 2009)*. For more detail, see *CID 30:4, 2000; JAVMA 219:1687, 2001; CID 37:96, 2003 (travel medicine advisory); Ln 363:959, 2004; EID 11:1921, 2005; MMWR 55 (RR-5), 2006.*

**Postexposure Rabies Immunization Schedule**

**IF NOT PREVIOUSLY VACCINATED**

| Treatment | Regimen[2] |
|---|---|
| Local wound cleaning | **All postexposure treatment should begin with immediate, thorough cleaning of all wounds with soap & water.** Then irrigate with a virucidal agent such as povidone-iodine solution if available. |
| Human rabies immune globulin (HRIG) | 20 IU per kg body weight given once on day 0. If anatomically feasible, the full dose should be infiltrated around the wound(s), the rest should be administered IM in the gluteal area. If the calculated dose of HRIG is insufficient to inject all the wounds, it should be diluted with normal saline to allow infiltration around additional wound areas. HRIG should **not** be administered in the **same syringe, or** into the **same anatomical site** as vaccine, or more than 7 days after the initiation of vaccine. Because HRIG may partially suppress active production of antibody, no more than the recommended dose should be given.[3] |
| Vaccine | Human diploid cell vaccine (HDCV), rabies vaccine adsorbed (RVA), or purified chick embryo cell vaccine (PCECV) 1 mL **IM (deltoid area[4])**, one each days 0, 3, 7, 14[5]. |

**IF PREVIOUSLY VACCINATED[6]**

| Treatment | Regimen[2] |
|---|---|
| Local wound cleaning | All postexposure treatment should begin with immediate, thorough cleaning of all wounds with soap **&** water. Then irrigate with a virucidal agent such as povidone-iodine solution if available. |
| HRIG | HRIG should **not** be administered |
| Vaccine | HDCV or PCEC, 1 mL **IM (deltoid area[4])**, one each on days 0 & 3 |

**CORRECT VACCINE ADMINISTRATION SITES**

| Age Group | Administration Site |
|---|---|
| Children & adults | **DELTOID[4]** only (**NEVER** in gluteus) |
| Infants & young children | Outer aspect of thigh (anterolateral thigh) may be used (**NEVER** in gluteus) |

[1] From *MMWR 48:RR-1, 1999; CID 30:4, 2000;* B. T. Matyas, Mass. Dept. of Public Health. *MMWR 57:1, 2008*
[2] These regimens are applicable for all age groups, including children.
[3] In most reported post-exposure treatment failures, only identified deficiency was failure to infiltrate wound(s) with HRIG *(CID 22:228, 1996)*. However, several failures reported from SE Asia in patients in whom WHO protocol followed *(CID 28:143, 1999)*.
[4] The **deltoid** area is the **only** acceptable site of vaccination for adults & older children. For infants & young children, outer aspect of thigh (anterolateral thigh) may be used. Vaccine should **NEVER** be administered in gluteal area.
[5] Note that this is a change from previous recommendation of 5 doses (days 0, 3, 7, 14 & 28) based on new data & recommendations from ACIP. Note that the number of doses for persons with altered immunocompetence remains unchanged (5 doses on days 0, 3, 7, 14 & 28) and recommendations for pre-exposure prophylaxis remain 3 doses administered on days 0, 7 and 21 or 28 *(MMWR 59 (RR-2), 2010)*.
[6] Any person with a history of pre-exposure vaccination with HDCV, RVA, PCECV; prior post-exposure prophylaxis with HDCV, PCEC or rabies vaccine adsorbed (RVA); or previous vaccination with any other type of rabies vaccine & a documented history of antibody response to the prior vaccination.

## TABLE 21 - SELECTED DIRECTORY OF RESOURCES

| ORGANIZATION | PHONE/FAX | WEBSITE(S) |
|---|---|---|
| **ANTIPARASITIC DRUGS & PARASITOLOGY INFORMATION** | | |
| CDC Drug Line | Weekdays: 404-639-3670 | http://www.cdc.gov/ncidod/srp/drugs/drug-service.html |
| | Evenings, weekends, holidays: 404-639-2888 | |
| DPDx: Lab ID of parasites | | www.dpd.cdc.gov/dpdx/default.htm |
| Malaria | daytime: 770-488-7788 | www.cdc.gov/malaria |
| | other: 770-488-7100 | |
| | US toll free: 855-856-4713 | |
| Expert Compound. Pharm. | 800-247-9767/Fax: 818-787-7256 | www.expertpharmacy.org |
| World Health Organization (WHO) | | www.who.int |
| Parasites & Health | | www.dpd.cdc.gov/dpdx/HTML/Para_Health.htm |
| **BIOTERRORISM** | | |
| Centers for Disease Control & Prevention | 770-488-7100 | www.bt.cdc.gov |
| Infectious Diseases Society of America | 703-299-0200 | www.idsociety.org |
| Johns Hopkins Center Civilian Biodefense | | www.jhsph.edu |
| Center for Biosecurity of the Univ. of Pittsburgh Med. Center | | www.upmc-biosecurity.org |
| US Army Medical Research Institute of Inf. Dis. | | www.usamriid.army.mil |
| **HEPATITIS B** | | |
| Hepatitis B Foundation | | www.hepb.org, www.natap.org |
| **HEPATITIS C** | | |
| CDC | | www.cdc.gov/ncidod/diseases/hepatitis/C |
| Individual | | http://hepatitis-central.com |
| | | www.natap.org |
| HCV Guidelines | | www.hcvguidelines.org |
| **HIV** | | |
| General | | |
| HIV InSite | | http://hivinsite.ucsf.edu |
| | | www.natap.org |
| Drug Interactions | | |
| Liverpool HIV Pharm. Group | | www.hiv-druginteractions.org |
| Other | | http://AIDS.medscape.com |
| Prophylaxis/Treatment of Opportunistic Infections; HIV Treatment | | www.aidsinfo.nih.gov |
| **IMMUNIZATIONS** | | |
| CDC, Natl. Immunization Program | 404-639-8200 | www.cdc.gov/vaccines/ |
| FDA, Vaccine Adverse Events | 800-822-7967 | www.fda.gov/cber/vaers/vaers.htm |
| National Network Immunization Info. | 877-341-6644 | www.immunizationinfo.org |
| Influenza vaccine, CDC | 404-639-8200 | www.cdc.gov/vaccines/ |
| Institute for Vaccine Safety | | www.vaccinesafety.edu |
| Immunization, "Ask the experts" | | www.immunize.org/asktheexperts |
| **OCCUPATIONAL EXPOSURE, BLOOD-BORNE PATHOGENS (HIV, HEPATITIS B & C)** | | |
| Clinicians Consultation Center | 888-448-4911 | www.ucsf.edu/hivcntr |
| PEPline (exposed clinicians) | | |
| WARMline (clinicians of HIV pts) | | |
| Perinatal HIV Hotline | 888-448-8765 | www.ucsf.edu/hivcntr |
| **Q-T$_c$ INTERVAL PROLONGATION BY DRUGS** | | www.qtdrugs.org; www.crediblemeds.org |
| **TRAVELERS' INFO: Immunizations, Malaria Prophylaxis, More** | | |
| Amer. Soc. Trop. Med. & Hyg. | | www.astmh.org |
| CDC, general | 877-394-8747 | http://www.cdc.gov/travel/default.asp |
| CDC, Malaria: | | www.cdc.gov/malaria |
| Prophylaxis | | http://www.cdc.gov/travel/default.asp |
| Medical Considerations Before Int'l Travel | | N Engl J Med 2016,375:247 |
| Pan American Health Organization | | www.paho.org |
| World Health Organization (WHO) | | www.who.int/home-page |

## TABLE 22A – ANTI-INFECTIVE DRUG-DRUG INTERACTIONS

For HIV drug interactions, see: https://www.hiv-druginteractions.org/. For Hepatitis C drug-drug interactions, see https://www.hep-druginteractions.org/checker

| Anti-Infective agent | Other Drug | Effect on concentration (or other effect) | Suggested management |
|---|---|---|---|
| Abacavir | Methadone | ↓ methadone | Monitor, adjust dosage |
| Amantadine | Alcohol | ↑ CNS effects | Monitor |
| | Anticholinergic agents | ↑ anticholinergic effects | Monitor |
| | Digoxin | ↑ digoxin | Monitor, adjust dosage |
| Aminoglycosides (parenteral) | Amphotericin B (deoxychol, lipid forms) | ↑ nephrotoxicity | Avoid co-administration |
| | Cisplatin | ↑ nephrotoxicity, ototoxicity | Avoid co-administration |
| | Cyclosporine | ↑ nephrotoxicity | Avoid co-administration |
| | Furosemide | ↑ ototoxicity | Monitor |
| | Neuromuscular blocking agents | ↑ apnea or respiratory paralysis | Monitor |
| | NSAIDs | ↑ nephrotoxicity | Monitor |
| | Non-polarizing muscle relaxants | ↑ apnea | Monitor |
| | Radiographic contrast | ↑ nephrotoxicity | Avoid co-administration |
| | Vancomycin | ↑ nephrotoxicity | Monitor |
| Aminoglycosides (oral)(kanamycin, neomycin) | Warfarin | ↑ warfarin | Monitor INR, adjust dosage |
| Ampho B (deoxychol, lipid forms) | Digoxin | ↑ toxicity of digoxin if pt hypokalemic | Monitor |
| Amoxicillin, ampicillin | Allopurinol | ↑ frequency of rash | Monitor |

### Antiretroviral Drug Combinations

| Other Drug | Combivir | Kaletra | Cimduo | Odefsey | Atripla | Juluca | Biktarvy | Descovy | Delstrigo | Genvoya | Symtuza (LO) | Triumeq | Stribild | Truvada | Evotaz | Prezcobix | Trizivir | Effect on concentration (or other effect) | Suggested management |
|---|---|---|---|---|---|---|---|---|---|---|---|---|---|---|---|---|---|---|---|
| Alfuzosin | X | X | | | | | | | | | | | | | X | X | | ↑ alfuzosin | Contraindicated |
| Amiodarone | | X | | | | | | | | X | | | | | X | X | | ↑ amiodarone | Monitor, adjust dosage |
| Antacids | | | | | | | X | | | X | | | X | | | | | ↓ INSTI component | Separate admin by 2 hr |
| Antacids | | | | | | | | | | | | X | | | | | | ↓ dolutegravir | Triumeq 2 hr pre or 6 hr post |
| Antacids | | | | X | | X | | | | | | | | | | | | ↓ dolutegravir and/or ↓ rilpivirine | Separate admin by 4-6 hr |
| Atazanavir | | | | | | | | | | | | | | | X | | | ↑ atazanavir | Give Evotaz 2 hr pre or post |
| Antiarrhythmic agents | | X | | | | | | | | | | | | | X | X | | ↑ antiarrhythmic agent | Monitor, adjust dosage |
| Apixaban | | X | | | | | | | | | | | | | X | X | | ↑ apixaban | Avoid co-administration |
| Artemether-lumefantrine | | X | | | | | | | | | | | | | | X | | ↓ artemether, ↓ DHA, ↓ lumefantrine | Avoid co-administration |
| Artemether-lumefantrine | | | | | X | | | | | | | | | | | | | ↓ artemether-lumefantrine | Monitor |
| Atazanavir/ritonavir | | | | | | | | | | | | | | | | | | Effect uncertain | Monitor or avoid |
| Atazanavir/ritonavir | X | | | | | | | | | | | | | X | | | | ↓ atazanavir, ↑ tenofovir | Monitor or avoid |
| Atorvastatin | | X | | | | | | | | | | | | | X | X | | ↑ atorvastatin | Monitor, adjust dosage |
| Atorvastatin | | | | | X | | | | | X | | | X | | | | | ↓ atorvastatin | Max atorvastatin 20 mg daily |
| Atorvastatin | | | | | | | | | | | | | | | | | | ↓ atorvastatin | Monitor, adjust dosage |
| Atovaquone | X | X | | | | | | | | | | | | | | | | ↓ atovaquone | Monitor, adjust dosage |

**TABLE 22A (2)**

Antiretroviral Drug Combinations *(continued)*

| Combivir | Kaletra | Cimduo | Odefsey | Atripla | Juluca | Biktarvy | Descovy | Delstrigo | Genvoya | Symfi (LO) | Triumeq | Stribild | Truvada | Evotaz | Prezcobix | Trizivir | Other Drug | Effect on concentration (or other effect) | Suggested management |
|---|---|---|---|---|---|---|---|---|---|---|---|---|---|---|---|---|---|---|---|
| × | | | | | | | | | | | | | | | | × | Atovaquone | ↑ zidovudine | Monitor |
| | × | | | | | | | | | | | | | × | × | | Atovaquone-proguanil | ↓ atovaquone, ↓ proguanil | Avoid co-administration |
| | × | | | | | | | | | | | | | × | × | | Avanafil | ↑ avanafil | Avoid co-administration |
| | × | | | | | | | | | | | | | × | × | | Bedaquiline | ↑ bedaquiline | Avoid co-administration |
| | × | | | | | | | | | | | | | × | × | | Bepridil | ↑ bepridil | Monitor, adjust dosage |
| | × | | | | | | | | × | | | × | | × | × | | Beta-blockers | ↑ beta-blockers | Monitor, adjust dosage |
| | × | | | | | | | | × | | | × | | × | × | | Bosentan | ↑ bosentan | Monitor, adjust dosage |
| | × | | | | | | | | | | | | | × | × | | Bosentan | ↓ protease inhibitor, ↓ cobicistat, ↑ bosentan | Monitor, adjust dosage |
| | × | | | | | | | | × | | | × | | × | × | | Buprenorphine | ↑ buprenorphine | Monitor, adjust dosage |
| | × | | | | | | | | | | | | | × | × | | Buprenorphine/naloxone | Effect uncertain | Monitor, adjust dosage |
| | × | | × | | | | | | | × | | | | × | × | | Bupropion | ↓ bupropion | Monitor, adjust dosage |
| | × | | | | | | | | × | | | × | | × | × | | Buspirone | ↑ buspirone | Monitor, adjust dosage |
| | | | | | | × | | | | | | | | | | | Calcium/iron containing supplements | ↓ bictegravir | Take drug + supps w/food |
| | | | | | | | | | | | × | | | | | | Calcium/iron containing supplements | ↓ dolutegravir | Triumeq 2 hr pre or 6 hr post |
| | × | | | | | | | | × | | | × | | × | × | | Calcium channel blockers | ↑ calcium channel blocker | Monitor, adjust dosage |
| | × | | | | | | | | × | | | × | | × | × | | Calcium channel blockers | ↑ calcium channel blocker | Monitor, adjust dosage |
| | | | | | | × | | | × | | | × | | × | × | | Carbamazepine | ↓ INSTI, ↓ cobicistat (↓ TAF in Genvoya) | Contraindicated |
| | | | | | | × | | | | | | | | | | | Carbamazepine | ↓ bictegravir and/or ↓ TAF | Avoid co-administration |
| | | | | × | | | | | | × | | | | | | | Carbamazepine | ↓ carbamazepine, ↓ efavirenz | Avoid co-administration |
| | | | | | × | | | | | | × | | | | | | Carbamazepine | ↓ dolutegravir | Give extra 50 mg DTG daily |
| | | | × | | | | | × | | | | | | | | | Carbamazepine | ↓ dolutegravir and/or ↓ rilpivirine | Contraindicated |
| | × | | | | | | | | | | | | | × | × | | Carbamazepine | ↓ protease inhibitor, ↓ cobicistat | Contraindicated |
| | | | | | | | | × | | | | | | | | | Carbamazepine | ↓ doravirine | Contraindicated |
| | × | | | | | | | | × | | | × | | × | × | | Clarithromycin | ↑ clarithromycin and/or ↑ cobicistat | Monitor, adjust dosage |
| | | | | × | | | | | | × | | | | | | | Clarithromycin | ↓ clarithromycin, ↑ 14-OH metabolite | Avoid co-administration |
| | | | × | | | | | × | | | | | | | | | Clarithromycin | ↑ rilpivirine | Avoid co-administration |
| | × | | | | | | | | | | | | | × | × | | Clarithromycin | ↑ protease inhibitor, ↑ cobicistat, ↑ clarithromycin | Avoid co-administration |
| | × | | | | | | | | × | | | × | | × | × | | Clonazepam | ↑ clonazepam | Monitor |
| | × | | | | | | | | × | | | × | | × | × | | Clorazepate | ↑ clorazepate | Monitor, adjust dosage |
| | × | | | | | | | | × | | | × | | × | × | | Colchicine | ↑ colchicine | Adjust dosage or avoid |
| | × | | | | | | | | × | | | × | | × | × | | Corticosteroids (not dex) | ↑ corticosteroid | Use non-3A4 substrate steroids |
| | × | | | | | | | | × | | | × | | × | × | | Cyclosporine | ↑ cyclosporine, ↑ EVG, ↑ cobicistat | Monitor, adjust dosage |
| | | | | | | | | | | | | | | | | × | Cyclosporine | ↓ cyclosporine | Monitor, adjust dosage |

## TABLE 22A (3)

**Antiretroviral Drug Combinations** *(continued)*

| Combivir | Kaletra | Cimduo | Odefsey | Atripla | Juluca | Biktarvy | Descovy | Delstrigo | Genvoya | Symfi (Lo) | Triumeq | Stribild | Truvada | Evotaz | Prezcobix | Trizivir | Other Drug | Effect on concentration (or other effect) | Suggested management |
|---|---|---|---|---|---|---|---|---|---|---|---|---|---|---|---|---|---|---|---|
|  | × |  |  |  |  |  |  |  |  |  |  |  |  | × | × |  | Cyclosporine | ↑ cyclosporine | Monitor, adjust dosage |
|  |  |  |  |  |  |  |  |  |  |  |  |  |  | × | × |  | Dabigatran | ↑ dabigatran | Avoid co-administration |
|  |  |  |  |  |  |  |  |  |  |  |  |  | × |  |  |  | Darunavir/ritonavir | ↑ tenofovir | Monitor |
|  | × |  |  |  |  |  |  |  |  |  |  |  |  | × | × |  | Dasatinib | ↑ dasatinib | Monitor, adjust dosage |
|  |  |  |  |  |  |  |  |  | × |  |  | × |  |  |  |  | Dexamethasone | ↑ dexamethasone, ↓ EVG, ↓ cobicistat | Consider alternate steroid |
|  |  |  | × |  |  |  |  |  |  |  |  |  |  |  |  |  | Dexamethasone | ↓ rilpivirine | Contraindicated |
|  | × |  |  |  |  |  |  |  |  |  |  |  |  | × | × |  | Dexamethasone | ↑ dexamethasone, ↓ lopinavir | Avoid co-administration |
|  |  |  |  |  |  |  |  |  |  |  |  |  |  | × | × |  | Dexamethasone | ↓ protease inhibitor, ↓ cobicistat, ↑ dexamethasone | Avoid co-administration |
|  | × |  |  |  |  |  |  |  |  |  |  |  |  | × | × |  | Diazepam | ↑ diazepam | Monitor, adjust dosage |
|  |  |  |  |  |  |  |  |  |  |  |  |  |  | × | × |  | Didanosine | ↑ didanosine | Monitor, adjust dosage |
|  | × |  |  |  |  |  |  |  |  |  |  |  |  | × | × |  | Didanosine EC | ↓ protease inhibitor, ↓ didanosine | Separate admin by 2 hr |
|  |  |  |  |  |  |  |  |  | × |  |  | × |  | × | × |  | Digoxin | ↑ digoxin | Monitor, adjust dosage |
|  |  |  |  |  |  |  |  |  |  |  |  |  |  | × | × |  | Diltiazem | ↓ diltiazem, metabolites | Monitor, adjust dosage |
|  |  |  |  |  |  |  |  |  |  |  |  |  |  | × | × |  | Disopyramide | Disopyramide | Monitor |
|  | × |  |  |  |  |  |  |  |  |  |  |  |  |  |  |  | Disulfiram | Disulfiram reaction | Avoid co-admin (Kaletra soln) |
|  |  |  |  |  |  | × |  |  | × |  |  | × |  |  |  |  | Dofetilide | ↑ dofetilide | Contraindicated |
| × |  |  |  |  |  |  |  |  |  |  |  |  |  |  |  | × | Doxorubicin | Antagonistic with zidovudine in vitro | Avoid co-administration |
|  |  |  |  |  |  |  |  |  |  |  |  |  |  | × | × |  | Dronedarone | ↑ dronedarone | Contraindicated |
|  |  |  |  |  |  |  |  |  | × |  |  | × |  | × | × |  | Drospirenone | ↑ drospirenone | Monitor, adjust dosage |
|  |  |  |  | × |  |  |  |  |  |  |  |  |  |  |  |  | Dolutegravir | ↓ dolutegravir | Give extra 50 mg DTG daily |
|  | × |  |  |  |  |  |  |  |  |  |  |  |  | × | × |  | Efavirenz | ↓ protease inhibitor, ↓ cobicistat | Avoid co-administration |
|  |  |  |  | × |  |  |  |  |  | × |  |  |  |  |  |  | Efavirenz | ↑ ALT | Contraindicated |
|  | × |  |  |  |  |  |  |  |  |  |  |  |  | × | × |  | Elbasvir/grazoprevir | ↓ grazoprevir | Contraindicated |
|  |  |  | × |  | × |  |  | × |  |  |  |  |  |  |  |  | Elbasvir/grazoprevir | ↓ doravirine | Contraindicated |
|  |  |  |  |  |  |  | × |  |  |  |  |  |  |  |  |  | Enzalutamide | ↑ ergot derivatives | Contraindicated |
|  | × |  |  |  |  |  |  |  |  |  |  |  |  | × | × |  | Ergot derivatives | ↑ rilpivirine | Avoid co-administration |
|  |  |  |  |  |  |  |  |  |  |  |  |  |  | × | × |  | Erythromycin | ↑ protease inhibitor, ↑ cobicistat, ↑ erythromycin | Avoid co-administration |
|  | × |  |  |  |  |  |  |  |  |  |  |  |  |  |  |  | Erythromycin | ↑ protease inhibitor, ↓ cobicistat | Monitor or avoid |
|  |  |  |  |  |  |  |  |  |  |  |  |  |  | × | × |  | Eslicarbazepine | ↑ protease inhibitor, ↓ cobicistat | Monitor, adjust dosage |
|  | × |  |  |  |  |  |  |  |  |  |  |  |  | × | × |  | Estazolam | ↑ estazolam | Monitor, adjust dosage |
|  |  |  | × |  | × |  |  |  |  |  |  |  |  |  |  |  | Ethinyl estradiol | ↓ ethinyl estradiol | Monitor, adjust dosage |
|  |  |  |  |  |  |  |  |  | × |  |  | × |  |  |  |  | Ethosuximide | ↑ ethosuximide, ↓ EVG, ↓ cobicistat (Gen, ↓ TAF) | Monitor, adjust dosage |
|  |  |  |  |  |  |  |  |  |  |  |  |  |  | × | × |  | Etravirine | ↓ protease inhibitor, ↓ cobicistat | Avoid co-administration |
|  |  |  |  |  |  |  |  |  |  |  |  |  |  | × | × |  | Everolimus | ↑ everolimus | Avoid co-administration |

**TABLE 22A (4)**

**Antiretroviral Drug Combinations** *(continued)*

| Anti-infective agent | | | | | | | | | | | | | | | | | Other Drug | Effect on concentration (or other effect) | Suggested management |
|---|---|---|---|---|---|---|---|---|---|---|---|---|---|---|---|---|---|---|---|
| Combivir | Kaletra | Cimduo | Odefsey | Atripla | Juluca | Biktarvy | Descovy | Delstrigo | Genvoya | Symfi (Lo) | Triumeq | Stribild | Truvada | Evotaz | Prezcobix | Trizivir | | | |
| | X | | | | | | | | | | | | | X | X | | Felodipine | ↑ felodipine | Monitor, adjust dosage |
| | X | | | | | | | | | | | | | X | X | | Fentanyl | ↑ fentanyl | Monitor, adjust dosage |
| | X | | | | | | | | | | | | | X | X | | Flecainide | ↑ flecainide | Monitor |
| | | | X | | | | | | | | | | | | | | Fluconazole | ↑ rilpivirine, ↑ TAF | Monitor |
| X | | | | | | | | | | | | | | | | X | Fluconazole | ↑ zidovudine | Monitor |
| | X | | | | | | | | | | | | | X | X | | Flurazepam | ↑ flurazepam | Monitor, adjust dosage |
| | X | | | | | | | | | | | | | X | X | | Fluvastatin | ↑ fluvastatin | Monitor, adjust dosage |
| | | | | | X | | | | | | X | | | | | | Fosamprenavir/ritonavir | ↓ dolutegravir | Give extra 50 mg DTG daily |
| | | | X | | | | | | | | | | | | | | H2-antagonists | ↓ rilpivirine | Give H2 12 hr pre or 4 hr post |
| | | | | | | | | | | | | | | X | X | | H2-antagonists | ↓ atazanavir (because of ↑ pH) | Limit H2 dose (see PI) |
| | X | | | | | | | | | | | | | X | | | Hormonal contraceptives | ↑ ethinyl estradiol, ↑ progestogen | Use non-hormonal method |
| | | | | X | | | | | | X | | | | | | | Hormonal contraceptives | ↓ ethinyl estradiol and/or ↓ progestogen | Use non-hormonal method |
| | | | | | | | X | | | | | | X | | | | Hormonal contraceptives | Effect uncertain | Use non-hormonal method |
| | X | | | | | | | | | | | | | X | X | | Indinavir | Hyperbilirubinemia | Contraindicated |
| X | | | | | | | | | | | | | | | | X | Indomethacin | ↑ zidovudine toxic metabolite | Monitor |
| | X | | | | | | | | | | | | | X | X | | Inhaled/nasal steroids | ↑ steroid (if a CYP3A4 substrate) | Avoid co-administration |
| | | | | | X | | | | | | X | | | | | | Iron (oral) | ↓ dolutegravir | Separate admin by 4-6 hr |
| | X | | | | | | | | | | | | | | | | Irinotecan | ↑ irinotecan | Contraindicated |
| | X | | | | | | | | | | | | | X | X | | Isavuconazole | ↑ isavuconazole | Avoid co-administration |
| | | | | | | | | | X | | | X | | | | | Itraconazole | ↑ itraconazole, ↑ EVG, ↑ cobicistat | Max itra dose 200 mg qd |
| | X | | | | | | | | | | | | | | | | Itraconazole | ↑ itraconazole | Monitor, adjust dosage |
| | | | | | | | X | | | | | | | | | | Itraconazole | ↑ itraconazole, ↓ OH-itraconazole | Avoid co-administration |
| | | | X | | | | | | | | | | | | | | Itraconazole | ↑ rilpivirine, ↑ TAF | Monitor |
| | X | | | | | | | | | | | | | X | X | | Itraconazole | ↑ protease inhibitor, ↑ cobicistat, ↑ itraconazole | Avoid co-administration |
| | | | | | | | | | X | | | X | | | | | Ketoconazole | ↑ ketoconazole, ↑ EVG, ↑ cobicistat | Max keto dose 200 mg qd |
| | X | | | | | | | | | | | | | | | | Ketoconazole | ↑ ketoconazole | Monitor, adjust dosage |
| | | | | | | | X | | | | | | | | | | Ketoconazole | ↓ ketoconazole | Monitor, adjust dosage |
| | | | X | | | | | | | | | | | | | | Ketoconazole | ↑ rilpivirine, ↑ TAF, ↓ ketoconazole | Monitor |
| | X | | | | | | | | | | | | | X | X | | Ketoconazole | ↑ protease inhibitor, ↑ cobicistat, ↑ ketoconazole | Avoid co-administration |
| | | | | X | | | | X | | X | | | | | | | Lamotrigine | ↓ lamotrigine | Monitor, adjust dosage |
| | X | | | | | | | | | | | | | | | | Lamotrigine | Effect uncertain | Monitor |
| | | | | | | X | | | | | | | | | | | Ledipasvir/sofosbuvir | ↑ tenofovir | Avoid co-administration |
| | X | | X | | | | X | | | | | | X | | | | Ledipasvir/sofosbuvir | ↑ tenofovir | Monitor or avoid |

**TABLE 22A (5)**

Antiretroviral Drug Combinations *(continued)*

| Trizivir | Prezcobix | Evotaz | Truvada | Stribild | Triumeq | Symfi (LO) | Genvoya | Delstrigo | Descovy | Biktarvy | Juluca | Atripla | Odefsey | Cimduo | Kaletra | Combivir | Other Drug | Effect on concentration (or other effect) | Suggested management |
|---|---|---|---|---|---|---|---|---|---|---|---|---|---|---|---|---|---|---|---|
|  | X |  |  |  |  |  |  |  |  |  |  |  |  |  | X |  | Lidocaine | ↑ lidocaine | Monitor, adjust dosage |
|  | X | X |  | X |  |  | X |  |  |  |  | X |  |  |  |  | Lopinavir/ritonavir | ↓ lopinavir, ↑ tenofovir | Monitor, adjust dosage |
|  |  |  | X |  |  |  |  |  |  |  |  |  |  |  |  |  | Lopinavir/ritonavir | ↑ tenofovir | Monitor |
|  | X | X |  | X |  |  | X |  |  |  |  |  |  |  | X |  | Lovastatin | ↑ lovastatin | Contraindicated |
|  | X | X |  | X |  |  | X |  |  |  |  |  |  |  | X |  | Lurasidone | ↑ lurasidone | Contraindicated |
|  |  |  |  |  |  |  |  |  |  | X |  | X |  |  |  |  | Maraviroc | ↓ maraviroc | See maraviroc PI for help |
|  | X | X |  |  |  |  |  |  |  |  |  |  |  |  | X |  | Maraviroc | ↑ maraviroc | Consider MVC 150 mg bid |
|  |  |  |  |  | X |  |  |  |  | X |  |  |  |  | X |  | Metformin | ↑ metformin | Monitor, adjust dosage |
|  | X | X |  |  |  |  |  |  |  |  |  |  |  |  | X |  | Methadone | ↓ methadone | Monitor, adjust dosage |
| X |  |  |  |  |  |  |  |  |  |  |  |  |  |  |  |  | Methadone | ↓ zidovudine | Monitor |
|  |  |  |  |  |  |  |  |  |  |  |  |  |  |  |  | X | Methadone | ↑ zidovudine, ↓ methadone | Monitor, adjust methadone |
|  |  |  |  |  | X |  |  |  |  |  |  | X |  |  |  |  | Methadone | ↓ methadone | Monitor, adjust dosage |
|  |  |  |  |  |  |  |  |  |  |  |  |  |  |  | X |  | Metronidazole | Effect uncertain Disulfiram-like reaction | Avoid co-admin (Kaletra soln) |
|  | X | X |  | X |  |  | X |  |  |  |  |  |  |  | X |  | Mexiletine | ↑ mexiletine | Monitor |
|  | X | X |  | X |  |  | X | X |  | X |  |  |  |  | X |  | Midazolam (IV) | ↑ midazolam | Monitor, adjust dosage |
|  | X | X |  | X |  |  | X | X |  | X |  |  |  |  | X |  | Midazolam (po) | ↑ midazolam | Contraindicated |
|  |  |  |  |  |  |  |  | X |  |  |  |  | X |  |  |  | Mitotane | ↓ doravirine | Contraindicated |
|  |  |  |  |  |  |  |  |  |  |  |  |  |  |  | X |  | Naloxone | ↓ naloxone | Monitor |
| X |  |  |  |  |  |  |  |  |  |  |  |  |  |  |  |  | Nelfinavir | ↓ zidovudine | Monitor |
|  |  |  |  |  | X |  |  |  |  |  | X |  |  |  |  |  | Nevirapine | ↓ dolutegravir | Avoid co-administration |
|  | X | X |  | X |  |  | X |  |  |  |  |  |  |  | X |  | Nevirapine | ↑ nevirapine, ↓ protease inhibitor? | Contraindicated |
|  | X | X |  | X |  |  | X |  |  |  |  |  |  |  | X |  | Nicardipine | ↑ nicardipine | Monitor, adjust dosage |
|  | X | X |  | X |  |  | X |  |  |  |  |  |  |  | X |  | Nifedipine | ↑ nifedipine | Monitor, adjust dosage |
|  | X | X |  | X |  |  | X |  |  |  |  |  |  |  | X |  | Nilotinib | ↑ nilotinib | Monitor, adjust dosage |
|  | X | X |  | X |  |  | X |  |  |  |  |  |  |  |  |  | Omeprazole | ↓ atazanavir (because of ↑ pH) | Limit omeprazole dose or avoid |
|  |  |  |  | X |  |  | X |  |  |  |  | X |  |  |  |  | Oxcarbazepine | ↓ elvitegravir, ↓ cobicistat | Use different anticonvulsant |
|  |  |  |  | X |  |  | X |  |  | X |  |  |  |  |  |  | Oxcarbazepine | ↓ INSTI and/or ↓ TAF | Avoid co-administration |
|  |  |  |  |  | X |  |  |  |  | X | X |  |  |  |  |  | Oxcarbazepine | ↓ dolutegravir and/or↓ rilpivirine | Contraindicated |
|  | X | X |  |  |  |  |  |  |  |  |  |  |  |  | X |  | Oxcarbazepine | ↓ protease inhibitor?, ↓ cobicistat | Monitor or avoid |
|  |  |  |  |  |  |  |  | X |  |  |  |  | X |  |  |  | Oxcarbazepine | ↓ doravirine | Contraindicated |
|  | X | X |  | X |  |  | X |  |  |  |  |  |  |  | X |  | Oxycodone | ↑ oxycodone | Monitor, adjust dosage |
|  | X | X |  | X |  |  | X |  |  |  |  |  |  |  | X |  | Perphenazine | ↑ perphenazine | Monitor, adjust dosage |
|  | X | X |  | X |  |  | X |  |  |  |  | X |  |  | X |  | Phenobarbital | ↓ EVG, ↓ cobicistat (Gen, ↓ TAF) | Contraindicated |

**TABLE 22A (6)**

**Antiretroviral Drug Combinations** *(continued)*

| Other Drug | Effect on concentration (or other effect) | Suggested management |
|---|---|---|
| Phenobarbital | ↓ protease inhibitor, ↓ cobicistat? | Contraindicated |
| Phenobarbital | ↓ phenobarbital, ↓ efavirenz | Monitor, adjust dosage |
| Phenobarbital | ↓ INSTI and/or ↓ TAF | Avoid co-administration |
| Phenobarbital | ↓ dolutegravir and/or ↓ NNRTI | Contraindicated |
| Phenytoin | ↓ EVG, ↓ cobicistat (Gen: ↓ TAF) | Contraindicated |
| Phenytoin | ↓ phenytoin, ↓ efavirenz | Monitor, adjust dosage |
| Phenytoin | ↓ INSTI and/or ↓ TAF | Avoid co-administration |
| Phenytoin | ↓ dolutegravir and/or ↓ rilpivirine | Contraindicated |
| Phenytoin | ↓ lopinavir, ↓ phenytoin | Avoid co-administration |
| Phenytoin | ↓ protease inhibitor, ↓ cobicistat? | Contraindicated |
| Phenytoin | ↓ doravirine | Contraindicated |
| Pimozide | ↑ pimozide | Contraindicated |
| Posaconazole | ↓ posaconazole | Avoid co-administration |
| Posaconazole | ↑ rilpivirine, ↑ TAF | Monitor |
| Pravastatin | ↓ pravastatin | Monitor, adjust dosage |
| Pravastatin | ↑ pravastatin | Monitor, adjust dosage |
| Probenecid | ↑ zidovudine | Monitor |
| Propafenone | ↑ propafenone | Monitor |
| Proton-pump inhibitors | ↓ rilpivirine | Contraindicated |
| Quetiapine | ↑ quetiapine | Adjust dosage or avoid |
| Quinidine | ↑ quinidine | Monitor, adjust dosage |
| Raltegravir | ↓ raltegravir | Monitor |
| Ranolazine | ↑ ranolazine | Contraindicated |
| Ribavirin | ↑ anemia | Avoid co-administration |
| Rifabutin | ↓ INSTI and/or ↓ cobi and/or ↓ TAF | Avoid co-administration |
| Rifabutin | ↑ rifabutin | Monitor, adjust dosage |
| Rifabutin | ↑ rifabutin | ↑ rif dosage by 50-100% |
| Rifabutin | ↑ rilpivirine | Give extra 25 mg RPV daily |
| Rifabutin | ↑ rilpivirine, ↓ TAF | Avoid co-administration |
| Rifabutin | ↓ doravirine | Extra 100 mg DOR 12 hr post |
| Rifampin | ↓ INSTI and/or ↓ NNRTI and/or ↓ cobi and/or ↓ TAF | Contraindicated |
| Rifampin | ↓ TAF | Avoid co-administration |
| Rifampin | ↓ dolutegravir | Give extra 50 mg DTG daily |

**TABLE 22A (7)**

Antiretroviral Drug Combinations (continued)

| Anti-infective agent | | | | | | | | | | | | | | | | | Other Drug | Effect on concentration (or other effect) | Suggested management |
|---|---|---|---|---|---|---|---|---|---|---|---|---|---|---|---|---|---|---|---|
| Combivir | Kaletra | Cimduo | Odefsey | Atripla | Juluca | Biktarvy | Descovy | Delstrigo | Genvoya | Symfi (LO) | Triumeq | Stribild | Truvada | Evotaz | Prezcobix | Trizivir | | | |
| | | | | X | | | | | | X | | | | | | | Rifampin | ↓ efavirenz | Avoid co-administration |
| | | | | X | | | | | | X | | | | | | | Rifampin | ↓ efavirenz | Consider extra efavirenz |
| | X | | | | | | | | | | | | | | | | Rifampin | ↓ lopinavir, ↓ ritonavir, ↑ rifampin | Contraindicated |
| X | | | | | | | | | | | | | | | | X | Rifampin | ↓ zidovudine | Monitor |
| | X | | | | | | | | | | | | | X | X | | Rifapentine | ↓ protease inhibitor, ↓ cobicistat? | Contraindicated |
| | | | X | | | X | X | | X | | X | X | | | | | Rifapentine | ↓ INSTI and/or ↓ cobicistat and/or ↓ TAF | Avoid co-administration |
| | | | | | X | | | X | | | X | | | | | | Rifapentine | ↓ dolutegravir and/or ↓ NNRTI | Contraindicated |
| | | | | | | | | | | | | | | | X | | Rifapentine | ↓ darunavir | Avoid co-administration |
| | X | | | | | | | | | | | | | X | X | | Risperidone | ↑ risperidone | Monitor, adjust dosage |
| | X | | | | | | | | | | | | | X | X | | Rivaroxaban | ↑ rivaroxaban | Avoid co-administration |
| | X | | | | | X | | | X | | | X | | | | | Rosuvastatin | ↑ rosuvastatin | Max rosuva 10 mg daily |
| | | | | | | | | | | | | | | X | X | | Rosuvastatin | ↑ rosuvastatin | Max rosuva 20 mg daily |
| | X | | | | | | | | | | | | | X | X | | Salmeterol | ↑ salmeterol | Avoid co-administration |
| | X | | | | | | | | | | | | | | | | Sertraline | ↓ sertraline | Monitor, adjust dosage |
| | X | | | | | | | | X | | | X | | X | X | | Sildenafil (for ED) | ↑ sildenafil | Monitor, adjust dosage |
| | X | | | | | | | | X | | | X | | X | X | | Sildenafil (for PAH) | ↑ sildenafil | Contraindicated |
| | X | | | | | | | | | | | | | | | | Simeprevir | ↓ simeprevir | Avoid co-administration |
| | X | | | | | | | | X | | | X | | X | X | | Simeprevir | ↑ simeprevir | Avoid co-administration |
| | X | | | | | | | | X | | | X | | X | X | | Simvastatin | ↑ simvastatin | Contraindicated |
| | | | | | | | | | | | | | | | | | Simvastatin | ↑ simvastatin | Monitor, adjust dosage |
| | X | | | | | | | | X | | | X | | X | X | | Sirolimus | ↑ sirolimus | Monitor, adjust dosage |
| | | | | X | | | | | | X | | | | | | | Sirolimus | ↓ sirolimus | Monitor, adjust dosage |
| | | | X | | | X | X | | X | | | X | X | | | | Sofosbuvir/velpatasvir | ↑ tenofovir | Monitor or avoid |
| | X | | | | | | | | | | | | | X | X | | Sofosbuvir/velpatasvir | ↑ tenofovir, ↓ velpatasvir | Avoid co-administration |
| | | | X | | | X | X | | X | | | X | X | | | | Sofosbuvir/velpatasvir/voxilaprevir | ↑ tenofovir | Monitor |
| X | | X | | | | | | | | | X | | X | | | X | Sorbitol | ↓ lamivudine | Avoid co-administration |
| | X | | | | | | | | | | | | | X | X | | SSRIs (not sertraline) | ↑ SSRI | Monitor, adjust dosage |
| | | | | X | | | | | | X | | | | | | | SSRIs | Effect uncertain | Monitor, adjust dosage |
| | | | X | X | X | X | | X | X | X | X | X | | | | | St. John's wort | ↓ INSTI and/or ↓ NNRTI and/or ↓ cobicistat and/or ↓ TAF | Contraindicated |
| | | | | | | X | | | | | X | | | | | | St. John's wort | ↓ INSTI and/or ↓ TAF | Avoid co-administration |
| | X | | | | | | | | | | | | | X | X | | St. John's wort | ↓ protease inhibitor, ↓ cobicistat? | Contraindicated |
| | | | | | | | | | | | X | | | | | | Sucralfate | ↓ dolutegravir | Triumeq 2 hr pre or 6 hr post |
| | X | | | | | | | | X | | | X | | X | X | | Tacrolimus | ↑ tacrolimus | Monitor, adjust dosage |

**TABLE 22A (8)**

**Antiretroviral Drug Combinations** *(continued)*

| Anti-infective agent / Antiretroviral agent *(continued)* | Other Drug | Effect on concentration (or other effect) | Suggested management |
|---|---|---|---|
| | Tacrolimus | ↓ tacrolimus | Monitor, adjust dosage |
| | Tadalafil (for PAH) | ↑ tadalafil | Monitor, adjust dosage |
| | Tadalafil (for ED) | ↑ tadalafil | Monitor, limit tadalafil dosage |
| | Telithromycin | ↑ rilpivirine | Avoid co-administration |
| | Telithromycin | ↑ protease inhibitor, ↑ cobicistat, ↑ telithromycin | Avoid co-administration |
| | Tenofovir | ↓ atazanavir, ↑ tenofovir | Monitor |
| | Thioridazine | ↑ thioridazine | Monitor, adjust dosage |
| | Ticagrelor | ↑ ticagrelor | Avoid co-administration |
| | Tipranavir/ritonavir | ↓ TAF | Avoid co-administration |
| | Tipranavir/ritonavir | ↑ dolutegravir | Give extra 50 mg DTG daily |
| | TMP-SMX | ↑ zidovudine | Monitor |
| | Tramadol | ↑ tramadol | Monitor, adjust dosage |
| | Trazodone | ↑ trazodone | Monitor, adjust dosage |
| | Triazolam | ↑ triazolam | Contraindicated |
| | Tricyclic antidepressants | ↑ TCA | Monitor, adjust dosage |
| | Valproic acid | ↓ valproic acid | Monitor, adjust dosage |
| | Valproic acid | ↑ zidovudine | Monitor |
| | Vardenafil (for ED) | ↑ vardenafil | Monitor, adjust dosage |
| | Venetoclax | ↑ venetoclax | Monitor, check venetoclax PI |
| | Viekira (Pak, XR) | ↑ ombitasvir, ↑ paritaprevir, ↑ ritonavir | Avoid co-administration |
| | Vinblastine | ↑ vinblastine | Monitor, avoid if necessary |
| | Vincristine | ↑ vincristine | Monitor, avoid if necessary |
| | Voriconazole | ↑ voriconazole, ↑ EVG, ↑ cobicistat | Avoid co-administration |
| | Voriconazole | ↑ voriconazole, ↑ efavirenz | Contraindicated |
| | Voriconazole | ↓ voriconazole | Avoid co-administration |
| | Voriconazole | ↑ atazanavir, ↑ cobicistat, ↓ voriconazole | Avoid co-administration |
| | Voriconazole | Effect uncertain | Avoid co-administration |
| | Warfarin | Effect uncertain | Monitor INR, adjust dosage |
| | Zolpidem | ↑ zolpidem | Monitor, adjust dosage |
| **Artemether-lumefantrine** | CYP3A4 inhibitors | ↑ artemether-lumefantrine | Monitor, adjust dosage |
| | CYP2D6 substrates | ↑ 2D6 substrate | Monitor, adjust dosage |
| **Atovaquone** | Metoclopramide | ↓ atovaquone | Monitor, adjust dosage |
| | Tetracycline | ↓ atovaquone | Monitor, adjust dosage |

The antiretroviral agent columns (marked with × in the original grid) are, left to right: Combivir, Kaletra, Cimduo, Odefsey, Atripla, Juluca, Biktarvy, Descovy, Descovy, Delstrigo, Genvoya, Symtuza (TO), Triumeq, Truvada, Stribild, Evotaz, Prezcobix, Trizivir.

**TABLE 22A (9)**

| Fluconazole | Isavuconazole | Itraconazole | Ketoconazole | Posaconazole | Voriconazole | Other Drug | Effect on concentration (or other effect) | Suggested management |
|---|---|---|---|---|---|---|---|---|
| X | | X | | | √ | Amitriptyline | ↑ amitriptyline | Monitor, adjust dosage |
| | X | | X | | | Atorvastatin | ↑ atorvastatin | Monitor, adjust dosage |
| | X | | | | | Bupropion | ↓ bupropion | Monitor, adjust dosage |
| X | | X | X | | X | Calcium channel blockers | ↑ calcium channel blocker | Monitor, adjust dosage |
| | X | X | X | X | X | Carbamazepine | ↓ azole | Avoid co-administration |
| X | | X | X | X | X | Cyclosporine | ↑ cyclosporine | Monitor, adjust dosage |
| | | X | X | | | Didanosine | ↓ absorption of azole | Avoid co-administration |
| | X | X | | | | Digoxin | ↑ digoxin | Monitor, adjust dosage |
| | X | X | X | X | X | Efavirenz | ↓ azole, ↑ efavirenz | Avoid co-administration |
| | X | X | X | X | | H2 blockers, antacids, sucralfate | ↓ absorption of azole | Avoid co-administration |
| X | X | X | X | X | X | Phenytoin | ↓ phenytoin, ↓ azole | Monitor, adjust dosage |
| | | X | X | | | Isoniazid | ↓ azole | Avoid co-administration |
| X | X | X | X | X | X | Lopinavir/ritonavir | ↑ azole, ↑ lopinavir/ritonavir | Monitor, adjust dosage |
| | X | X | X | X | X | Lovastatin, simvastatin | ↑ statin | Avoid co-administration |
| | | X | | | | Maraviroc | ↑ maraviroc | Monitor, adjust dosage |
| | | X | | | X | Methadone | ↑ methadone | Monitor, adjust dosage |
| | | | | X | | Metoclopramide | ↑ posaconazole (susp form only) | Monitor, adjust dosage |
| X | X | X | X | X | X | Midazolam, triazolam | ↑ midazolam, triazolam | Monitor, adjust dosage |
| | | | | X | | Mycophenolate | ↑ mycophenolate | Monitor, adjust dosage |
| X | | X | X | | X | Oral hypoglycemics | ↑ oral hypoglycemic | Avoid co-administration |
| | X | X | X | X | X | Pimozide | ↑ pimozide | Avoid co-administration |
| | X | X | X | X | X | Protease inhibitors | ↑ protease inhibitor | Avoid co-administration |
| | | | | X | | Proton pump inhibitors | ↓ azole, ↑ PPI (posa-susp form only) | Avoid co-administration |
| | | | | X | | Proton pump inhibitors | ↑ PPI (posa, tab form only) | Monitor, adjust dosage |
| | | | | | X | Proton pump inhibitors | ↓ voriconazole, ↑ PPI | Avoid co-administration |
| | X | X | | | | Rituximab | Inhibits action of rituximab | Avoid co-administration |
| X | X | X | X | X | X | Sirolimus | ↑ sirolimus | Avoid co-administration |
| X | X | X | X | X | X | Tacrolimus | ↑ tacrolimus | Monitor, adjust dosage |
| | | X | X | | | Theophylline | ↑ theophylline | Monitor, adjust dosage |
| | | X | | | | Trazodone | ↑ trazodone | Monitor, adjust dosage |
| X | | X | X | | | Warfarin | ↑ warfarin, ↑ INR | Monitor INR, adjust dosage |
| X | | | | | X | Zidovudine | ↑ zidovudine | Avoid co-administration |

**TABLE 22A (10)**

| Anti-infective agent | Other Drug | Effect on concentration (or other effect) | Suggested management |
|---|---|---|---|
| Bedaquiline | Rifampin | ↓ bedaquiline | Avoid co-administration |
| | Ketoconazole | ↑ bedaquiline | Avoid co-administration |
| Caspofungin | Cyclosporine | ↑ caspofungin | Monitor |
| | Tacrolimus | ↓ tacrolimus | Monitor, adjust dosage |
| | Other CYP inducers | ↓ caspofungin | Consider ↑ caspo dosage |
| Cephalexin | Metformin | ↑ metformin | Monitor, adjust dosage |
| Chloramphenicol | Phenytoin | ↑ phenytoin | Monitor, adjust dosage |
| | Iron salts, Vitamin B12 | ↓ response to iron salts, vitamin B12 | Monitor |
| | HIV Protease inhibitors | ↑ chloramphenicol, protease inhibitors | Avoid co-administration |
| Clindamycin | Kaolin | ↓ absorption of clindamycin | Avoid co-administration |
| | Atracurium | ↑ neuromuscular blockade | Avoid co-administration |
| | St John's wort | ↓ clindamycin | Monitor, adjust dosage |
| Cycloserine | Ethanol | ↑ neurotoxicity | Monitor |
| | INH, ethionamide | ↑ neurotoxicity | Monitor |
| Dapsone | Didanosine | ↓ absorption of dapsone | Avoid co-administration |
| | Oral contraceptives | ↓ effectiveness of oral contraceptives | Use alternate method |
| | Pyrimethamine | ↑ marrow toxicity | Monitor |
| | Zidovudine | ↑ marrow toxicity | Monitor |
| Daptomycin | HMG-CoA inhibitors (statins) | ↑ muscle toxicity | Monitor or avoid |
| Didanosine (dd) | Allopurinol | ↑ didanosine | Avoid co-administration |
| | Ethanol | ↑ risk of pancreatitis | Monitor |
| | Fluoroquinolones | ↓ FQ absorption | Avoid co-administration |
| | Drugs needing low pH for absorption | ↓ absorption | Avoid co-administration |
| | Methadone | ↓ didanosine | Avoid co-administration |
| | Pentamidine | ↑ risk of pancreatitis | Monitor |
| | Ribavirin | ↑ mitochondrial toxicity | Avoid co-administration |
| | Tenofovir | ↑ didanosine | Adjust didanosine dosage |
| Doripenem | Probenecid | ↑ doripenem | Adjust dosage or avoid |
| | Valproic acid | ↓ valproic acid | Monitor, adjust dosage |
| Doxycycline | Aluminum, bismuth, iron, magnesium salts | ↓ doxycycline absorption | Avoid co-administration |
| | Barbiturates | ↓ doxycycline | Avoid co-administration |
| | Carbamazepine | ↓ doxycycline | Avoid co-administration |
| | Digoxin | ↑ digoxin | Monitor, adjust dosage |
| | Phenytoin | ↓ doxycycline | Avoid co-administration |
| | Warfarin | ↑ warfarin | Monitor INR, adjust dosage |
| Eravacycline | Strong CYP3A4 inducer | ↓ eravacycline | ↑ dose to 1.5 mg/kg q12h |
| | Warfarin | ↑ INR | Monitor INR, adjust dosage |

**TABLE 22A (11)**

| Anti-infective agent | Ciprofloxacin | Gatifloxacin | Gemifloxacin | Levofloxacin | Moxifloxacin | Ofloxacin | Other Drug | Effect on concentration (or other effect) | Suggested management |
|---|---|---|---|---|---|---|---|---|---|
| Ertapenem | | | | | | | Probenecid | ↑ ertapenem | Monitor or avoid |
| | | | | | | | Valproic acid | ↓ valproic acid | Monitor, adjust dosage |
| Ethambutol | | | | | | | Aluminum salts | ↓ absorption of ethambutol, aluminum salts | Avoid co-administration |
| Flucloxacillin | | | | | | | Warfarin | ↓ warfarin | Monitor INR, adjust dosage |
| | | | | | | | Voriconazole | ↓ voriconazole | Monitor, adjust dosage |
| **Fluoroquinolones** | | | | | | | | | |
| | × | × | | × | × | × | Antiarrhythmics (procainamide, amiodarone) | ↑ QT interval | Monitor |
| | | × | | | × | | Insulin, oral hypoglycemics | Hypo- or hyperglycemia | Monitor |
| | × | | | | | × | Caffeine | ↑ caffeine | Monitor |
| | × | | | | | × | Cimetidine | ↑ fluoroquinolone | Monitor, adjust dosage |
| | × | | | × | | × | Cyclosporine | ↑ cyclosporine | Avoid co-administration |
| | × | | × | × | × | × | Didanosine | ↓ absorption of FQ | Avoid co-administration |
| | × | × | × | × | × | × | Cations (Al, Ca, Fe, Mg, Zn) | ↓ absorption of FQ | Monitor, adjust dosage |
| | | × | | | | | Methadone | ↑ methadone | Monitor |
| | × | | | | | × | NSAIDs | ↑ neurotoxicity | Monitor |
| | × | | | | | | Phenytoin | ↑ or ↓ phenytoin | Monitor |
| | × | × | × | × | | × | Probenecid | ↓ renal clearance of FQ | Monitor, adjust dosage |
| | × | | | | | | Rasagiline | ↑ rasagiline | Monitor, adjust dosage |
| | | | | | × | | Rifampin | ↓ moxifloxacin | Adjust dosage or avoid |
| | × | × | | × | | × | Sucralfate | ↓ absorption of FQ | Avoid co-administration |
| | × | | | | | | Theophylline | ↑ theophylline | Monitor, adjust dosage |
| | × | | | | | | Thyroid hormone | ↓ thyroid hormone | Monitor or avoid |
| | × | | | | | | Tizanidine | ↑ tizanidine | Avoid co-administration |
| | × | | | × | × | × | Warfarin | ↑ warfarin | Monitor INR, adjust dosage |
| Fusidic acid | | | | | | | Atorvastatin | ↑ atorvastatin (↑ risk of rhabdomyolysis) | Avoid co-administration |
| | | | | | | | Rifampin | ↑ rifampin, ↓ fusidic acid | Monitor or avoid |
| | | | | | | | Ritonavir | ↑ fusidic acid | Monitor or avoid |
| | | | | | | | Simvastatin | ↑ simvastatin (↑ risk of rhabdomyolysis) | Avoid co-administration |
| Ganciclovir | | | | | | | Imipenem | ↑ risk of seizures | Monitor |
| | | | | | | | Probenecid | ↑ ganciclovir | Monitor, adjust dosage |
| | | | | | | | Zidovudine | ↓ ganciclovir, ↑ zidovudine | Adjust dosage or avoid |

**TABLE 22A (12)**

**Griseofulvin**

| Other Drug | Effect on concentration (or other effect) | Suggested management |
|---|---|---|
| Barbiturates | ↓ griseofulvin | Adjust dosage or avoid |
| Cyclosporine | ↓ cyclosporine | Monitor, adjust dosage |
| Ethinyl estradiol | ↓ ethinyl estradiol | Avoid co-administration |
| Salicylates | ↓ salicylates | Monitor, adjust dosage |
| Warfarin | ↓ warfarin | Monitor INR, adjust dosage |

**Hepatitis C antivirals**

| Other Drug | Effect on concentration (or other effect) | Epclusa | Zepatier | Daclatasvir | Simeprevir | Sofosbuvir | Sofosbuvir / Ledipasvir | Technivie | Viekira Pak | Mavyret | Vosevi | Suggested management |
|---|---|---|---|---|---|---|---|---|---|---|---|---|
| Alfuzosin | Potential for hypotension | | | | | | | × | × | | | Avoid co-administration |
| Alprazolam | ↑ alprazolam | | | | | | | × | × | | | Monitor, adjust dosage |
| Amiodarone | Bradycardia | × | | | | × | × | | | | × | Avoid co-administration |
| Amlodipine | ↑ amlodipine | | | | | | | × | × | | | Monitor, adjust dosage |
| Antacids | ↓ ledipasvir | | | | | | × | | | | | Separate administration |
| Antacids | ↓ velpatasvir | × | | | | | | | | | × | Separate administration |
| Atazanavir | ↑ glecaprevir, ↑ pibrentasvir | | | | | | | | | × | | Contraindicated |
| Atazanavir | ↑ voxilaprevir | | | | | | | | | | × | Avoid co-administration |
| Atazanavir / ritonavir | ↑ hep C drug | | × | × | | | | | | | | Avoid co-administration |
| Atazanavir / ritonavir | ↑ paritaprevir | | | | | | | × | × | | | Monitor, adjust dosage |
| Atorvastatin | ↑ atorvastatin | × | × | | | | × | | | | × | Avoid co-administration |
| Atorvastatin | ↑ atorvastatin | | | | | | | × | × | | | Monitor, adjust dosage |
| Bepridil | ↑ bepridil | | | | | | | × | × | | | Monitor, adjust dosage |
| Bosentan | ↑ hep C drug | × | | | × | | | | | | | Adjust dosage or avoid |
| Buprenorphine | ↑ buprenorphine | | | | | | | × | × | | | Monitor, adjust dosage |
| Carbamazepine | ↓ hep C drug(s) | × | × | × | × | × | × | × | × | × | × | Avoid co-administration |
| Ciprofloxacin | ↑ daclatasvir | | | × | | | | | | | | Avoid co-administration |
| Clarithromycin | ↑ daclatasvir | | | × | | | | | | | | Avoid co-administration |
| Cobicistat | ↑ simeprevir | | | | × | | | | | | | Avoid co-administration |
| Cyclosporine | ↑ simeprevir | | | | × | | | | | | | Avoid co-administration |
| Cyclosporine | ↑ cyclosporine | | | | × | | × | | | | | Adjust dosage or avoid |
| Cyclosporine | ↑ grazoprevir | | × | | | | | | | | | Avoid co-administration |
| Cyclosporine | ↑ voxilaprevir | | | | | | | | | | × | Avoid co-administration |
| Cyclosporine | ↑ glecaprevir, ↑ pibrentasvir | | | | | | | | | × | | Avoid if stable cyclo >100 mg/d |
| Dabigatran | ↑ dabigatran | × | | | | | | | | | | Avoid co-administration |
| Dabigatran | ↑ dabigatran | | | | | | | | | × | | Monitor, adjust dosage |
| Darunavir | ↑ glecaprevir | | | | | | | | | × | | Avoid co-administration |
| Darunavir/ritonavir | ↑ hep C drug | | × | × | | | | | | | × | Avoid co-administration |

**TABLE 22A (13)**

Hepatitis C antivirals *(continued)*

| Epclusa | Zepatier | Daclatasvir | Simeprevir | Sofosbuvir | Sofosbuvir / Ledipasvir | Technivie | Viekira Pak | Mavyret | Vosevi | Other Drug | Effect on concentration (or other effect) | Suggested management |
|---|---|---|---|---|---|---|---|---|---|---|---|---|
| | | | | | | × | × | | × | Darunavir/ritonavir | ↓ darunavir/ritonavir | Avoid co-administration |
| | × | | | | | | | | | Darunavir/ritonavir | ↑ grazoprevir | Avoid co-administration |
| | | × | × | | | | × | × | | Dexamethasone | ↓ hep C drug | Avoid co-administration |
| | × | | | | × | × | × | × | | Digoxin | ↑ digoxin | Monitor, adjust dosage |
| | | × | | | | | | | | Diltiazem | ↑ daclatasvir | Avoid co-administration |
| | | | | | | × | × | | | Diltiazem | ↑ diltiazem | Monitor, adjust dosage |
| | | × | × | | | | | | | Disopyramide | ↑ disopyramide | Monitor, adjust dosage |
| × | × | | | | | | | | × | Disopyramide | ↓ hep C drug(s) | Avoid co-administration |
| | | × | × | | | | | | | Efavirenz | Increased LFTs | Monitor |
| | | | × | | | × | × | | | Ergot derivatives | Ergot toxicity | Avoid co-administration |
| | | × | | | | | | | | Erythromycin | ↑ daclatasvir | Avoid co-administration |
| | | | × | | | | | | | Erythromycin | ↑ simeprevir, erythromycin | Monitor |
| | | | | | | × | × | | | Ethinyl estradiol | ALT elevations | Avoid co-administration |
| | | × | × | | | | | | | Ethinyl estradiol | Effects uncertain | Avoid co-administration |
| × | × | | | | | | | | × | Etravirine | ↓ hep C drug | Avoid co-administration |
| | | | | | × | | | | | Famotidine | ↓ ledipasvir | Max fam 40 mg q12h |
| × | | | | | | | | | × | Famotidine | ↓ velpatasvir | Max fam 40 mg q12h |
| | | | | | | × | × | | | Felodipine | ↑ felodipine | Monitor, adjust dosage |
| | | | × | | | × | × | | | Flecainide | ↑ flecainide | Monitor, adjust dosage |
| | | | | | | × | × | × | | Fluconazole | ↑ hep C drug | Avoid co-administration |
| | | | | | × | × | × | | | Fluticasone nasal | ↑ fluticasone | Monitor, adjust dosage |
| | | × | × | | | | | | | Fluvastatin | ↑ fluvastatin | Monitor, adjust dosage |
| | | | | | | × | × | | | Furosemide | ↑ furosemide | Monitor, adjust dosage |
| | × | | | | | | × | | | Gemfibrozil | ↑ dasabuvir | Avoid co-administration |
| × | | | | | | | | | × | H2-antagonists | ↓ velpatasvir | Max fam 40 mg q12h (or equiv) |
| | | × | × | | | | | | | Itraconazole | ↑ hep C drug | Avoid co-administration |
| | | | | | | × | × | | | Ketoconazole | ↑ hep C drug | Monitor, adjust dosage |
| | | × | × | | | | | | | Ketoconazole | ↑ ketoconazole | Monitor, adjust dosage |
| | | | | | | × | × | | | Lidocaine | ↑ lidocaine | Monitor, adjust dosage |
| | | | | | | | | × | | Lopinavir/ritonavir | ↑ plbrentasvir | Avoid co-administration |
| | | × | × | | | | | | | Lopinavir/ritonavir | ↑ paritaprevir | Avoid co-administration |
| | × | | | | | | | | | Lopinavir/ritonavir | ↑ grazoprevir | Avoid co-administration |
| | | | | | | | | | × | Lopinavir/ritonavir | ↑ voxilaprevir | Avoid co-administration |

**TABLE 22A (14)**

**Hepatitis C antivirals** *(continued)*

| Epclusa | Zepatier | Daclatasvir | Simeprevir | Sofosbuvir | Ledipasvir / Sofosbuvir | Technivie | Viekira Pak | Mavyret | Vosevi | Other Drug | Effect on concentration (or other effect) | Suggested management |
|---|---|---|---|---|---|---|---|---|---|---|---|---|
|  |  |  |  |  |  |  |  |  | × | Lovastatin | ↑ lovastatin | Monitor, adjust dosage |
|  |  |  | × |  |  | × | × |  |  | Lovastatin | ↑ lovastatin | Avoid co-administration |
|  |  |  | × |  |  |  |  |  |  | Mexiletine | ↑ mexiletine | Monitor, adjust dosage |
|  |  |  | × |  |  | × | × |  |  | Midazolam | ↑ midazolam | Monitor, adjust dosage |
|  | × |  |  |  |  |  |  |  |  | Modafinil | ↓ zepatier | Avoid co-administration |
|  |  | × |  |  |  |  |  |  |  | Nafcillin | ↓ daclatasvir | Avoid co-administration |
|  | × |  |  |  |  |  |  |  |  | Nafcillin | ↓ zepatier | Avoid co-administration |
|  |  |  | × |  |  |  |  |  |  | Nicardipine | ↑ nicardipine | Monitor, adjust dosage |
|  |  |  | × |  |  |  |  |  |  | Nifedipine | ↑ nifedipine | Monitor, adjust dosage |
|  |  |  | × |  |  |  |  |  |  | Nisoldipine | ↑ nisoldipine | Monitor, adjust dosage |
| × |  |  |  |  | × |  |  |  |  | Omeprazole | ↓ ledipasvir | Max omep 20 mg q24h |
| × |  |  |  |  |  |  |  |  |  | Omeprazole | ↓ velpatasvir | Avoid co-administration |
|  |  |  | × |  |  |  |  |  |  | Omeprazole | ↓ omeprazole | Monitor, adjust dosage |
| × | × |  | × |  |  | × | × |  | × | Oxcarbazepine | ↓ hep C drug | Avoid co-administration |
| × | × |  | × |  |  | × | × |  | × | Phenytoin | ↓ hep C drug | Avoid co-administration |
| × | × |  | × |  |  | × | × |  | × | Phenobarbital | ↓ hep C drug | Avoid co-administration |
|  |  |  |  |  |  |  |  |  |  | Pimozide | Cardiac arrhythmias | Monitor |
|  |  |  | × |  |  |  |  |  |  | Pitavastatin | ↑ pitavastatin | Monitor, adjust dosage |
|  |  |  |  |  |  |  | × |  |  | Pitavastatin | ↑ pitavastatin | Avoid co-administration |
|  |  | × |  |  |  | × | × |  |  | Posaconazole | ↑ hep C drug | Avoid co-administration |
|  |  |  | × |  |  |  |  |  | × | Pravastatin | ↑ pravastatin | Monitor, adjust dosage |
|  |  |  |  |  |  | × | × |  |  | Pravastatin | ↑ pravastatin | ↓ pravastatin dose by 50% |
|  |  |  | × |  |  |  |  |  |  | Propafenone | ↑ propafenone | Monitor, adjust dosage |
|  |  |  | × |  |  |  |  |  |  | Quetiapine | ↑ quetiapine | Monitor, adjust dosage |
|  |  |  | × |  |  |  |  |  |  | Quinidine | ↑ quinidine | Monitor, adjust dosage |
| × | × |  | × | × | × | × | × |  | × | Rifampin | ↓ hep C drug | Avoid co-administration |
|  |  |  |  |  |  |  |  | × |  | Rifampin | ↓ glecaprevir, ↓ pibrentasvir | Contraindicated |
| × | × |  | × | × | × | × | × |  | × | Rifabutin | ↓ hep C drug | Avoid co-administration |
| × | × |  |  | × | × |  |  | × |  | Rifapentine | ↓ hep C drug | Avoid co-administration |
|  |  |  | × |  |  | × | × |  |  | Rilpivirine | ↑ rilpivirine | Monitor, adjust dosage |
| × | × |  | × | × | × |  |  | × | × | Rosuvastatin | ↑rosuvastatin | Avoid co-administration |
| × |  |  |  |  |  |  |  |  |  | Rosuvastatin | ↑rosuvastatin | Monitor, adjust dosage |
|  |  |  | × |  |  | × | × |  |  | Salmeterol | ↑ salmeterol | Avoid co-administration |

**TABLE 22A (15)**

Anti-infective agent (continued)

**Hepatitis C antivirals** *(continued)*

| Epclusa | Zepatier | Daclatasvir | Simeprevir | Sofosbuvir | Sofosbuvir / Daclatasvir | Technivie | Viekira Pak | Mavyret | Vosevi | Other Drug | Effect on concentration (or other effect) | Suggested management |
|---|---|---|---|---|---|---|---|---|---|---|---|---|
| | × | | | | | | | | | Saquinavir | ↑ grazoprevir | Avoid co-administration |
| × | | × | × | | | × | × | × | × | Sildenafil | ↑ sildenafil | Monitor, adjust dosage |
| | × | | × | | | × | × | × | | Simvastatin | ↑ simvastatin | Monitor, adjust dosage |
| | | | | | | × | × | × | | Simvastatin | ↑ simvastatin | Avoid co-administration |
| | | | | | | × | × | | | Sirolimus | ↓ or ↑ sirolimus | Monitor, adjust dosage |
| × | × | × | × | × | × | × | × | × | × | St. John's wort | ↓ hep C drug(s) | Avoid co-administration |
| × | × | | × | | | × | × | × | × | Tacrolimus | ↑ tacrolimus | Monitor, adjust dosage |
| | | | × | | | | | | | Tadalafil | ↑ tadalafil | Monitor, adjust dosage |
| × | | | | | | × | × | | × | Tenofovir DF | ↑ tenofovir DF | Avoid co-administration |
| | | × | × | | × | × | × | | | Tipranavir/ritonavir | ↓ or ↑ hep C drug | Avoid co-administration |
| × | | | | × | × | | | | × | Tipranavir/ritonavir | ↓ sofosbuvir, ↓ velpatasvir | Avoid co-administration |
| | × | | | | | | | | | Tipranavir/ritonavir | ↑ grazoprevir | Avoid co-administration |
| × | | | | | | | | | × | Topotecan | ↑ topotecan | Avoid co-administration |
| | | | × | | | × | × | | | Triazolam | ↑ triazolam | Avoid co-administration |
| | | | × | | | | | | | Vardenafil | ↑ vardenafil | Monitor, adjust dosage |
| | | × | | | | | | | | Verapamil | ↑ daclatasvir | Avoid co-administration |
| | | | × | | × | | | | | Verapamil | ↑ verapamil | Monitor, adjust dosage |
| | | × | | | | | | | | Voriconazole | ↑ hep C drug | Avoid co-administration |
| | × | | × | | × | × | × | | | Voriconazole | ↓ voriconazole | Avoid co-administration |

**Imipenem**

| | | | | | | | | | | Other Drug | Effect on concentration (or other effect) | Suggested management |
|---|---|---|---|---|---|---|---|---|---|---|---|---|
| | | | | | | | | | | BCG | ↓ effectiveness of BCG | Avoid co-administration |
| | | | | | | | | | | Ganciclovir | ↑ seizure risk | Monitor |
| | | | | | | | | | | Probenecid | ↑ imipenem | Monitor, adjust dosage |
| | | | | | | | | | | Valproic acid | ↓ valproic acid | Monitor, adjust dosage |

**Integrase Strand Transfer Inhibitors (INSTI)**

| Dolutegravir | Raltegravir | Other Drug | Effect on concentration (or other effect) | Suggested management |
|---|---|---|---|---|
| × | × | Antacids (polyvalent cations) | ↓ INSTI | Space dosing or avoid |
| × | | Carbamazepine | ↓ dolutegravir | Monitor, adjust dosage |
| × | | Dofetilide | ↑ dofetilide | Avoid co-administration |
| × | | Efavirenz | ↓ dolutegravir | Avoid co-administration |
| × | × | Etravirine | ↓ INSTI | Avoid co-administration |
| × | | Fosamprenavir/ritonavir | ↓ dolutegravir | Monitor, adjust dosage |
| × | | Metformin | ↑ metformin | Monitor, adjust dosage |
| × | | Nevirapine | ↓ dolutegravir | Monitor, adjust dosage |

**TABLE 22A (16)**

| Anti-infective agent | | | | | Other Drug | Effect on concentration (or other effect) | Suggested management |
|---|---|---|---|---|---|---|---|
| **Integrase Strand Transfer Inhibitors (INSTI)** *(continued)* | | | | | | | |
| Dolutegravir | Raltegravir | | | | | | |
| x | | | | | Oxcarbazepine | ↓ dolutegravir | Avoid co-administration |
| x | | | | | Phenobarbital | ↓ dolutegravir | Avoid co-administration |
| x | | | | | Phenytoin | ↓ dolutegravir | Avoid co-administration |
| x | | | | | Primidone | ↓ dolutegravir | Avoid co-administration |
| x | x | | | | Rifampin | ↓ INSTI | Avoid co-administration |
| x | | | | | St. John's wort | ↓ dolutegravir | Avoid co-administration |
| x | x | | | | Sucralfate | ↓ INSTI | Space dosing or avoid |
| x | | | | | Tipranavir/ritonavir | ↓ dolutegravir | Monitor, adjust dosage |
| | x | | | | Tipranavir/ritonavir | ↓ raltegravir | Avoid HD combination |
| Isoniazid | | | | | Alcohol | ↑ risk of hepatic injury | Monitor |
| | | | | | Aluminum salts | ↓ absorption of INH | Avoid co-administration |
| | | | | | Carbamazepine | ↑ carbamazepine | Monitor, adjust dosage |
| | | | | | Itraconazole, ketoconazole | ↓ isoniazid | Monitor, adjust dosage |
| | | | | | Phenytoin | ↑ phenytoin | Monitor, adjust dosage |
| | | | | | Oral hypoglycemics | ↓ oral hypoglycemics | Monitor, adjust dosage |
| Linezolid | | | | | Adrenergic agents | Risk of hypertension | Monitor |
| | | | | | Aged, fermented, pickled or smoked foods | Risk of hypertension | Monitor |
| | | | | | Meperidine | Risk of serotonin syndrome | Monitor |
| | | | | | Rasagiline | Risk of serotonin syndrome | Monitor |
| | | | | | Rifampin | ↓ linezolid | Monitor, adjust dosage |
| | | | | | Serotonergic drugs (SSRIs) | Risk of serotonin syndrome | Monitor |
| **Macrolides** | | | | | | | |
| Erythromycin | Azithromycin | Clarithromycin | | | | | |
| x | | x | | | Carbamazepine | ↑ carbamazepine | Avoid co-administration |
| x | | x | | | Cimetidine | ↑ cimetidine | Monitor, adjust dosage |
| x | | x | | | Clozapine | ↑ clozapine | Monitor, adjust dosage |
| x | | x | | | Colchicine | ↑ colchicine | Avoid co-administration |
| x | | x | | | Corticosteroids | ↑ corticosteroids | Monitor, adjust dosage |
| x | x | x | | | Cyclosporine | ↑ cyclosporine | Monitor, adjust dosage |
| x | x | x | | | Digoxin | ↑ digoxin | Monitor, adjust dosage |
| x | | x | | | Ergot alkaloids | ↑ ergot alkaloids | Monitor, adjust dosage |
| x | | x | | | Lovastatin | ↑ lovastatin | Monitor, adjust dosage |
| x | | x | | | Maraviroc | ↑ maraviroc | Monitor, adjust dosage |
| x | | x | | | Midazolam | ↑ midazolam | Monitor, adjust dosage |
| x | | x | | | Phenytoin | ↑ phenytoin | Monitor, adjust dosage |
| x | x | x | | | Pimozide | ↑ QT interval | Monitor |

## TABLE 22A (17)

| Anti-Infective agent | | | Other Drug | Effect on concentration (or other effect) | Suggested management |
|---|---|---|---|---|---|
| Erythromycin | Azithromycin | Clarithromycin | | | |
| **Macrolides** (continued) | | | | | |
| x | | x | Simvastatin | ↑ simvastatin | Monitor, adjust dosage |
| x | | x | Tacrolimus | ↑ tacrolimus | Monitor, adjust dosage |
| x | | x | Theophylline | ↑ theophylline | Monitor, adjust dosage |
| x | | x | Triazolam | ↑ triazolam | Monitor, adjust dosage |
| x | | x | Valproic acid | ↑ valproic acid | Monitor, adjust dosage |
| x | | x | Warfarin | ↑ warfarin | Monitor INR, adjust dosage |
| x | | x | Zidovudine | ↓ zidovudine | Monitor, adjust dosage |
| Maraviroc | | | Nefazodone | ↑ maraviroc | Monitor, adjust dosage |
| | | | Carbamazepine | ↓ maraviroc | Avoid co-administration |
| | | | Efavirenz | ↓ maraviroc | Avoid co-administration |
| | | | Phenobarbital | ↓ maraviroc | Avoid co-administration |
| | | | Phenytoin | ↓ maraviroc | Avoid co-administration |
| | | | Rifampin | ↓ maraviroc | Avoid co-administration |
| Mefloquine | | | Beta blockers | ↑ arrhythmias | Avoid co-administration |
| | | | Calcium channel blockers | ↑ arrhythmias | Avoid co-administration |
| | | | Halofantrine | QT prolongation | Avoid co-administration |
| | | | Protease inhibitors | ↓ mefloquine | Avoid co-administration |
| | | | Quinidine, quinine | ↑ arrhythmias | Avoid co-administration |
| | | | Valproic acid | ↓ valproic acid | Monitor, adjust dosage |
| Meropenem | | | BCG | ↓ effectiveness of BCG | Avoid co-administration |
| | | | Ganciclovir | ↑ seizure risk | Monitor |
| | | | Probenecid | ↑ meropenem | Monitor, adjust dosage |
| | | | Valproic acid | ↓ valproic acid | Monitor, adjust dosage |
| Methenamine mand/hipp | | | Drugs that ↑ urine pH | ↓ antibacterial effect | Acidify urine |
| Metronidazole | | | Alcohol | Disulfiram-like reaction | Avoid co-administration |
| | | | Cyclosporine | ↑ cyclosporine | Monitor, adjust dosage |
| | | | Disulfiram | Acute toxic psychosis | Monitor |
| | | | Lithium | ↑ lithium | Monitor, adjust dosage |
| | | | Warfarin | ↑ warfarin | Monitor INR, adjust dosage |
| | | | Phenobarbital | ↑ phenobarbital | Monitor, adjust dosage |
| | | | Phenytoin | ↑ phenytoin | Monitor, adjust dosage |
| Micafungin | | | Itraconazole | ↑ itraconazole | Monitor, adjust dosage |
| | | | Nifedipine | ↑ nifedipine | Monitor, adjust dosage |
| | | | Sirolimus | ↑ sirolimus | Monitor, adjust dosage |
| Nafcillin | | | Warfarin | ↓ warfarin effect | Monitor INR, adjust dosage |
| Nitrofurantoin | | | Antacids | ↓ nitrofurantoin | Monitor, adjust dosage |

**TABLE 22A (18)**

| Non-Nucleoside RTIs | | | | | Other Drug | Effect on concentration (or other effect) | Suggested management |
|---|---|---|---|---|---|---|---|
| Doravirine | Efavirenz | Etravirine | Nevirapine | Rilpivirine | | | |
| x | | | | x | Alprazolam | ↓ or ↑ alprazolam | Monitor or avoid |
| | x | x | x | | Amiodarone | ↑ NNRTI, ↓ or ↑ amiodarone | Avoid co-administration |
| | x | x | x | | Amlodipine | ↓ or ↑ amlodipine | Monitor, adjust dosage |
| | x | x | x | | Atorvastatin | ↓ or ↑ atorvastatin | Monitor |
| | x | x | x | x | Carbamazepine | ↓ NNRTI, ↓ or ↑ carbamazepine | Avoid co-administration |
| x | | | | | Carbamazepine | ↓ doravirine | Contraindicated |
| x | x | x | x | | Clarithromycin | ↓ or ↑ clari metabolite, ↑ NNRTI | Monitor, adjust dosage |
| | | | | x | Clarithromycin | ↑ rilpivirine | Monitor, adjust dosage |
| x | | | | | Cyclosporine | ↓ or ↑ cyclosporine | Avoid co-administration |
| | x | x | x | | Dexamethasone | ↓ NNRTI, ↑ or ↓ dexamethasone | Avoid co-administration |
| | | | | x | Dexamethasone | ↓ rilpivirine | Avoid co-administration |
| x | | | | | Efavirenz | ↓ doravirine | Avoid co-administration |
| x | | | | | Enzalutamide | ↓ doravirine | Contraindicated |
| | x | x | x | | Ergotamine | ↓ or ↑ ergotamine | Avoid co-administration |
| x | | | | | Etravirine | ↓ doravirine | Avoid co-administration |
| | | | | x | Gastric acid suppressors | ↓ NNRTI | Avoid co-administration |
| | x | x | x | | Itraconazole | ↓ itraconazole, ↑ NNRTI | Avoid co-administration |
| | | | | x | Itraconazole | ↑ rilpivirine | Avoid co-administration |
| | x | x | x | | Ketoconazole | ↓ ketoconazole, ↑ NNRTI | Avoid co-administration |
| | | | | x | Ketoconazole | ↑ rilpivirine | Avoid co-administration |
| | x | x | x | | Lidocaine | ↓ or ↑ lidocaine | Avoid co-administration |
| x | | | | x | Lidocaine | ↓ or ↑ lidocaine | Monitor |
| | x | x | x | | Lovastatin | ↑ or ↓ lovastatin | Avoid co-administration |
| | x | x | x | | Mefloquine | ↑ or ↓ mefloquine | Monitor or avoid |
| x | | | | x | Midazolam | ↓ or ↑ midazolam | Contraindicated |
| x | | | | | Mitotane | ↓ doravirine | Avoid co-administration |
| x | | | | | Nevirapine | ↓ doravirine | Avoid co-administration |
| | x | x | x | | Opioids: fentanyl, methadone | ↑ or ↓ opioid | Monitor |
| | x | x | x | | Oral contraceptives | ↑ or ↓ oral contraceptive | Use alternative method |
| x | | | | | Oxcarbazepine | ↓ doravirine | Contraindicated |
| | x | x | | | PDE5 inhibitors | ↑ or ↓ PDE5 inhibitor | Monitor, adjust dosage |
| | x | x | x | | Phenobarbital | ↓ NNRTI, ↓ or ↑ phenobarbital | Avoid co-administration |
| x | | | | | Phenobarbital | ↓ doravirine | Contraindicated |
| | x | x | x | | Phenytoin | ↓ NNRTI, ↓ or ↑ phenytoin | Avoid co-administration |
| x | | | | | Phenytoin | ↓ doravirine | Contraindicated |
| | | | | x | Phenytoin | ↑ or ↓ phenytoin | Avoid co-administration |
| | x | x | x | | Pimozide | ↑ or ↑ pimozide | Contraindicated |
| | x | x | x | | Posaconazole | ↓ posaconazole, ↑ NNRTI | Avoid co-administration |

# TABLE 22A (19)

**Non-Nucleoside RTIs** *(continued)*

| Anti-infective agent | | | | | Other Drug | Effect on concentration (or other effect) | Suggested management |
|---|---|---|---|---|---|---|---|
| Doravirine | Efavirenz | Etravirine | Nevirapine | Rilpivirine | | | |
| | | | | x | Posaconazole | ↑ rilpivirine | Avoid co-administration |
| | x | x | | | Rifabutin | ↑ or ↓ rifabutin, ↓ NNRTI | Avoid co-administration |
| x | | | | | Rifabutin | ↓ doravirine | ↑DOR to 100 mg q12h |
| | | | | x | Rifabutin | ↓ rilpivirine | Avoid co-administration |
| | | | | x | Rifampin | ↓ rilpivirine | Avoid co-administration |
| x | | | | | Rifampin | ↓ doravirine | Contraindicated |
| x | | | | | Rifapentine | ↓ doravirine | Contraindicated |
| | x | x | x | | Sirolimus | ↓ or ↑ sirolimus | Avoid co-administration |
| | x | x | x | | Simvastatin | ↓ or ↑ simvastatin | Monitor |
| | x | x | x | x | St. John's wort | ↓ NNRTI | Avoid co-administration |
| x | | | | | St. John's wort | ↓ doravirine | Contraindicated |
| | x | x | x | | Tacrolimus | ↓ or ↑ tacrolimus | Avoid co-administration |
| | x | x | x | | Triazolam | ↓ or ↑ triazolam | Monitor or avoid |
| | x | x | x | | Verapamil | ↓ or ↑ verapamil, ↑ NNRTI | Avoid co-administration |
| | | | | x | Verapamil | ↑ rilpivirine | Monitor, adjust dosage |
| | x | x | x | | Voriconazole | ↓ voriconazole, ↑ NNRTI | Avoid co-administration |
| | | | | x | Voriconazole | ↑ rilpivirine | Avoid co-administration |
| | x | x | x | | Warfarin | ↓ or ↑ warfarin | Monitor INR, adjust dosage |
| Omadacycline | | | | | Antacids (Al, Mg, Ca, bismuth subsalicylate | ↓ omadacycline | Separate administration by 4 hr |
| | | | | | Iron-containing preparations | ↓ omadacycline | Separate administration by 4 hr |
| | | | | | Verapamil | ↓ omadacycline | Monitor |
| | | | | | Warfarin | ↑ INR | Monitor INR, adjust dosage |
| Oritavancin | | | | | Warfarin | ↑ warfarin | Monitor INR, adjust dosage |
| Pentamidine (IV) | | | | | Amphotericin B | ↑ risk of nephrotoxicity | Monitor |
| Piperacillin-Tazobactam | | | | | Methotrexate | ↑ methotrexate | Monitor or avoid |
| Pivmecillinam | | | | | Probenecid | ↑ mecillinam | Monitor, adjust dosage |
| | | | | | Valproic acid | Enhanced carnitine depletion | Avoid co-administration |
| Polymyxin B, E (colistin) | | | | | Curare paralytics | Neuromuscular blockade | Avoid co-administration |
| | | | | | Aminoglycosides, amphotericin B, vancomycin | ↑ nephrotoxicity risk | Avoid co-administration |
| Primaquine | | | | | Drugs causing hemolysis in G6PD-deficiency | ↑ risk of hemolysis | Monitor or avoid |
| Pristinamycin | | | | | Cyclosporine | ↑ cyclosporine | Monitor, adjust dosage |
| | | | | | Tacrolimus | ↑ tacrolimus | Monitor, adjust dosage |

**TABLE 22A (20)**

| Protease inhibitors | | | | | | | | Other Drug | Effect on concentration (or other effect) | Suggested management |
|---|---|---|---|---|---|---|---|---|---|---|
| Atazanavir/r | Darunavir/r | Fosamprenavir/r | Indinavir/r | Lopinavir/r | Nelfinavir | Saquinavir/r | Tipranavir/r | | | |
| × | × | × | × | × | × | × | × | Amiodarone | ↑ PI, ↑ amiodarone | Monitor or avoid |
| × | × | × | × | × | × | × | × | Amitriptyline | ↑ amitriptyline | Adjust dosage or avoid |
| × | × | × | × | × | × | × | × | Amlodipine | ↑ amlodipine | Adjust dosage or avoid |
| × | × | × | × | × | × | × | × | Antacids | ↓ PI | Avoid co-administration |
| × | × | × | × | × | × | × | × | Bepridil | ↑ bepridil | Adjust dosage or avoid |
| × | × | × | × | × | × | × | × | Carbamazepine | ↓ PI, ↑ carbamazepine | Adjust dosage or avoid |
| × | × | × | × | × | × | × | × | Citalopram | ↓ citalopram | Adjust dosage or avoid |
| × | × | × | × | × | × | × | × | Clarithromycin | ↑ PI, ↑ clarithromycin | Adjust dosage or avoid |
| × | × | × | × | × | × | × | × | Cyclosporine | ↑ PI, ↑ cyclosporine | Adjust dosage or avoid |
| × | × | × | × | × | × | × | × | Dapsone | ↑ dapsone | Adjust dosage or avoid |
| × | × | × | × | × | × | × | × | Desipramine | ↑ desipramine | Adjust dosage or avoid |
| × | × | × | × | × | × | × | × | Dexamethasone | ↓ PI, ↑ dexamethasone | Avoid co-administration |
| × | × | × | × | × | × | × | × | Diazepam | ↑ diazepam | Monitor |
| × | × | × | × | × | × | × | × | Digoxin | ↓ or ↑ digoxin | Monitor |
| × | × | × | × | × | × | × | × | Diltiazem | ↑ PI, ↑ diltiazem | Adjust dosage or avoid |
| × | × | × | × | × | × | × | × | Diphenhydramine | ↑ diphenhydramine | Adjust dosage or avoid |
| × | × | × | × | × | × | × | × | Ergotamine | ↑ ergotamine | Avoid co-administration |
| × | × | × | × | × | × | × | × | Ethinyl estradiol | ↓ ethinyl estradiol | Avoid co-administration |
| × | × | × | × | × | × | × | × | Famotidine | ↓ PI | Avoid co-administration |
| × | × | × | × | × | × | × | × | Fentanyl | ↑ fentanyl | Monitor, adjust dosage |
| × | × | × | × | × | × | × | × | Flecainide | ↑ flecainide | Monitor, adjust dosage |
| × | × | × | × | × | × | × | × | Fluoxetine | ↓ or ↑ fluoxetine | Monitor |
| × | × | × | × | × | × | × | × | Imipramine | ↑ imipramine | Adjust dosage or avoid |
| × | × | × | × | × | × | × | × | Irinotecan | ↑ irinotecan | Avoid co-administration |
| × | × | × | × | × | × | × | × | Itraconazole | ↑ PI, ↑ itraconazole | Avoid co-administration |
| | × | × | × | × | × | × | | Itraconazole | ↑ itraconazole | Avoid co-administration |
| × | × | × | × | × | × | × | × | Lidocaine | ↑ lidocaine | Monitor, adjust dosage |
| × | × | × | × | × | × | × | × | Loratadine | ↑ loratadine | Monitor, adjust dosage |
| × | × | × | × | × | × | × | × | Lovastatin | ↑ lovastatin | Avoid co-administration |
| × | × | × | × | × | × | × | × | Maraviroc | ↑ maraviroc | Avoid co-administration |
| × | × | × | × | × | × | × | × | Methadone | ↓ methadone | Monitor, adjust dosage |

**TABLE 22A (21)**

### Protease inhibitors (continued)

| Atazanavir/r | Darunavir/r | Fosamprenavir/r | Indinavir/r | Lopinavir/r | Nelfinavir | Saquinavir/r | Tipranavir/r | Other Drug | Effect on concentration (or other effect) | Suggested management |
|---|---|---|---|---|---|---|---|---|---|---|
| × | × | × | × |  |  |  | × | Metronidazole | Possible disulfiram reaction | Monitor |
| × | × | × |  | × |  | × | × | Mexiletine | ↑ mexiletine | Monitor, adjust dosage |
| × | × | × | × | × | × | × | × | Midazolam | ↑ midazolam | Avoid co-administration |
| × | × |  | × | × |  | × | × | Nifedipine | ↑ nifedipine | Monitor, adjust dosage |
| × | × | × |  | × |  | × | × | Nortriptyline | ↑ nortriptyline | Adjust dosage or avoid |
| × |  |  |  |  |  |  |  | Omeprazole | ↓ atazanavir, ↑ omeprazole | Avoid co-administration |
|  | × |  |  |  |  |  |  | Omeprazole | ↓ omeprazole | Monitor, adjust dosage |
|  |  |  |  |  |  | × | × | Omeprazole | ↓ PI | Avoid co-administration |
| × | × | × |  | × |  |  | × | Paroxetine | ↓ paroxetine | Adjust dosage or avoid |
| × | × | × | × | × | × | × | × | Phenytoin | ↓ PI, ↓ phenytoin | Avoid co-administration |
| × | × | × | × | × | × | × | × | Pimozide | ↑ pimozide | Avoid co-administration |
| × | × | × | × | × |  | × | × | Posaconazole | ↑ PI | Avoid co-administration |
| × | × | × |  | × |  | × | × | Prednisone | ↑ prednisone | Adjust dosage or avoid |
| × |  |  |  |  |  |  | × | Ranitidine | ↓ PI | Avoid co-administration |
| × | × | × | × | × | × | × | × | Rifabutin | ↓ PI, ↓ or ↑ rifabutin | Avoid co-administration |
| × | × | × | × | × | × | × | × | Rifampin | ↓ PI, ↓ or ↑ rifabutin | Avoid co-administration |
| × | × | × | × | × | × | × | × | Rifapentine | ↓ rifapentine | Avoid co-administration |
| × | × | × |  | × |  | × | × | Sertraline | ↓ sertraline | Monitor, adjust dosage |
| × | × | × | × | × | × | × | × | Sildenafil | ↑ sildenafil | Adjust dosage or avoid |
| × | × | × | × | × |  | × | × | Sirolimus | ↑ sirolimus | Monitor, adjust dosage |
| × | × | × | × | × | × | × | × | Simvastatin | ↑ simvastatin | Avoid co-administration |
| × | × | × | × | × | × | × | × | St. John's wort | ↓ PI | Avoid co-administration |
| × | × | × | × | × |  | × | × | Tacrolimus | ↑ tacrolimus | Monitor, adjust dosage |
| × | × | × | × | × | × | × | × | Tadalafil | ↑ tadalafil | Adjust dosage or avoid |
| × |  |  |  | × |  |  | × | Theophylline | ↓ theophylline | Monitor, adjust dosage |
| × | × | × | × | × | × | × | × | Triazolam | ↑ triazolam | Monitor or avoid |
| × | × | × | × | × | × | × | × | Vardenafil | ↑ vardenafil | Adjust dosage or avoid |
| × | × | × | × | × |  | × | × | Verapamil | ↑ PI, ↑ verapamil | Adjust dosage or avoid |
| × | × | × | × | × | × | × | × | Voriconazole | ↓ or ↑ voriconazole | Avoid co-administration |
| × | × | × | × | × | × | × | × | Warfarin | ↓ or ↑ warfarin | Monitor INR, adjust dosage |

**TABLE 22A (22)**

| Anti-infective agent | Other Drug | Effect on concentration (or other effect) | Suggested management |
|---|---|---|---|
| Pyrimethamine | Lorazepam | ↑ risk of hepatotoxicity | Monitor |
|  | TMP-SMX | ↑ risk of marrow suppression | Monitor |
|  | Zidovudine | ↑ risk of marrow suppression | Monitor |
| Quinine | Digoxin | ↑ arrhythmias | Monitor, adjust dosage |
|  | Mefloquine | ↑ arrhythmias | Monitor |
|  | Warfarin | ↑ warfarin | Monitor INR, adjust dosage |
| Quinupristin-Dalfopristin | Calcium channel blockers | ↑ calcium channel blocker | Monitor, adjust dosage |
|  | Carbamazepine | ↑ carbamazepine | Monitor, adjust dosage |
|  | Cyclosporine | ↑ cyclosporine | Monitor, adjust dosage |
|  | Diazepam | ↑ diazepam | Monitor, adjust dosage |
|  | Docetaxel | ↑ docetaxel | Avoid co-administration |
|  | Lidocaine | ↑ lidocaine | Monitor, adjust dosage |
|  | Methylprednisolone | ↑ methylprednisolone | Monitor, adjust dosage |
|  | Midazolam | ↑ midazolam | Monitor, adjust dosage |
|  | Paclitaxel | ↑ paclitaxel | Avoid co-administration |
|  | Statins metabolized by CYP3A4 | ↑ statin | Monitor, adjust dosage |
|  | Tacrolimus | ↑ tacrolimus | Monitor, adjust dosage |
|  | Vincristine | ↑ vincristine | Avoid co-administration |
| Ribavirin | Didanosine | ↑ didanosine | Avoid co-administration |
|  | Stavudine | ↓ stavudine | Avoid co-administration |
|  | Zidovudine | ↓ zidovudine | Avoid co-administration |

**Rifamycins**

| Rifabutin | Rifampin | Rifapentine | Other Drug | Effect on concentration (or other effect) | Suggested management |
|---|---|---|---|---|---|
| x | x | x | Amitriptyline | ↓ amitriptyline | Adjust dosage or avoid |
|  | x |  | Antacids | ↓ rifampin | Adjust dosage or avoid |
| x | x |  | Atovaquone | ↑ rifamycin, ↓ atovaquone | Adjust dosage or avoid |
|  | x |  | Caspofungin | ↓ caspofungin | Adjust dosage or avoid |
|  | x |  | Chlorpropamide | ↓ chlorpropamide | Adjust dosage or avoid |
|  | x |  | Clarithromycin | ↓ clarithromycin | Adjust dosage or avoid |
| x |  |  | Clarithromycin | ↑ rifamycin, ↓ clarithromycin | Adjust dosage or avoid |
|  | x |  | Cyclosporine | ↓ cyclosporine | Adjust dosage or avoid |
| x |  |  | Cyclosporine | ↑ rifamycin, ↓ cyclosporine | Adjust dosage or avoid |
|  | x |  | Dapsone | ↓ dapsone | Adjust dosage or avoid |
|  | x |  | Desipramine | ↓ desipramine | Adjust dosage or avoid |
|  | x | x | Dexamethasone | ↓ dexamethasone | Adjust dosage or avoid |
| x |  |  | Dexamethasone | ↓ rifamycin, ↓ dexamethasone | Adjust dosage or avoid |
| x | x |  | Diazepam | ↓ diazepam | Adjust dosage or avoid |
| x | x |  | Digoxin | ↓ digoxin | Adjust dosage or avoid |

**TABLE 22A (23)**

**Rifamycins** (*continued*)

| Anti-infective agent | | | Other Drug | Effect on concentration (or other effect) | Suggested management |
|---|---|---|---|---|---|
| Rifabutin | Rifampin | Rifapentine | | | |
| | | x | Diltiazem | ↓ diltiazem | Adjust dosage or avoid |
| x | x | | Diltiazem | ↑ rifampin, ↓ diltiazem | Adjust dosage or avoid |
| x | x | | Disopyramide | ↓ disopyramide | Adjust dosage or avoid |
| | x | | Ethinyl estradiol | ↑ rifabutin, ↓ ethinyl estradiol | Avoid co-administration |
| x | | x | Ethinyl estradiol | ↓ ethinyl estradiol | Adjust dosage or avoid |
| x | | | Fluconazole | ↑ rifabutin, ↓ fluconazole | Adjust dosage or avoid |
| | x | x | Fluconazole | ↓ fluconazole | Adjust dosage or avoid |
| | x | | Fluvastatin | ↓ fluvastatin | Adjust dosage or avoid |
| | x | | Fusidic acid | ↑ rifampin, ↓ fusidic acid | Monitor |
| x | x | | Haloperidol | ↓ haloperidol | Adjust dosage or avoid |
| x | x | | Imipramine | ↓ imipramine | Adjust dosage or avoid |
| | x | | Isavuconazole | ↓ isavuconazole | Avoid co-administration |
| x | x | | Itraconazole | ↓ itraconazole, ↑ rifabutin | Avoid co-administration |
| | x | | Linezolid | ↓ linezolid | Adjust dosage or avoid |
| x | x | x | Methadone | ↓ methadone | Adjust dosage or avoid |
| | x | | Metoprolol | ↓ metoprolol | Adjust dosage or avoid |
| | x | | Moxifloxacin | ↓ moxifloxacin | Monitor, adjust dosage |
| x | x | | Nifedipine | ↓ nifedipine | Monitor, adjust dosage |
| x | x | | Nortriptyline | ↓ nortriptyline | Monitor, adjust dosage |
| x | x | | Phenytoin | ↓ phenytoin | Monitor, adjust dosage |
| x | | | Phenytoin | ↓ rifabutin | Monitor, adjust dosage |
| x | x | | Posaconazole | ↓ rifabutin | Adjust dosage or avoid |
| | x | x | Prednisone | ↓ prednisone | Monitor, adjust dosage |
| | x | | Propranolol | ↓ propranolol | Monitor, adjust dosage |
| x | x | | Quinidine | ↓ quinidine | Monitor, adjust dosage |
| | x | | Quinidine | ↑ rifampin, ↓ quinidine | Monitor, adjust dosage |
| | x | | Raltegravir | ↓ raltegravir | Adjust dosage or avoid |
| x | x | | Tacrolimus | ↓ tacrolimus | Monitor, adjust dosage |
| | x | | Tacrolimus | ↑ rifampin, ↓ tacrolimus | Monitor, adjust dosage |
| | x | | Telithromycin | ↓ telithromycin | Adjust dosage or avoid |
| | x | | Terbinafine | ↓ terbinafine | Adjust dosage or avoid |
| x | x | x | Theophylline | ↓ theophylline | Monitor, adjust dosage |
| | x | | Tinidazole | ↓ tinidazole | Adjust dosage or avoid |
| x | x | | Triazolam | ↓ triazolam | Monitor, adjust dosage |
| | x | | Trimethoprim-Sulfamethoxazole | ↑ rifampin? ↓ TMP-SMX (likely) | Adjust dosage or avoid |
| x | x | | Voriconazole | ↑ rifamycin, ↓ voriconazole | Avoid co-administration |

**TABLE 22A (24)**

| Anti-infective agent | | | Other Drug | Effect on concentration (or other effect) | Suggested management |
|---|---|---|---|---|---|
| Rifabutin | Rifampin | Rifapentine | | | |
| **Rifamycins** (continued) | | | | | |
| x | x | x | Warfarin | ↓ warfarin | Avoid co-administration |
| x | x | | Zidovudine | ↓ zidovudine | Avoid co-administration |
| Sarecycline | | | Antacids (Al, Ca, Mg) | ↓ sarecycline | Separate dosing |
| | | | Bismuth subsalicylate | ↓ sarecycline | Separate dosing |
| | | | Digoxin | ↑ digoxin | Monitor, adjust dosage |
| | | | Iron-containing preparations | ↓ sarecycline | Separate dosing |
| | | | Penicillin | ↓ penicillin bactericidal activity | Avoid co-administration |
| | | | Retinoids | ↑ intracranial pressure | Avoid co-administration |
| | | | Warfarin | ↑ INR | Monitor INR, adjust dosage |
| Tafenoquine | | | Dofetilide | ↑ dofetilide | Monitor, adjust dosage |
| | | | Metformin | ↑ metformin | Monitor, adjust dosage |
| Tecovirimat | | | Midazolam | ↓ midazolam | Monitor, adjust dosage |
| | | | Repaglinide | ↑ repaglinide | Monitor blood glucose |
| Telithromycin | | | Carbamazepine | ↓ telithromycin | Adjust dosage or avoid |
| | | | Digoxin | ↑ digoxin | Monitor, adjust dosage |
| | | | Ergot alkaloids | ↑ ergot alkaloids | Avoid co-administration |
| | | | Itraconazole, ketoconazole | ↑ telithromycin | Adjust dosage or avoid |
| | | | Metoprolol | ↑ metoprolol | Monitor, adjust dosage |
| | | | Midazolam | ↑ midazolam | Monitor, adjust dosage |
| | | | Warfarin | ↑ warfarin | Monitor INR, adjust dosage |
| | | | Phenobarbital, phenytoin | ↓ telithromycin | Adjust dosage or avoid |
| | | | Pimozide | ↑ pimozide | Adjust dosage or avoid |
| | | | Simvastatin | ↑ simvastatin | Monitor, adjust dosage |
| | | | Sotalol | ↓ sotalol | Monitor, adjust dosage |
| | | | Theophylline | ↑ theophylline | Monitor, adjust dosage |
| Terbinafine | | | Cimetidine | ↑ terbinafine | Adjust dosage or avoid |
| | | | Phenobarbital | ↓ terbinafine | Adjust dosage or avoid |
| Tetracyclines | | | Atovaquone | ↓ atovaquone | Adjust dosage or avoid |
| | | | Digoxin | ↑ digoxin | Monitor, adjust dosage |
| | | | Methoxyflurane | ↑ methoxyflurane | Monitor, adjust dosage |
| | | | Sucralfate | ↓ tetracycline absorption | Separate by 2-3 hrs |
| Tigecycline | | | Digoxin | ↓ digoxin | Monitor, adjust dosage |
| | | | Oral contraceptives | ↓ oral contraceptives | Use alternate method |
| | | | Warfarin | ↑ warfarin | Monitor INR, adjust dosage |
| Tinidazole | | | Alcohol | Disulfiram-like reaction | Monitor |
| | | | Azole antifungals | ↑ tinidazole | Monitor, adjust dosage |

**TABLE 22A (25)**

| Anti-infective agent | Other Drug | Effect on concentration (or other effect) | Suggested management |
|---|---|---|---|
| Trimethoprim | ACE inhibitors | ↑ serum K+ | Avoid co-administration |
| | Amantadine | ↑ amantadine | Monitor, adjust dosage |
| | Dapsone | ↑ trimethoprim, ↑ dapsone | Monitor, adjust dosage |
| | Methotrexate | ↑ methotrexate | Monitor, adjust dosage |
| | Phenytoin | ↑ phenytoin | Monitor, adjust dosage |
| | Potassium-sparing diuretics | ↑ serum K+ | Monitor |
| | Procainamide | ↑ procainamide, ↑ NAPA | Monitor, adjust dosage |
| | Repaglinide | ↑ repaglinide | Monitor blood glucose |
| Trimethoprim-Sulfamethoxazole | 6-mercaptopurine | ↓ 6-mercaptopurine | Monitor, adjust dosage |
| | ACE inhibitors | ↑ serum K+ | Monitor |
| | Amantadine | ↑ amantadine | Monitor, adjust dosage |
| | Cyclosporine | ↓ cyclosporine | Monitor, adjust dosage |
| | Loperamide | ↑ loperamide | Monitor, adjust dosage |
| | Methotrexate | ↑ methotrexate | Monitor, adjust dosage |
| | Oral contraceptives | ↓ oral contraceptives | Use alternate method |
| | Phenytoin | ↑ phenytoin | Monitor, adjust dosage |
| | Pimozide | ↓ pimozide | Monitor, adjust dosage |
| | Spironolactone | ↑ serum K+ | Monitor |
| | Sulfonylureas | ↑ sulfonylureas | Monitor blood glucose |
| | Warfarin | ↑ warfarin | Monitor INR, adjust dosage |
| Zidovudine (ZDV, AZT) | Atovaquone | ↑ zidovudine | Monitor |
| | Doxorubicin | Antagonistic in vitro | Avoid co-administration |
| | Fluconazole | ↑ zidovudine | Monitor |
| | Indomethacin | ↑ zidovudine toxic metabolite | Monitor |
| | Methadone | ↑ zidovudine | Monitor |
| | Nelfinavir | ↓ zidovudine | Monitor |
| | Probenecid | ↑ zidovudine | Monitor |
| | Ribavirin | ↑ anemia | Avoid co-administration |
| | Rifampin | ↓ zidovudine | Monitor |
| | TMP-SMX | ↑ zidovudine | Monitor |
| | Valproic acid | ↑ zidovudine | Monitor |

## TABLE 22B - DRUG-DRUG INTERACTIONS BETWEEN NON-NUCLEOSIDE REVERSE TRANSCRIPTASE INHIBITORS (NNRTIS) AND PROTEASE INHIBITORS
(Adapted from Guidelines for the Use of Antiretroviral Agents in HIV-Infected Adults & Adolescents; see www.aidsinfo.nih.gov)

| NAME (Abbreviation, Trade Name) | Atazanavir (ATV, Reyataz) | Darunavir (DRV, Prezista) | Fosamprenavir (FOS-APV, Lexiva) | Indinavir (IDV, Crixivan) | Lopinavir/Ritonavir (LP/R, Kaletra) | Nelfinavir (NFV, Viracept) | Saquinavir (SQV, Invirase) | Tipranavir (TPV) |
|---|---|---|---|---|---|---|---|---|
| **Delavirdine** (DLV, Rescriptor) | No data | No data | **Co-administration not recommended** | IDV levels ↑ 40%; Dose: IDV 600 mg q8h, DLV standard | Expect LP levels to ↑. No dose data | NFV levels ↑ 2X; DLV levels ↓ 50%. Dose: No data | SQV levels ↑ 5X. Dose: SQV 800 mg q8h, DLV standard | No data |
| **Efavirenz** (EFZ, Sustiva) | ATV AUC ↓ 74%; Dose: EFZ standard; ATA/RTV 300/100 mg q24h with food | Standard doses of both drugs | FOS-APV levels ↓; Dose: EFZ standard; FOS-APV 1400 mg + RTV 300 mg q24h or 700 mg FOS-APV + 100 mg RTV q12h | Levels: IDV ↓ 31%. Dose: IDV 1000 mg q8h, EFZ standard | Level of LP ↓ 40%. Dose: LP/R 533/133 mg q12h, EFZ standard | Standard doses | Level: SQV ↓ 62%. Dose: SQV 400 mg + RTV 400 mg q12h | No dose change necessary |
| **Etravirine** (ETR, Intelence) | ↑ ATV & ↑ ETR levels. | Standard doses of both drugs | ↑ levels of FOS-APV. | ↓ level of IDV. | ↑ levels of ETR, ↓ **levels of LP/R.** | ↑ levels of NFV. | ↓ ETR levels 33%, SQV/R no change. Standard dose of both drugs. | ↓ levels of ETR, ↑ levels of TPV & RTV. **Avoid combination.** |
| **Nevirapine** (NVP, Viramune) | Avoid combination. ATZ increases NVP concentrations >25%; NVP increases ATZ AUC by 42% | Standard doses of both drugs | Use with caution. NVP AUC increased 14% (700/100 Fos/rit); NVP AUC inc 29% (Fos 1400 mg bid). | IDV levels ↓ 28%. Dose: IDV 1000 mg q8h or combine with RTV; NVP standard | LP levels ↓ 53%. Dose: LP/R 533/133 mg q12h; NVP standard | Standard doses | Dose: SQV + RTV 400/400 mg, both q12h | Standard doses |

## TABLE 23 - LIST OF GENERIC AND COMMON TRADE NAMES

### GENERIC NAME: TRADE NAMES

Abacavir: Ziagen
Abacavir + Lamivudine: Epzicom
Abacavir + Lamivudine + Dolutegravir: Triumeq
Abacavir + Lamivudine + Zidovudine: Trizivir
Acyclovir: Zovirax
Adefovir: Hepsera
Albendazole: Albenza
Amantadine: Symmetrel
Amikacin: Amikin
Amikacin liposomal: Arikayce
Amoxicillin: Amoxil, Polymox
Amoxicillin extended release: Moxatag
Amox./clav.: Augmentin, Augmentin ES-600; Augmentin XR
Amphotericin B: Fungizone
Ampho B-liposomal: AmBisome
Ampho B-lipid complex: Abelcet
Ampicillin: Omnipen, Polycillin
Ampicillin + Sulbactam: Unasyn
Artemether + Lumefantrine: Coartem
Atazanavir: Reyataz
Atovaquone: Mepron
Atovaquone + Proguanil: Malarone
Azithromycin: Zithromax
Azithromycin ER: Zmax
Aztreonam: Azactam, Cayston
Baloxavir marboxil: Xofluza
Bedaquiline: Sirturo
Benznidazole: Exeltis, Abarax
Bezlotoxumab: Zinplava
Bictegravir + FTC + TAF: Biktarvy
Boceprevir: Victrelis
Caspofungin: Cancidas
Cefaclor: Ceclor, Ceclor CD
Cefadroxil: Duricef
Cefazolin: Ancef, Kefzol
Cefdinir: Omnicef
Cefditoren pivoxil: Spectracef
Cefepime: Maxipime
Cefixime[AUS]: Suprax

Cefoperazone + Sulbactam: Sulperazon[AUS/UK]
Cefonicid: Monocid
Cefotaxime: Claforan
Cefotetan: Cefotan
Cefoxitin: Mefoxin
Cefpodoxime proxetil: Vantin
Cefprozil: Cefzil
Ceftaroline: Teflaro
Ceftazidime: Fortaz, Tazicef, Tazidime
Ceftazidime + Avibactam: Avycaz
Ceftibuten: Cedax
Ceftizoxime: Cefizox
Ceftobiprole: Zeftera
Ceftolozane + Tazobactam: Zerbaxa
Ceftriaxone: Rocephin
Cefuroxime: Zinacef, Ceftin
Cephalexin: Keflex
Cephradine: Anspor, Velosef
Chloroquine: Aralen
Cidofovir: Vistide
Ciprofloxacin: Cipro, Cipro XR
Clarithromycin: Biaxin, Biaxin XL
Clindamycin: Cleocin
Clofazimine: Lamprene
Clotrimazole: Lotrimin, Mycelex
Cloxacillin: Tegopen
Colistimethate: Coly-Mycin M
Cycloserine: Seromycin
Daclatasvir: Daklinza
Daptomycin: Cubicin
Dalbavancin: Dalvance
Darunavir: Prezista
Darunavir + FTC + COBI + TAF: Symtuza
Delafloxacin: Baxdela
Delavirdine: Rescriptor
Dicloxacillin: Dynapen
Didanosine: Videx
Diethylcarbamazine: Hetrazan
Diloxanide furoate: Furamide
Dolutegravir: Tivicay
Doravirine + 3TC + TDF: Delstrigo
Doripenem: Doribax

Doxycycline: Vibramycin
Efavirenz: Sustiva
Efavirenz + Emtricitabine + Tenofovir: Atripla
Elbasvir + Grazoprevir: Zepatier
Elvitegravir: Vitekta
Elvitegravir + Cobicistat + Emtricitabine + Tenofovir: Stribild
Elvitegravir + Cobicistat + Emtricitabine + Tenofovir AF: Genvoya
Emtricitabine: Emtriva
Emtricitabine + Tenofovir: Truvada
Emtricitabine + Rilpivirine + Tenofovir: Complera
Enfuvirtide (T-20): Fuzeon
Entecavir: Baraclude
Eravacycline: Xerava
Ertapenem: Invanz
Erythromycin(s): Ilotycin
Erythro succinate: Pediamycin
*Estolate*: Ilosone *Erythro*
Erythro + Sulfisoxazole: Pediazole
Ethambutol: Myambutol
Ethionamide: Trecator
Etravirine: Intelence
Famciclovir: Famvir
Fidaxomicin: Dificid
Fluconazole: Diflucan
Flucytosine: Ancobon
Fosamprenavir: Lexiva
Fosfomycin: Monurol
Fusidic acid: Takista
Ganciclovir: Cytovene
Gatifloxacin: Tequin
Gemifloxacin: Factive
Gentamicin: Garamycin
Grazoprevir + Elbasvir: Zepatier
Griseofulvin: Fulvicin
Halofantrine: Halfan
Ibalizumab-uiyk: Trogarzo
Idoxuridine: Dendrid, Stoxil

INH + RIF: Rifamate
INH + RIF + PZA: Rifater
Interferon alfa-2A: Roferon A
Interferon, pegylated: PEG-Intron, Pegasys
Interferon + Ribavirin: Rebetron
Imipenem + Cilastatin: Primaxin, Tienam
Imiquimod: Aldara
Indinavir: Crixivan
Isavuconazonium sulfate: Cresemba
Itraconazole: Sporanox
Iodoquinol: Yodoxin
Ivermectin: Stromectol, Sklice
Ketoconazole: Nizoral
Lamivudine: Epivir, Epivir-HBV
Lamivudine + Abacavir: Epzicom
Ledipasvir + Sofosbuvir: Harvoni
Letermovir: Prevymis
Levofloxacin: Levaquin
Linezolid: Zyvox
Lomefloxacin: Maxaquin
Lopinavir + Ritonavir: Kaletra
Loracarbef: Lorabid
Maraviroc: Selzentry
Mebendazole: Vermox
Mefloquine: Lariam
Meropenem: Merrem
Meropenem + vaborbactam: Vabomere
Mesalamine: Asacol, Pentasa
Methenamine: Hiprex, Mandelamine
Metronidazole: Flagyl
Micafungin: Mycamine
Minocycline: Minocin
Moxifloxacin: Avelox
Mupirocin: Bactroban
Nafcillin: Unipen
Nelfinavir: Viracept
Nevirapine: Viramune
Nitazoxanide: Alinia
Nitrofurantoin: Macrobid, Macrodantin
Nystatin: Mycostatin

Ofloxacin: Floxin
Olysio: Simeprevir
Olysio + Sovaldi: Nuzira
Oritavancin: Orbactiv
Oseltamivir: Tamiflu
Oxacillin: Prostaphlin
Palivizumab: Synagis
Paritaprevir + Ritonavir + Ombitasvir: Technivie
Paritaprevir + Ritonavir + Ombitasvir + Dasabuvir: Viekira Pak
Paromomycin: Humatin
Pentamidine: NebuPent, Pentam 300
Peramivir: Rapivab
Piperacillin + Tazobactam: Zosyn, Tazocin
Piperazine: Antepar
Plazomicin: Zemdri
Podophyllotoxin: Condylox
Polymyxin B: Poly-Rx
Posaconazole: Noxafil
Praziquantel: Biltricide
Primaquine: Primachine
Proguanil: Paludrine
Pruliflloxacin: Sword
Pyrantel pamoate: Antiminth
Pyrimethamine: Daraprim
Pyrimethamine + Sulfadoxine: Fansidar
Quinupristin + Dalfopristin: Synercid
Raltegravir: Isentress
Retapamulin: Altabax
Ribavirin: Virazole, Rebetol
Rifabutin: Mycobutin
Rifampin: Rifadin, Rimactane
Rifapentine: Priftin
Rifaximin: Xifaxan
Rilpivirine: Edurant
Rimantadine: Flumadine
Ritonavir: Norvir
Saquinavir: Invirase
Secnidazole: Solosec
Spectinomycin: Trobicin
Stavudine: Zerit

Stibogluconate: Pentostam
Silver sulfadiazine: Silvadene
Sofosbuvir: Sovaldi
Sofosbuvir + Velpatasvir: Epclusa
Sulfamethoxazole: Gantanol
Sulfasalazine: Azulfidine
Sulfisoxazole: Gantrisin
Tafenoquine: Krintafel, Arakoda
Tecovirimat: Tpoxx
Tedizolid: Sivextro
Telaprevir: Incivek
Telavancin: Vibativ
Telbivudine: Tyzeka
Telithromycin: Ketek
Temocillin: Negaban, Temopen
Tenofovir AF-FTC: Descovy
Tenofovir alafenamide: Vemlidy
Tenofovir DF: Viread
Terbinafine: Lamisil
Thalidomide: Thalomid
Thiabendazole: Mintezol
Tigecycline: Tygacil
Tinidazole: Tindamax
Tipranavir: Aptivus
Tobramycin: Nebcin
Tretinoin: Retin A
Trifluridine: Viroptic
Trimethoprim: Primsol
Trimethoprim + Sulfamethoxazole: Bactrim, Septra
Valacyclovir: Valtrex
Valganciclovir: Valcyte
Velpatasvir + Sofosbuvir: Epclusa
Voriconazole: Vfend
Zalcitabine: HIVID
Zanamivir: Relenza
Zidovudine (ZDV): Retrovir
Zidovudine + 3TC: Combivir
Zidovudine + 3TC + Abacavir: Trizivir

## TABLE 23 (2)
### LIST OF COMMON TRADE AND GENERIC NAMES

**TRADE NAMES: GENERIC NAME**

| Trade Name | Generic Name |
|---|---|
| Abelcet | Ampho B-lipid complex |
| Aldara | Imiquimod |
| Albenza | Albendazole |
| Alinia | Nitazoxanide |
| Altabax | Retapamulin |
| AmBisome | Amphe B-liposomal |
| Amoxil | Amoxicillin |
| Ancef | Cefazolin |
| Ancobon | Flucytosine |
| Anspor | Cephradine |
| Antepar | Piperazine |
| Antiminth | Pyrantel pamoate |
| Aptivus | Tipranavir |
| Aralen | Chloroquine |
| Arakoda | Tafenoquine |
| Arikayce | Amikacin liposomal |
| Asacol | Mesalamine |
| Atripla | Efavirenz + Emtricitabine + Tenofovir |
| Augmentin, Augmentin ES-600, Augmentin XR | Amox./clav. |
| Avelox | Moxifloxacin |
| Avycaz | Ceftazidime + Avibactam |
| Azactam | Aztreonam |
| Azulfidine | Sulfasalazine |
| Bactroban | Mupirocin |
| Baraclude | Entecavir |
| Baxdela | Delafloxacin |
| Biaxin, Biaxin XL | Clarithromycin |
| Biktarvy | Bictegravir + FTC + TAF |
| Biltricide | Praziquantel |
| Cancidas | Caspofungin |
| Cayston | Aztreonam (inhaled) |
| Ceclor, Ceclor CD | Cefaclor |
| Cedax | Ceftibuten |
| Cefizox | Ceftizoxime |
| Cefotan | Cefotetan |
| Ceftin | Cefuroxime axetil |
| Cefzil | Cefprozil |
| Cipro, Cipro XR | Ciprofloxacin & extended release |
| Claforan | Cefotaxime |
| Coartem | Artemether + Lumefantrine |
| Coly-Mycin M | Colistimethate |
| Combivir | Zidovudine + 3TC |
| Complera | Emtricitabine + Tenofovir + Rilpivirine |
| Cresemba | Isavuconazonium sulfate |
| Crixivan | Indinavir |
| Cubicin | Daptomycin |
| Cytovene | Ganciclovir |
| Daklinza | Daclatasvir |
| Dalvance | Dalbavancin |
| Daraprim | Pyrimethamine |
| Descovy | Tenofovir AF-FTC |
| Delstrigo | Doravirine + 3TC + TDF |
| Dificid | Fidaxomicin |
| Diflucan | Fluconazole |
| Doribax | Doripenem |
| Duricef | Cefadroxil |
| Dynapen | Dicloxacillin |
| Edurant | Rilpivirine |
| Emtriva | Emtricitabine |
| Epclusa | Velpatasvir + Sofosbuvir |
| Epivir, Epivir-HBV | Lamivudine |
| Epzicom | Abacavir + Lamivudine |
| Eraxis | Anidulafungin |
| Factive | Gemifloxacin |
| Famvir | Famciclovir |
| Fansidar | Pyrimethamine + Sulfadoxine |
| Flagyl | Metronidazole |
| Floxin | Ofloxacin |
| Flumadine | Rimantadine |
| Fortaz | Ceftazidime |
| Foscavir | Foscarnet |
| Fortovase | Saquinavir |
| Fungizone | Amphotericin B |
| Furadantin | Nitrofurantoin |
| Fuzeon | Enfuvirtide (T-20) |
| Gantanol | Sulfamethoxazole |
| Gantrisin | Sulfisoxazole |
| Garamycin | Gentamicin |
| Genvoya | Elvitegravir + Cobicistat + Emtricitabine + Tenofovir |
| Halfan | Halofantrine |
| Harvoni | Ledipasvir + Sofosbuvir |
| Hepsera | Adefovir |
| Herplex | Idoxuridine |
| Hiprex | Methenamine hippurate |
| HIVID | Zalcitabine |
| Humatin | Paromomycin |
| Ilosone | Erythromycin estolate |
| Ilotycin | Erythromycin |
| Incivek | Telaprevir |
| Intelence | Etravirine |
| Intron A | Interferon alfa |
| Invanz | Ertapenem |
| Invirase | Saquinavir |
| Isentress | Raltegravir |
| Kaletra | Lopinavir + Ritonavir |
| Kantrex | Kanamycin |
| Keflex | Cephalexin |
| Ketek | Telithromycin |
| Krintafel | Tafenoquine |
| Lamisil | Terbinafine |
| Lamprene | Clofazimine |
| Lariam | Mefloquine |
| Levaquin | Levofloxacin |
| Lexiva | Fosamprenavir |
| Lorabid | Loracarbef |
| Macrobid, Macrobid | Nitrofurantoin |
| Malarone | Atovaquone + Proguanil |
| Mandelamine | Methenamine mandelate |
| Maxaquin | Lomefloxacin |
| Maxipime | Cefepime |
| Mefoxin | Cefoxitin |
| Mepron | Atovaquone |
| Merrem | Meropenem |
| Minocin | Minocycline |
| Mintezol | Thiabendazole |
| Monocid | Cefonicid |
| Monurol | Fosfomycin |
| Moxatag | Amoxicillin extended release |
| Myambutol | Ethambutol |
| Mycamine | Micafungin |
| Mycobutin | Rifabutin |
| Mycostatin | Nystatin |
| Nebcin | Tobramycin |
| NebuPent | Pentamidine |
| Nizoral | Ketoconazole |
| Norvir | Ritonavir |
| Noxafil | Posaconazole |
| Nuzyra | Omadacycline |
| Olysio | Simeprevir |
| Omnicef | Cefdinir |
| Omnipen | Ampicillin |
| Orbactiv | Oritavancin |
| Pediamycin | Erythro. ethyl succinate |
| Pediazole | Erythro. ethyl succinate + sulfisoxazole |
| Pegasys, PEG-Intron | Interferon, pegylated |
| Pentam 300 | Pentamidine |
| Pentasa | Mesalamine |
| Polycillin | Ampicillin |
| Polymox | Amoxicillin |
| Poly-Rx | Polymyxin B |
| Prezista | Darunavir |
| Prevymis | Letermovir |
| Priftin | Rifapentine |
| Primaxin | Imipenem + Cilastatin |
| Primsol | Trimethoprim |
| Prostaphlin | Oxacillin |
| Rapivab | Peramivir |
| Rebetol | Ribavirin |
| Rebetron | Interferon + Ribavirin |
| Relenza | Zanamivir |
| Rescriptor | Delavirdine |
| Retin-A | Tretinoin |
| Retrovir | Zidovudine (ZDV) |
| Rifadin | Rifampin |
| Rifamate | INH + RIF |
| Rifater | INH + RIF + PZA |
| Rimactane | Rifampin |
| Rocephin | Ceftriaxone |
| Selzentry | Maraviroc |
| Septra | Trimethoprim + Sulfamethoxazole |
| Seromycin | Cycloserine |
| Silvadene | Silver sulfadiazine |
| Sirturo | Bedaquiline |
| Sivextro | Tedizolid |
| Sklice | Ivermectin lotion |
| Solosec | Secnidazole |
| Sovaldi | Sofosbuvir |
| Spectracef | Cefditoren pivoxil |
| Sporanox | Itraconazole |
| Stoxil | Idoxuridine |
| Stribild | Elvitegravir + Cobicistat + Emtricitabine + Tenofovir |
| Stromectol | Ivermectin |
| Sulfamylon | Mafenide |
| Sulperazone[aus] | Cefoperazone + Sulbactam |
| Suprax | Cefixime[aus] |
| Sustiva | Efavirenz |
| Symmetrel | Amantadine |
| Symtuza | Darunavir + Cobi + FTC + TAF |
| Synagis | Palivizumab |
| Synercid | Quinupristin + Dalfopristin |
| Taksta | Fusidic acid |
| Tamiflu | Oseltamivir |
| Tazicef | Ceftazidime |
| Technivie | Ombitasvir + Paritaprevir + Ritonavir |
| Teflaro | Ceftaroline |
| Tegopen | Cloxacillin |
| Tequin | Gatifloxacin |
| Tienam | Imipenem |
| Tinactin | Tolnaftate |
| Tindamax | Tinidazole |
| Tivicay | Dolutegravir |
| Tobi | Tobramycin |
| Trecator SC | Ethionamide |
| Triumeq | Abacavir + Lamivudine + Dolutegravir |
| Trizivir | Zidovudine + 3TC + Abacavir |
| Trobicin | Spectinomycin |
| Truvada | Emtricitabine + Tenofovir |
| Tygacil | Tigecycline |
| Tyzeka | Telbivudine |
| Unasyn | Ampicillin/sulbactam |
| Unipen | Nafcillin |
| Vabomere | Meropenem + vaborbactam |
| Valcyte | Valganciclovir |
| Valtrex | Valacyclovir |
| Vancocin | Vancomycin |
| Vantin | Cefpodoxime proxetil |
| Velosef | Cephradine |
| Vemlidy | Tenofovir alafenamide |
| Vermox | Mebendazole |
| Vfend | Voriconazole |
| Vibativ | Telavancin |
| Vibramycin | Doxycycline |
| Victrelis | Boceprevir |
| Videx | Didanosine |
| Viekira Pak | Paritaprevir + Ritonavir + Ombitasvir + Dasabuvir |
| Viracept | Nelfinavir |
| Viramune | Nevirapine |
| Virazole | Ribavirin |
| Viread | Tenofovir |
| Vistide | Cidofovir |
| Vitekta | Elvitegravir |
| Xerava | Eravacycline |
| Xifaxan | Rifaximin |
| Xofluza | Baloxavir marboxil |
| Yodoxin | Iodoquinol |
| Zemdri | Plazomicin |
| Zerit | Stavudine |
| Zeftera | Ceftobiprole |
| Zepatier | Elbasvir + Grazoprevir |
| Zerbaxa | Ceftolozane + Tazobactam |
| Ziagen | Abacavir |
| Zinacef | Cefuroxime |
| Zinplava | Bezlotoxumab |
| Zithromax | Azithromycin |
| Zmax | Azithromycin ER |
| Zovirax | Acyclovir |
| Zosyn | Piperacillin + Tazobactam |
| Zyvox | Linezolid |